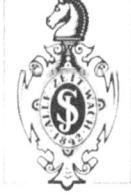

C.S.B. Galasko · I. Isherwood (Eds.)

Imaging Techniques in Orthopaedics

With 296 Figures

Springer-Verlag
London Berlin Heidelberg New York
Paris Tokyo

C.S.B. Galasko, MSc, ChM, FRCS (Eng), FRCS (Ed)
Professor of Orthopaedic Surgery, University of Manchester, Consultant Orthopaedic Surgeon,
Salford Health Authority, Department of Orthopaedic Surgery, Clinical Sciences Building,
Hope Hospital, Eccles Old Road, Salford M6 8HD, UK

I. Isherwood, MD, FRCP, FRCR, FFRRSCI
Professor of Diagnostic Radiology, University of Manchester, Department of Diagnostic
Radiology, Stopford Building, Oxford Road, Manchester M13 9PT, UK

Cover illustrations are taken from within this book.

British Library Cataloguing in Publication Data
Imaging techniques in orthopaedics.
1. Medicine. Orthopaedics. Applications of imaging.   I. Galasko, C.S.B. (Charles Samuel Bernard)
II. Isherwood, Ian   617'.3

Library of Congress Cataloging-in-Publication Data
Imaging techniques in orthopaedics.
Includes bibliographies and index.
1. Radiography in orthopedics. I. Galasko, C. S. B. (Charles Samuel Bernard) II. Isherwood, Ian. [DNLM: 1. Bone
Disease—diagnosis.   2.   Diagnostic imaging.   3.   Orthopedics—methods.   WE   141   I31]   RD734.5.R33I45
1989   617'.3   88-24862

ISBN-13: 978-1-4471-1642-4   e-ISBN-13: 978-1-4471-1640-0
DOI: 10.1007/978-1-4471-1640-0

2128/3830–543210   Printed on acid-free paper

Preface

Recent years have witnessed major developments in diagnostic imaging methods. The facilities for these new methods are sometimes expensive, and not always accessible, yet they continue to improve and to change. It is essential that those concerned with orthopaedic imaging should appreciate not only recent developments but also the changes likely to occur during the next few years. It is also important that the indications, contraindications, uses and complications for each individual imaging technique should be understood. This book is an attempt to provide such information for orthopaedic surgeons, diagnostic radiologists, and other clinicians, particularly those in training or those who are involved in management of patients with disorders of the musculoskeletal system. In the first part of the book the different imaging techniques are discussed, with emphasis on advantages and disadvantages, indications and contraindications. In the second part, authors have been asked to discuss ways in which specific groups of disorders might be investigated. It is hoped that the reader will obtain from this section a balanced view of the different diagnostic imaging methods, the indications for their use, and the sequence in which they might be carried out.

The Editors are grateful to all authors for the time and work they have put into their individual chapters. They are also grateful to the publishers, in particular Michael Jackson, for help given in the preparation of this book.

Manchester
June 1988

C.S.B. Galasko
I. Isherwood

Contents

List of Contributors

PART 1 RADIOLOGICAL TECHNIQUES ix

1 Conventional Radiography of the Appendicular Skeleton
D.J. Stoker and D. Horsfield 3

2 Angiography of the Appendicular Skeleton
Anne P. Hemingway and A. Adam 19

3 Arthrography
B.J. Preston 35

4 Conventional Radiography of the Axial Skeleton
W.P. Butt 51

5 Myelography
J.V. Occleshaw 77

6 Epidurography
I. Emery and G. Hamilton 89

7 Angiography of the Axial Skeleton
G. Forbes 95

8 Discography
J.T. Patton 107

9 Facet Arthrography
I.W. McCall 117

10 Computed Tomography
W.St.C. Forbes 123

11 Digital Orthopaedic Radiography: Vascular and Non-vascular
W.D. Foley and C.R. Wilson 145

12 Magnetic Resonance Imaging (MRI)
J.P.R. Jenkins and I. Isherwood 159

13 Skeletal Scintigraphy
C.S.B. Galasko 181

14 Isotope Techniques in the Investigation of Diseases of Joints
    M.V. Merrick 207

15 Ultrasound of the Axial Skeleton
    R.W. Porter 221

16 Appendicular Ultrasound
    D. Rickards 231

PART 2 BONE MINERAL STUDIES

17 Bone Measurement by Conventional Radiographic Techniques
    A. Horsman 243

18 Photon Absorptiometry
    P. Tothill 251

19 Quantitative Computed Tomography (QCT)
    J. E. Adams 259

PART 3 CLINICAL INDICATIONS

20 Musculoskeletal Trauma
    H. Stein 271

21 Primary Tumours of Bone and Soft Tissue
    F.H. Sim, T.H. Berquist and R.A. McLeod 283

22 Metastatic Tumours
    C.S.B. Galasko and I. Isherwood 293

23 Infection
    D.R.A. Davies 307

24 Skeletal Dysplasias
    J.F. Crossan 313

25 Back Pain
    R.C. Mulholland 325

26 Spinal Deformity
    J.E. Lonstein 335

27 Disorders in Childhood
    C.S.B. Galasko 345

28 Osteonecrosis
    P.J. Gregg 363

Subject Index 371

Contributors

A. Adam, MB, BS, MRCP, FRCR
Consultant Radiologist, Department of Diagnostic Radiology, Royal Postgraduate Medical School, Hammersmith Hospital, Du Cane Road, London W12 0HS, UK

Judith E. Adams, MBBS, FRCP, FRCR
Senior Lecturer, University of Manchester and Honorary Consultant Radiologist, Manchester Royal Infirmary, Department of Diagnostic Radiology, Stopford Building, Oxford Road, Manchester M13 9PT, UK

T.H. Berquist, MD
Consultant, Department of Diagnostic Radiology, Mayo Clinic and Mayo Foundation and Associate Professor of Radiology, Mayo Medical School, Mayo Clinic, Rochester, MI 55905, USA

W.P. Butt, FRCR, FRCP
Consultant Radiologist, Department of Diagnostic Radiology, St. James's University Hospital, Beckett Street, Leeds LS9 7TF, UK

J.F. Crossan, BSc, FRCS
Consultant Orthopaedic Surgeon, Victoria Infirmary, Glasgow G42 9TY, UK

D.R.A. Davies, MD, FRCS (Ed)
Consultant Orthopaedic Surgeon, Park Hospital, Davyhulme, Manchester M31 3SL, UK

I.H. Emery, MBChB, FRCS (Ed), MChOrth
Consultant Orthopaedic Surgeon, Department of Orthopaedic and Traumatic Surgery, Royal Lancaster Infirmary, Ashton Road, Lancaster, UK

W.D. Foley, MD, BS, DMRD, FRACR
Professor of Radiology, Milwaukee County Medical Complex, 8700 West Wisconsin Avenue, Milwaukee, WI 53226, USA

G. Forbes, MD
Associate Professor of Radiology, Mayo Medical School and Consultant in Neuroradiology, Mayo Clinic, Department of Diagnostic Radiology, Mayo Clinic, Rochester, MI 55905, USA

W. St. C. Forbes, MA, MB, BCh, DMRD, FRCR
Consultant Neuroradiologist, Hope Hospital, Eccles Old Road, Salford M6 8HD, UK

C.S.B. Galasko, MSc, ChM, FRCS (Eng), FRCS (Ed)
Professor of Orthopaedic Surgery, University of Manchester, Honorary Consultant Orthopaedic Surgeon, Salford Health Authority, Department of Orthopaedic Surgery, University of Manchester, Clinical Sciences Building, Hope Hospital, Eccles Old Road, Salford M6 8HD, UK

P.J. Gregg, MD, FRCS
Professor of Orthopaedic Surgery, University of Leicester, Department of Orthopaedic Surgery, Clinical Sciences Building, Glenfield General Hospital, Groby Road, Leicester LE3 9QP, UK

E.A.G. Hamilton, MB, ChB, DMRD
Consultant Radiologist, Department of Radiology, Royal Lancaster Infirmary, Lancaster LA1
4RP, UK

Anne P. Hemingway, BSc, MB, BS, MRCP, DMRD, FRCR
Kodak Professor of Radiology, Academic Department of Radiology, Floor P, Royal Hallamshire
Hospital, Glossop Road, Sheffield S10 2JF, UK

D. Horsfield, DCR(R), FETC, SRR(R)
Superintendent Radiographer, X-Ray Department, Royal National Orthopaedic Hospital, 45–51
Bolsover Street, London W1P 8AQ, UK

A. Horsman, MA, PhD
MRC External Scientific Staff, Department of Medical Physics, The General Infirmary, Leeds
LS1 3EX, UK

I. Isherwood, MD, FRCP, FRCR, FFR RSCI (Hon)
Professor of Diagnostic Radiology, Department of Diagnostic Radiology, University of Manchester, Stopford Building, Oxford Road, Manchester M13 9PT, UK

J.P.R. Jenkins, MBChB, MRCP, DMRD, FRCR
Senior Lecturer in Diagnostic Radiology, University of Manchester, Department of Diagnostic
Radiology, University of Manchester Medical School, Stopford Building, Oxford Road, Manches-
ter M13 9PT, UK

J.E. Lonstein, MB, BCh
Minnesota Spine Center, 606 24th Avenue, So. Minneapolis, MI 55427, USA

I.W. McCall, MBChB, DMRD, FRCR
Consultant Radiologist, The Robert Jones and Agnes Hunt Orthopaedic Hospital, Oswestry,
Shropshire SY10 7AG, UK

R.A. McLeod, MD
Consultant, Department of Diagnostic Radiology, Mayo Clinic and Mayo Foundation, and Professor of Radiology, Mayo Medical School, Rochester, MI 55905, USA

M.V. Merrick, MSc, FRCP(E), FRCR
Consultant in Nuclear Medicine and Senior Lecturer in Medicine and Medical Radiology,
Western General Hospital, Edinburgh EH4 2XU, UK

R.C. Mulholland, MB, BS, FRCS
Consultant Orthopaedic Surgeon, Harlow Wood Orthopaedic Hospital, Mansfield Road,
Mansfield, UK

J.V. Occleshaw, BSc, MD, FRCR
Consultant Radiologist (Neuroradiology), Manchester Royal Infirmary and Withington Hospital, Manchester Royal Infirmary, Oxford Road, Manchester M13 9WL, UK

J.T. Patton, FRCR, FRCP (Ed)
Consultant Radiologist, Department of Radiology, Manchester Royal Infirmary, Oxford Road,
Manchester M13 9WL, UK

R.W. Porter, MD, FRCS, FRCSE
Consultant Orthopaedic Surgeon, Doncaster Royal Infirmary, Armthorpe Road, Doncaster
DN2 5LT, UK

B.J. Preston, FRCR
Consultant Radiologist, Radiology Department, University Hospital, Queen's Medical Centre,
Nottingham NG7 2UH, UK

D. Rickards, FRCR, FFR(D)SA
Consultant Radiologist, Department of Radiology, The Middlesex Hospital, London W1N 8AA,
UK and Department of Radiology, The Institute of Urology, London WC1, UK

F.H. Sim, MD
Consultant, Department of Orthopedics, Mayo Clinic and Mayo Foundation and Professor of Orthopedic Surgery, Mayo Medical School, Rochester, MI 55905, USA

H. Stein, MD, DPhil
Associate Professor of Orthopaedic Surgery at the Medical Faculty of the Technion, Haifa and Director, Department of Orthopaedic Surgery A, Rambam Medical Center, Haifa, Israel

D.J. Stoker, FRCP, FRCR
Consultant Radiologist, Royal National Orthopaedic Hospital, 45–51 Bolsover Street, London W1P 8AQ, UK

P. Tothill, BSc, PhD, FInstP, CPhys, FRSE
Reader in Medical Physics, Department of Medical Physics, Western General Hospital, Edinburgh EH4 2XU, UK

C.R. Wilson, PhD
Associate Professor of Radiology, Department of Radiology, Medical College of Wisconsin, 8700 W. Wisconsin Avenue, Milwaukee, WI 53226, USA

Part 1 :

Radiological Techniques

1 Conventional Radiography of the Appendicular Skeleton

D.J. Stoker and D. Horsfield

Introduction	3
Film Processing	4
Hand	4
Standard Projections	4
Wrist and Carpus	5
Standard Projections	5
Forearm and Elbow	6
Standard Projections	6
Humerus, Shoulder, Shoulder Girdle and Sternum	7
Standard Projections	7
Scapula	8
Clavicle	9
Sternum	9
Pelvis	9
Standard Projections	9
Hip Joint	11
Standard Projections	11
Femur	12
Standard Projections	12
Leg	12
Standard Projections	13
Ankle Joint	13
Standard Projections	13
Foot	14
Standard Projections	14
Lower Limb Length	15
Basic Principle of Measurement Technique	16
Stereoradiography	16
References	17
Further Reading	17

Introduction

The objective of good orthodox radiography is to demonstrate the part under examination to its best advantage. Clearly, this often depends upon the reason for the examination being requested, but it is necessary in a busy department to undertake routine examinations in a standard way for reasons of time, expense, lack of clinical information and serial comparison. Standard views therefore have been evolved to offer a good compromise in the demonstration of any part, because the nature of the abnormality may not be known prior to the examination. Standard views are the bedrock of radiographic practice; however they are only truly standard to the department under consideration although many, perhaps over 90%, with perhaps inconsequential variation, are used in daily practice in all departments throughout the United Kingdom. Standard views therefore serve to standardize the quality of radiography. They must, however, not be regarded as the only possible projections. In many cases, e.g. uncomplicated trauma, they will suffice. In others, they will not achieve the objective of demonstrating the region of interest and the referring doctor must then seek the advice of the radiologist or radiographer to see whether some other projection is needed.

The basic principle of radiographic projection, in that the image is a two-dimensional one of a three-dimensional object, is to obtain two views at right angles so that the superimposition of adjoining shadows is obviated to the greatest degree or at least recognized as being present. In some areas, notably the foot and the ribs where bony overlap is the rule, in cases of suspected trauma an oblique projection is usually considered to be more useful.

Film Processing

In modern radiology departments the automatic film processor is now an integral piece of equipment. It has helped in achieving a greater throughput of patients by reducing the time needed for development; much of the drudgery of the darkroom has been eliminated. As the vast majority of processors work on a roller transport system, the total time that the film spends in the processor cannot be varied. With the modern 90-second processing cycle, the chemical concentrations, pH and temperature are all crucial. Small variations in any of these factors may produce a noticeable variation in film quality. Standardized automation aims at producing consistently good results with minimal loss of overall quality compared to hand processing. As a consequence of introducing a 90-second cycle, the processing chemistry has been altered greatly to adapt to the much shortened periods in which contact with the film occurs. In automatic systems the chemicals operate at higher temperatures, in greater concentrations and with a different pH. This has the effect of increasing the photographic contrast of the films developed in automatic processors. If the manufacturer's instructions are followed and the processor is correctly set and used regularly, only minimal alterations are likely to be necessary.

The introduction and gradual acceptance of more efficient rare-earth intensifying screens has also had an effect on the quality of the final image in films produced today. The increase in the "speed" of these film/screen combinations and the consequent reduction in the radiation dose to the patient is commendable. However, the result is that the images produced today can show even higher photographic contrast. To improve the efficiency of the intensifying screens and to reduce the contrast, manufacturers recommend a technique using a higher kilovoltage. This does seem to be effective; it also helps in reducing the dose of radiation to the patient.

To be able to visualize both bone and soft tissue on one film is the objective in musculoskeletal radiology. Careful manipulation of the techniques and products available today will provide acceptable results. Correct management of these factors may increase image quality quite markedly. Reduction of the temperature of the developer in an automatic processor is probably the single most effective variation. When the temperature of the developer drops, a considerable improvement in the quality of the image can result. This is a consequence of reduction in the level of background fogging together with a clearer demonstration of the soft tissues. The gamma of the system is reduced, having the effect of extending the range of the grey scale and in reducing contrast. An additional effect is the extension of the latitude of exposure and a reduction in quantum mottle.

Editors' note: In order to make good a lower developing temperature for conventional radiography, the exposure of the film has to be increased. For a reduction of 2.3°C, an increase of 25% for old film is required and, for new-technology film, 5%–10% – a substantial increase in radiation dose to the patient. However, against this has to be set an increase in quality and reduction in repeat examinations.

Hand

Standard Projections

The routine basic radiographic projections of the whole hand or individual fingers include postero-anterior (PA) i.e. forearm pronated, lateral and postero-anterior oblique. For the thumb, an additional antero-posterior (AP) view is also available.

Patients with restricted movement of their upper limbs may find the conventional positioning for such routine examination of their hands impossible to achieve. By flexing the elbows and placing both hands palm down with the fingers pointing in opposite directions (ulnar border of one hand against radial border of the other) the examination may be performed satisfactorily. This projection is undesirable as a routine view as it is difficult for the radiologist to compare the two hands.

Norgaard's ("Ball-catching") Projection

This may be used to demonstrate early erosive changes of the metacarpal heads not usually visible on standard projections. The hands are placed in

Wrist and Carpus

Standard Projections

The basic projections are postero-anterior (PA) and lateral, though flexion and extension views may be included.

An immaculately true lateral is required to allow any deduction about ulnar subluxation. This projection thus requires careful positioning.

If lateral projections of both wrists are required they may be obtained with one exposure by placing both hands in the lateral position with fingers extended and bringing them together so that the palmar surfaces touch.

Scaphoid

Injuries to the scaphoid may not be clearly visualized unless separation of bony fragments has occurred. Many fractures are demonstrated better on repeat examination after a delay of 10 days. It has become standard practice to take a number of routine projections of the scaphoid to try to demonstrate the bony injury. Usually a combination of the following are undertaken: PA wrist in ulnar deviation, PA oblique wrist in ulnar deviation, AP oblique wrist in ulnar deviation and PA wrist – 30° projection in ulnar deviation.

Lunate

The lunate is best demonstrated on the standard PA and lateral views of the wrist. Specific views are not required, although the scaphoid views above may be valuable in specific situations.

Trapezium: PA oblique projection with ulnar deviation

To identify minor injury it is usually advisable to take radiographs of both the sound and the injured limb for comparison. Both hands are placed in pronation with the thumbs touching and positioned to raise the medial border of the carpus to an angle of 30°.

Other Carpal Bones

Specific investigations may be required to suit the problem. A fracture of the hook of the hamate is

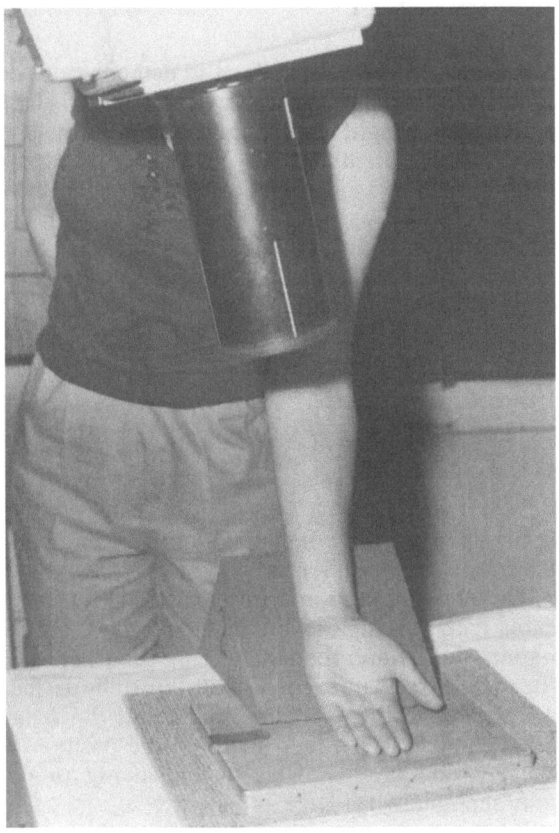

Fig. 1.1. Brewerton's projection for the metacarpo-phalangeal joints. Observe the limited flexion at the metacarpo-phalangeal joints and the angulation of the X-ray tube.

incomplete supination, i.e. 35–45°, with the medial borders almost touching. Each hand is supported on a 45° pad with thumbs fully extended.

Although certainly not a routine projection, the "ball-catching" view can be extremely valuable in detecting early erosions. In many departments it is undertaken without careful attention to position.

Brewerton's View

Early erosions of the metacarpal heads and the bases of the phalanges may be demonstrated more clearly on this projection (Figure 1.1). With the patient standing, the hand is placed in supination. The fingers are placed on the film and the metacarpals are flexed to 45° or 65°; the tube is angled 20° towards the thumb.

This projection is required only rarely in rheumatological practice; on occasion it can be very rewarding.

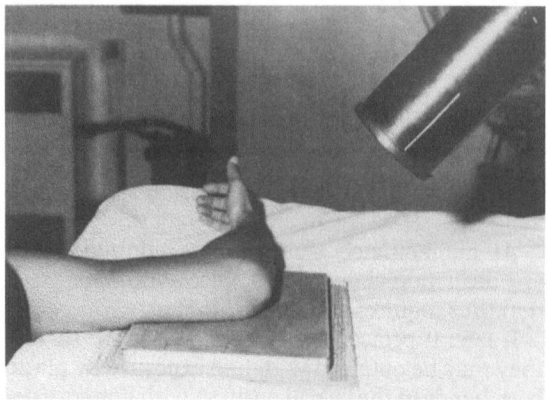

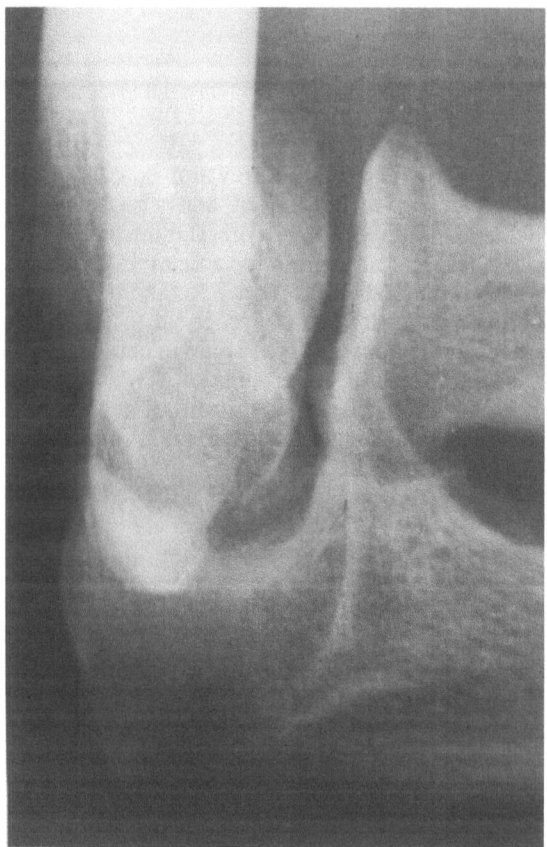

Fig. 1.2. **a** Angled projection to show head of radius and capitulum. **b** Film of Fig. 1.2a. The radial head and capitulum are elongated but overlap is reduced to a minimum.

often shown best on a lateral tomographic section. Computed tomography (CT) has great value in the difficult case.

Carpal Tunnel

The carpal tunnel is examined to demonstrate the presence of any bony anomaly or soft tissue calcification which might involve or compress the median nerve or the digital flexor tendons which pass through it. The most useful radiograph is an axial projection. In essence it is only one projection but the method of achieving that depends upon the individual radiographer.

Forearm and Elbow

Standard Projections

Standard projections include antero-posterior and lateral views for either part.

The lateral projection of the elbow has been advocated with varying degrees of supination and pronation of the hand thereby altering the position of the radial head. The exact position is usually decided on clinical grounds. It is essential that the radial head should not be seen in the same position in the AP and lateral views by employing pronation/supination.

Injuries to the elbow joint often leave the patient with some fixed flexion at the joint. Under such conditions the basic technique needs to be modified in order to compensate for this. An axial projection may be used to demonstrate the olecranon process. More usually it is employed to demonstrate the general alignment of the distal humerus and proximal forearm. Alternatively, the radio-humeral joint can be demonstrated by tilting the X-ray beam proximally along the axis of the arm. Occasionally circumstances dictate that the preceding technique is reversed to obtain a supero-inferior projection. In some cases this position may be altered slightly to provide a useful projection of the radial head. Any pathological changes in the bony sulcus of the ulnar groove or in the adjoining soft tissues may be demonstrated by either supero-inferior or axial projections.

Oblique projections of the elbow joint may be required to demonstrate loose bodies and periarticular calcification. Occasionally an AP projection of the radial head is necessary. This view also shows the proximal radio-ulnar joint in its entirety.

A special projection for the capitulum/head of the radius (Fig. 1.2) with the X-ray beam angled 45° to the shoulder in the long axis of the humerus is often helpful when a fracture of the radial head is suspected, i.e. a positive fat pad sign on the routine

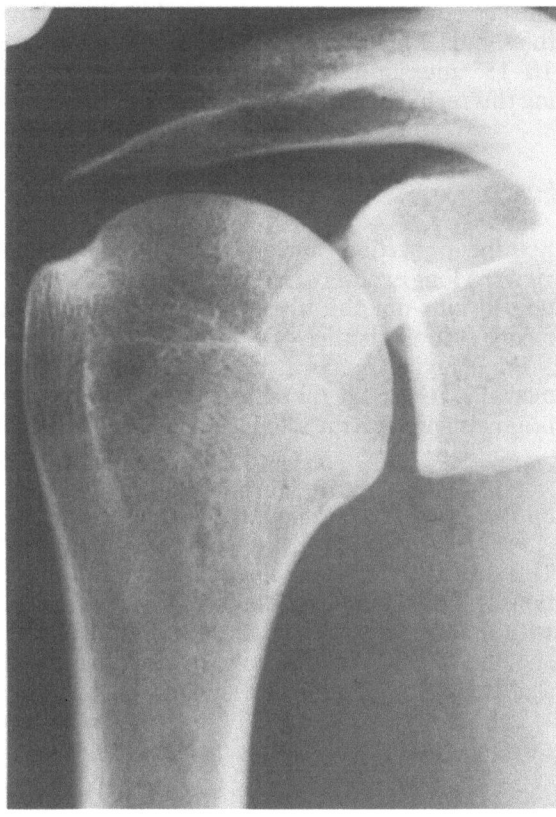

Fig. 1.3. True antero-posterior projection of the shoulder joint showing the glenoid process in profile.

AP and lateral projections, but with no evidence of bony injury. Our experience indicates that it is not necessary to undertake this additional projection routinely in cases of injury to the elbow.

Humerus, Shoulder, Shoulder Girdle and Sternum

Standard Projections

The humerus may be examined in the supine or erect position. The radiographic principles are the same. The choice of position really depends upon which position is easier for the patient. The standard projections include an AP and a lateral projection.

A transthoracic view is undertaken only to overcome physical difficulties; it may be obtained in the erect or sitting position. The patient is rotated so that the injured arm is against a vertical film stand throughout its length. This projection should be accepted only in exceptional circumstances. It is possible usually to obtain a more informative alternative view.

An AP projection of the shoulder may be undertaken in the erect, sitting or supine position depending on the patient's ability to achieve the position without discomfort. The erect or sitting positions are usually easier for the patient but entail a larger object-film distance. Conversely, the difficulty in positioning the supine position is often outweighed by the reduced object-film distance and the reduced likelihood of patient movement. The patient lies in the supine position on the radiography table. The unaffected side is raised until the affected shoulder is touching the film; the head is turned to the affected side. The precise amount of rotation depends on the build of the individual patient; it must be at least 25°, but 45° or greater may be required. This projection (Fig. 1.3) should be employed as the only standard AP projection. In some departments, notably in the United States, an unrotated standard AP projection, which is of very limited value, is used.

An axial projection of the shoulder may be obtained either supero-inferiorly or infero-superiorly in the erect or supine position, depending on the patient's condition. A curved cassette is only required in the supero-inferior position. The modified axial view (Wallace and Hellier 1983) or Stripp axial (see below) should be used when a standard axial radiograph cannot be taken, because it is too uncomfortable, for example following a comminuted fracture of the proximal humerus or fracture dislocation.

Stryker's Projection

This is mainly used to demonstrate the characteristic humeral notch (hatchet defect) following anterior dislocation of the shoulder (Fig. 1.4). The patient is supine with the affected shoulder positioned centrally. The patient's hand is placed on the side of his head with the elbow directed towards the ceiling so that the humerus is perpendicular to the film. The X-ray beam is angulated 30° cranially, having previously been centred to the coracoid process. Both shoulders should be examined for comparison. This projection has proved to be the most useful and reproducible one in demonstrating the humeral notch in recurrent anterior dislocation (Stoker 1982).

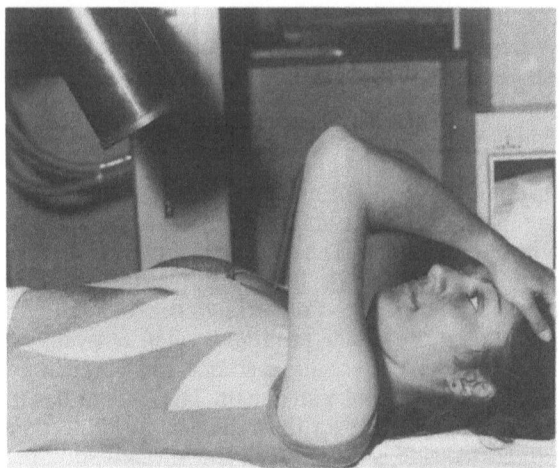

Fig. 1.4. Stryker's projection. The increased cephalad angulation of the tube (shown here) is preferable to that of the original description.

Upon completion of the routine radiographic examination of the shoulder, further projections may be required to demonstrate the exact anatomical location of calcific deposits within a specific tendon.

Supraspinatus is generally demonstrated in an AP view of the shoulder, when the calcification lies wholly or partially above the humeral head.

Infraspinatus, although often evident on the routine AP and axial projections, is more clearly demonstrated in the AP projection by placing the arm in full lateral rotation with a 25° caudal tilt on the X-ray tube.

Teres minor is best demonstrated in an AP position of the shoulder with the humerus in full medial rotation.

Calcification in *subscapularis* may be detected on the AP view as a density overlying the humeral head. A clearer demonstration can be achieved by repeating the axial projection with the arm in pronation and supination. The calcification should be clearly visible on the supination film, but overlapping the humeral head in pronation.

Bicipital Groove

The patient may be examined in the erect, sitting or supine position. The supine position is often preferable as there is less likelihood of patient movement and it is easier to support the film cassette. On initial examination both sides are examined for comparison. The shoulder is palpated and the arm positioned so that the bicipital groove is uppermost. A

film cassette is supported in a vertical position above the shoulder joint with a horizontal X-ray beam. A 10–15° anterior angulation may assist in visualizing this region better.

Scapula

Routine projections include the AP and lateral views. A long exposure time is used in the AP projection to blur out the ribs which may overlap the medial scapular border.

Use of an oblique X-ray beam projects the thorax medially. In the lateral projection, obliquity of the beam also projects the scapula away from the ribs.

Special Axial Projection (Stripp Axial)

This may be used when conventional axial projections are unobtainable. The patient sits on a stool with the film cassette placed at 35° on the affected shoulder (Fig. 1.5). The patient leans backwards slightly, rotating the affected shoulder backwards.

This projection, devised by Stripp, has proved extremely valuable in selected patients.

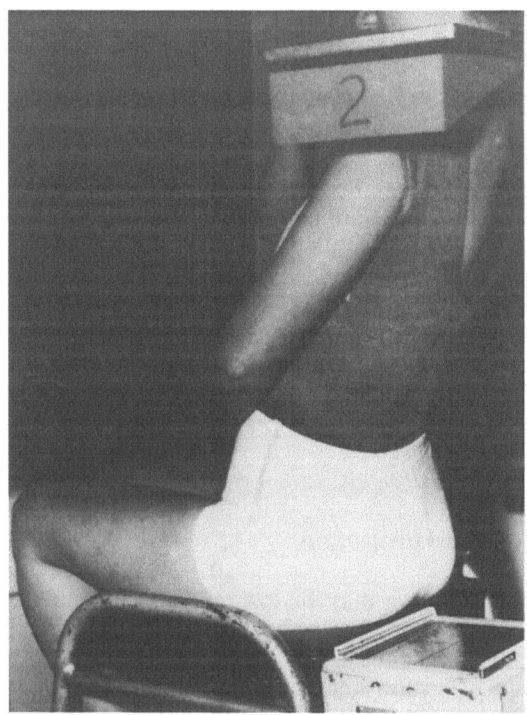

Fig. 1.5. Stripp axial projection of scapula and shoulder joint. This valuable projection will usually succeed when all else fails, e.g. in a patient with limited motion at the shoulder who is unable to stand.

Suprascapular Fossa

This oblique projection may be obtained with the patient in the erect position, but magnification and patient movement make it easier to obtain in the supine position.

The affected shoulder is raised 15° with a 30° caudal tilt of the X-ray tube. The exposure is made on arrested respiration.

Coracoid Process

The coracoid process is usually adequately demonstrated on the lateral scapular or Stryker's projection, but lesions or injuries of its base may require an additional projection with the arm raised and the affected side raised 15°.

Acromion

An AP or axial projection of the shoulder also shows the acromion well. A supplementary projection is achieved with the patient positioned as for a lateral scapular projection but with the forearm raised and rested on the top of the head.

Projections for the acromio-clavicular joints also specifically demonstrate part or all of the acromion.

Clavicle

Routine projections include AP and infero-superior views.

A frontal projection of the clavicle may be obtained in the erect, prone or supine positions, either by an AP or PA technique. It is more usual to use the AP projection in the erect or supine position, as both of these provide an additional projection of the shoulder joint.

The infero-superior projection is sometimes referred to as the lateral view of the clavicle. The X-ray tube is lowered and inverted and the radiograph is obtained usually with the patient erect during arrested respiration. This valuable second projection of the clavicle is used infrequently in many departments.

Acromio-clavicular Joint

An AP projection is normally obtained in the erect position and the joints on both sides examined for comparison.

To demonstrate subluxation weight-bearing with equal weights (usually 2 kg) in each hand is carried out. The weights must not be actively held up; the shoulders are relaxed, arms by the sides and the weights allowed to pull them down. The film is taken during arrested respiration.

The last two projections usually show the lateral end of the clavicle superimposed over the acromion process and therefore provide only comparative alignment. Demonstration of the joint space and the lateral end of the clavicle requires an additional projection with the X-ray beam angulated 25° cranially and 10° laterally.

The acromio-clavicular joints are demonstrated poorly in many radiological departments. This last projection is specific and most valuable.

Sterno-clavicular Joints

These joints may be examined in the AP or PA projections, and in the prone/supine or erect positions. Both joints should be included for comparison in each projection.

Tomography may provide better visualization of any pathology in this area and often proves to be the primary radiographic examination of choice in difficult subjects.

A lateral projection is rarely of any clinical value.

Sternum

Lateral and PA projections – the latter with beam angulation where required – are usually obtained.

Tomography of the sternum is required however if any doubt of a pathological process exists after inspection of the plain films.

Pelvis

Standard Projections

The size and shape of the adult bony pelvis varies with the sex and build of the patient. The highest points of the pelvis are the posterior elements of the two iliac crests and the lowest, the two ischial tuberosities. All these landmarks must be included on a standard AP projection.

The ankles are placed approximately 6″ apart and the feet rotated medially until the toes touch. This has the effect of internally rotating the femora, eliminating the normal anteversion and producing a true *en face* projection of the femoral neck.

Most orthopaedic requests for radiological examination of the pelvis are for assessment of the hip joints, most commonly in respect of degenerative joint disease. In these circumstances the surgeon is really interested in the hip joint concerned and the proximal end of the femoral shaft. On subsequent examinations the surgeon may need a demonstration of the whole of a hip prosthesis on the same film. In such cases the patient is positioned as for a radiographic examination of the pelvis, and the affected hip positioned centrally.

Lateral Pelvimetry

A lateral projection of the pelvis may be undertaken in the horizontal or, more usually, the erect position. A radio-opaque ruler is held or taped between the patient's thighs and included on the film so that accurate measurement of the mid-pelvic diameter can be made. As the projection encompasses the most dense part of the body, a substantial increase in radiographic exposure is necessary.

The increased use and value of ultrasonography has significantly reduced the need for X-ray pelvimetry.

Ilium

The iliac fossae and crests are demonstrated on the AP projection of the pelvis. To obtain a flatter projection of the blade of the ilium, the patient is rotated 45° to the side of interest.

Symphysis Pubis

In certain situations it may be necessary to demonstrate disorder or subluxation at the symphysis pubis. The examination is undertaken in the AP erect position.

When instability is suspected, two radiographs are taken with the patient standing with his weight on each leg in turn. These so-called "flamingo" views allow the demonstration of movement and hence instability at the symphysis often associated with stress sclerosis of the bony margins.

After surgical fusion of an unstable symphysis, the conventional frontal projection does not demonstrate adequately the site of the fusion. A supplementary axial projection is therefore necessary and is obtained with the patient seated and reclining at an angle of 60°. A vertical central ray is

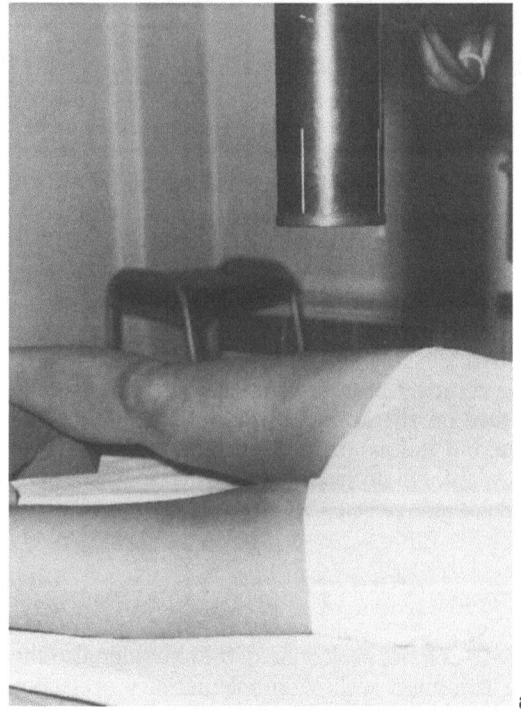

a

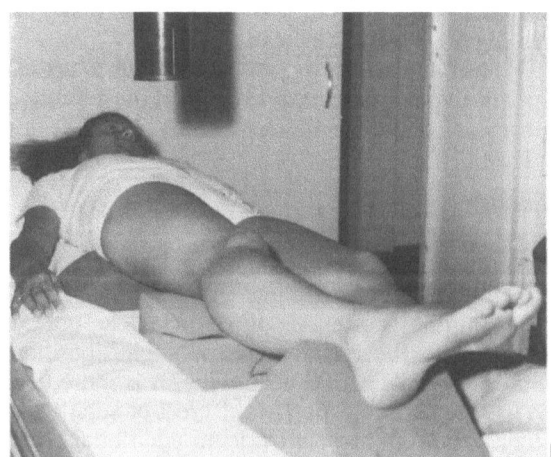

b

Fig. 1.6. a Judet projection of left ilium – posterior oblique. **b** Judet projection of right ilium – anterior oblique.

employed. The ischio-pubic rami are superimposed and the obturator foramina observed on the resultant radiograph. This projection is essential to confirm eccentric ankylosis of the symphysis.

Sacro-iliac Joints

The sacro-iliac joints may be demonstrated radiographically by a number of means. The most effective and simple examination is an AP projection of both joints at the same time with the patient supine.

The use of a PA projection with caudal angulation has a theoretical advantage in that the divergence of the X-ray beam follows the line of the joint. In practice it offers no advantage as the joints are further from the film.

If a more precise and detailed projection is required, individual oblique views may be obtained to demonstrate each joint in turn. Due to individual variation, no specific angle of obliquity can be given but it lies in the range of 15–25°.

If a minor degree of subluxation of a sacro-iliac joint is suspected, the conventional radiographic examination is unlikely to be of any value. In these circumstances the examination should be carried out in the erect position using a horizontal central beam angled 25° cranially.

Acetabulum

The usual projection to demonstrate the outer rim of an individual acetabulum is a prone 45° oblique projection.

The brothers Judet of Paris described anterior and posterior oblique projections (Fig. 1.6) which are of great value in the demonstration of fractures of the acetabulum. It should be noted, however, that these projections are not undertaken in the Accident Department without medical supervision.

Acetabular fractures are best demonstrated by computed tomography when available (Chap. 20). By this means not only is anatomical detail shown with the greatest accuracy, but unsuspected intra-articular bony fragments may be revealed; the ability to identify and remove such loose bodies protects the hip joint from progressive damage.

Hip Joint

Because of the proximity of the gonads to the proximal end of the femur, every means available (technique, shielding, avoidance of unnecessary examination) must be employed to reduce gonadal irradiation, while at the same time demonstrating the whole part under examination.

Standard Projections

Standard projections of the hip include AP and lateral views. In the former both hips are usually examined together but an AP projection of a single hip joint may be required.

Numerous methods are available to obtain a lateral projection of the hip joint. Each is dictated by the patient's condition, and his/her ability to move into the required position, the preference of the clinician and the need for a true lateral projection of the acetabulum as well as of the femoral head and neck.

"Frog" Lateral

Here both hips, flexed and rotated laterally, are exposed simultaneously on the same film for comparison. This projection is of use in children, particularly in Perthes' disease or in suspected slipped capital femoral epiphysis. Adults usually cannot obtain the degree of femoral abduction necessary.

Note that this projection does not alter the position of the acetabulum; only the femoral position is lateral.

Supine Horizontal Beam Lateral (Smith-Petersen)

This view with the sound limb flexed at the hip and knee is the projection of choice in patients with a suspected fracture of the neck of the femur. A slightly modified version is used during operative fixation of fractures of the femoral neck and the same principle is used during image intensifying procedures. This projection gives a true lateral view of the acetabulum.

Sitting Horizontal Beam Lateral

This projection with the sound limb abducted at the hip produces a radiograph comparable to the supine horizontal beam lateral. It has the advantages that it only needs slight movement of the X-ray tube and only slightly more exposure than for the AP projection.

Some patients may need support from a back rest when sitting up. If the patient leans back, providing he or she is comfortable and not likely to slip off the table, the quality of the film will not be affected.

In some cases, a lateral projection of the hip will be required on a patient who cannot achieve the

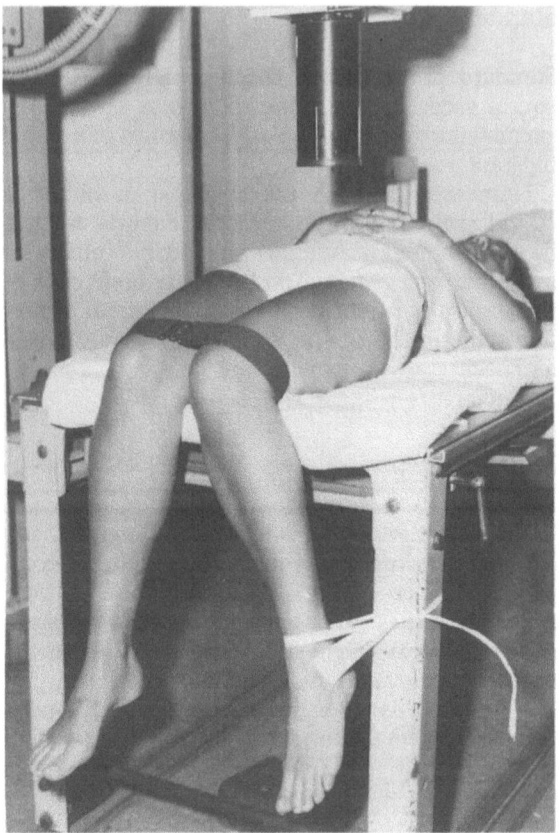

Fig. 1.7. Billing's antero-posterior projection. Velcro bands are normally used to maintain the position.

correct position for any of the techniques described above. Here the radiographic technique employed must be individually adapted to achieve a useful result.

Billing Projections

Since the mid-1940s a number of authors have described special radiographic techniques to demonstrate slipped femoral capital epiphysis. The technique proposed by Billing (1954) has found most favour.

Billing described an AP and two lateral projections, either of which can be used to demonstrate the angle between the epiphysis and the femoral neck. In addition to slipping of the epiphysis, it is possible to measure accurately the angle between the femoral neck and the diaphysis and the anteversion angle.

As an increased incidence of bilateral slip is well recognized, both hips should be examined for comparison. Such an examination also provides a baseline examination for future serial views of the "normal" hip.

Anteroposterior. The longitudinal axis of the femur is positioned parallel to the table top with the hip medially rotated 20° (Fig. 1.7) (Billing and Eklof 1984).

"Ideal" Lateral View. The hip is abducted and 90° laterally rotated with the femoral shaft at 25° to the X-ray table.

Alternative Lateral View. This projection must be used when the "S" angle, relating the axis of the femoral shaft and the plane of the growth plate on the AP view, falls outside the range 15–35°. The technique is the same as the "ideal" lateral with the femoral shaft elevated to an angle equal to the S-angle as measured on the AP film. (The S-angle is equal to 90° minus the angle between the femoral shaft and the plane of the growth plate.)

The axes of the femoral diaphysis and neck and the plane of the epiphyseal cartilage can be drawn on the resultant radiographs and the angle of anteversion determined from Billing's nomogram. In the lateral projection, the angle relating the axis of the femoral neck to the plane of the growth plate (eppa) normally lies between 84° and 90°. Values less than 78° indicate slipping of the epiphysis, those between 84° and 78° are suspect and such patients require close observation.

Femur

Standard Projections

Standard projections include AP and lateral views. In the former the film must be long enough to include the knee joint.

A 5° cranial tilt of the X-ray beam often helps to obtain a true lateral projection at the knee joint.

Leg

Torsion injuries to the ankle joint and the distal end of the tibia may produce a compensatory injury of the proximal shaft of the fibula or the proximal tibiofibular joint. Correct location and alignment of such a fracture requires examination of the knee and ankle joints on the same film. As the commonly employed 18 × 43 cm cassette will not include the whole leg in the majority of adults, it is usually necessary to employ the diagonal length of a 35 × 43 cm cassette.

Standard Projections

Standard projections include AP, lateral and oblique views.

In patients with a deformity of the limb, the leg can be positioned by using the tibial tubercle rather than the malleoli as a landmark.

As a result of divergence of the X-ray beam, the ankle joint may not be shown clearly in the lateral projection. A 5° compensatory cranial tilt of the X-ray tube may then be helpful.

Antero-posterior and lateral oblique projections are necessary to demonstrate the proximal tibio-fibular joint.

Knee

In addition to conventional AP and lateral projections it may be necessary to examine the knee in forced adduction and abduction (varus and valgus stress) to demonstrate any widening of the joint compartments due to defective collateral ligaments. A suitably protected (lead gloves and apron) medical officer provides the stress necessary and the radiographer exposes the film at a pre-arranged signal. Valgus and varus stress are applied in turn, ensuring that the knee is *not* fully extended as it is then often quite stable. If the knee is painful, e.g. following recent trauma, the examination should be carried out under a general anaesthetic.

To investigate AP subluxation the patient can be examined in the erect or supine position with the leg outstretched, supported at the ankle and relaxed, but often the examination is best carried out under general anaesthesia. The effects of gravity and slight hyperextension upon the knee are tested.

Any patient with a suspected varus or valgus deformity should have the AP projection of the knees exposed in the erect position. Such weight-bearing views with the feet 6″ apart are rightly being requested frequently or routinely. They offer a truer picture of alignment at the knee.

An intercondylar projection obtained with the patient prone and the knee flexed (Fig. 1.8) is employed to demonstrate the whole of the femoral condyles and any loose bodies within the inter-

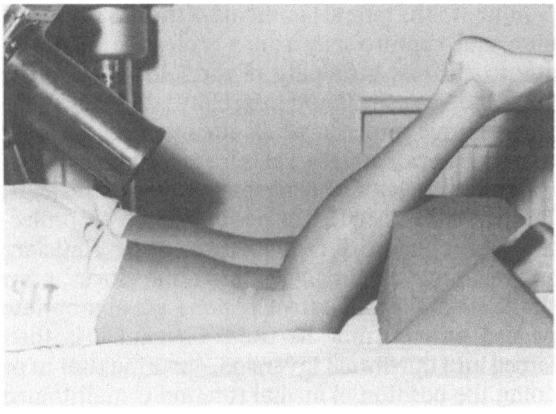

Fig. 1.8. Intercondylar projection of femur ("tunnel" view).

condylar notch. If the lower pole of the patella is demonstrated on the radiograph in the notch, the angle of flexion of the knee can be reduced.

Patella

To obtain better detail of the patella, PA, oblique and infero-superior ("skyline") projections can be obtained.

The knee is flexed approximately 35° for the last projection. A lead rubber sheet is held in position directly behind the cassette to reduce the radiation dose to the patient's trunk. With the knee fixed, however, angulation is critical and the experienced radiographer will modify the angulation of the X-ray beam to suit the individual anatomical situation.

Specific multiple axial views of the patella may be obtained with the knees flexed to 30°, 60°, and 90° respectively. Such views have been fashionable, but rarely provide information of clinical value except possibly in some cases of patellar subluxation.

Ankle Joint

Standard Projections

Standard projections include AP, lateral and oblique views. The standard AP view should be taken with the leg at 20° internal rotation to demonstrate the distal tibio-fibular syndesmosis.

Injury to the lateral ligaments of the ankle is common and rupture may cause prolonged disability due to chronic instability of the joint. The radiographic demonstration of instability is usually a simple dynamic procedure. If attempted soon after injury, general anaesthesia is frequently required to allow the application of adequate stress to the joint. The patient is placed in the position for an AP projection of the ankle. A radiologist or other clinician, suitably protected in a lead apron and gloves, grips the foot in the mid-tarsal region; an appropriate padded wrench may be used. The ankle is then forced into maximum inversion, ensuring that in so doing the position of medial rotation is maintained while the exposure is made. Both ankles must be examined to allow comparison. A line is drawn along the distal subarticular border of the tibia and similarly on the upper border of the dome of the talus. The angle between these represents the degree of talar tilt. The following findings provide a rough working guide:

a. A tilt of 5 to 15° more than the uninjured side suggests a rupture of the anterior talofibular ligament
b. A tilt of 15 to 30° suggests rupture of the anterior talofibular ligament and the calcaneofibular ligament
c. A tilt of 30° or more suggests complete rupture of all three ligaments.

The range of normal variation, however, is wide and where abnormal tilt is seen in both ankles, this can reflect either the patient's normal laxity or previous bilateral tears of the lateral ligamentous complex.

If the results of forced inversion views are inconclusive and there is a specific clinical problem, the ankle is raised from the table-top and supported. A weight is placed on the patient's leg for 30 seconds and a horizontal beam lateral projection then obtained. Both ankles must be examined for comparison. An abnormality is said to be present if there is a difference of 3 mm or more in the posterior talotibial separation. Forced eversion films may also be required.

Patients suffering from congenital talipes equino varus present numerous technical difficulties. The success of the examination depends largely on the relaying of information to the radiographer undertaking the examination. When a lateral ankle is requested, it must include the whole foot. When an AP ankle is requested it also should show the whole foot. The AP projection should preferably be undertaken in a weight-bearing position. In all cases the position of the malleoli is paramount, regardless of the position of the foot due to the deformity. If the malleoli are equidistant from the film for the AP ankle and superimposed for the lateral then the position is correct and the examination successful.

Foot

The stability of the foot is maintained by a number of arches in different planes. Considerable variations in thickness and therefore in radiographic density exist. When a film-screen combination is used, it is often advisable to employ a high kilovoltage technique to reduce excessive photographic contrast in the resultant radiograph.

Standard Projections

Standard projections include AP (dorsi-plantar), oblique and lateral (medio-lateral or lateral-medial) views.

Weight-bearing projections in the dorsi-plantar or lateral positions can be obtained with the patient standing; both feet are examined and the patients' weight distributed evenly down each leg. For specific anatomical accuracy, each foot may be examined separately, with separate films and centring to the individual foot. A simultaneous lateral projection has few advantages and considerable disadvantages in interpretation and comparison. It is not recommended.

Hallux

Localized dorsi-plantar and lateral projections can be obtained. If hallux valgus is demonstrated, the projections can be supplemented by a weight-bearing dorsi-plantar view. The sesamoid bones are shown well in the routine lateral hallux projection and can also be shown tangentially in axial projections.

Calcaneus

The calcaneus is well demonstrated on lateral and axial projections.

An axial projection with a 30° cranial tilt of the X-ray beam demonstrates the talo-calcaneal joint. Greater degrees of angulation tend only to elongate the calcaneus.

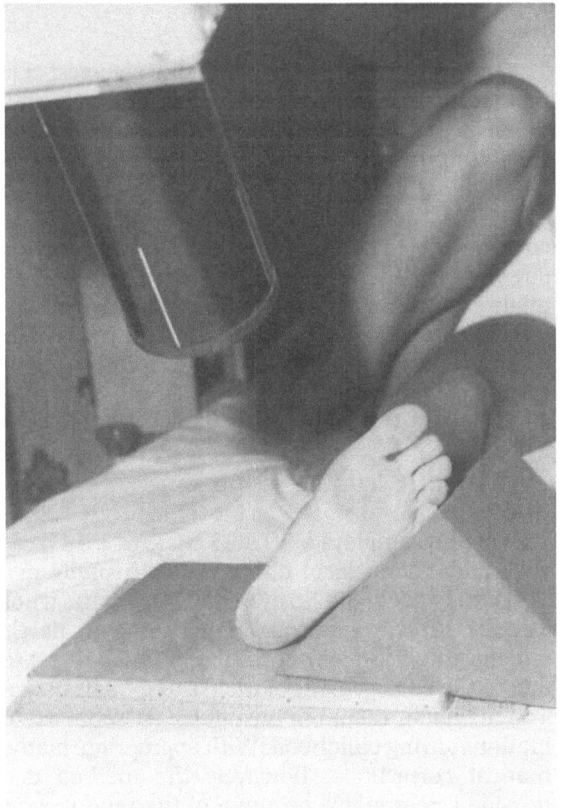 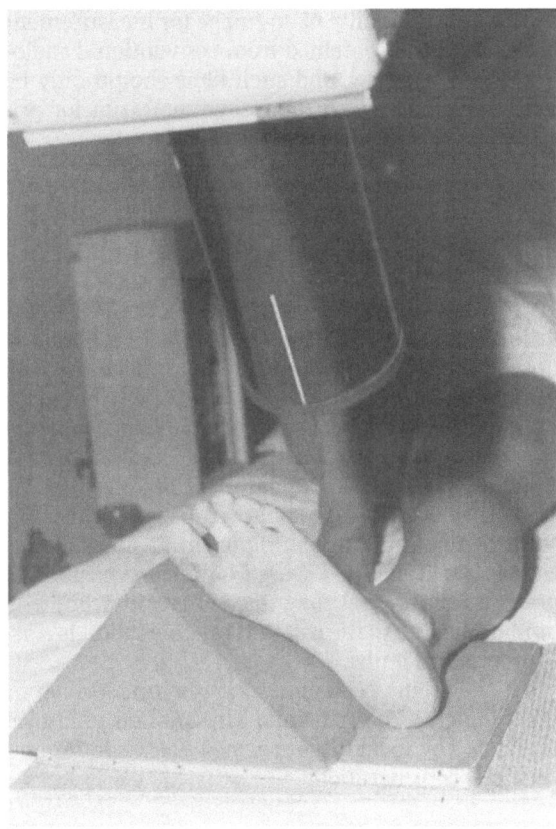

a   b

Fig. 1.9a,b. Complementary views to demonstrate subtalar joints. These together often give more information than Anthonsen's projection.

Standing Axial Projection (Harris). This projection is employed principally to demonstrate congenital abnormalities such as talo-calcaneal bars. It may also be used as an additional projection for a fractured calcaneus.

If demonstration is inadequate a CT examination is indicated.

Subtalar Joint

Projections to demonstrate the subtalar joints involve a double angulation of the X-ray tube. Modification of the lateral projection (Anthonsen) or of the axial (medial and lateral oblique, Fig. 1.9) can be employed.

One of the problems with all subtalar projections is that they work very well with a normal joint, but as soon as the joint is deformed or narrowed it is difficult to demonstrate anatomical detail. The value of CT for anatomical detail in this region is unsurpassed.

Lower Limb Length

A number of techniques can be employed to produce radiographs from which measurements of limb length may be obtained. The method used in any department will be dependent upon the local expertise and the facilities available. It is commonly recognized that any method used must allow accurate comparative measurements at a single examination. The method must also provide an accuracy similar for varying lengths of limb, and with sufficient detail to demonstrate the epiphyseal plates and any bony abnormalities. In all the radiographic techniques employed, positioning of the patient is constant. Most techniques may be undertaken in either erect or supine positions. The supine position is preferred as it can be achieved by all patients with less likelihood of movement. The ankles are placed approximately 15 cm (6″) apart and the pelvis symmetrically positioned. Gonadal protection should be used in all cases.

The overall quality of an image for measurement is less than that obtained from conventional radiographic techniques, and such films should only be used for measurement and alignment, not for primary diagnostic purposes.

Basic Principle of Measurement Technique

To obtain accurate measurements of limb length, little or no longitudinal foreshortening or magnification of the limbs must occur. To achieve this the vertical central ray must always be centred directly over the ends of the bones. Magnification can be reduced by the use of a large (110 cm) focus-film distance. With certain apparatus this distance can be further extended. It is important for continuing studies that once a technique protocol has been established it should be used on each occasion. In practice, the actual magnification of the limbs is immaterial due to the fact that magnification is constant for both limbs.

The following techniques may be undertaken in most imaging departments. The method of choice is dictated by local expertise, available facilities and financial considerations.

Scanography

Scanography is probably the most widely used method for measurement of limb length. The technique requires a slit-beam diaphragm with an aperture of 1/16th of an inch, fitted to the X-ray tube, a long film cassette (90 × 35 cm), and a motorized X-ray tube column capable of movement in the long axis of the X-ray table. During exposure, the X-ray tube traverses the whole length of the film, effectively scanning the entire lower limb. As this technique allows the X-ray beam to intersect the bone ends perpendicularly, comparative limb lengths can be measured.

A modified scanogram with three separate exposures over the hips, knees and ankles can be undertaken when a long cassette but not a motorized tube is available. The modified scanogram is reproducible and accurate but has two disadvantages; firstly, it does not demonstrate the diaphyses and, secondly, separate exposures of each limb may be required where there is gross discrepancy in length.

The number of exposures on each film can be increased to six but the disadvantages are the potential for patient movement and the effect of X-ray scatter giving rise to radiographs of low quality.

Mini-scanogram

The mini-scanogram is currently the cheapest of all methods for measuring limb length. The only additional piece of equipment required is an orthopaedic rule, with a radio-opaque scale. The rule is placed longitudinally down the centre of the X-ray table. The lower two thirds of a 35 × 43 cm cassette are covered by lead rubber, and a vertical beam centred directly over the hip joints. Further exposures are made at the knee and ankle joints in turn, uncovering the corresponding areas of the film. As with the other orthoradiographic techniques, the diaphyses are not demonstrated.

The Marquet Method

This method employs a 90 × 35 cm (36″ × 14″) cassette and a long focal film distance (usually over 180 cm) to allow the X-ray beam to cover the whole cassette in one exposure. Unfortunately, as the patient grows, the object to film distance increases due to the enlargement of the posterior soft tissues. The method is therefore unsuitable for serial examinations during childhood. With appropriate mathematical corrections, however, the method does provide a reasonable estimate of the relative bone lengths at a single attendance.

Stereoradiography

This technique employs a shift in position of the X-ray tube to provide two images which, when viewed together, provide a three-dimensional effect. Two films are always required, and are together referred to as a stereoscopic pair.

To produce a stereoscopic pair, it is essential that the patient remains stationary whilst the X-ray tube is shifted between exposures to be equidistant on each side of the central point. The ideal total shift should be that of the interpupillary distance, and is usually about 6 cm. To obtain optimal results, identical film-screen combinations and exposures are used and the films are processed together.

Stereoscopic pairs may be viewed by using the Wheatstone stereoscope, or, more commonly, by using prismatic binoculars. Both methods employ a mirror system, so to view the image in its true perspective, the films must be mounted in the reverse position. The film with shift to the left is mounted on the left and that with shift to the right is mounted on the right.

The correct stereoscopic viewing distance is equal to the focus-film distance used to expose the films, but most observers need to experiment and vary the distance to achieve a three-dimensional effect. It should be noted that 10% to 15% of the population is unable to perceive the stereoscopic effect at all.

Stereophotogrammetry has been used to study micromotion, for example in early joint loosening (Ryd 1986).

Acknowledgements. The authors wish to acknowledge the radiographic expertise over the years of William Stripp, for many years Superintendent Radiographer at the Royal National Orthopaedic Hospital. We thank Dirk de Camp, Medical Photographic Department of the Institute of Orthopaedics, Bolsover Street, London for preparing the illustrations and Miss Veronika Aurens for secretarial assistance. Our thanks are also due to Miss Penny Stocks and Mrs. Elaine Scotter for help with the illustrations.

References

Billing L (1954) Roentgen examination of the proximal femur end in children and adolescents. Standardized technique also suitable for determination of collum-, anteversion-, and epiphyseal angles. Study of slipped epiphysis and coxa plana. Acta Radiol Suppl 110:1–80

Billing L, Eklof O (1984) Slip of the capital femoral epiphysis: revival of a method of assessment. Pediatr Radiol 14:413–418

Ryd L (1986) Micromotion in knee arthroplasty. Acta Orthop Scand Suppl 220

Stoker DJ (1982) The radiology of the humeral defect in anterior dislocation of the shoulder – a comparative study. In: Bayley IW, Kessel L (eds) Shoulder surgery. Springer-Verlag, Berlin, pp 84–86

Wallace WA, Hellier M (1983) Improving radiographs of the injured shoulder. Radiography 49:229–233

Further Reading

Swallow RA, Naylor E (eds) (1986) Clark's positioning in radiography, 11th edn. Heinemann, London

2 Angiography of the Appendicular Skeleton

Anne P. Hemingway and A. Adam

Arteriography 19
  Technique 19
  Appearances on Arteriography 21
  Diagnostic Applications: Congenital Lesions 22
  Diagnostic Applications: Acquired Lesions 24
  Therapeutic Applications 25
Venography 28
  Anatomy 28
  Technique 28
  Appearances on Venography 32
  Indications 32
References 34

The value of angiography in the investigation of diseases of the intrathoracic, intra-abdominal and intracranial organs and of the peripheral vascular system is well established (Allison 1986a), but the techniques have had a more limited role in orthopaedic practice. Nevertheless angiography, correctly used, can make a major contribution to clinical decisions regarding the treatment of bone tumours and is certainly extremely valuable in certain cases of skeletal trauma. Recent developments, such as the availability of low-osmolality contrast media and digital subtraction techniques, have increased the safety and flexibility of the technique. The great advances in interventional radiology have also expanded the role of angiography in the treatment of bone tumours and traumatic lesions.

Arteriography

Arteriography can be divided into two broad categories: diagnostic investigations and therapeutic procedures. The basic techniques involved are similar in both groups, but specialist expertise and equipment are needed to undertake many of the therapeutic manoeuvres.

Technique

Conventional Angiographic Techniques

Access to the arterial tree can be afforded from a number of sites, but the most commonly used route is via the femoral artery. Procedures are almost invariably performed under local anaesthetic and light sedation. The femoral artery is catheterized using a needle, guidewire and catheter exchange technique as described by Seldinger (1953). Since this first description there have been enormous advances in technology relating to guidewire and catheter manufacture. A range of catheter and guidewire shapes and sizes are now available which enable the selective and superselective catheterization of virtually every vascular territory in the human body. Occasionally for either anatomical or technical reasons it is necessary to enter the vascular tree via either the brachial or axillary arteries. Following the introduction of a catheter into the arterial tree it can then be guided, under fluoroscopic control, into the area of the body to be examined. Once the catheter is appropriately sited contrast medium is injected through the catheter either by hand or using a mechanical pump, and radiographic exposures are made in rapid sequence, the information being recorded on film. It is important to visualize both the arterial and venous circulations as valuable information is often provided by the venous phase of the arteriogram.

Once these films have been developed and reviewed it may prove necessary to subject them to a further photographic process known as *subtraction*. By this process all background information, such as images of bones and soft tissues, is subtracted, leaving just an image of the blood vessels being examined. This technique is of particular value in orthopaedic angiography where the density of bone can obscure fine vascular detail.

Digital Subtraction Angiography (DSA)

The full implications for radiology of computer technology and digitalization have yet to be realized. One of the areas in which the technique has already made an impact and become established is digital subtraction angiography (DSA), also known as digital vascular imaging (DVI).

For DSA an initial mask is obtained fluoroscopically before the injection of contrast medium. This image is then subtracted electronically from the images obtained after the injection of contrast medium. The procedure results in the elimination of unwanted detail and affords the additional advantage of greater sensitivity to the detection of the iodine signal in blood vessels from relatively dilute concentrations of contrast material (Meaney and Weinstein 1986). Digital subtraction techniques may be used to obtain arterial images following a venous injection of contrast medium (iv DSA) or following selective arterial injection (ia DSA) and for direct venography.

Intravenous Digital Subtraction Angiography (iv DSA). There is, as yet, no agreement on whether central injection of contrast medium into the superior vena cava or right atrium, or peripheral injection into an upper extremity vein (basilic or cephalic vein) is better. Currently, most institutions use a central injection (Boxt 1983; Clark and Alexander 1983). It is possible that in the absence of known cardiac disease a peripherally placed catheter is sufficient in most patients for the evaluation of the aorta and its major branches, but a central injection is more likely to produce a diagnostic examination and should always be favoured if visualization of more distal arteries (i.e. second- and third-order branches) is required (Neiman et al. 1985). If a peripheral injection is to be made a short cannula is inserted into an antecubital vein. If a central injection is to be employed, usually a catheter is passed into the superior vena cava or right atrium via the brachial vein, although the femoral vein may also be used. It is essential that the patient is completely immobile during the injection, and in the case of young children or uncooperative adults a general anaesthetic is usually necessary.

The major advantages of iv DSA are ease of examination, safety, rapidity of diagnosis, and decreased necessity for technical skill. The major disadvantages relate to the intravenous injection of large amounts of contrast material and motion artefacts (Meaney and Weinstein 1986). In addition the spatial resolution of iv DSA is inferior to that of conventional angiography and this results in less sharp images and loss of some vessel detail. Another feature of iv DSA is the simultaneous opacification of vessels in a particular area of the body, resulting in superimposition and consequent difficulties in the detailed assessment of the vascular supply of a particular lesion.

Intravenous DSA has been used in the preoperative evaluation of bone tumours and has been found useful in ascertaining the nature of the lesion, its extension to soft tissues and joints, and the presence of arteriovenous shunts. The overall accuracy of the technique varies from 89% to 92% depending on the feature evaluated (Simonetti et al. 1985). Intravenous DSA has been found unreliable in the detection of vascular injury following trauma to the extremities (Goodman et al. 1984).

Intra-arterial DSA (ia DSA). The major disadvantage of this technique compared with iv DSA is the necessity for an arterial puncture. Nevertheless the greater contrast sensitivity of DSA allows the use of much smaller volumes of contrast media than are used in conventional angiography. Contrast can be delivered by hand injection via small-calibre catheters. Intra-arterial DSA provides excellent image detail and is particularly useful in the performance of interventional procedures such as embolization and angioplasty. The immediate availability of the subtracted images for review on the fluoroscopic monitor is a great advantage during angiographic embolization and significantly reduces the time necessary for its performance. The small amount of contrast material needed in ia DSA increases the patient's comfort during what is frequently a prolonged interventional procedure and reduces the danger of impairment of renal function. The use of fewer X-ray films than in conventional angiography means that ia DSA is less costly. A very useful facility during ia DSA is the use of "roadmapping" of vessels, which enables continuous fluoroscopic display of arterial anatomy during

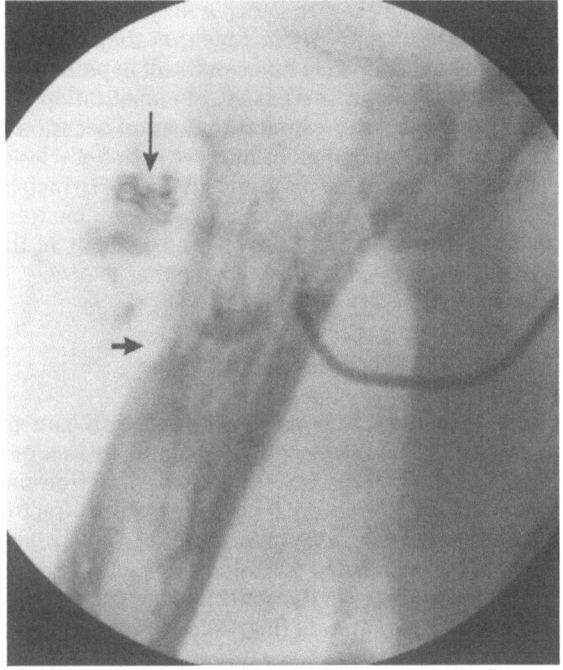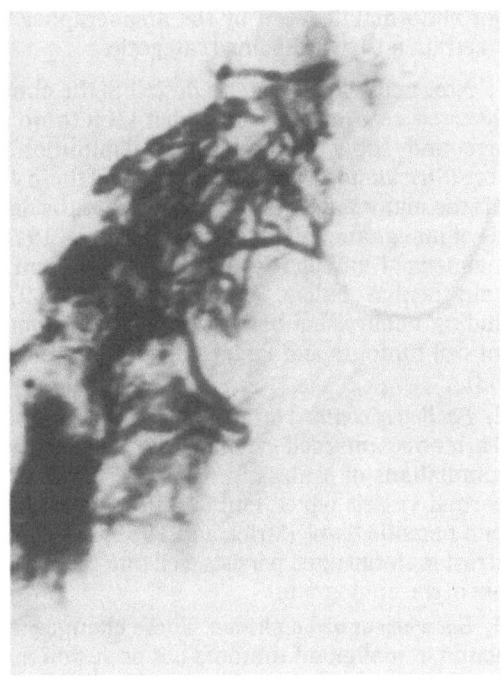

Fig. 2.1. a A film of the upper humerus in a 19-year-old male with an extensive arteriovenous malformation which is eroding bone (*short arrow*). The lesion is being treated by arterial embolization using steel coils (*long arrow*). **b** Selective digital subtraction angiogram showing part of the extensive malformation.

manipulation of catheters and guidewires (Chang et al. 1984). Thus the relationship of the guidewires and catheters to the vessels being negotiated can be continuously monitored (Kubal et al. 1983) – a very useful facility, especially in therapeutic procedures.

Indications. Intravenous DSA may be sufficient to assess the vascularity of a tumour mass or to demonstrate any large arteries involved in trauma, but intra-arterial DSA is necessary if visualization of small vessels is required. The technique is especially valuable in arterial embolization as it eliminates unwanted detail and allows accurate and rapid assessment of the results of this form of therapy. Arterial DSA is also extremely useful for the performance of indirect venography as it allows excellent images of draining veins to be obtained following the intra-arterial injection of small quantities of contrast medium.

Contrast Media

The high-osmolality contrast media which have been used in the past for angiographic studies are being superseded rapidly by a new generation of low-osmolality media such as Iohexol, Iopamidol and Ioxaglate. These are not only safer but are sub-

jectively more pleasant for the patient (Dawson et al. 1983; Adam et al. 1985). The new media are particularly useful in angiographic studies of the distal arteries of the extremities as these investigations are very painful when conventional media are employed and general anaesthesia may be necessary. The new media have also proved themselves to be of great value in complex interventional procedures when it may be necessary to inject large volumes of contrast into vulnerable vascular beds.

Pharmacoangiography

Pharmacoangiography is sometimes helpful during angiographic studies of bone or soft tissue tumours. Vasoconstrictor agents such as adrenaline, angiotensin (Ekelund et al. 1977) and vasopressin, and vasodilator agents such as tolazoline (Kadir et al. 1979), histamine, papaverine, reserpine and prostaglandins, have been employed during such studies.

Appearances on Arteriography

The detailed arteriographic appearances in bone lesions is beyond the scope of this chapter, but the major abnormalities seen by the angiographer fall into certain fairly well-defined categories:

1. *Neovascularity.* This term describes the abnormal vessels seen in tumours which keep to no set course and show no progressive diminution in calibre (Strickland 1959). The presence of these vessels is the major angiographic criterion for the diagnosis of malignancy (Voegeli and Uehlinger 1976), but abnormal vascularity may also be present in certain benign lesions (Viamonte et al. 1973) including aneurysmal bone cysts, osteoblastomas, giant cell tumours and Paget's disease (Tegtmeyer 1983).

2. *Pooling of contrast medium.* Malignant tumours and arteriovenous malformations may show patchy accumulations of contrast medium, resulting from abnormal vessels which end in amorphous spaces within necrotic tissue (Strickland 1959). Pooling of contrast material often persists well into the venous phase of the angiogram.

3. *Encasement and occlusion.* These changes may be found in malignant tumours but occlusion may, of course, also be seen in traumatic, embolic and atheromatous lesions, as well as in some cases of vasculitis.

4. *Tumour blush.* Diffuse staining by contrast material is a non-specific finding which does not in itself indicate malignancy and may be seen in several benign tumours. A similar appearance may be produced by contrast medium pouring from a traumatized artery.

5. *Displacement of vessels.* This may be seen in bone tumours but may also be produced by a haematoma or bone fragment causing an artery to alter its course.

6. *Compression of vessels.* This may be produced by any mass, including benign or malignant tumours and haematomas.

7. *Enlargement of vessels.* This change is seen when the vessel involved is supplying an area of markedly increased vascularity.

Diagnostic Applications: Congenital Lesions

The developments of DSA and new contrast media, together with advances in orthopaedic practice, have increased the number of indications for diagnostic angiographic procedures.

Primary Vascular Abnormalities

Primary vascular abnormalities may directly affect bone and may therefore present in an orthopaedic clinic. The most important lesions that can behave in this fashion are *arteriovenous malformations.* Some of these lesions are so massive that they cause erosion of bone (Fig. 2.1) that can result in pathological fracture. Prior to the advent of embolization techniques (see below) amputation was on occasion the only treatment option for massive peripheral lesions which were eroding bone and giving rise to incipient cardiac failure. Angiography plays a major role in the diagnosis of these lesions, assessment of their extent, and suitability for either surgery or embolization.

Primary Orthopaedic Abnormalities

Abnormalities such as *neurofibromatosis* can produce major bony deformity. This may be as a result of the primary dysplasia or as a result of trauma or pseudojoint formation. Following trauma, fractures may show malunion or non-union. This may be related to associated vascular damage. Assessment of the vascularity of the abnormal area can be useful in planning treatment (Fig. 2.2).

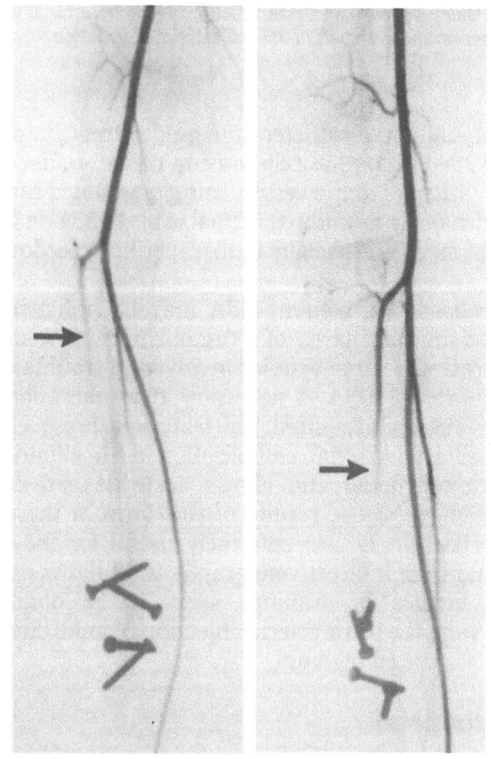

a   b

Fig. 2.2a,b. Anteroposterior and lateral views of an arteriogram showing the calf vessels in a child with neurofibromatosis. A fracture of the tibia had failed to heal after internal fixation resulting in a pseudoarthrosis. The anterior tibial artery (*arrow*) failed to fill below the level of the fracture even on delayed films.

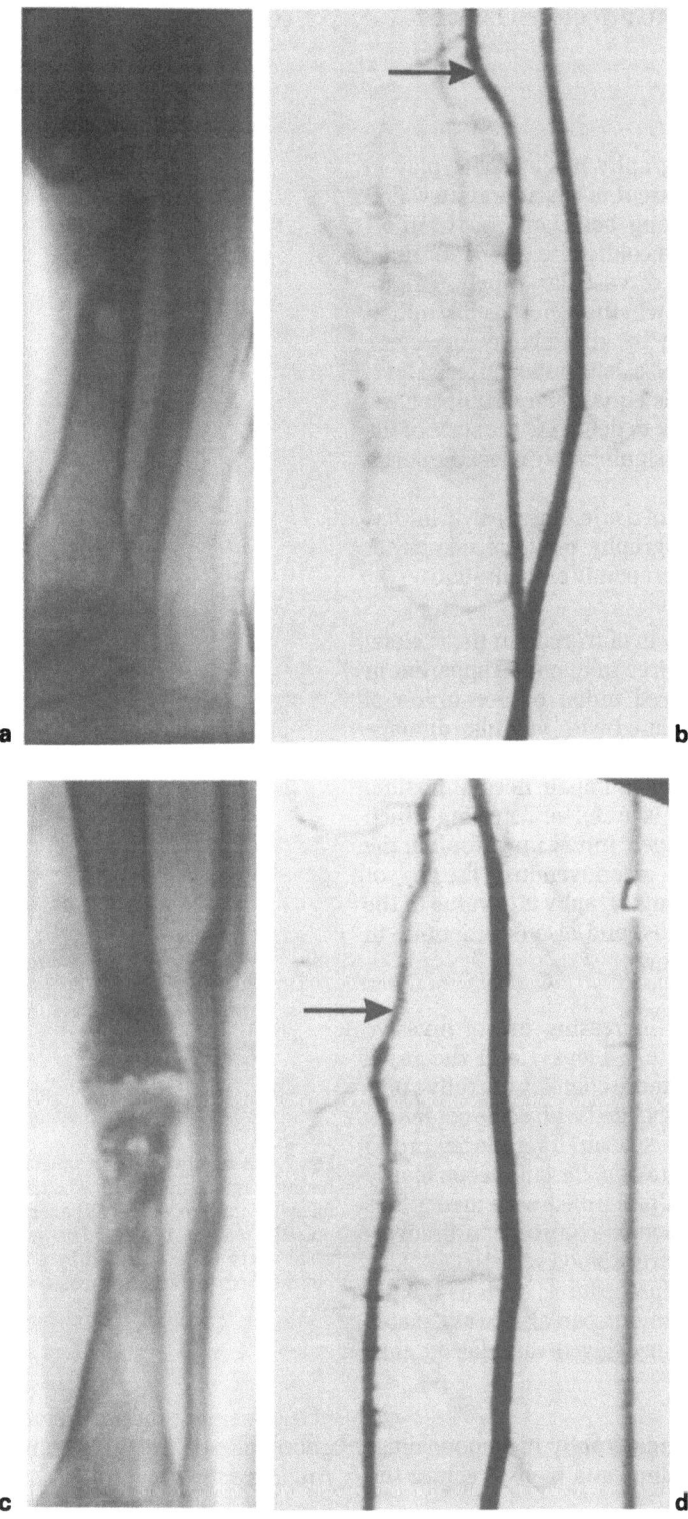

Fig. 2.3a–d. Digital subtraction angiograms (b and d) showing the calf vessels in a patient with non-union of a tibial fracture (a and c). The anterior tibial artery (*arrow*) is irregular and displaced by the bone deformity and neovascularity is seen in the region of the fracture.

Diagnostic Applications: Acquired Lesions

Trauma

Acute Diagnosis. Angiography has a role to play in the assessment of the extent of vascular injury. Following fracture to a long bone, one of the most feared complications is a cold, pulseless foot or hand indicating impairment of vascular supply. Angiography will determine whether there is disruption of the vessel, occlusion by an embolus, or severe vascular spasm; it will also determine the exact level of the abnormality. It is equally important for the angiographer to attempt to delineate the state of the distal vessels as this can significantly affect the surgical approach.

The technique is also of use in major pelvic injury, when diagnostic angiography may precede either definitive surgery or therapeutic embolization.

Delayed Effects. The effects of trauma to the skeletal system or the vascular tree may not be apparent in the acute phase. Delayed union or non-union of fractures may be associated with vascular damage which did not put the viability of the limb in jeopardy but is sufficient to impair normal healing (Fig. 2.3). Angiography is useful for detecting which vessels have been damaged. Injury may result in the development of an arteriovenous fistula or aneurysm formation; angiography is of value in the diagnosis of these lesions, and also occasionally in their treatment (see below).

Iatrogenic Trauma. The increasing use of invasive diagnostic techniques (e.g. biopsy) and the rapid development of several more complex operative procedures is inevitably associated with some complications. Plaster of Paris casts can, if misplaced or too tight, cause vascular damage. Percutaneous biopsy procedures, even when performed with meticulous care and under fluoroscopic control, can inadvertently damage neighbouring blood vessels (Fig. 2.4), and "routine" surgical procedures, such as hip pin and plate, or hip replacement, can also be associated with either immediate or delayed vascular damage (Fig. 2.5).

Tumours. The role of angiography in tumour diagnosis is modest. Plain films and biopsy remain the mainstay in this field.

Angiography should never be regarded as *diagnostic*; appearances may be suggestive of a particular tumour but the pathological diagnosis depends on tissue histology. If attempts at "confident" diag-

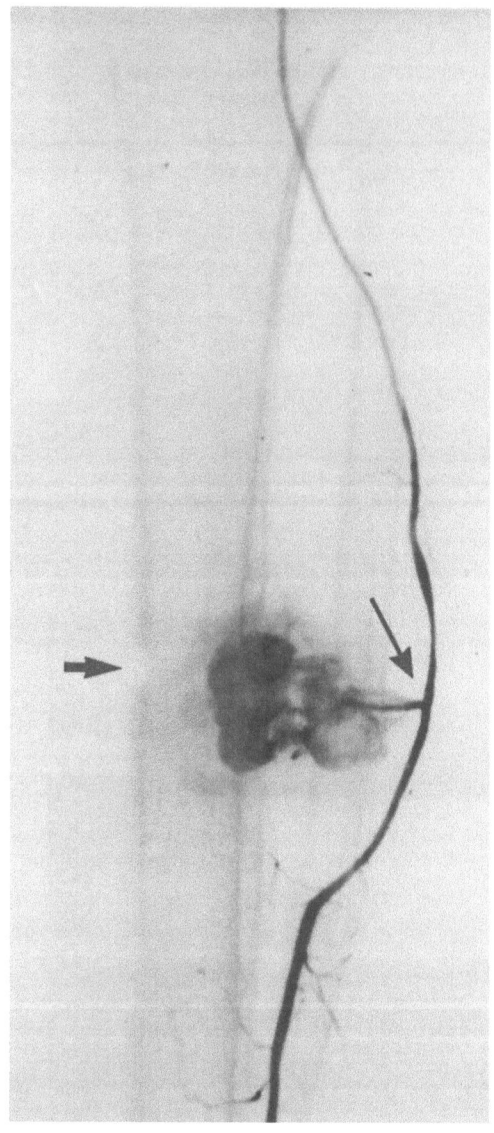

Fig. 2.4. A selective anterior tibial arteriogram in a patient who had undergone an operative bone biopsy (*short arrow*). Shortly following this procedure the patient complained of an enlarging pulsatile mass in the calf. The angiogram shows the anterior tibial artery to be displaced by a large haematoma and blood pouring from a defect in its medial wall (*long arrow*).

noses are made on the basis of angiographic appearances alone, mistakes can be made (Fig. 2.6). Angiography may, however, "suggest" an alternative diagnosis to that which is suspected clinically (Fig. 2.7).

The value of angiography lies in the delineation of vascular anatomy and assessment of tumour extent prior to biopsy, surgery or embolization.

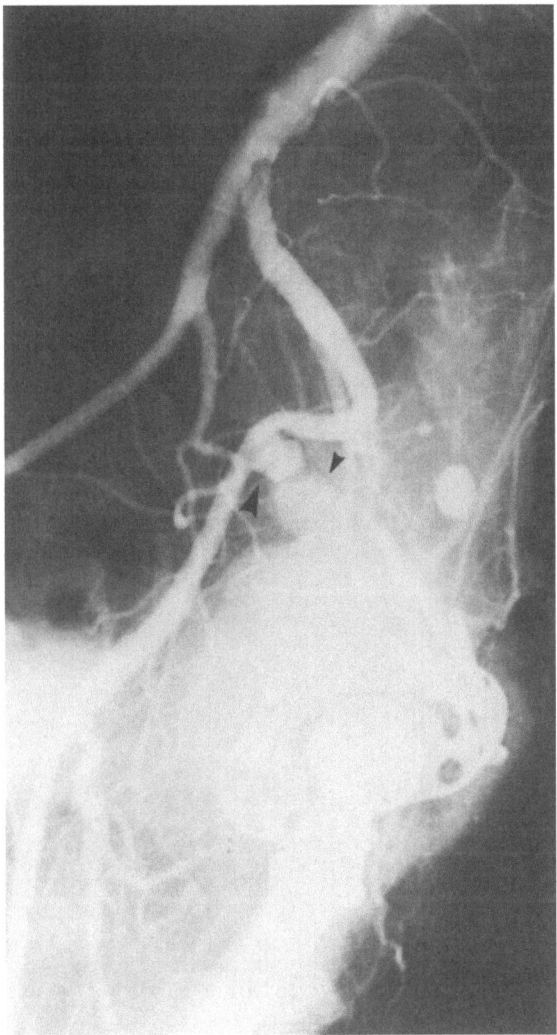

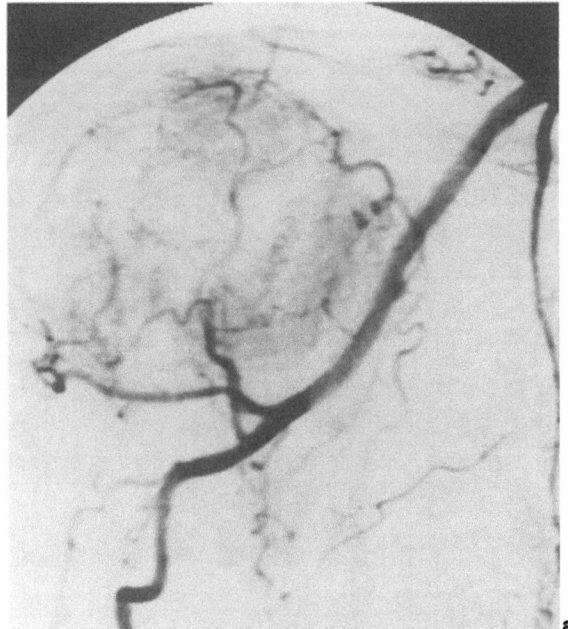

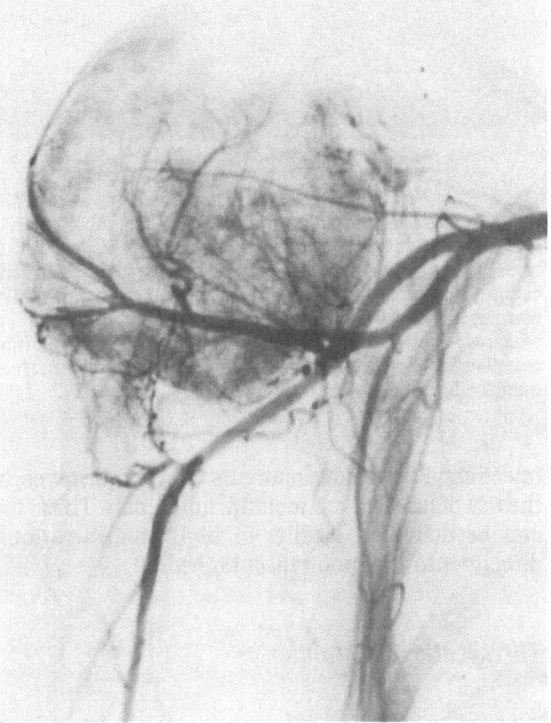

Fig. 2.5. Aneurysm of the external iliac artery following hip replacement. The exothermic reaction of the bone cement (*small arrowhead*) used in the prosthesis has caused an aneurysm in the neighbouring vessel (*large arrowhead*).

Therapeutic Applications

Infusion

There is increasing use of selective placement of catheters close to tumours for the local infusion of chemotherapeutic agents. It is hoped that by this technique high local concentrations of the drug can be delivered to the tumour with the minimum of systemic side-effects. We have noted that many cytotoxic agents are highly irritant to vessels and severe local pain and arterial spasm may follow their

Fig. 2.6. a A digital subtraction angiogram of the axillary artery in a female presenting with a large mass related to the right shoulder. Angiographically the appearances suggest the presence of a neoplastic process, but at surgery this proved to be a haematoma with no evidence of malignancy. b. A subclavian arteriogram in a young girl with a giant cell tumour of the humerus (see also Fig. 2.9). The similarities between a and b are striking.

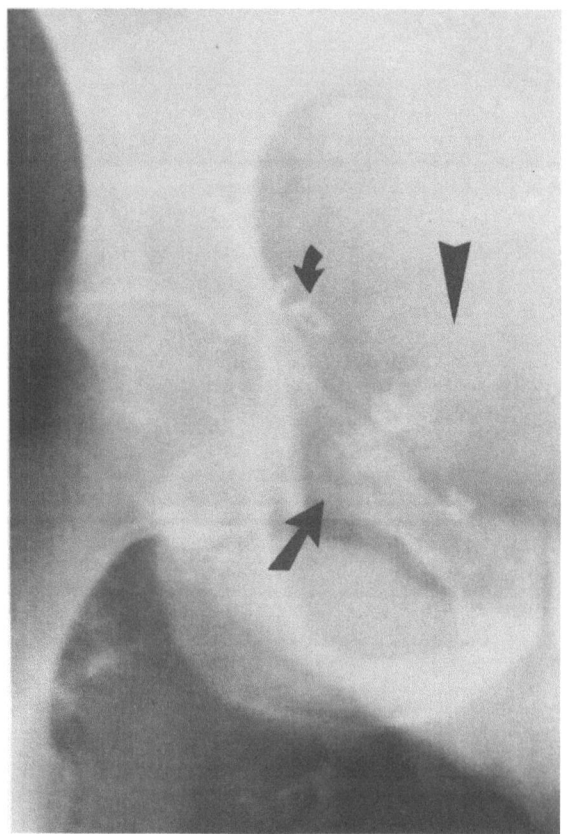

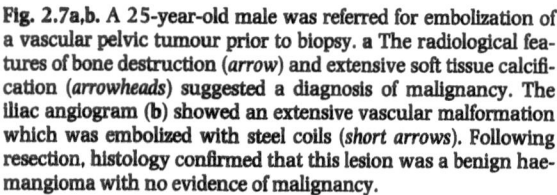

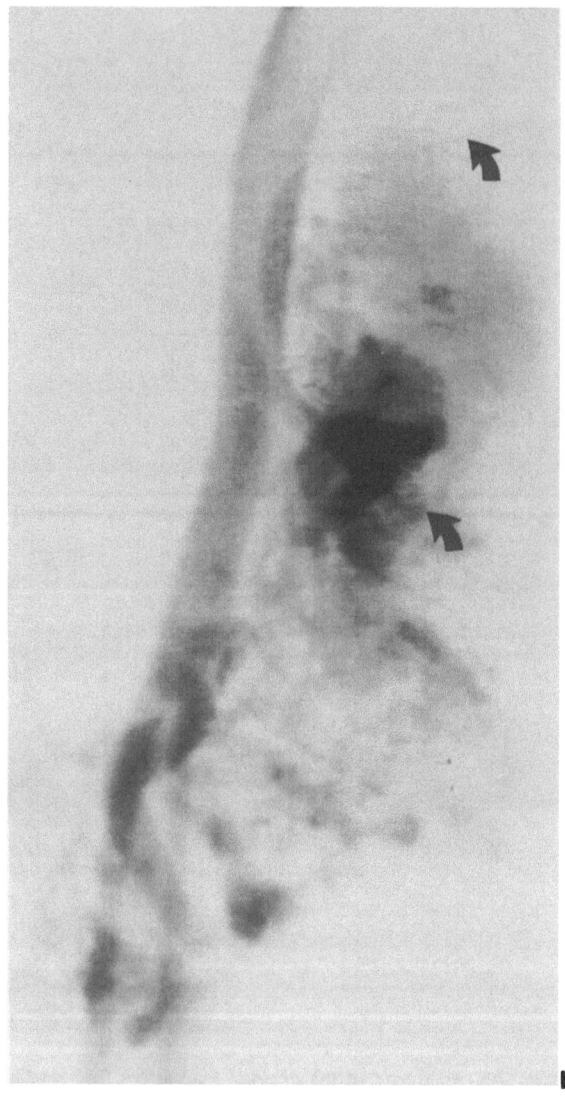

Fig. 2.7a,b. A 25-year-old male was referred for embolization of a vascular pelvic tumour prior to biopsy. a The radiological features of bone destruction (*arrow*) and extensive soft tissue calcification (*arrowheads*) suggested a diagnosis of malignancy. The iliac angiogram (b) showed an extensive vascular malformation which was embolized with steel coils (*short arrows*). Following resection, histology confirmed that this lesion was a benign haemangioma with no evidence of malignancy.

injection. Rapid developments are taking place in the use of labelled monoclonal antibodies. These too can be delivered locally, in high concentrations, directly into a tumour vascular bed.

Therapeutic Embolization

A large number of different materials have been used to embolize blood vessels. Ideally, an embolic substance should be non-toxic, thrombogenic, easy to inject down vascular catheters, radio-opaque, rapid and permanent in effect, sterile and readily available (Allison 1986b). None of the currently available substances meets these requirements and the choice of material depends on the nature of the embolism required and the preference and experience of the operator.

The materials that we use most commonly are sterile absorbable gelatin sponge (Sterispon, Gelfoam), lyophilized human dura mater and steel coils. Sterispon is readily available and easy to use but may sometimes produce only a temporary effect and in situations where permanent obliteration of blood flow is required dura mater, steel coils (Fig. 2.8) or, occasionally, liquid emboli such as absolute alcohol are used (Tegtmeyer 1983).

A detailed description of angiographic technique is beyond the scope of this chapter but a few principles should be noted (Allison 1986b):

1. Embolization should be preceded by high-quality angiography to define precisely the vascular

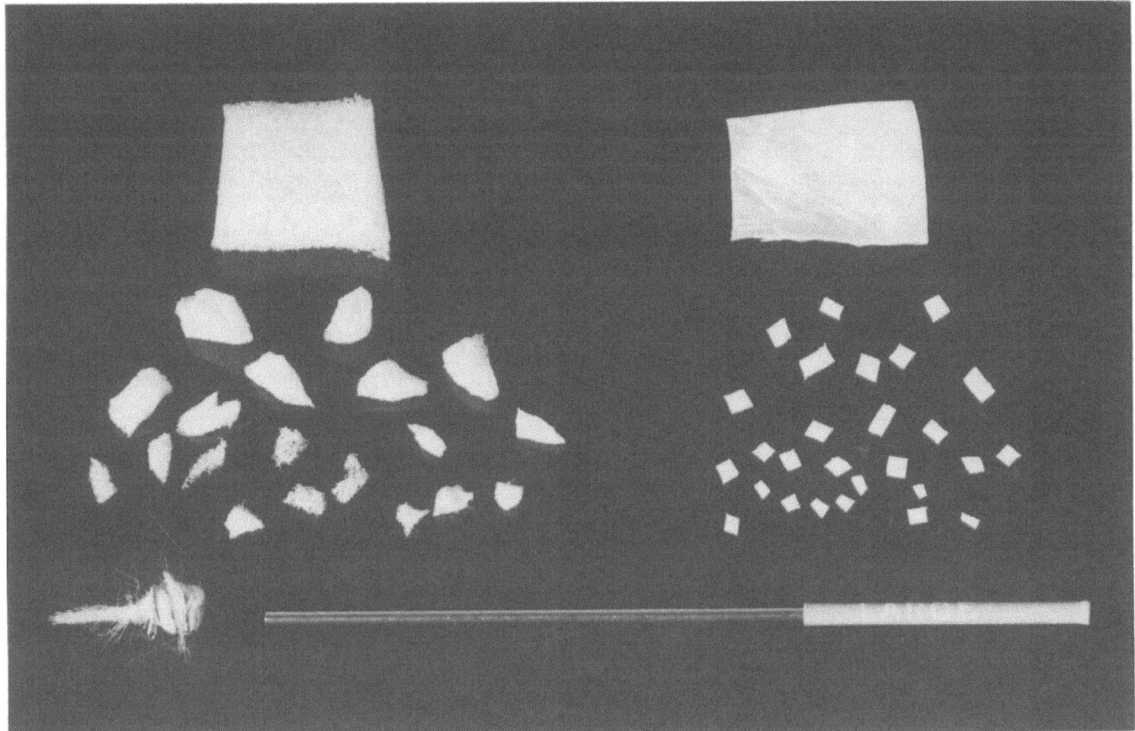

Fig. 2.8. Commonly used embolization materials: Sterispon (*left*), human dura mater (*right*) and steel coil and introducer (*below*).

territory of the lesion under consideration and its anastomotic communications. Subtraction films or, preferably, DSA may be very helpful, especially in lesions of the extremities where overlap by adjacent bones is likely to occur.

2. Embolizing catheters should be positioned as selectively as possible to avoid unintentional embolization of adjacent vascular territories. Special catheter systems such as steerable catheters or coaxial catheters may be necessary to achieve the required degree of selectivity.

3. The likely route of any "overspill" of emboli should be noted during preliminary angiography. Reflux of emboli into other vessels occurs very easily as flow progressively diminishes in the embolized bed; this hazard is best avoided by injecting emboli in small quantities at a time under constant fluoroscopic control.

4. Non-opaque emboli should be mixed with contrast medium so that they are visible as filling defects during injection. Video-recording of the injection sequence may be helpful in the accurate identification of the route followed by the emboli. If DSA is available the subtracted vascular images can be instantly reviewed and a "road map" of a selectively catheterized artery used to guide the operator.

5. In the case of peripheral vessels of the extremities particular care is required, especially if there is pre-existing vascular insufficiency.

6. It may be necessary to use a balloon catheter in some situations, either to reduce flow through the bed to be embolized, or as a temporary obstruction to flow in nearby vessels supplying normal structures when there is a potential danger of emboli entering such vessels.

Indications for Embolization

Therapeutic arterial embolization of bone or soft tissue tumours has been used in several clinical situations:

1. Pre-biopsy to reduce vascularity sufficiently to enable an adequate biopsy to be taken for full examination (see Fig. 2.7).

2. Pre-operatively to reduce tumour bulk and vascularity (Feldman et al. 1975) prior to tumour resection. This technique has proved to be of value in our unit prior to limb preservation surgery for malignant or potentially malignant lesions such as osteoclastoma and osteogenic sarcoma (Fig. 2.9).

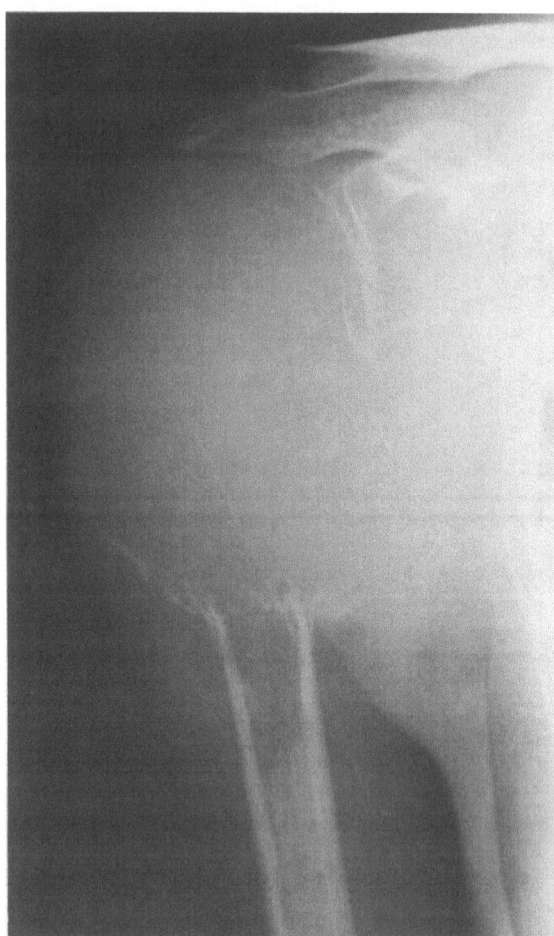

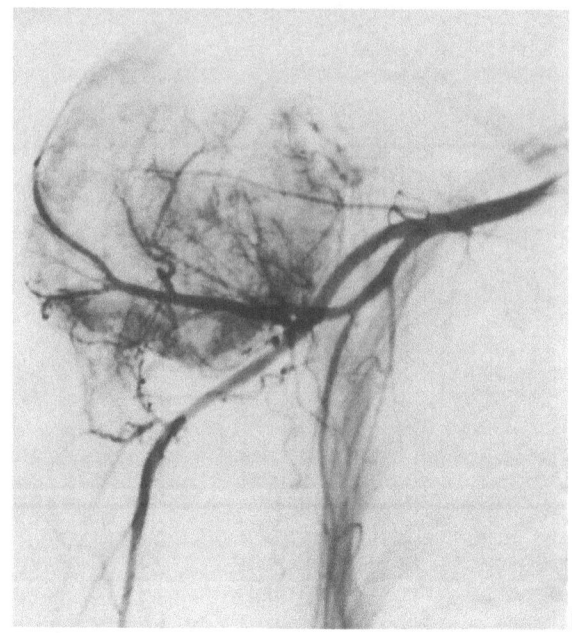

Fig. 2.9

3. For palliation of inoperable neoplasms to reduce pain and tumour bulk (Feldman et al. 1975; Wallace et al. 1979).

4. For the definitive management of benign vascular tumours such as haemangiomas (Stanley and Cubillo 1975) (Fig. 2.10).The technique is also of value in cases of trauma in controlling haemorrhage in the acute phase – for example in massive pelvic injury. Embolization can also be utilized to treat the delayed effects of trauma such as arteriovenous fistula and aneurysm formation.

Venography

Anatomy

The veins of the lower limb can be divided into deep and superficial systems. There are three pairs of deep veins in the calf, which accompany the arteries. These veins unite just below the knee to form the popliteal vein; this continues as the femoral vein, which accompanies the femoral artery. Multiple superficial veins are present in the calf and are linked to the deep venous system via paired, valved communicating veins. The normal direction of flow is from the superficial to the deep system.

In the upper limb there is also a deep and superficial system of veins, both of which drain into the axillary vein. Paired deep veins accompany the ulnar, radial and brachial arteries. Multiple intercommunicating veins lie in the subcutaneous tissues. Two major superficial veins, the cephalic and basilic veins, communicate in the antecubital fossa via the median cubital vein. The basilic vein joins the deep brachial veins to become the axillary vein.

Technique

Lower Extremity Venography

The standard technique used for lower extremity venography is ascending phlebography (Hemingway 1986; Lea Thomas and Browse 1985). Contrast medium is injected into a cannula in the dorsum of the foot. A tourniquet at the ankle prevents filling of the superficial veins and directs

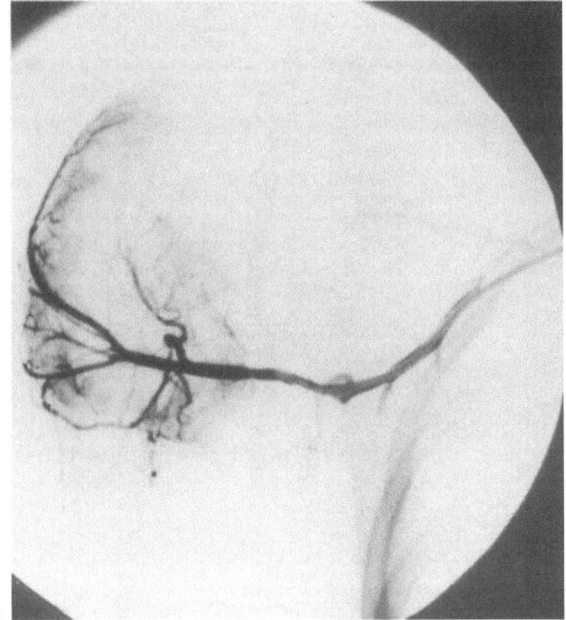

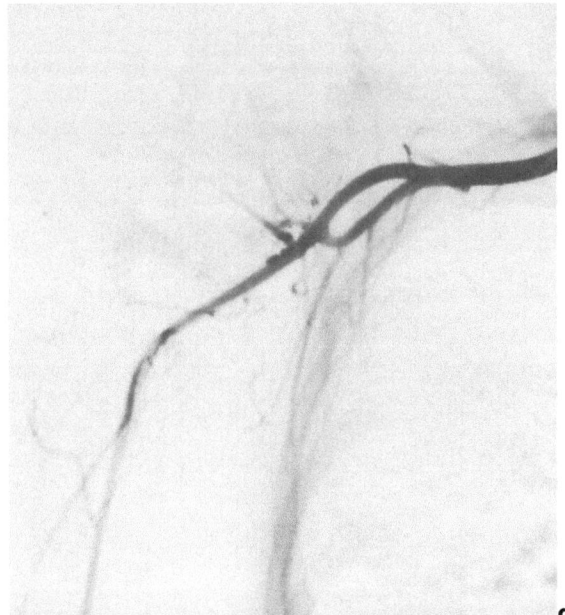

c

d

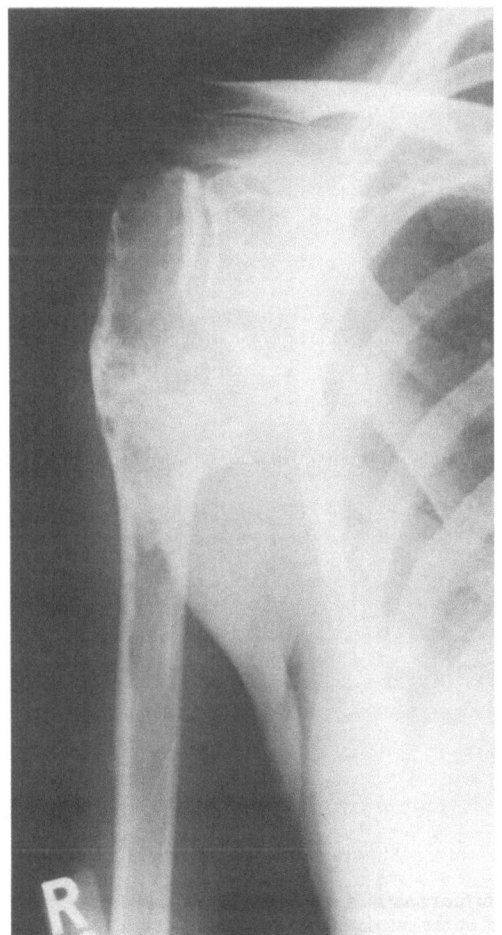

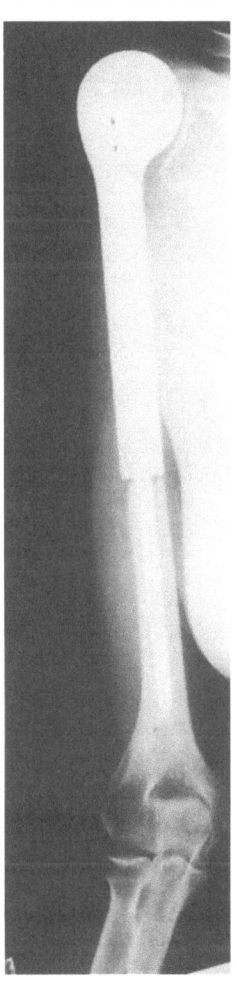

Fig. 2.9a–f. Embolization of a humeral giant cell tumour in a 17-year-old female which had proved resistant to radiotherapy. a Plain radiograph showing soft tissue mass and extensive bone destruction by a giant cell tumour. b Axillary arteriogram showing tumour circulation. c Selective catheterization of one of the principal feeding vessels to the lesion. This and the other feeding arteries were occluded. d Post-embolization arteriogram. e Plain radiograph taken 3 months after the embolization. Note the disappearance of the soft tissue mass and the regrowth of bone in the humeral head. f The improvement engendered by embolization enabled reconstructive surgery to be performed. A shoulder replacement was successfully carried out.

e

f

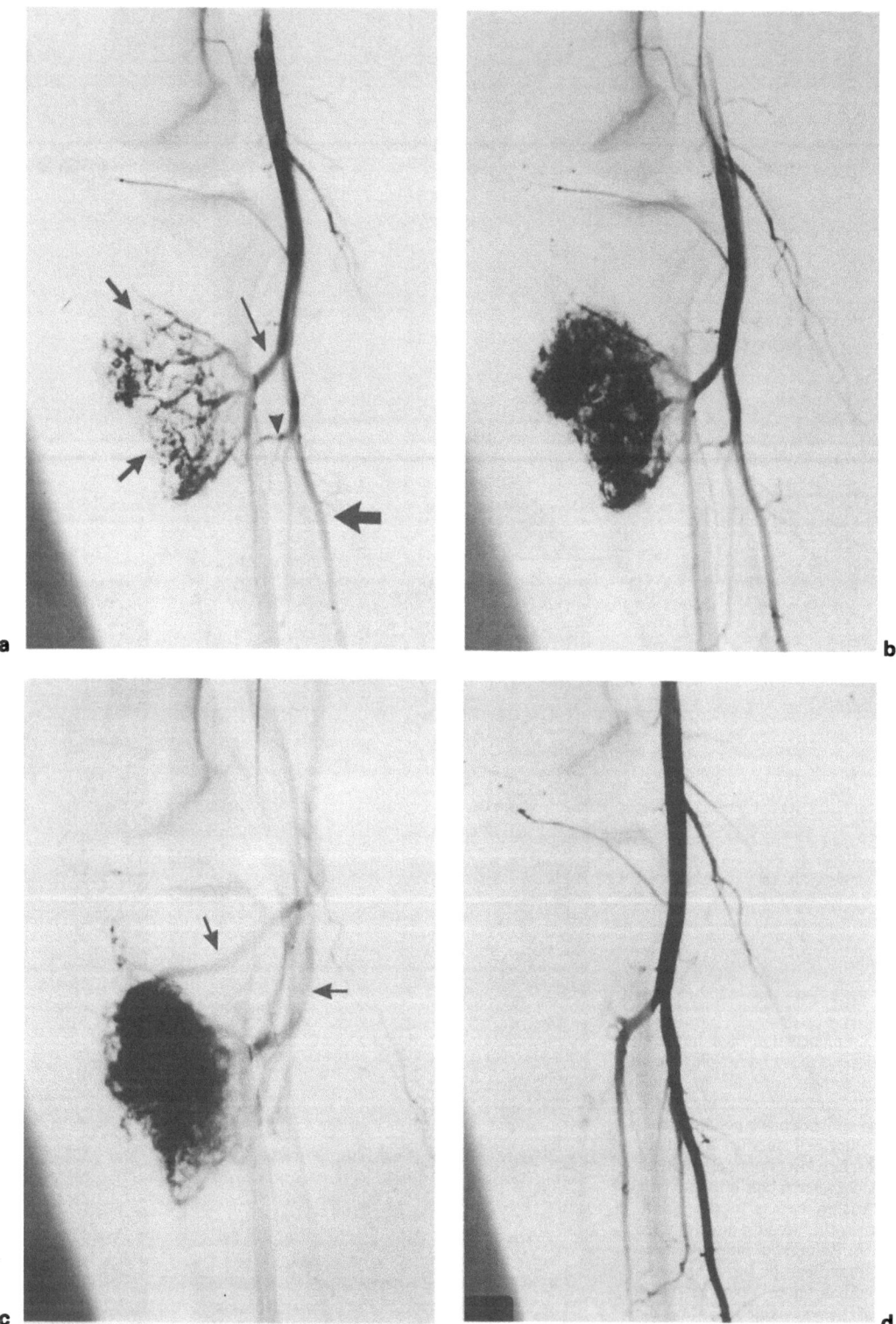

Fig. 2.10a–d. Haemangioma of the upper tibia. **a,b** Early arterial lateral film following a popliteal artery injection shows the vascular tumour (*short arrows*) supplied by the anterior tibial artery (*long arrow*) and twigs from the peroneal artery (*arrowhead*). The posterior tibial artery is not involved (*broad arrow*). **c** A few seconds later large veins are seen draining the lesion (*short arrows*). **d** After embolization a repeat arteriogram shows abolition of the blood supply to the lesion.

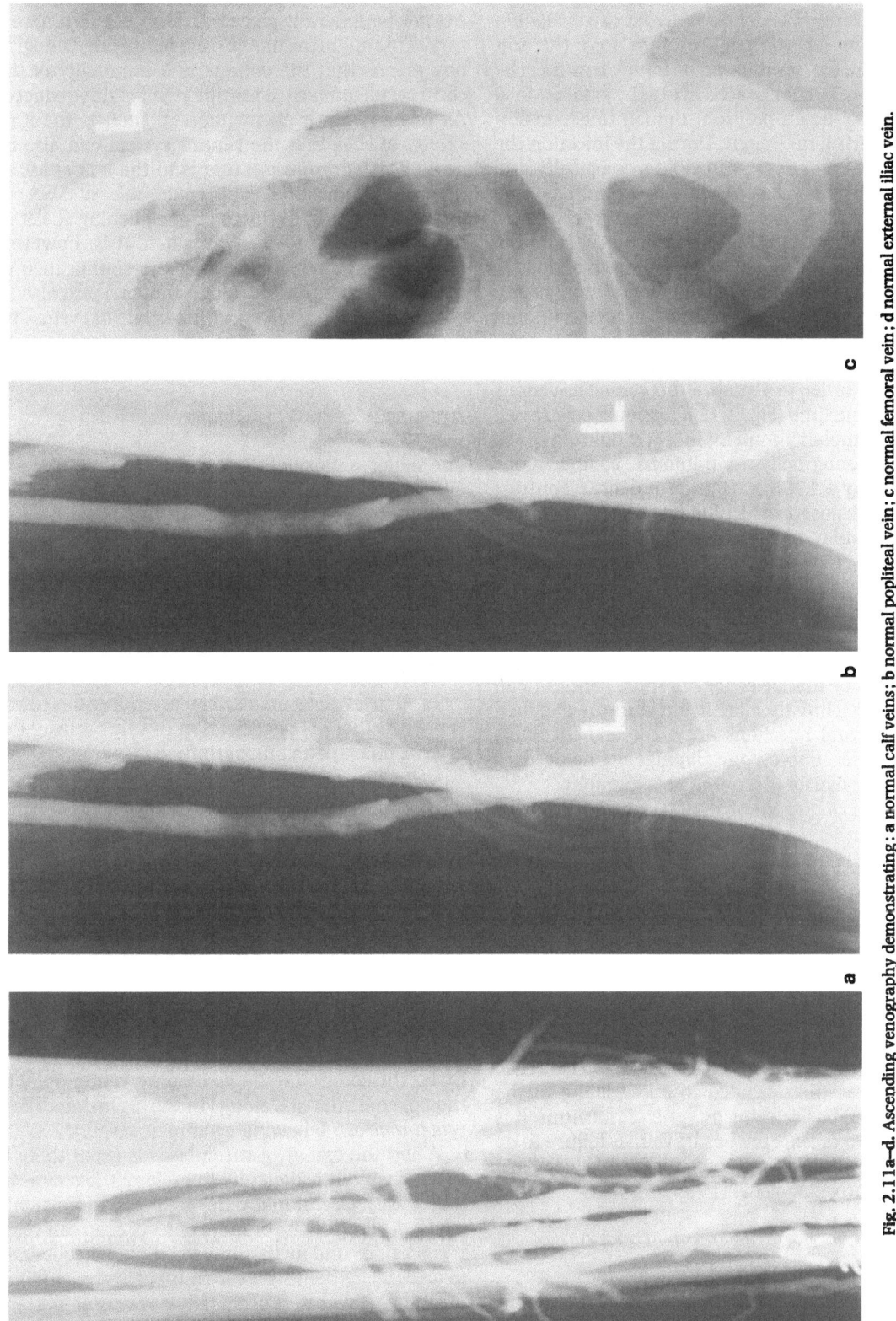

Fig. 2.11a–d. Ascending venography demonstrating: a normal calf veins; b normal popliteal vein; c normal femoral vein; d normal external iliac vein.

the contrast medium into the deep veins (Allison 1981). Care must be taken to avoid extravasation of hyperosmolar contrast medium into the soft tissues of the foot, as this can be highly irritant. The examination is commenced with the patient in a 30°–60° foot-down position, the leg under examination bearing no weight. During the injection the veins of the calf are examined fluoroscopically and spot radiographs taken in various projections. The popliteal, femoral and iliac veins and the inferior vena cava are then examined; the opacification of these vessels may be enhanced by raising the calf, restoring the patient to the supine position, asking him or her to perform a Valsalva manoeuvre, and releasing the tourniquet (if used). It may be necessary to give more than one injection of contrast medium in order to visualize the complete venous system in one limb (Fig. 2.11). It should be stressed that low-osmolality contrast media should *always* be used for venography to minimize complications (Hemingway 1986). High-osmolality contrast media predispose to phlebitis by causing irritation of the vascular endothelium (Allison 1981; Lea Thomas and Browse 1985; Hemingway 1986).

Intraosseous phlebography is rarely employed. It is painful and is best performed under general anaesthetic. It is indicated when the percutaneous method is impossible or contraindicated by oedema or fracture of the lower leg. A short cannula can be introduced into the calcaneum or the medial malleolus. Manual injections are made and the same procedure for fluoroscopy filming is employed as described above for ascending phlebography.

Upper Limb Venography

When the veins of the arm are to be examined a 19 or 21 gauge butterfly needle is placed in a vein on the dorsum of the hand and contrast medium is injected. To opacify the deep veins a tourniquet should be placed just above the elbow. The flow of contrast medium is assessed fluoroscopically and spot radiographs are taken of areas of interest. The tourniquet is then deflated to allow filling of the cephalic and basilic veins by contrast medium. It is important to opacify the basilic vein as failure to do so can give the false impression of axillary vein thrombosis (Neiman et al. 1985).

DSA for Direct and Indirect Venography

Using DSA it is possible to obtain excellent images of the veins of the extremities following injection of dilute contrast material. Only a hand injection into a small, peripherally placed butterfly needle is necessary. This augmentation of images during venography means that the volume and osmolality of the contrast medium used may be significantly reduced. As has already been mentioned, such is the sensitivity of DSA that the venous system can also be demonstrated *indirectly*, that is in the late phase of an arterial injection. The exact role of DSA in indirect venography in the appendicular skeleton has not yet been fully investigated. It is, however, of importance when assessing the significance of shunts in arteriovenous malformations and also in detecting compression or invasion of veins by tumours.

Appearances on Venography

The major abnormalities seen on venography are as follows:

1. *Displacement of veins.* This may be due to any large mass adjacent to the relevant vessel, such as a neoplasm or a haematoma. In the case of bone tumours the relation of large veins to the neoplasm may be relevant if a radical local resection is being considered, because the surgeon will have to deal with these vessels.

2. *Arteriovenous shunts.* If an arteriovenous shunt is present there is opacification of veins during the arterial phase of an angiogram.

3. *Tumour invasion of veins.* This uncommon finding is a sign of malignancy.

4. *Large abnormal draining veins.* These are seen in hypervascular tumours. It is important that these abnormal vessels should be identified in order to enable the surgeon to ligate them early during the course of an operation, thus preventing tumour embolization.

Indications

By far the commonest indication for venography in the appendicular skeleton is in the exclusion of *deep vein thrombosis* following trauma or surgery.

When the extent of thrombosis is great there is usually very little difficulty in making the diagnosis (Fig. 2.12). Occasionally the signs are more subtle – lack of filling of one or more pairs of deep calf veins is suspicious and further images should be obtained to assess whether this is the result of just poor filling or of the veins being occluded. It is very important to ascertain the upper limit of the clot as large amounts of loose thrombus in the iliac vein or

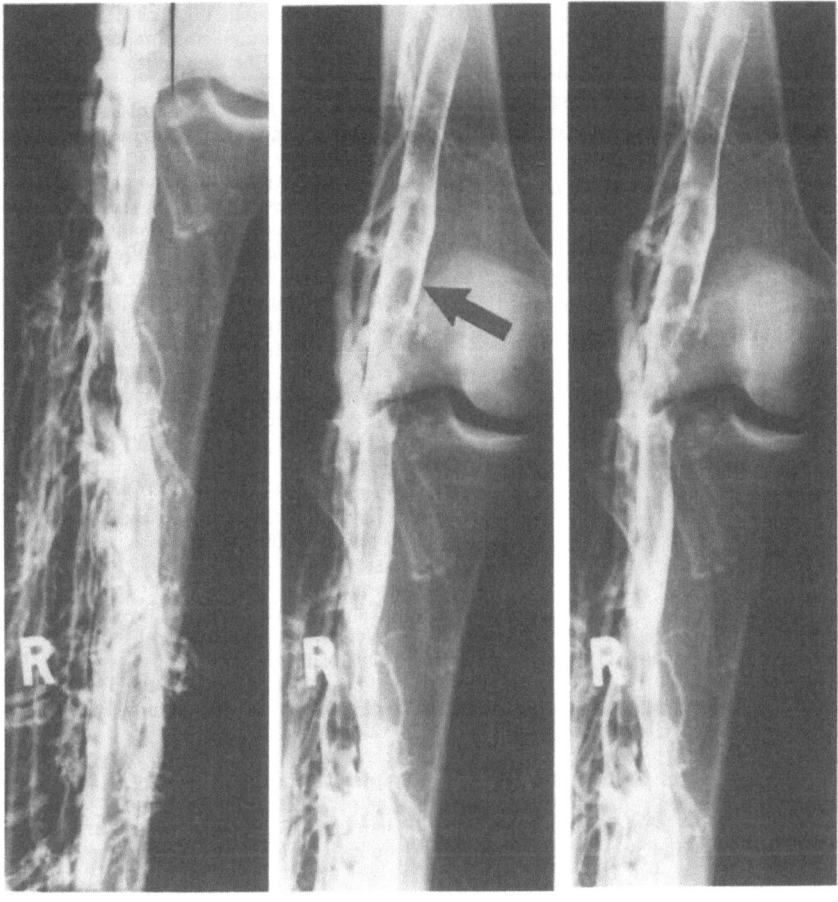

Fig. 2.12a–c. Lower limb venogram. Extensive filling defects (*arrow*) due to thrombus are seen in the calf and popliteal veins and the femoral vein.

inferior vena cava may warrant surgical intervention rather than anticoagulant therapy alone.

Deep vein thrombosis and recurrent pulmonary emboli in a patient who has suffered recent major trauma or undergone surgery can pose a therapeutic dilemma. Anticoagulants, while helping the embolic phenomena, may adversely affect the patient because of the increased risk of haemorrhage. This small group of patients provides one of the few indications for the insertion of *vena cava filters*. These devices are inserted percutaneously in the inferior vena cava, below the level of the renal veins. Their sieve-like construction then allows the passage of blood but blocks further migration of emboli. Recent design modifications in these devices have made them much less cumbersome to handle than the earlier models, which had to be inserted via a jugular venotomy and negotiated through the right atrium into the inferior vena cava. The newer

devices can be inserted percutaneously via the femoral vein.

Less frequently, venography may be required in the assessment of acute major trauma.

As has already been mentioned, indirect venography is also an essential part of an angiographic study of arteriovenous malformations and tumours.

Finally the ability to negotiate the venous system is important for any angiographer and interventionalist working in a unit where large numbers of central venous monitoring and feeding lines are inserted. This is particularly true in major trauma centres. Occasionally these lines fracture or become disconnected and migrate into the central venous system, usually the pulmonary arterial tree. They cannot be left behind because of the very high risk of complications such as infection, perforation and arrhythmias. Percutaneous extraction of these "lost lines" is the preferred means of removing them, the only alternative being open chest surgery. A variety of instruments including snares, baskets and grasping forceps have been described which can be inserted percutaneously and used to "grab" the lost line under fluoroscopic control (Tegtmeyer 1983).

Acknowledgements. We are very grateful to Churchill Livingstone for permission to reproduce Figs. 2.2a and b, 2.4, 2.5, 2.6b, 2.9, 2.10 and 2.11, which are from *Diagnostic Radiology: An Anglo-American Textbook of Imaging,* ed. R. G. Grainger and D. J. Allison (Churchill Livingstone, Edinburgh, 1986).

References

Adam A, Hemingway AP, Allison DJ (1985) Iohexol and diatrizoate: comparison in visceral arteriography. Radiology 155:529

Allison DJ (1981) Radiology in diagnosis of venous thromboembolism. In: Pitney WR (ed) Venous and arterial thrombosis. Churchill Livingstone, Edinburgh, pp 444–455

Allison DJ (1986a) Arteriography. In: Grainger RG, Allison DJ (eds) Diagnostic radiology: an Anglo-American textbook of imaging. Churchill Livingstone, Edinburgh, pp 1984–2059

Allison DJ (1986b) Interventional radiology. In: Grainger RG, Allison DJ (eds) Diagnostic radiology: an Anglo-American textbook of imaging. Churchill Livingstone, Edinburgh, pp 2121–2165

Boxt LM (1983) Intravenous digital subtraction angiography of the thoracic and abdominal aorta. Cardiovasc Intervent Radiol 6:205–213

Chang R, Kaufman SL, Kadir S, Mitchell SE, White RI Jr (1984) Digital subtraction angiography in interventional radiology. AJR 142:363–366

Clark RA, Alexander ES (1983) Digital subtraction angiography of the renal arteries: prospective comparison with conventional arteriography. Invest Radiol 18:6–10

Dawson P, Grainger RG, Pitfield J (1983) The new low-osmolar contrast media: a simple guide. Clin Radiol 34:221–226

Ekelund L, Laurin S, Lunderquist A (1977) Comparison of a vasoconstrictor and a vasodilator in pharmacoangiography of bone and soft tissue tumours. Radiology 122:95–99

Feldman F, Casarella WJ, Dick HM, Hollander BA (1975) Selective intra-arterial embolization of bone tumors: a useful adjunct in the management of selected lesions. AJR 123:130–139

Goodman PC, Jeffrey RB, Brant-Zawadzki M (1984) Digital subtraction angiography in extremity trauma. Radiology 153:61–64

Hemingway AP (1986) Venography. In: Grainger RG, Allison DJ (eds) Diagnostic radiology: an Anglo-American textbook of imaging. Churchill Livingstone, Edinburgh, pp 2061–2097

Kadir S, Athanasoulis CA, Waltman AC (1979) Tolazoline-augmented arteriography in the evaluation of bone and soft tissue tumours. Radiology 133:792–795

Kubal WS, Crummy AB, Turnipseed WD (1983) The utility of digital subtraction arteriography in peripheral vascular disease. Cardiovasc Intervent Radiol 6:241–249

Lea Thomas M, Browse NL (1985) Venography of the lower extremity. In: Naiman HL, Yao JST (eds) Angiography of vascular disease. Churchill Livingstone, New York, pp 421–480

Meaney TF, Weinstein MA (1986) Digital subtraction angiography. In: Grainger RG, Allison DJ (eds) Diagnostic radiology: an Anglo-American textbook of imaging. Churchill Livingstone, Edinburgh, pp 2099–2111

Neiman HL (1985) Techniques of angiography. In: Neiman HL, Yao JST (eds) Angiography of vascular disease. Churchill Livingstone, New York, pp 1–26

Neiman HL, Mintzer RA, Vogelzany RL (1985) Digital subtraction angiography. In: Neiman HL, Yao JST (eds) Angiography of vascular disease. Churchill Livingstone, New York, pp 27–56

Seldinger SL (1953) Catheter replacement of the needle in percutaneous arteriography: a new technique. Acta Radiol (Stockh) 39:368–376

Simonetti G, Passariello R, Rossi P et al. (1985) Digital angiography in the evaluation of orthopedic tumors. Cardiovasc Intervent Radiol 8:83–88

Stanley RJ, Cubillo E (1975) Non-surgical treatment of arteriovenous malformations of the trunk and limb by transcatheter arterial embolization. Radiology 115:609–612

Strickland B (1959) The value of arteriography in the diagnosis of bone tumours. Br J Radiol 52:705–713

Tegtmeyer CJ (1983) Angiography of bones, joints and soft tissues. In: Abrams HL (ed) Abrams angiography. Vascular and interventional radiology, 3rd edn. Little, Brown, Boston, pp 1937–1977

Viamonte M Jr, Roen S, LePage J (1973) Non-specificity of abnormal vascularity in the angiographic diagnosis of malignant neoplasms. Radiology 106:59–63

Voegeli E, Uehlinger E (1976) Arteriography in bone tumours. Skeletal Radiol 1:3–14

Wallace S, Granmayeh M, de Santos LA et al. (1979) Arterial occlusion of pelvic bone tumours. Cancer 43:322–328

3 Arthrography

B.J. Preston

Introduction 35
Knee Arthrography 36
   Indications 36
   Arthroscopy and Arthrography 40
Shoulder Arthrography 40
   Indications 41
Hip Arthrography 43
   Children 43
   Adults 44
Elbow Arthrography 44
Wrist Arthrography 44
   Indications 44
Hand Arthrography 45
Ankle Arthrography 45
   Indications 45
Foot Arthrography 46
Arthrographic Evaluation of Total Joint Replacement 46
Facet Arthrography 47
Traction Arthrography 47
Ganglionography 47
Tenography 47
   Peroneal Tenography 47
   Tenography of Sheaths of Hand and Wrist 48
Bursography 48
References 48

Introduction

Arthrography has developed so much over the last two decades that it is now widely practised. This has come about by a better understanding and realization of the role of the procedure, and by improved techniques and equipment. Over the last two years the use of arthrography combined with CT scanning in certain situations has added a further impetus to its development.

In the majority of situations arthrography should be done in the radiology department where there is access to a good image intensifier and equipment to produce high quality images. Contrast media containing iodine are usually employed but would be contra-indicated in patients with known sensitivity to iodine. In patients with such a history air could be employed but with a decrease in accuracy of the procedure. Local sepsis is a contra-indication to arthrography.

All joints should be punctured using an aseptic technique. The length of the needle employed will depend on how superficial or deep the joint is situated. Usually a 20 or 22-gauge needle is used but if it is necessary to aspirate a haemarthrosis prior to the injection of contrast a 19-gauge needle may be considered to be more appropriate. Short bevelled needles are employed to minimize any periarticular injection of contrast.

It is of value to perform all procedures under screen control in order to:

1. Aid in determining the site of puncture using a long radio-opaque pointer

2. Assess if a satisfactory puncture has been made. When it is thought that the needle is in the joint a little contrast can be injected into the joint either directly through the needle or indirectly through a

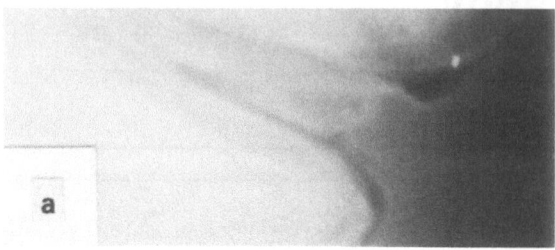 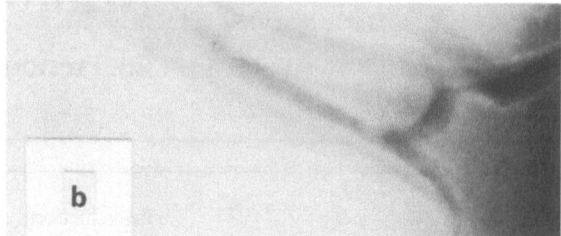

Fig. 3.1a,b. Vertical tear of the medial meniscus. **a** The tear is only recognized by the positive contrast tracking between the surfaces. **b** When distraction and a valgus stress are applied the fragments separate and the tear is recognizable as a vertical gap with the surfaces coated by contrast.

fine bore connecting tube. If the needle tip is within the joint the contrast will flow away from the needle into the recesses of the joint, but if the puncture is unsatisfactory the contrast will remain in the region of the tip of the needle as a dense irregular opacity

3. Observe the rate of flow of contrast through a tear in the capsule of a joint. This may give some idea of the size of the defect

Knee Arthrography

Arthrography of the knee is the most widely performed arthrographic investigation. This is because the knee is frequently injured, clinical examination and plain films do not lead to a precise diagnosis, and from a realization that removal of a meniscus leads to premature degenerative arthritis and ligamentous laxity.

A double contrast technique is employed except for the detection of a rupture of a popliteal cyst when a single contrast method is usually sufficient. Double contrast studies have been developed and popularized over the last two decades by Andren and Wehlin 1960, Butt and McIntyre 1969, Freiberger and Kaye 1979, Stoker 1980, and Dalinka 1980.

Indications

The majority of knee arthrograms are done to detect abnormalities of the menisci e.g. tear or discoid form. They are also used to detect loose bodies and chondral lesions and to evaluate ligaments and synovium.

Tears of the Menisci

The radiographic signs of a meniscal tear will depend on the degree of displacement of the fragments. If there is insufficient displacement the tear will appear as a radiolucent defect due to the air within the meniscus and the edges of the tear will be coated with the positive contrast. If the tear is a short closed one or the appropriate stress has not been applied to open up the gap only positive contrast will be seen extending into the meniscus (Fig. 3.1a,b).

Tears of the menisci are essentially of two types, namely vertical and horizontal. Vertical tears which may be perpendicular or oblique to the edges of the meniscus, are along either the long axis of the meniscus or the radial axis. Vertical tears along the axis of the meniscus may be short or long. Long vertical tears which allow displacement of the central fragment are known as "bucket handle" tears. Radial tears are easy to miss because the tear is perpendicular to the X-ray beam and the meniscus on either side is normal. However, radial tears are frequently associated with a small vertical tear extending along the long axis of the meniscus and this is easier to detect. Such a combined tear is known as a "parrot beak" tear. A radial tear should be suspected if a meniscus remains adherent to the condylar surface in spite of adequate stress manoeuvres. Peripheral detachment is another type of vertical tear and may be complete or incomplete. In the medial meniscus the tear takes place through the outermost part of the meniscus or the menisco-capsular junction. Peripheral detachment of the lateral meniscus will cause rupture of one or both struts on either side of the popliteus tendon sheaths. If the detachment is total and both bands are torn, this is usually obvious, but if only one of the bands is ruptured this is more difficult to detect leading on occasion to a false negative result.

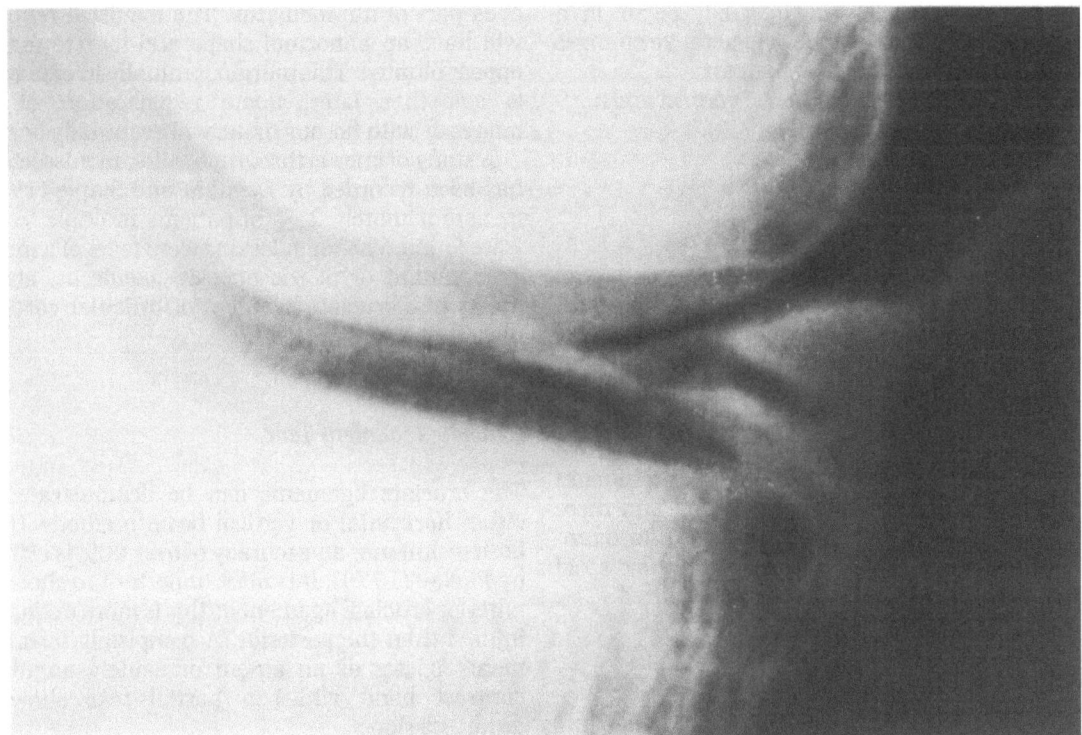

Fig. 3.2. Horizontal tear of the medial meniscus.

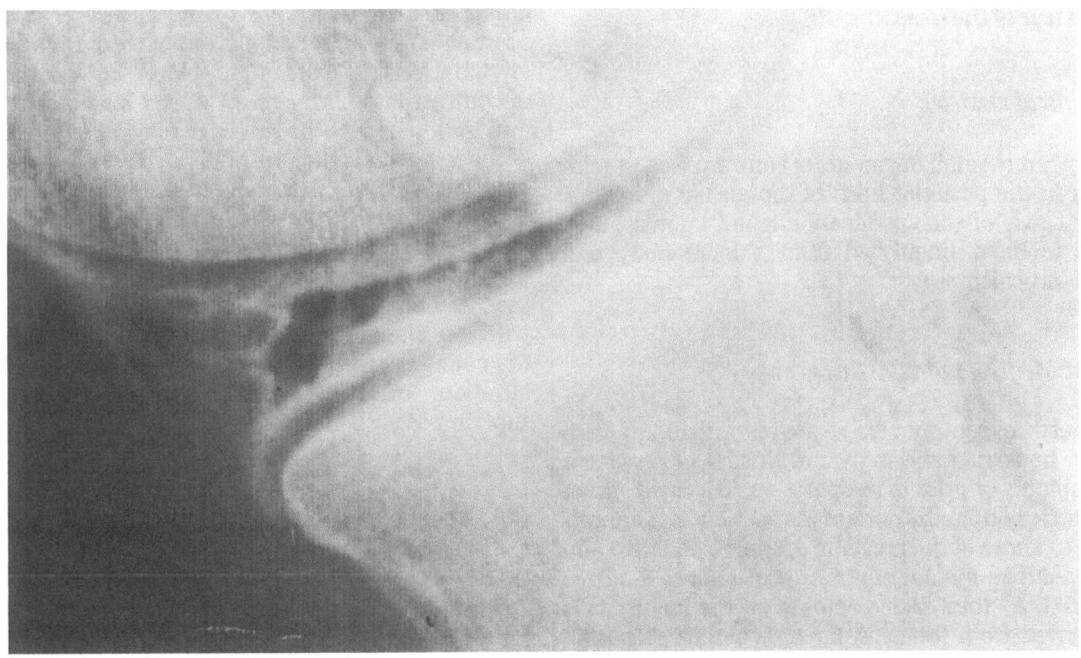

Fig. 3.3. Complex tear of medial meniscus.

Horizontal tears (Fig. 3.2) usually occur in a meniscus that has undergone degenerative changes and are thus seen in the older patient.

Complex tears, a combination of vertical and horizontal tears, may also occur (Fig. 3.3).

The Discoid Meniscus

A discoid abnormality usually affects the lateral meniscus and extremely rarely the medial side. Arthrographically a discoid meniscus appears larger than normal extending towards the intercondylar notch, usually with parallel surfaces and a rectangular, rather than triangular cross section.

Any discoid meniscus must be carefully examined for tears – a difficult problem (Stoker 1980), because the patient may resist normal stressing and there may be difficulty in bringing the meniscus into profile. If a discoid meniscus is grossly torn the discoid nature of the meniscus may not be recognized.

Meniscal Cysts

These are normally situated on the lateral meniscus and detected clinically as a swelling in the line of the meniscus. The origin of these cysts is debatable and there are traumatic, developmental and degenerative theories. Meniscal cysts are not lined by synovial epithelium and are thus not true cysts. The purpose of an arthrogram is to detect an associated tear of the meniscus.

Meniscal Ossicles

Very rarely small fragments of bone are seen in relation to the posterior horn of the medial meniscus. The cause of such ossification is not known but it has to be distinguished from a loose body and chondrocalcinosis.

Post Meniscectomy Arthrogram

An arthrogram may be requested in patients who have had a meniscectomy and is usual for persistent symptoms or prior to re-operation. The arthrogram is carried out in the normal manner but it is important to know of the previous operative findings, and procedure. Meniscectomies are either total or partial. At total meniscectomy all the meniscus is removed from the capsular attachment. A partial meniscectomy consists of the removal of the free segment of a bucket handle tear or resection of the dam-

aged part of the meniscus. The meniscal remnant will have an abnormal shape and its free margin appear blunted. This margin is initially irregular but is smoother later. Some regeneration of the meniscus with fibrous tissue will eventually occur.

A study of knee arthrography after meniscectomy has been recorded by Debnam and Staple (1974). In approximately 25% of patients multiple lesions were found. The main lesions were tears of a meniscal remnant or of the opposite meniscus, abnormality of a cruciate ligament or articular cartilage ulceration.

Cruciate Ligament Tears

The cruciate ligaments can be demonstrated by either horizontal or vertical beam methods. Using both techniques an accuracy of over 90% is claimed by Pavlov (1979). It is most important to show the anterior cruciate ligament as this is more frequently injured than the posterior. A completely torn ligament appears as an absent or acutely angulated contrast band whilst a partial tear shows a decreased slope.

Chondromalacia Patellae

The main symptom of chondromalacia patellae is anterior knee pain and it occurs typically in young adults. Plain radiographs of the knee are usually normal. The early findings on arthrography are swelling of the cartilage and increased absorption of contrast into cartilage. At a later stage thinning and irregularity of the cartilage may be found. One of the problems is that only a limited part of the articular cartilage of the patella is seen adequately on a routine view. Even with multiple views, lesions may be missed. More recently, CT following arthrography has been described (Boven et al. 1982) in the detection of changes due to chondromalacia patellae. The authors state that using this method the changes can be more reliably detected by visualization of the articular cartilage without superimposed shadows.

Osteochondritis Dissecans, Chondral and Osteochondral Fractures

Arthrography can be employed in these conditions for assessing articular cartilage and detecting associated lesions such as loose bodies and meniscal tears. CT scanning with conventional arthrography

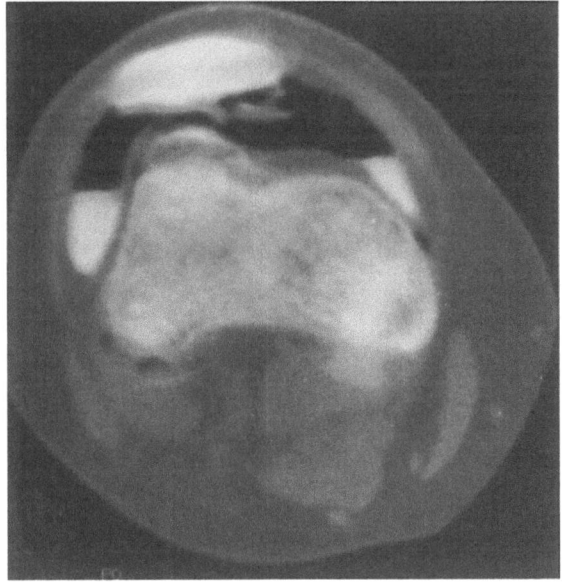

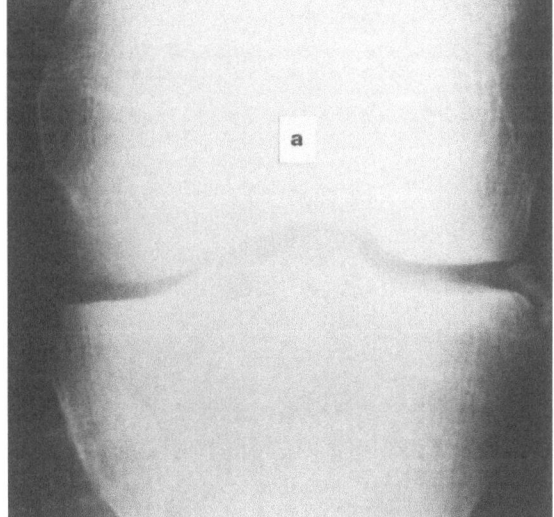

Fig. 3.4. CT arthrogram showing separated chondral fragment of the patella. This was poorly demonstrated by conventional arthrography.

is of value in the visualization of the articular cartilage of the patella (Fig. 3.4).

Loose Bodies

Arthrography is useful for determining the presence of a loose body within the joint (Fig. 3.5). Loose bodies are quite easily seen in the suprapatellar, lateral and posterior aspects of the knee joint but are more difficult to detect in the intercondylar region because of the confusing shadows of the cruciate ligaments and gas bubbles. If a loose body is seen then its nature must be ascertained.

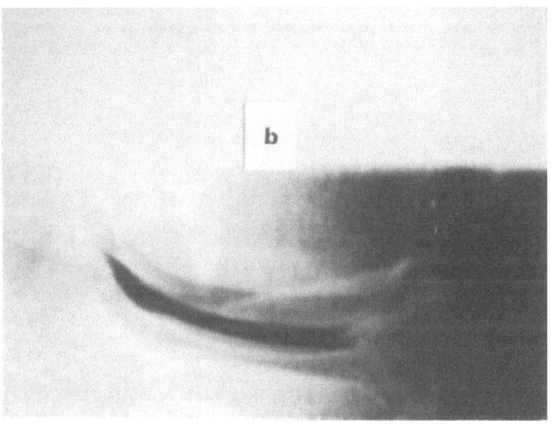

Fig. 3.5a,b. Plain films (a) and arthrogram (b) of loose body in the knee joint. The initial plain film shows an opacity which mimics part of the medial meniscus but the arthrogram shows it to be a loose body lying beneath a normal medial meniscus.

Rheumatoid Arthritis

Popliteal cysts are a feature of rheumatoid arthritis and other connective tissue disorders. They may present as a mass, cause pain and tenderness, and interfere with venous blood flow causing oedema. These cysts may rupture causing symptoms which mimic deep vein thrombosis. Either a single or double contrast technique is used. A ruptured or dissecting cyst is identified by extravasation of contrast between the muscle bundles and an irregular edge (Fig. 3.6). Usually contrast passes into the calf but it may also pass upwards into the posterior aspect

of the thigh. Other changes which may be noted include a joint of increased capacity, multiple filling defects due to hypertrophy of the synovium and fibrous bodies, irregularity, thinning and disappearance of articular cartilage and menisci, and occasionally lymphatic filling.

Synovial Lesions

Occasionally arthrography will detect synovial lesions such as pigmented villonodular synovitis (Fig. 3.7) and synovial chondromatosis.

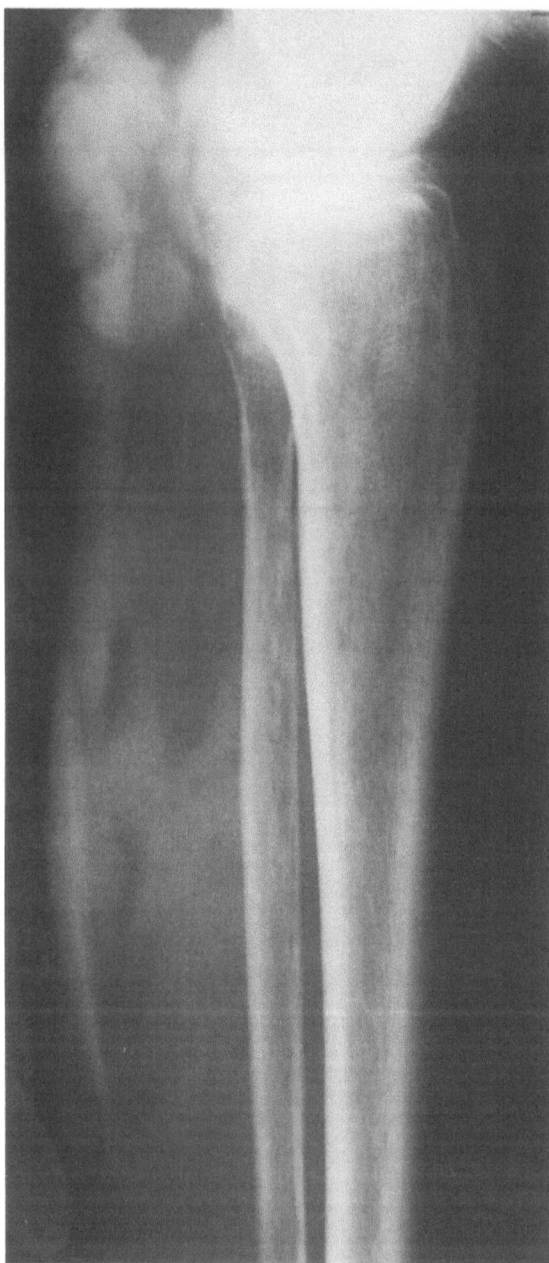

Fig. 3.6. Rupture of a popliteal cyst. Contrast is seen extravasating into the soft tissues of the calf.

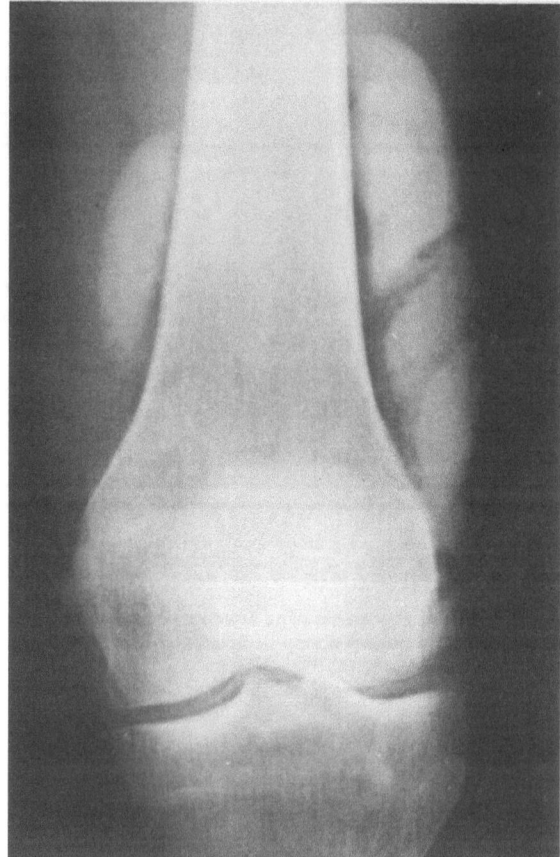

Fig. 3.7. Pigmented villonodular synovitis: the arthrographic feature of this condition is multiple filling defects coming from the synovium, in this case in the suprapatellar pouch.

entirety whilst the posterior horn is more difficult to visualize at arthroscopy. The posterior horn of the lateral meniscus is more difficult to assess by arthrography because of its mobility and the intervening sheath of the popliteus tendon. Arthroscopy is effective in detecting articular cartilage and cruciate ligament abnormalities.

Shoulder Arthrography

Plain films only occasionally reveal the nature of pain and limitation of movement at the shoulder joint and are used primarily to exclude neoplasm, infection and the inflammatory arthropathies. Arthrography is used to provide information about the joint and surrounding soft tissues. Thus it is indicated for detecting and assessing tears of the rotator

Arthroscopy and Arthrography

Arthroscopy, particularly of the knee joint, is an established procedure and is frequently compared with arthrography. Arthrography is good at demonstrating the medial meniscus throughout its

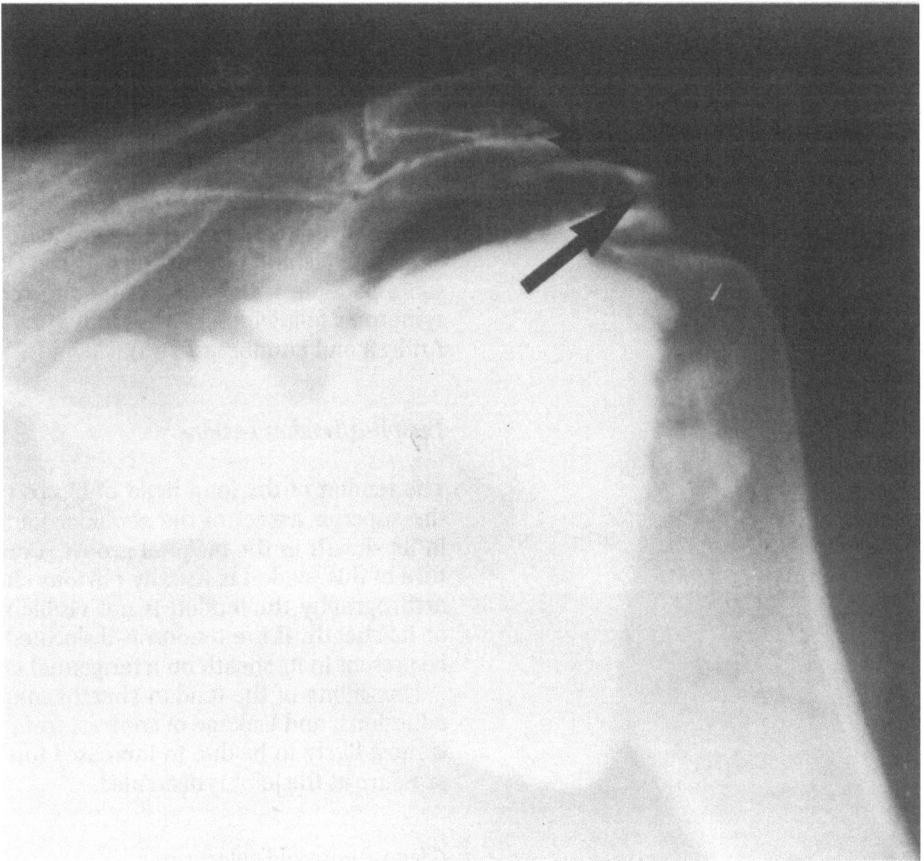

Fig. 3.8. Complete tear in rotator cuff. Contrast is noted in the gleno-humeral joint and the subacromial bursa. The arrow shows contrast in the tear of the supraspinatus tendon.

cuff, capsulitis, instability, loose bodies, rheumatoid arthritis and synovial tumours.

In the majority of instances a double contrast technique is used (Preston and Jackson 1976, 1977). It is important to use screen control both to confirm that the joint has been satisfactorily punctured, and if there is a tear of the rotator cuff, to obtain some idea of its size by observing the rate of leakage of contrast from the joint into the subacromial bursa. With the double contrast technique approximately 5-ml positive contrast and 10-ml air are employed, i.e. a total of 15-ml. Occasionally, it is only possible to inject a smaller quantity of contrast though in some cases of rheumatoid arthritis a larger amount may be necessary. One of the main advantages of the double contrast technique is that it shows the superior aspect of the joint extremely well and this is the site where most tears of the rotator cuff occur.

Indications

Complete Tears of the Rotator Cuff

Contrast passing from the gleno-humeral joint into the subacromial bursa indicates a complete tear of the rotator cuff. It is important to note the radiolucent band between the contrast medium in the subacromial bursa and that in the upper part of the shoulder joint as this represents the rotator cuff. If this band is broad the tear is probably small (Fig. 3.8), but if it is narrow it indicates that there is either a large tear in the rotator cuff or the cuff is thinned.

Incomplete Tears

The diagnosis of an incomplete tear of the rotator cuff is recognized by the passage of contrast into the

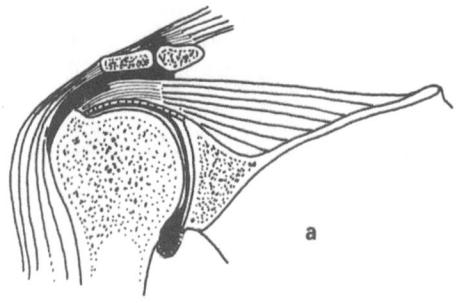

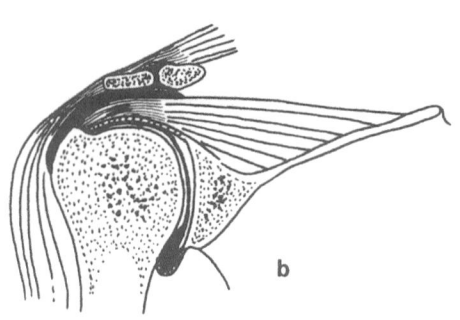

of contrast, approximately 3–5 ml. The main arthrographic feature is contracture of the synovium with the axillary and subscapularis recesses being particularly small. Contrast may leak from the joint as a manifestation of overdistension. Occasionally some patients with capsulitis obtain relief of their symptoms following arthrography (Neviaser 1962, Andren and Lundberg 1965).

Bicipital Tendon Lesions

The tendon of the long head of biceps runs across the superior aspect of the shoulder joint and then in its sheath in the bicipital groove. Complete rupture of this tendon is usually obvious clinically. On arthrography the tendon is not visible in the joint or its sheath. If the tendon is dislocated it will not be present in its sheath on a tangential view.

Non-filling of the tendon sheaths may be due to adhesions, and leakage of contrast from the sheath is most likely to be due to increased intra-articular pressure as the joint is distended.

Gleno-humeral Dislocations

Two types of arthrographic patterns have been demonstrated by Reeves (1966) in patients with acute anterior dislocations – a capsular tear, and labral or capsular detachment. With a capsular tear the contrast dispersed anteriorly into the soft tissues in an irregular manner. A repeat arthrogram some days later showed that the tear had healed and none of these patients developed recurrent dislocation. Anterior labral or capsular detachment was recognized by observing the contrast passing beneath the subscapularis region into a false pouch. If this finding was still present on a repeat arthrogram three weeks later recurrent dislocation developed without significant injury.

Rupture of the rotator cuff may occur together with an acute anterior dislocation.

Arthrograms in recurrent anterior dislocation will demonstrate an enlarged entrance into the subscapularis recess so that the inferior axillary recess merges with the subscapularis recess. Detachment and distortion of the anterior glenoid labrum may also occur. This is not usually detected with standard arthrographic techniques but can be shown easily by arthrography combined with CT scanning.

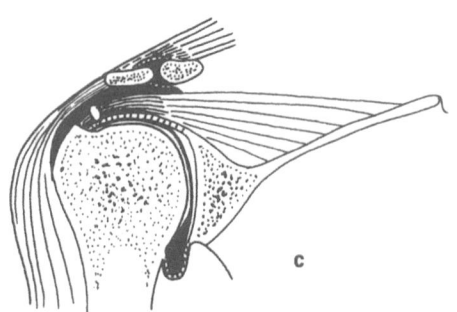

rotator cuff without filling of the subacromial bursa. Incomplete tears of the rotator cuff would not be detected if the tear was on the bursal side of the cuff (Fig. 3.9a), a deep central tear of the rotator cuff (Fig. 3.9b), or had healed leaving a fibrous nodule (Fig. 3.9c).

Capsulitis

In this condition the joint may be more difficult to puncture than usual and only accept a small volume

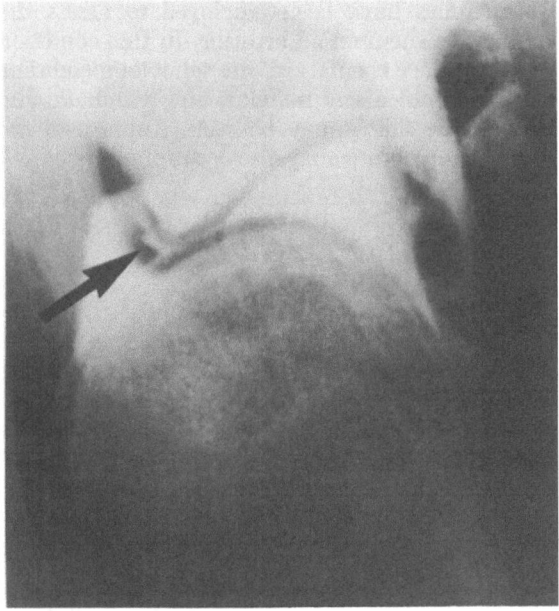

Fig. 3.10. Tear of posterior aspect of glenoid labrum. The arrow points to contrast extending into the tear.

Patients with recurrent posterior dislocation have a large posterior pouch with increased joint capacity, and the posterior glenoid labrum is torn (Fig. 3.10), ill-defined or absent.

Rheumatoid Arthritis

The arthrographic features which may be seen in rheumatoid arthritis are joint enlargement, nodular defects within the joint due to synovial hypertrophy, complete and incomplete tears of the rotator cuff, capsulitis, large synovial cysts and filling of peri-articular lymphatics and lymph nodes.

Miscellaneous

Arthrography is also employed for the detection of loose bodies, synovial chondromatosis and pigmented villo-nodular synovitis.

Hip Arthrography

Children

Hip arthrography in children is usually performed to assess the salient points of an already-diagnosed disease. Thus it is done for the evaluation of congenital dislocation, other dysplasias, and Perthes disease. Occasionally, arthrography is employed for the investigation of monarticular arthritis and trauma.

In congenital dislocation failure to reduce the femoral head is usually due to interposition of the limbus between the femoral head and the acetabulum, or by a thickened ligamentum teres in the acetabulum. An interposed limbus is seen as a radiolucent filling defect between the supero-lateral aspect of the acetabulum and the femoral head. An enlarged ligamentum teres appears as a band-like radiolucent filling defect in the acetabulum extending to the femoral head.

The arthrographic features of subluxation are less than half coverage of the femoral head by the acetabulum and elevation of the limbus thorn (Goldman 1979). In dislocation, the femoral head is displaced supero-laterally and is completely uncovered by the acetabulum and the capsule of the hip has an hour-glass deformity.

Arthrography in Perthes disease is used for detecting femoro-acetabular incongruity and to find the optimal position for obtaining cover of the femoral head prior to osteotomy. A good result is expected if the femoral head and acetabulum maintain their normal shape during the disease process of fragmentation and repair. The arthrographic findings in those hips with a poor prognosis have been listed by Goldman (1979), and are: an abnormal shape of the cartilagenous femoral capital epiphysis with a decrease in its height, persistent enlargement and irregularity of the contour of the cartilagenous femoral head, compression of the limbus and/or narrowing of the supero-lateral aspect of the joint space, femoro-acetabular incongruity as shown by pooling of contrast between the femoral head and acetabulum, and poor coverage of the femoral head by the acetabulum.

Arthrography is employed in the acute stages of septic arthritis to confirm the correct siting of the needle during aspiration and may be used in the late stages for assessment of the extent of the cartilagenous destruction.

Other conditions of the hip in which arthrography is occasionally employed are proximal focal femoral deficiency, dislocations due to neuro-muscular disorders, chondrolysis, Still's disease and loose bodies. In proximal focal femoral deficiency arthrography will demonstrate the presence or absence of the cartilagenous femoral head in the acetabulum.

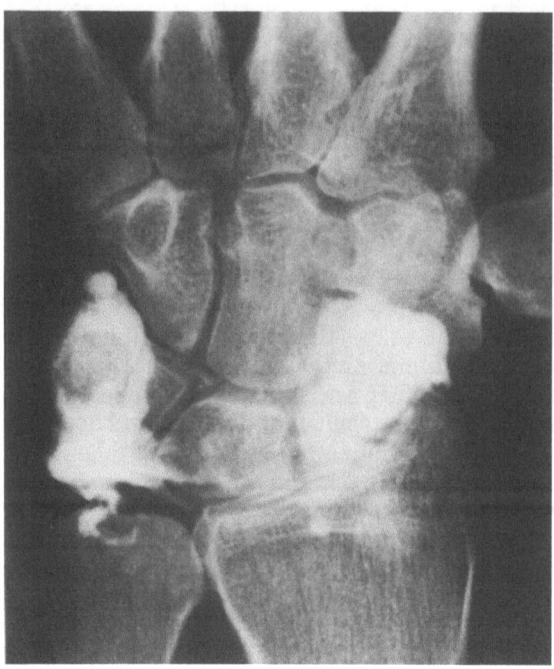

Fig. 3.11. Wrist arthrogram: contrast is seen tracking from the radio-carpal compartment through a defect in the triangular fibro-cartilage.

Adults

Arthrography of the hip is rarely requested because of its limited value but may be indicated in septic arthritis, and in the detection of loose bodies and synovial lesions.

Elbow Arthrography

Indications for this procedure are locking due to chondral and osteochondral fragments, and the assessment of articular cartilage, arthropathies, and synovial disorders.

Single and double contrast techniques are used and tomography has been incorporated into the latter method by Eto, Anderson and Harley (1975).

An osteochondral or chondral fragment will appear as a filling defect and both the number and site of origin should be confirmed. Small fragments are best detected by arthrotomography. Single con-

trast studies have been employed to assess the changes of rheumatoid arthritis. In this condition the joint space is enlarged, the synovial membrane is hypertrophied and nodular, and lymphatic and lymph-node filling may be seen. Rupture of the synovial membrane may also occasionally occur.

Wrist Arthrography

The wrist extends from the lower radius and ulna to the base of the metacarpals and includes the following joints (compartments): radio-carpal, inferior radio-ulnar, mid-carpal, pisiform-triquetral, carpometacarpal and inter-metacarpal.

The radio-carpal joint is the largest of these compartments and a wrist arthrogram will refer to this joint. The radio-carpal joint is separated from the inferior radio-ulnar joint by the triangular fibrocartilage. Communications between these compartments are related to traumatic and degenerative changes. The pisiform-triquetral joint is found frequently to communicate with the radio-carpal compartment due to incomplete attachment of the meniscus homologue to the triquetrum and this is considered to be a variation of normal.

Indications

Post Traumatic Disability

Tears of the triangular fibro-cartilage are recorded by the passage of contrast from the radio-carpal to the inferior radio-ulnar compartment (Fig. 3.11). It is a finding which has to be interpreted in conjunction with the patient's symptoms and signs as its incidence increases with age. Other findings in patients with disability after trauma are other intercompartmental communications, mild synovial irregularity and tendon opacification (Resnick 1974). Arthrography is occasionally indicated to determine if a bony fragment around the joint is lying loose within the joint.

Miscellaneous Conditions

Other indications for performing a wrist arthrogram are ganglia, rheumatoid arthritis and pigmented villo-nodular synovitis. Wrist ganglia are outlined in approximately two thirds of cases during wrist arthrography (Andren and Eiken 1971), and a narrow tortuous communication between the radiocarpal joint and ganglion may be shown.

Hand Arthrography

The small joints of the hands are rarely investigated by arthrography because the additional information obtainable appears to have little effect on further management.

Resnick and Danzig (1976) described the arthrographic findings in gamekeepers' thumb, a condition where radial stress produces damage to the ulnar collateral ligament, volar plate and joint capsule of the metacarpo-phalangeal joint. The arthrographic findings are extravasation of contrast along the ulnar aspect of the joint and a filling defect due to interposition of the dorsal aponeurosis between the torn ligament and its phalangeal attachment.

Ankle Arthrography

Arthrography of the ankle is employed in the assessment of ligament injuries particularly the lateral, chondral and osteochondral fractures, osteochondritis dissecans and capsulitis.

A single contrast technique is employed with contrast introduced through a 22-gauge needle introduced anteriorly between the tendons of tibialis anterior and extensor hallucis longus. Tomography can be helpful for assessing cartilage abnormalities.

Indications

Lateral Ligament Tears

In acute injuries where there is no fracture, arthrography is done to detect tears of the lateral ligament. This ligament has three main components, the anterior talo-fibular ligament, the calcaneofibular and posterior talo-fibular ligaments. A tear of the anterior talo-fibular ligament results in contrast passing anterior and lateral to the malleolus. Rupture of the calcaneo-fibular ligament enables contrast to pass into the peroneal tendon sheath as the inner aspect of this sheath is intimately related

to the ligament. It must be remembered that the tendon sheaths of the flexor hallucis longus and flexor digitorum longus which are on the medial aspect of the ankle may fill normally. A further variation of normal is filling of the posterior subtalar joint.

Rupture of the calcaneo-fibular ligament is usually associated with a tear of the anterior talo-fibular ligament. Thus arthrographic signs of both injuries will be present.

Tears of the posterior talo-fibular ligament are less frequently encountered and when they occur are usually in conjunction with rupture of the other two bands of the lateral ligaments. The arthrographic findings are essentially those discussed above with contrast passing posteriorly.

The investigation should be carried out as soon as possible after injury, ideally within 48 hours, to avoid false negative procedures by a tear becoming sealed by blood clot. A false negative result may also be produced by the preferential leakage of contrast from the joint at the site of one large tear. This tends to occur when the anterior talo-fibular ligament and calcaneo-fibular ligaments are torn with excessive leakage into the subcutaneous tissue through the tear of the more anterior ligament and failure of the peroneal tendon sheath to outline. The problem can be overcome by using a tourniquet, by injecting more contrast and by gentle exercise of the ankle. An alternative is a peroneal tenogram.

Occasionally a little contrast is seen in the peroneal tendon sheath without evidence of contrast in the extrasynovial tissues due probably to an old rupture of the calcaneo-fibular ligament.

Medial (Deltoid) Ligament Tears

Arthrography is rarely done for a tear of this ligament but if it is, extravasation of contrast around the medial malleolus will indicate a rupture.

Distal Anterior Tibio-fibular Ligament

A tear of this ligament may occur in isolation or in association with other ligament ruptures and is identified by extravasation of contrast anterior to the tibio-fibular syndesmosis and proximally in the syndesmosis for a distance greater than 2.5 cm.

Loose Bodies

Small bony fragments are commonly seen around the ankle and are usually due to avulsion fractures or accessory ossicles lying outside the joint. Occasionally they may be thought to be loose bodies causing symptoms. Arthrography can resolve whether they are lying inside or outside the joint. Screening prior to the arthrogram and after the injection of contrast is very valuable in order to ascertain the extent and type of motion of a loose body and also to aid radiographic positioning. Hudson (1984) found that freely-floating loose bodies had a tumbling motion whilst less freely mobile densities were attached to the synovial lining or wedged between articular surfaces. Intra-articular fragments will be completely or almost completely surrounded by contrast. Opacities outside the joint move in a more limited and linear fashion and are not surrounded by contrast.

Osteochondritis Dissecans

The articular cartilage can be assessed by arthrography and this may be of value in determining whether the cartilage is intact or separated in cases of osteochondritis dissecans. Arthrography can also detect the presence of a chondral fracture which will not be seen on the plain films. The broad radiolucent line of the articular cartilage is disrupted if there is a detachment of an osteochondral or chondral fragment.

Miscellaneous Conditions

Rarely, arthrography may be employed for assessment of such conditions as rheumatoid arthritis and ganglia.

Adhesive capsulitis is a condition in which movements of the ankle are decreased following trauma and has been described by Goldman et al. (1976). The arthrographic findings are a decrease in joint capacity, obliteration of the normal anterior and posterior recesses and extravasation of contrast along the needle track.

Foot Arthrography

Arthrography of the posterior subtalar joint can be used in the investigation of the sinus tarsi syndrome which is characterized by a feeling of instability of the ankle and pain over the lateral opening of the sinus tarsi. Taillard et al. (1981) noted in acute lesions that a haemarthrosis was frequently present

and there was extravasation of contrast and absence of the small synovial recesses. In chronic lesions the main findings were absence of filling of the small synovial recesses along the interosseus ligament, stoppage of flow of the contrast when it reached the sinus tarsi and failure of filling of the lateral recesses.

Arthrography of the anterior subtalar joint is rarely requested but can be performed for investigation of tarsal coalition, post traumatic disability and club foot. This joint extends anteriorly into the talo-navicular joint such that it is really the talo-calcaneo-navicular joint. The sustentaculum tali is the part of the calcaneum which articulates with the talus. If this part of the joint is not outlined by contrast a tarsal coalition is present.

Combined arthrography of the tibio-talar and talo-calcaneo-navicular joint has been performed by Hjelmstedt and Sahlstedt (1978) in infants to outline the talus in disorders such as club foot.

Arthrographic Evaluation of Total Joint Replacement

The detection of loosening and infection of prosthetic replacements by arthrography has been advocated although in our centre we rely almost exclusively on serial plain films and scintigraphy.

Arthrography for assessment of pain following total hip replacement was introduced by Salvati, Freiberger and Wilson (1971). Salvati et al. (1974) subsequently devised a subtraction technique which is the method that is usually employed.

The arthrographic findings of loosening or infection are extension of contrast between the cement and bone or between the prosthesis and bone, and contrast filled cavities and sinuses. Extension of contrast for 1 cm or less along the cement–bone interface at the supero-lateral or infero-medial aspects of the acetabulum and at the top of the femoral component does not indicate total loosening (Ghelman and Freiberger 1979). This latter point is important and may explain some of the false positive results in some of the earlier papers. False negative results may be due to inadequate amount of contrast being injected, the prevention of contrast passing along the bone–cement interface by granulation tissue and a poor distribution of contrast due to preferential filling of a large abscess cavity or sinus track.

Arthrography for the detection of loosening of components in other joint replacements is occasionally employed and the same radiographic principles apply as in the hip. In the abnormal total knee replacement arthrography is of value for assessing the tibial component but of less value for the femoral component because the cement–bone interface at this region is obscured on the antero-posterior view.

Facet Arthrography

Intervertebral disc degeneration and prolapse do not explain all low back and leg pain. Injections of the posterior facet joints of the lower lumbar spine first by contrast to ascertain the correct position of the needle, and then by local anaesthetic, have been found useful as a diagnostic-therapeutic procedure (Mooney and Robertson 1976). The lower three facet joints on the side of the pain were routinely injected unless the preliminary plain films showed unilateral one level degeneration and then only that joint was injected. Long-term relief was obtained in one fifth of patients with low back pain and sciatica and partial relief in another one third.

Traction Arthrography

The phenomenon of gas appearing within a joint and outlining part of the articular cartilage when traction is applied to a limb is well known. It is seen most frequently in the shoulders of children undergoing chest radiography when the arms are outstretched. It has limited application and is not widely used. It has been employed to detect effusions by Martel et al. (1971) in the hip and by Yousefzadeh (1979) in the wrist and metacarpo-phalangeal joints. The gas within a joint will appear as a radiolucent band and this will exclude an effusion. Provided sufficient traction is applied to increase the joint space then the absence of gas will indicate that an effusion is probably present.

Ganglionography

Ganglia are outpouches from synovial joints and tendon sheaths. Ganglionography is performed by inserting a wide bore needle into a ganglion under local anaesthetic using an aseptic technique. Some of the contents of the ganglion are aspirated and

then contrast is injected and appropriate radiographs taken.

A study of ganglia around the wrist was made by Andren and Eiken (1971) who performed carpal arthrography and ganglionography. Arthrography led to filling of the ganglion and identification of a communicating duct in approximately two thirds of cases. Ganglionography did not cause the passage of contrast into a joint. Thus it was postulated that there is a one-way valve mechanism preventing contrast passing from the ganglion into the joint but allowing contrast to pass from the joint into the ganglion. However, in a case reported by Daffner and Whitfield (1977) injection of a ganglion on the lateral aspect of the calcaneum led to filling of the peroneal tendon sheaths.

Tenography

Tenography is the injection of contrast into tendon sheaths and is performed around the ankle and rarely in the hand.

Peroneal Tenography

A peroneal tenogram is usually carried out to assess the integrity of the calcaneo-fibular ligament which is the middle component of the lateral ligament of the ankle. The calcaneo-fibular ligament of the ankle joint is related to the deep surface of the peroneal tendon sheath and rupture of this ligament is associated with a tear of the peroneal tendon sheaths. Thus, if contrast is injected into the tendon sheath and passes into the ankle joint (Fig. 3.12) it will indicate a tear of the calcaneo-fibular ligament. This technique has been employed by Evans and Freyno (1979) and Blanshard et al. (1986). It may be a more accurate method of detecting a calcaneo-fibular ligament rupture than an ankle arthrogram, as in this latter procedure it is possible for contrast to pass preferentially through a tear in the antero-lateral aspect of the capsule. It is important to do the peroneal tenogram as soon as possible after the injury as tears become sealed with blood clots. Films after manipulation should also be done if the initial radiographs are negative as there may be delayed flow of contrast into the ankle joint. Peroneal tenography has been performed in patients with a painful hindfoot following calcaneal fractures. The findings have been documented by

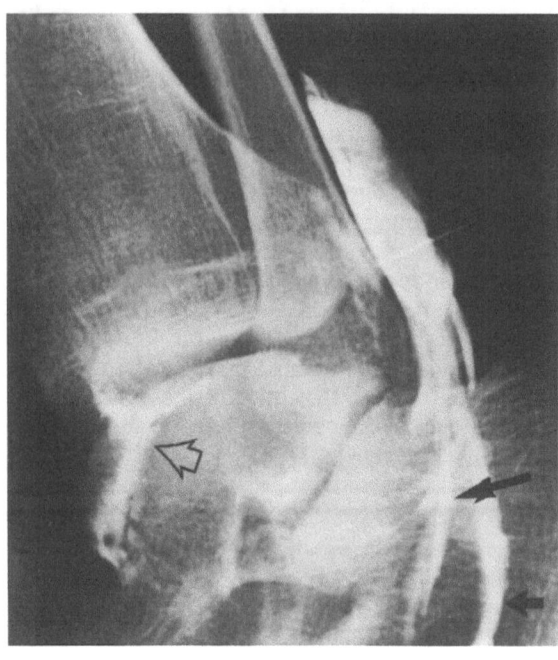

Fig. 3.12. Peroneal tenogram showing contrast in the ankle (*open arrow*) having passed from the peroneal tendon sheath. The *short arrow* is pointing to the peroneus longus and the *long arrow* to the peroneus brevis.

Bursography

Bursography is the technique of injecting contrast directly into a bursa. The technique can have occasional value in the investigation of a mass around a joint. The outlining of a bursa will exclude any soft tissue tumour.

A bursa may fill following an arthrogram and examples of this are the subacromial bursa after shoulder arthrography and the iliopsoas bursa after hip arthrography.

References

Resnick and Goergen (1975), and are extrinsic compression and irregularity of the sheath, lateral and/or anterior displacement, complete obstruction of contrast flow and tendon rupture.

Tenography of Sheaths of Hand and Wrist

Tenography of the flexor and extensor tendon sheaths of the wrist and hand is rarely performed because of its limited clinical application. It has been mainly used for assessing rheumatoid disease and enlargement of the synovial sheaths, hypertrophy of the synovium, rupture of tendon sheaths and communications with joints have all been demonstrated.

Tenography has also been applied to the diagnosis and prognosis of flexor tendon rupture (Semple 1970) and assessing the synovial tendon sheath within the carpal tunnel to determine any local mechanical factor producing the carpal tunnel syndrome (Resnick 1975).

Andren L, Eiken O (1971) Arthrographic studies of wrist ganglions. J Bone Joint Surg [Am] 53:299–302

Andren L, Lundberg BJ (1965) Treatment of rigid shoulders by joint distension during arthrography. Acta Orthop Scand 36:45–53

Andren L, Wehlin L (1960). Double contrast arthrography of the knee with horizontal roentgen ray beam. Acta Orthop Scand 29:307–314

Blanshard KS, Finlay DBL, Scott DJA, Ley CC, Siggins D, Allen MJ (1986) A radiological analysis of lateral ligament injuries of the ankle. Clin Radiol 37:247–251

Boven F, Bellemans M, Geurts J, DeBoeck H, Potvliege R (1982) The value of computed tomography scanning in chondromalacia patellae. Skeletal Radiol 8:183–185

Butt WP, McIntyre JL (1969) Double contrast arthrography of the knee. Radiology 92:487–499

Daffner RH, Whitfield PW (1977) Recurrent ganglion cyst. The value of preoperative ganglionography. AJR 129:345–346

Dalinka MK (1980) Knee arthrography. Springer-Verlag, New York

Debnam JW, Staple TW (1974) Arthrography of the knee after meniscectomy. Radiology 113:67–71

Eto RT, Anderson PW, Harley JD (1975) Elbow arthrography with the application of tomography. Radiology 115:283–288

Evans GA, Freyno SD (1979) The stress tenogram in the diagnosis of ruptures of the lateral ligament of the ankle. J Bone Joint Surg [Br] 61:347–351

Freiberger RH, Kaye JJ (eds) (1979) Arthrography. Appleton-Century Crofts, New York

Ghelman B, Freiberger RH (1979) The adult hip. In: Freiberger RH, Kaye JJ (eds) Arthrography. Appleton-Century Crofts, New York

Goldman AB (1979) Hip arthrography in infants and children. In: Freiberger RH, Kaye JJ (eds) Arthrography. Appleton-Century Crofts, New York

Goldman AB, Katz MC, Freiberger RH (1976) Post-traumatic adhesive capsulitis of the ankle. Arthrographic diagnosis. AJR 127:585:588

Hjelmstedt A, Sahlstedt B (1978) Simultaneous arthrography of the talo-crural and talo-navicular joints in children. IV. Measurements on congenital club feet. Acta Radiol [Diagn] (Stockh) 19:223–236

Hudson TM (1984) Joint fluoroscopy before arthrography. Detection and evaluation of loose bodies. Skeletal Radiol 12:199–203

Martel W, Poznanski AK, Kuhns LR (1971) Further observations on the value of traction during roentgenography of the hip. Invest Radiol 6:1–8

Mooney V, Robertson J (1976) The facet syndrome. Clin Orthop 115:149–156

Neviaser JS (1962) Arthrography of the shoulder joint; study of findings in adhesive capsulitis of the shoulder. J Bone Joint Surg [Am] 44:1321–1330

Pavlov H (1979) The cruciate ligaments in arthrography. In: Freiberger RH, Kaye JJ (eds) Arthrography. Appleton-Century Crofts, New York

Preston BJ, Jackson JP (1976) Shoulder arthrography. Br J Radiol 49:288

Preston BJ, Jackson JP (1977) Investigation of shoulder disability by arthrography. Clin Radiol 28:259–266

Reeves B (1966) Arthrography of the shoulder. J Bone Joint Surg [Br] 48:424–435

Resnick D (1974) Arthrography in the evaluation of arthritic disorders of the wrist. Radiology 113:331–340

Resnick D (1975) Roentgenographic anatomy of the tendon sheaths of the hand and wrist: tenography. AJR 124:44–51

Resnick D, Danzig LA (1976) Arthrographic evaluation of injuries of the first metacarpo-phalangeal joint; game-keepers' thumb. AJR 126:1046–1052

Resnick D, Goergen TG (1975) Peroneal tenography in previous calcaneal fractures. Radiology 115:211–213

Salvati EA, Freiberger RH, Wilson PD Jr (1971) Arthrography for complications of total hip replacement. A review of thirty-one arthrograms. J Bone Joint Surg [Am] 53:701–709

Salvati EA, Ghelman B, McLaren T, Wilson PD Jr (1974) Subtraction technique in arthrography for loosening of total hip replacement fixed with radio-opaque cement. Clin Orthop 101:105–109

Semple JC (1970) Radiographic appearances of normal flexor tendon sheaths in the hand. Br J Radiol 43:271–273

Stoker DJ (1980) Knee arthrography. Chapman and Hall, London

Taillard W, Meyer J, Garcia J, Blanc Y (1981) The sinus tarsi syndrome. Int Orthop 5:117–130

Yousefzadeh DK (1979) The value of traction during roentgenography of the wrist and metacarpo-phalangeal joints. Skeletal Radiol 4:29–33

4 Conventional Radiography of the Axial Skeleton

W. P. Butt

Introduction 51
Standard Anteroposterior and Lateral Views of the Area of Interest 52
  Occiput, C1 and C2 52
  C2 to C7 53
  Cervico-Thoracic Junction 57
  Thoracic Spine 58
  Thoraco-Lumbar Junction 60
  Lumbo-Sacral Junction, Sacrum and Sacro-Iliac Joints 61
  Pelvis 62
Additional Radiography 62
  Screening 62
  Tomography 62
Specific Radiographic Challenges 63
  Spondylolysis 63
  Inflammatory Spondylitis 64
  Facet Injuries 64
  Scoliosis 67
  Acetabular Injuries 67
Radiographic Signs of Bone and Joint Disorder 67
  Loss of Cortical Integrity 70
  Fracture 70
  Rotation 72
  Repair 72
  Loss of Subchondral Cortex 72
  Malalignment 72
  Spasm 74
Errors in Diagnosis "Caused" by Radiography 74
  Errors Due to an Inadequate or Incomplete Examination 74
  Errors Due to the Inherent Deficiencies of Radiography 75
References 75

Introduction

Conventional radiography has been with us for so long that we have forgotten the reasons for the examinations which are now performed routinely. "Antero-posterior and lateral" views were chosen because it was felt that they would demonstrate, or exclude, the cardinal signs of bone and joint disorder. Special views and techniques were developed to assess known abnormalities or to demonstrate or exclude specific entities. It is futile in practice, and incorrect in theory, to use the latter type of examination to do the work of the former. For example, oblique projections of the spine cannot compensate for an inadequate lateral film (Fig. 4.12); nor can a good lateral projection compensate for no frontal (Fig. 4.1).

The anatomical divisions of the spine into cervical, thoracic and lumbar are radiographically awkward and, apart from tradition, have no reason for

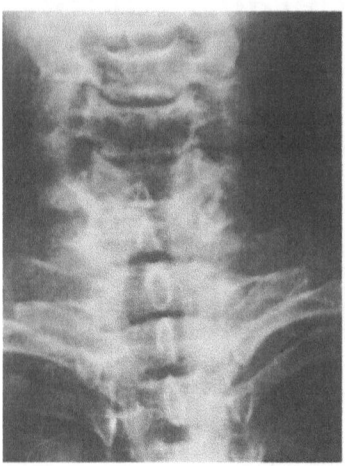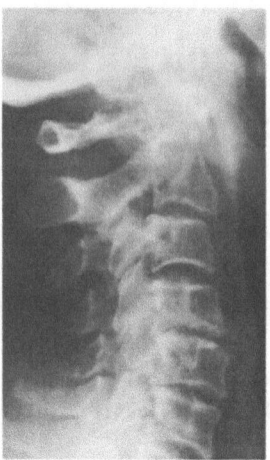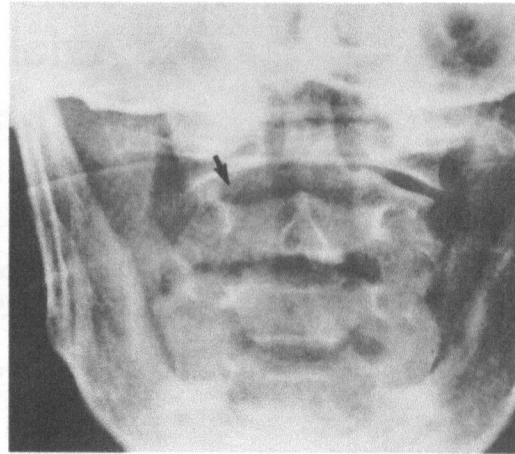

Fig. 4.1. An open mouth view is an essential film in radiography of the cervical spine. This view demonstrates destruction of the body of C2. One cardinal radiological sign of bone disorder is loss of cortical integrity (*arrow*).

their existence. The junctional areas (e.g. lower dorsal/upper lumbar) are radiographic units from the points of view of pathology, projection and exposure factors and may differ from the central areas of the anatomical divisions from the same points of view. Unfortunately, tradition will prevail and the interpreter of the radiographs must realize that adequate (i.e. antero-posterior and lateral) views will not be obtained in junctional areas on the standard examinations. Films obtained perpendicular to the table top may not be perpendicular to the spine, and a frontal film with no angulation will frequently show no vertebral bodies and project the laminae in such a way as to mimic vertebral bodies. It is the duty of the interpreter, and not of the radiographer, to be certain that frontal and lateral films have been obtained of the *area of interest*.

A word must be said about the significance of abnormal radiographic findings. General medical usage decrees that "significant" means that an abnormality requires treatment or that the prognosis will be affected. To these two meanings one must add the significance of a radiographic abnormality (e.g. abnormal alignment). In this situation, "significant" means an adequate explanation for the abnormality must be found, while the medical significance of the radiographic abnormality will depend on the explanation of the abnormality and not on the abnormality itself. Understanding the difference will help to avoid the conflict that frequently occurs between a radiologist's and a clinician's opinion of a given abnormality.

Standard Antero-posterior and Lateral Views of the Area of Interest

Occiput, C1 and C2

Antero-posterior Projection

A frontal film of the cervical spine will not provide an antero-posterior projection of the occiput to C2. An open mouth view is as necessary a film in the routine investigation of the cervical spine as is the lateral. For example, only the open mouth view will demonstrate the reasonably common occurrence of metastases in the lateral part of the body of C2 with collapse of C1 into C2 (Fig. 4.1).

The standard open mouth projection will superimpose the alveolus of the upper jaw on the occiput. If this occurs and the odontoid is not demonstrated, an explanation must be found. It must be emphasized that this does not necessarily mean that a significant clinical entity is present but rather that the cause for the failure of demonstration must be found. Usually hyperextension of the neck is the explanation, but basilar invagination and other anomalies are frequent enough to underline the necessity of explaining the observation.

Symmetry is anticipated and if it is not present a satisfactory explanation must be found. Rotation of C1 on C2 (Fig. 4.2) is a normal occurrence in response to muscle spasm and does *not* indicate C1/C2 disease.

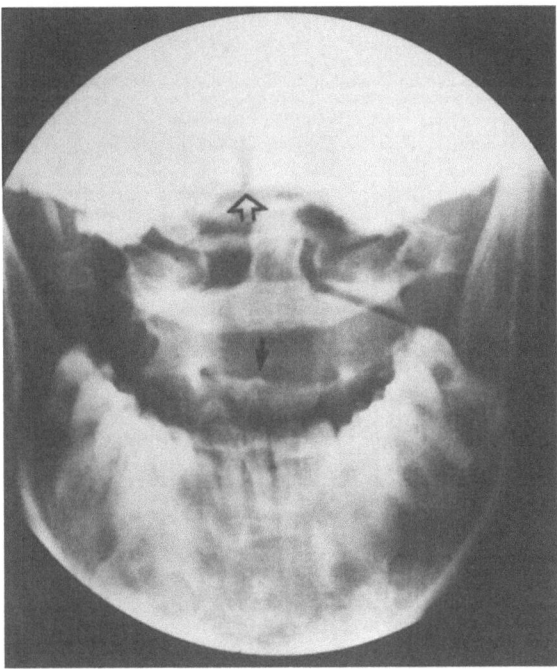

Fig. 4.2. The *solid arrow* points to the spinous process of C2 lying to the right, indicating that C2 is turned to the left. The *open arrow* points to the incisor teeth on the right, indicating that the head is turned to the right. Therefore rotation of C1 on C2 must have occurred. This is a normal response to muscle spasm and is almost always caused by a lesion somewhere other than C1/C2. Notice that the right lateral mass of C1 is smaller and more dense than the left and although the space between it and the odontoid is greater than that on the left side it is not displaced laterally in relation to the lateral margin of C2. Increased density and decreased size are characteristic appearances of a rotated oval of bone.

A number of lines, none of which is likely to remain in the reader's memory, have been drawn on frontal films in an attempt to relate the normal anatomical structures. One should make a habit of verifying the accepted measurements rather than remembering them.

Lateral Projection

Most people remember McGregor's line, which extends from the back of the hard palate to the foraminal cortex of the occipital bone at the foramen magnum, and know that the tip of the odontoid should lie not more than 5–8 mm above that line. Most radiologists do not realize that this is one of those radiographically significant but clinically indeterminate observations which requires an explanation before its clinical significance can be established. An odontoid which lies higher than the normal range may not be symptomatic, may not require treatment and may not influence prognosis.

Lines which are more commonly distorted and which are more useful clinically than McGregor's line are the alignment of the fronts of the vertebral bodies in relation to the anterior arch of C1 and the alignment of the posterior arches of C1 and C2. Comparing the component parts of Fig. 4.3 will show that the anterior arch of C1 normally lies in front of the anterior surface of the vertebral bodies below it because it is, in effect, a sesamoid bone in the anterior longitudinal ligament and is not the developmental body of C1. If the anterior arch of C1 does lie in the same plane as the fronts of the vertebral bodies below that level the odontoid must be deficient, absent or fractured.

The posterior arch of C1 should lie slightly anterior to the posterior arch of C2 and, unless the neck is hyperextended, there should not be smooth continuity of these posterior arches. Fig. 4.3 compares the normal with a posteriorly displaced C1.

The stability of the C1/C2 articulation is assessed by changes that occur in the relationship of the anterior arch of C1 to the odontoid on flexion and extension films in the lateral projection. It is generally accepted that an adult cannot have more than 3 mm between these two surfaces and maintain normal anatomical stability. It is also accepted that a distance greater than 1 cm means that there is no ligament holding the odontoid to the atlas or to the occiput. Note that this measurement is, again, one with radiographic significance. The cause for a greatly widened space must be determined before its clinical relevance is known. Many patients do not require treatment for and have no symptoms from an increase in the space between the odontoid and the anterior arch of C1. No negative significance can be assigned to the odontoid touching the anterior arch of C1 in the absence of flexion films (Fig. 4.4).

C2 to C7

Antero-posterior Projection

The standard AP projection of the cervical spine shows few vertebral bodies and frequently no vertebral bodies at all. What appears to be vertebral body on many frontal films is, in fact, lamina. Fig. 4.5 demonstrates this point nicely by showing the transition from visualization of the vertebral body to visualization of the lamina occurring in the middle of one vertebral body. If the joints of Luschka are demonstrated it can be accepted that a frontal film of the vertebral bodies has been obtained.

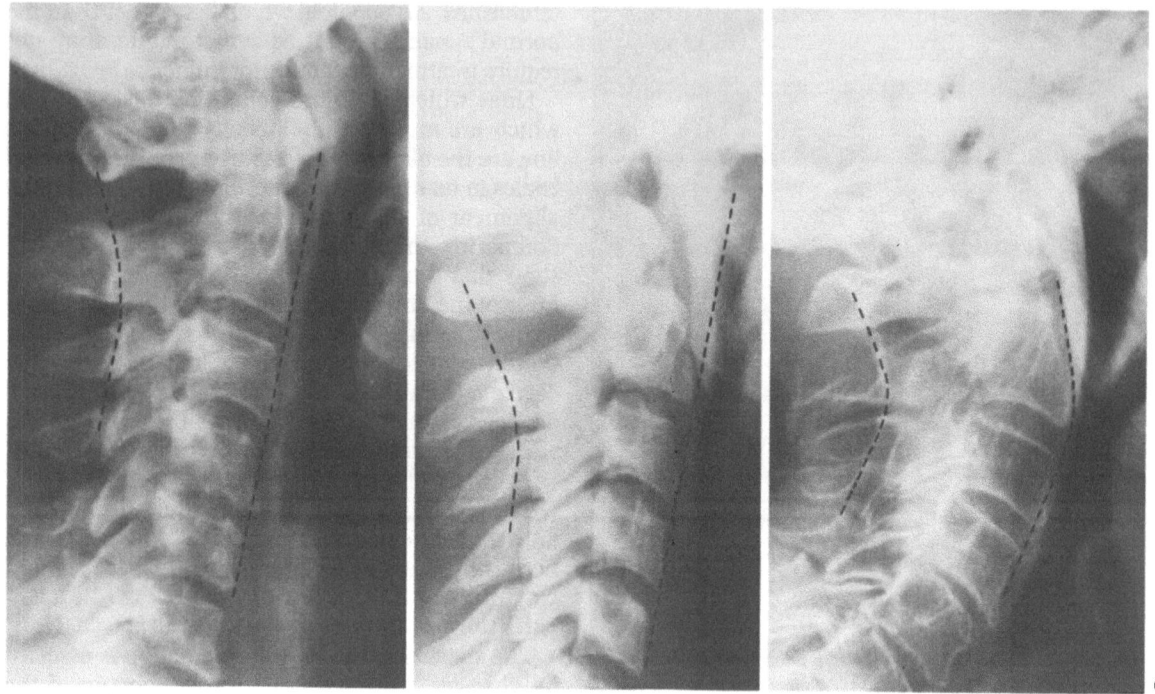

a, b   c

Fig. 4.3a–c. In the normal cervical spine (**a**) a smooth continuation of the line joining the bases of the spinous processes should pass behind the anterior surface of the posterior arch of C1 and a continuation of the anterior longitudinal ligament should meet or pass just in front of the anterior arch of C1. The anterior arch of C1 is not the vertebral body of C1 and should not lie in the same plane as the other vertebral bodies. In **b**, C1 is clearly displaced posteriorly. In **c**, C1 is also displaced posteriorly but it is not as easy to appreciate.

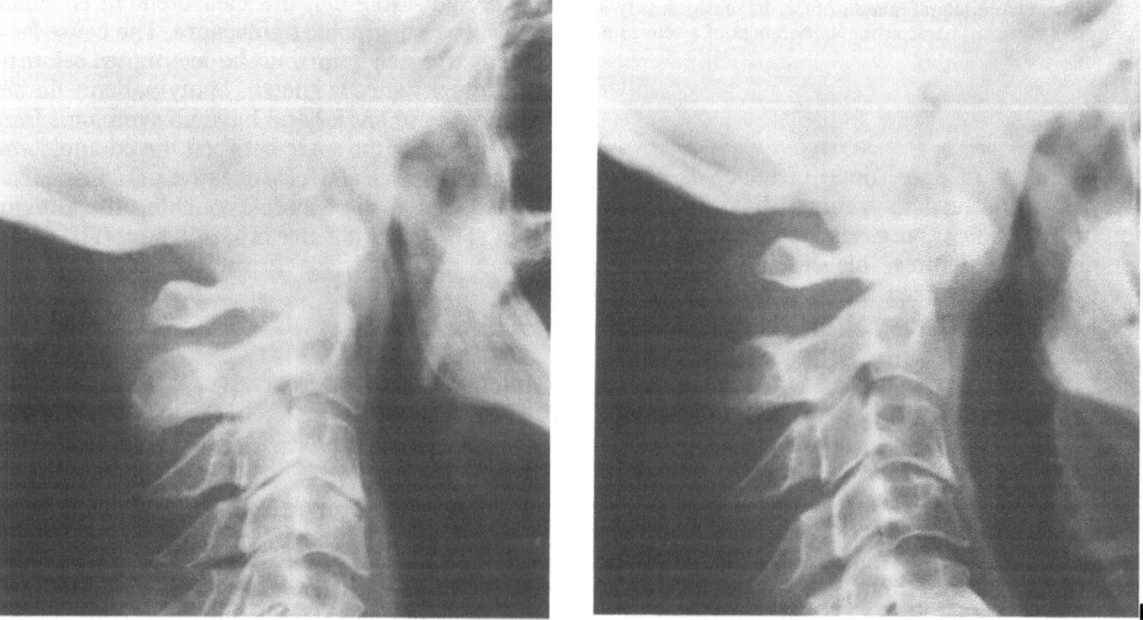

a   b

Fig. 4.4a,b. Radiography of the cervical spine in patients with rheumatoid arthritis is incomplete without a lateral flexion film. A case can be made for obtaining these films routinely in patients with rheumatoid arthritis who are to undergo surgery. Many patients such as the one illustrated here have atlanto-axial instability without symptoms. **a** straight lateral; **b** in flexion.

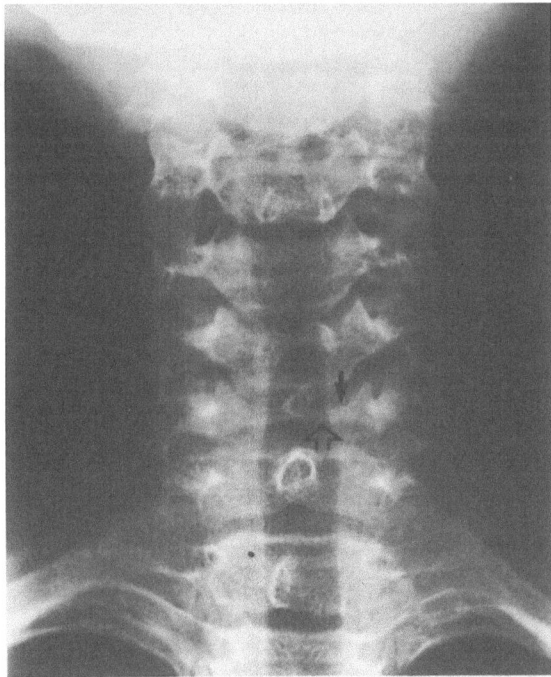

Fig. 4.5. A frontal film which is perpendicular to the table top is frequently not perpendicular to the spine, causing laminae to simulate vertebral bodies. The apparent flattening of C6 is illusory and is due to the upper border of the vertebral body (*solid arrow*) being truly vertebral body whereas the lower border (*open arrow*) is lamina. Frequently no vertebral bodies and only laminae are seen on a frontal film.

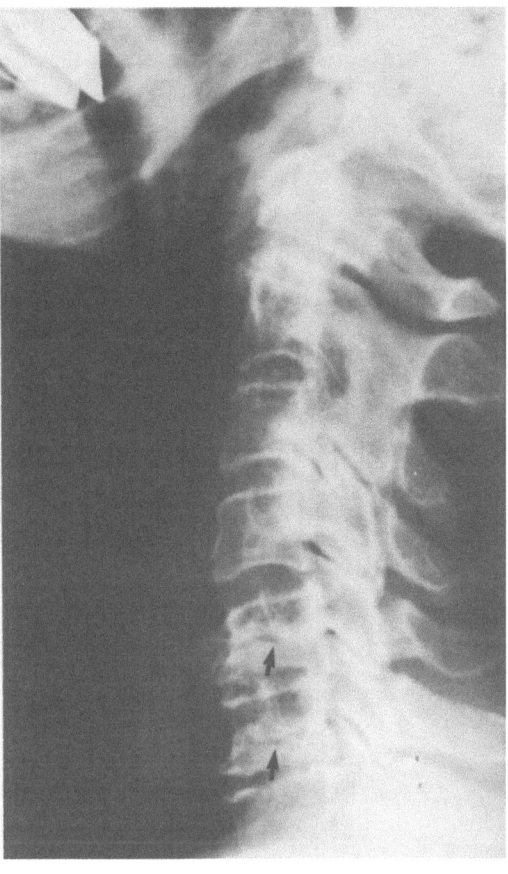

Fig. 4.6. If the joints of Luschka are osteoarthritic, the marginal osteophytes may be projected over the vertebral body on a lateral radiograph, simulating a fracture.

Lateral Projection

The standard lateral radiograph of the cervical spine is adequate to show C2 to C7 in most cases and additional radiographs are usually not necessary. On this projection some anatomical features are worth noting. The joints of Luschka, if osteophytic, may present as a radiolucent line paralleling the disc space across the inferior part of the vertebral body (Fig. 4.6), and this "pseudo-fracture" has trapped the unwary.

The prevertebral soft tissues receive much attention and there is no doubt that a massive retropharyngeal haematoma can be diagnosed (Fig. 4.7). What is not as commonly understood is that a normal prevertebral space can coexist with extensive vertebral injury and that there is no negative significance to normal prevertebral soft tissues. Great variation in the prevertebral space occurs in the same patient depending on the phase of respiration and the position in which the radiographs were obtained. Because of that, retropharyngeal swelling must be viewed with considerable tolerance in the patient who is crying, recumbent, intubated, young, or struggling. Localized swelling is much less likely to be due to innocuous causes, but even that can occur normally (Fig. 4.8).

Minor malalignments of the vertebral bodies are common because gliding of one vertebra on another is a normal movement. Anything that interferes with balance of the spine will interfere with this gliding or fix it in a glided position, and in this author's experience little significance can be attached to the radiological finding of minor malalignment.

Additional Projections

Abel Views. Frontal films of the lateral masses can be obtained by angling the incident beam approximately 45° cephalocaudad AP. If the head is not rotated the mandible and facial bones may be projected over the lateral masses and some degree of

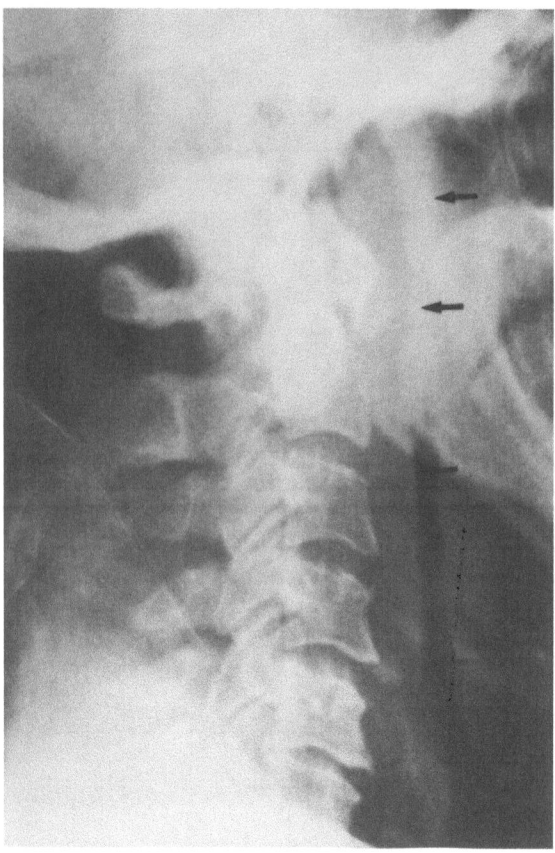

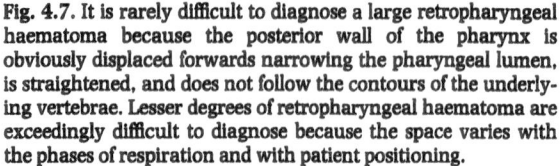

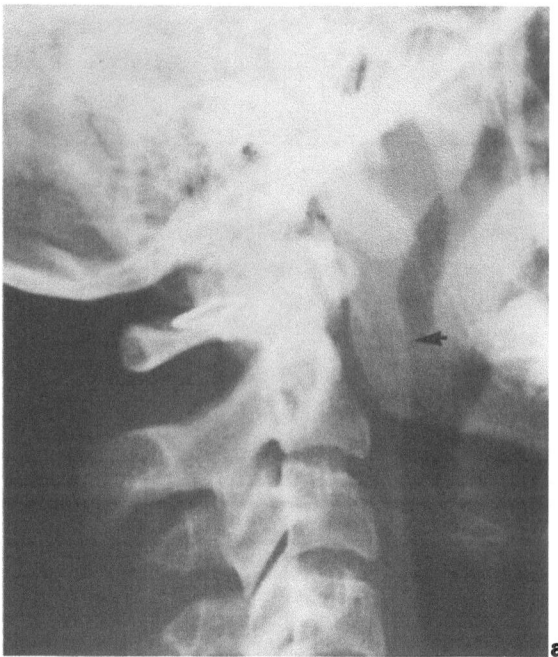

Fig. 4.7. It is rarely difficult to diagnose a large retropharyngeal haematoma because the posterior wall of the pharynx is obviously displaced forwards narrowing the pharyngeal lumen, is straightened, and does not follow the contours of the underlying vertebrae. Lesser degrees of retropharyngeal haematoma are exceedingly difficult to diagnose because the space varies with the phases of respiration and with patient positioning.

head rotation may assist in demonstrating these masses to best advantage (Fig. 4.9). It may be necessary to vary the incident angulation depending on whether the upper part of the neck or the lower part of the neck is being investigated.

Off Lateral Projection. Because the facets are superimposed on a lateral radiograph, a slightly off lateral projection shows the individual column of facets on each side to better advantage. Fifteen degrees of rotation is sufficient (Fig. 4.10).

Flexion and Extension. Lateral films in flexion and extension, with or without videotape recording, tend to be cyclically popular but this author finds them of little use. If a specific question of stability arises, then clearly attempts to demonstrate instability by radiographs during movement will be

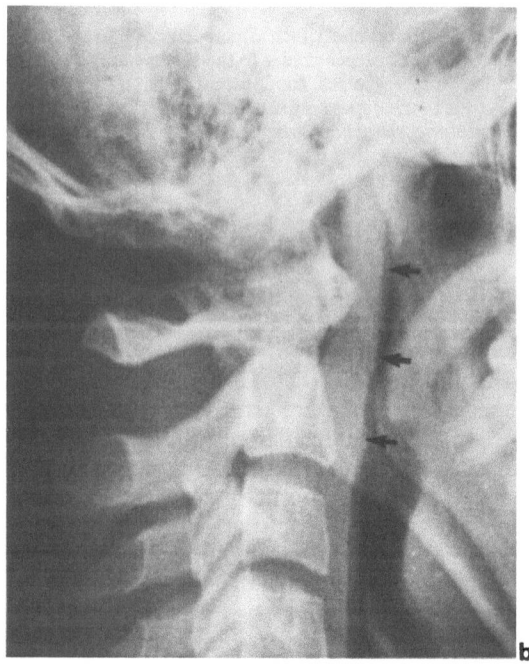

Fig. 4.8a,b. Localized retropharyngeal soft tissue swelling is usually due to injury (a), but can occur in the normal (b). Again, caution is advised in diagnosing haematoma.

valuable. However, to expect flexion and extension films to solve a mysterious complaint is to invite disappointment.

Oblique Projection. Most oblique projections are obtained by rotating the patient's head in relation to the shoulders, and this should be discouraged. Proper oblique views of the cervical spine are obtained by rotating the patient or changing the angulation of the incident beam with the patient's head and shoulders remaining in the usual alignment. Rotating the head can reduce pathological displacements (Fig. 4.10c) and will not allow comparison of one intervertebral foramen with another because each is seen in a different projection.

Cervico-Thoracic Junction

Antero-posterior Projection

AP projections of the cervico-thoracic junction are usually easily obtained, but require different radiographic exposure from frontal films of the cervical spine or frontal films of the dorsal spine. Angulation of the incident beam is essential if films of the vertebral bodies are to be obtained (Fig. 4.11).

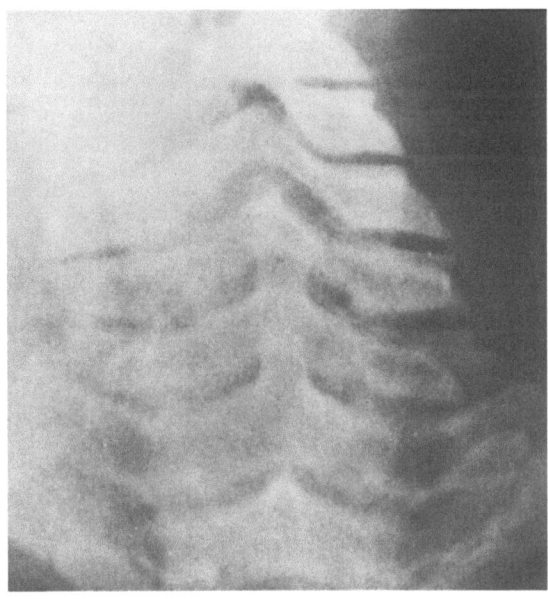

Fig. 4.9. Frontal films of the lateral masses (Abel views) require steep angulation.

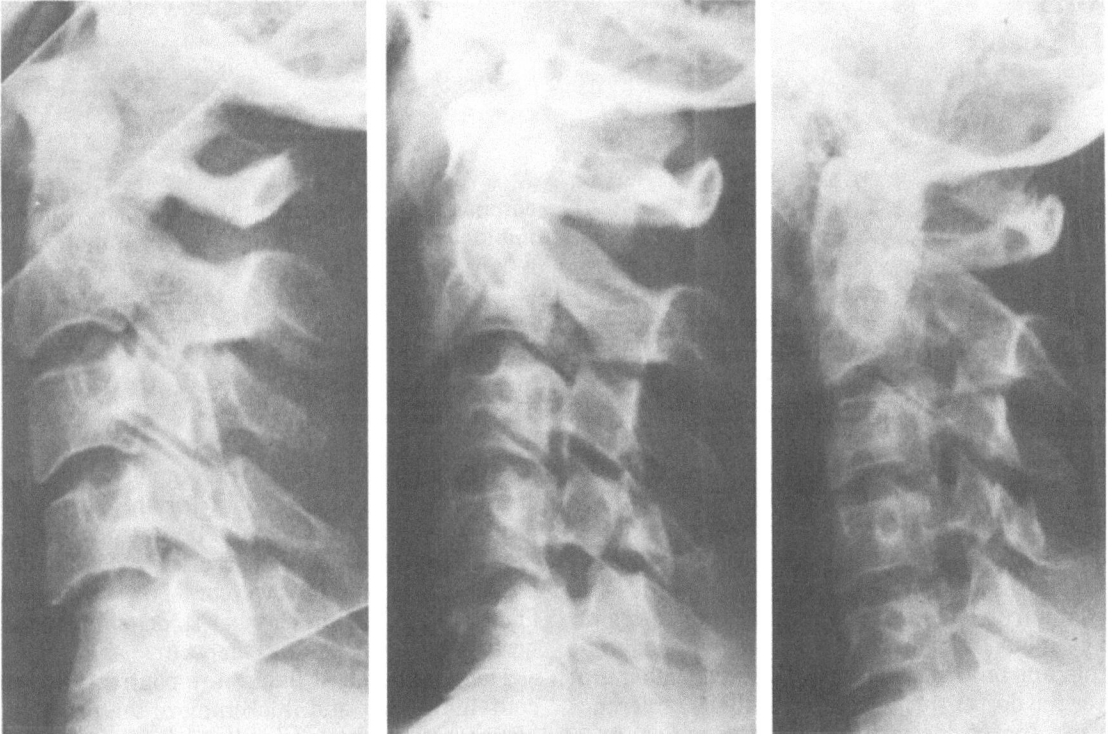

a   b, c

Fig. 4.10a. Lateral films of the cervical spine superimpose the lateral masses making it difficult to appreciate the cause of the displacement of C4 on C5. b A 15° off lateral oblique film projects one column of masses behind the other, clearly demonstrating the fracture with displacement of the lateral mass of C4. c It is important not to obtain the oblique view by rotating the head because that may reduce the displacement, making diagnosis difficult.

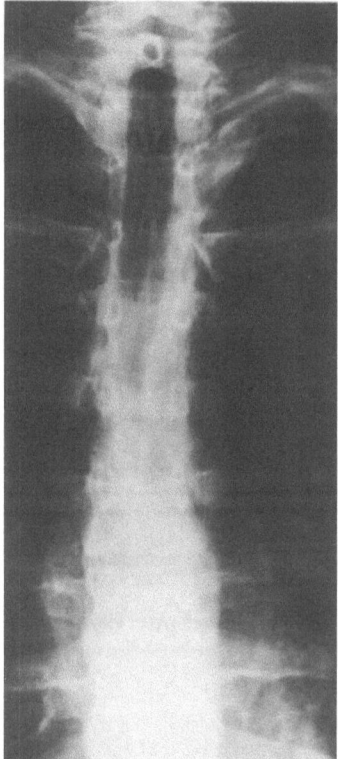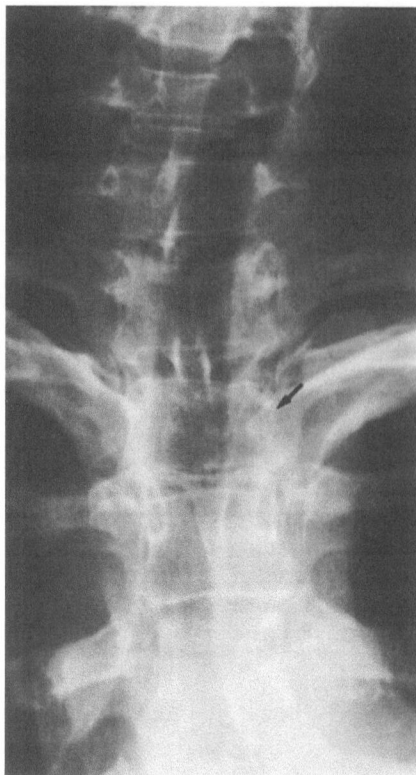

a   b

Fig. 4.11a,b. A frontal film of the cervico-dorsal junction which is obtained perpendicular to the table top will not demonstrate the vertebral bodies whereas an inclined frontal film parallel to the discs will. In this case the angled film demonstrates early destruction and collapse of the left side of T2. Note, once again, that the earliest sign of bone disorder is loss of cortical integrity (*arrow*).

Lateral Projection

Nothing induces more despair than attempting lateral films of the cervico-thoracic junction. From the number of recommended projections one can infer that no particular projection is successful in all patients. It must be accepted that on occasion films of this region cannot be obtained. In general terms there are two methods of attempting lateral radiographs. The first displaces the shoulder girdles away from the spine either by anterior traction or by angling the incident beam to project one shoulder behind and one in front of the spinal column. Unfortunately the latter variant means that the projection is not a true lateral. The other technique attempts to even out the radiographic density of the area by projecting one arm over the neck and the other arm over the dorsal spine. It is this author's preference to put the offside arm up, because radiographic magnification will tend to blur out the detail of the elevated humerus so that it will not produce an image on the film in the way that it does if the arm near the film is raised. It should not need to be

emphasized that a film of the cervical spine that does not include C7 is not an adequate examination (Fig. 4.12).

Thoracic Spine

It is virtually impossible to obtain adequate frontal radiographs of the entire thoracic spine with a single projection and one should not hesitate to use coned angled films of any suspicious area.

The demonstration of vertebral bodies may be difficult and, as in the cervical spine, simulation of vertebral body by lamina can occur.

The paravertebral tissues are contrasted by air-containing lung and thickening of the tissues can be seen. Any displacement of the paravertebral pleura on the right side (Fig. 4.13) must be viewed with concern, and localized displacement cannot be accepted without a satisfactory explanation. On the left, the aorta tends to pull the paravertebral pleura

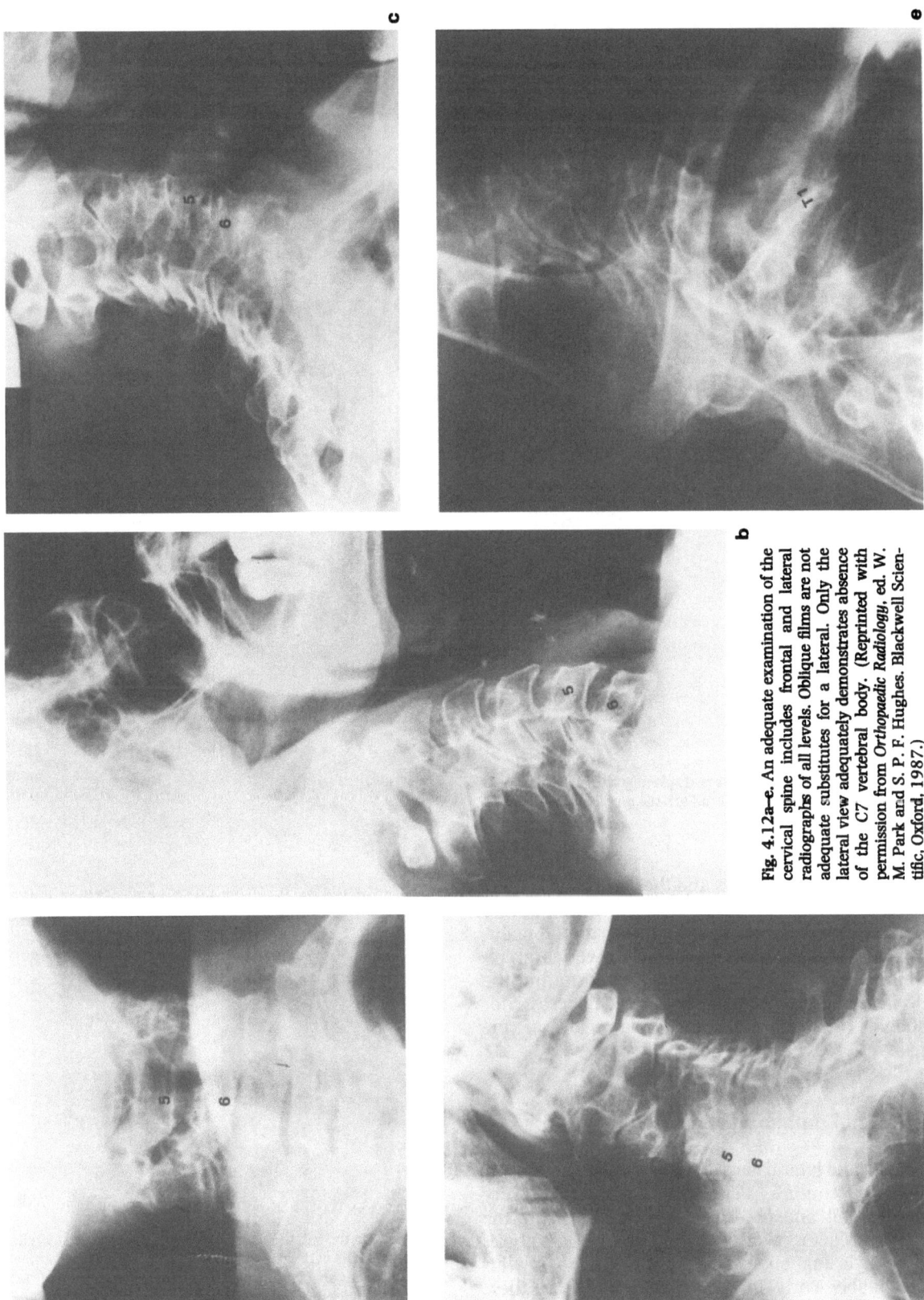

Fig. 4.12a–e. An adequate examination of the cervical spine includes frontal and lateral radiographs of all levels. Oblique films are not adequate substitutes for a lateral. Only the lateral view adequately demonstrates absence of the C7 vertebral body. (Reprinted with permission from *Orthopaedic Radiology*, ed. W. M. Park and S. P. F. Hughes. Blackwell Scientific, Oxford, 1987.)

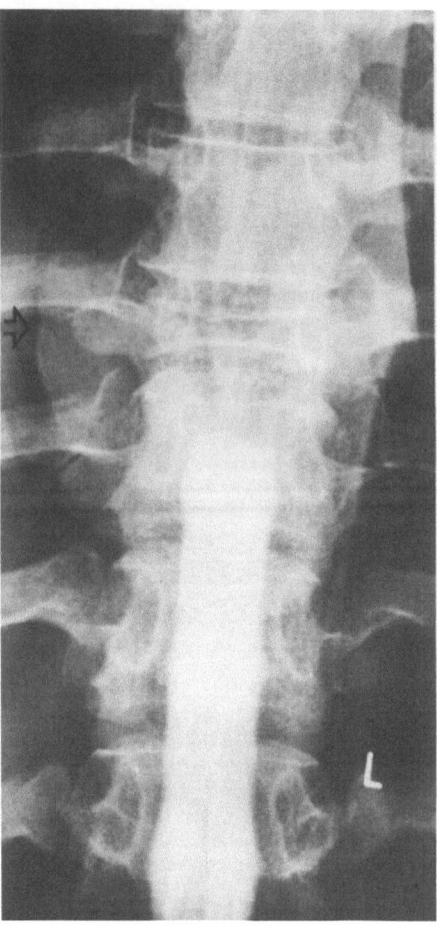

Fig. 4.13. Paravertebral masses displacing the right paravertebral pleura usually present no diagnostic problems.

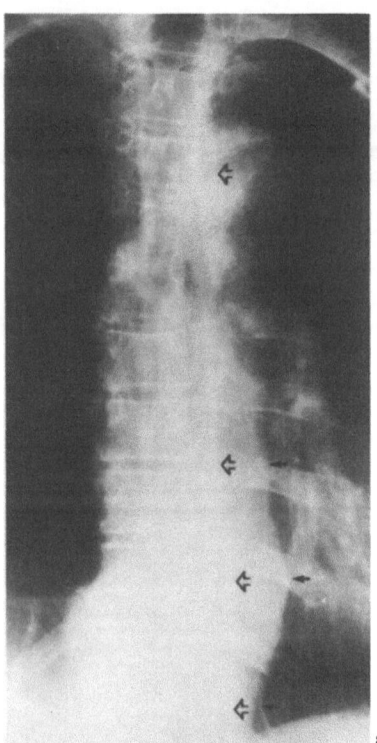

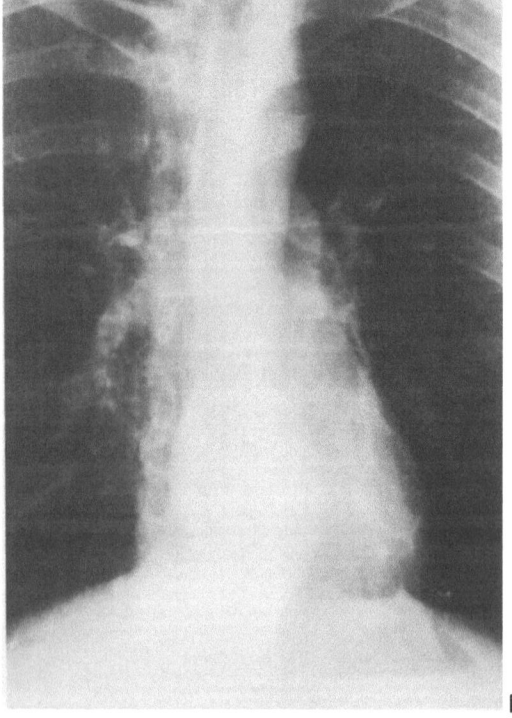

with it when it elongates and the paraspinal pleural reflection (Fig. 4.14) tends, with advancing age, to parallel the course of the aorta rather than remaining parallel to the lateral surface of the vertebral column. Nevertheless the paths of the aorta and the displaced paravertebral pleura should not cross, nor should there be localized displacement of the paravertebral pleura.

Thoraco-Lumbar Junction

Frontal and lateral films of the thoraco-lumbar junction are routine projections available in every department and need no comment. They are the only satisfactory way of making a positive diagnosis of ankylosing spondylitis or Reiter's spondylitis reasonably early in the clinical course of these diseases.

Fig. 4.14. a On the left, the paravertebral pleura (*open arrow*) can be pulled from the vertebrae by the elongating aorta (*closed arrow*) so that it roughly parallels the aorta. b The normal left paravertebral pleural density must not cross the aorta or have a localized bulge. (Reproduced by courtesy of Dr S. Millward.)

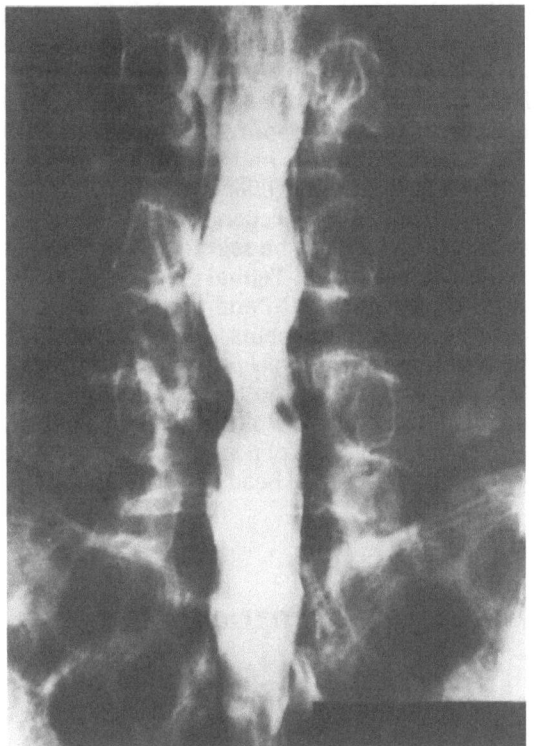
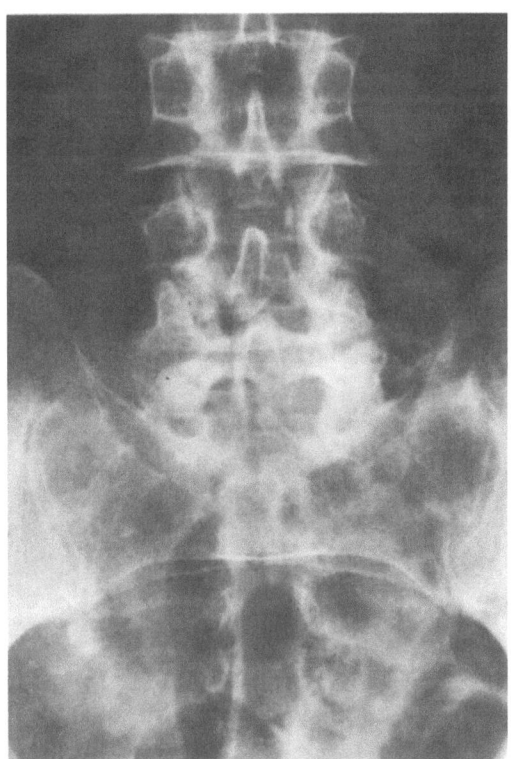

Fig. 4.15a,b. An inclined beam is necessary to obtain a frontal film of L5. Note how the metastasis to the base of the right pedicle of L5 (a) is invisible on the standard frontal radiograph. (Reprinted with permission from *Orthopaedic Radiology*, ed. W. M. Park and S. P. F. Hughes. Blackwell Scientific, Oxford, 1987.)

Lumbar Spine

The paravertebral soft tissues are not contrasted by air, and paravertebral masses are usually *not* visible. If the mass is calcified or if it is in a plane which will interfere with the psoas shadow it may be seen. A normal psoas shadow does *not* exclude a paravertebral soft tissue mass.

Adequate frontal films of L1 and L5 will not be obtained on a standard frontal film of the lumbar spine. Lesions of L5 in particular may not be diagnosable unless an inclined frontal film of that vertebra is obtained.

Flexion and Extension Films

This author does not find flexion and extension films of the lumbar spine to be of any value in general diagnosis. Once again, a need for specific information about mobility of a single level in order to answer a specific clinical question justifies the films.

Lumbo-Sacral Junction, Sacrum and Sacro-Iliac Joints

The optimum radiographic projection for demonstrating the lumbo-sacral junction, the sacrum and the sacro-iliac joints is an inclined AP projection with approximately 25° angulation towards the head. This projection is parallel to the L5/S1 disc space and provides a frontal film of L5 (Fig. 4.15). It is also an adequate frontal projection of the sacrum and will demonstrate the anterior sacral arches, which are the key to the diagnosis of sacral disease (Fig. 4.16). This projection will separate the front and back of the sacro-iliac joints thereby showing early disease which commonly begins anteriorly. It is quite possible to convert an abnormal sacro-iliac joint into a normal one radiographically by rotating the patient or projecting the normal posterior joint over an abnormal anterior joint by using a postero-anterior projection.

Oblique films of the sacro-iliac joints have their place, but this is not in the diagnosis of the presence

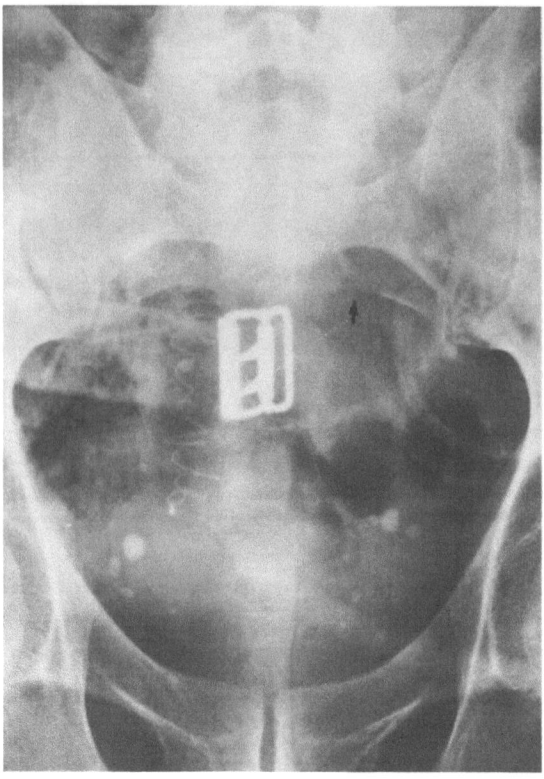

Fig. 4.16. The anterior sacral arches are the key to diagnosing sacral disease. Once again, lack of cortical bone (*arrow*) is the sign of bone disorder.

of diseases of the sacro-iliac joints. They are ideally suited to demonstrating that an abnormality seen on other films lies either on one side or the other of the joint. The classic example is osteitis condensans ilii, which may appear to be on both sides of the sacro-iliac joint on a frontal film but can be shown to be only iliac on an oblique film.

Lateral spot films of the lumbo-sacral junction are now routine in most departments. Young readers will not realize that these spot films were as uncommon in the past as inclined frontal films are today. One can only hope that the future, when inclined frontal films will be recognized as an essential part of routine radiography of the lumbar spine, comes quickly.

Pelvis

A basic tenet of radiography is that the minimum radiographic investigation requires two films at right-angles. How often does one see a lateral film of the pelvis? It is assumed, entirely without justification, that lesions of the pelvis, and injuries in particular, can be seen on a frontal film. This "frontal" film, obtained with a beam perpendicular to the table top, is angled approximately 40° across the main axis of the pelvis and it is not surprising that displacements are often difficult to appreciate on this single, rather odd projection. Extra projections are available and should be selected according to the information required. Pennal views (Fig. 4.17a,b.) are taken parallel with, and perpendicular to, the pelvic inlet. Displacements of the pelvic rim and encroachment on the pelvic inlet are much easier to appreciate on this view than on the standard frontal film. A lateral view of the pelvis including the acetabulum (Fig. 4.17c) permits assessment of congruence of the femoral head and acetabulum.

Additional Radiography

Screening

Fluoroscopic screening to assess motion or to assist in positioning can be invaluable. One should resist the temptation to depend on a fluoroscopic image alone and ensure that a permanent record is kept. Anything appreciable on screening should be recordable on standard media, either videotape or spot film, and if it is not the "impression" is of doubtful validity.

Tomography

Tomography is a technique which records a plane of interest in the body by reducing the demonstration of structures in the other planes. Tomography does not show structures which are invisible on standard radiographs nor does it increase the demonstration of any structure. The entire effect is due to decreasing the definition of structures that are recorded, but doing so disproportionately. It is particularly valuable in the spine because the complex anatomy of each individual vertebra ensures that overlap of one part by another is almost universal. At present, tomography is under-used, and there should be no objection to its use in clarifying an observation or improving the demonstration of something known to exist. There is no place for the use of tomography as a screening procedure to exclude abnormalities. A typical example of its value is demonstrated in Fig. 4.18, where a burst fracture

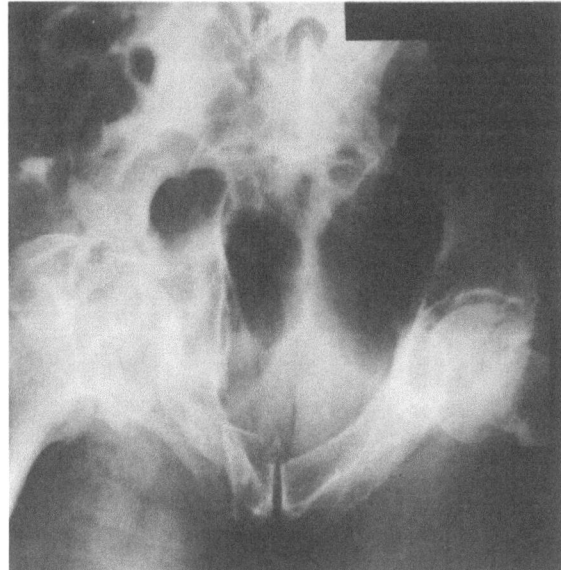

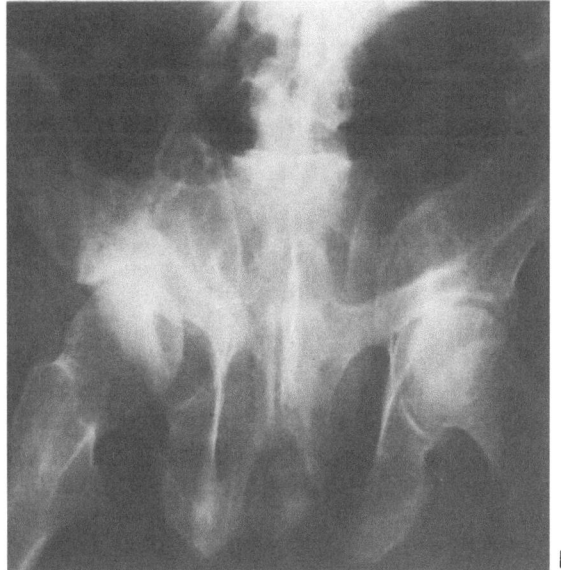

is known and a retropulsed fragment suspected. Although the retropulsed fragment is visible on the standard lateral film (Fig. 4.18a) its presence would not be appreciated because of overlying bone structures. "Removal" of the bone overlap allows the retropulsed fragment to be seen clearly (Fig. 4.18b). Figs. 4.19, 4.21, 4.27 and 4.28 are other examples of the value of tomography.

Specific Radiographic Challenges

Spondylolysis

Spondylolysis without spondylolisthesis is a radiographic challenge because the plane of the lysis through the pars interarticularis varies from patient to patient and no standard projection can be guaranteed to show it. The lysis may be seen on lateral, frontal and/or oblique films or on none of the standard projections. False positive lytic defects can be simulated by projection of the adjacent osteoarthritic facet joints over the pars interarticularis and for similar reasons spondylolytic defects can be hidden by the facets. Currently 60° oblique tomography is considered to be the investigation of choice and it seems to be entirely reliable (Fig. 4.19).

The investigation of the patient with spondylolysis and root pain is a challenge because hypertrophic repair about the lysis can compress the same nerve that would be compressed by a disc hernia

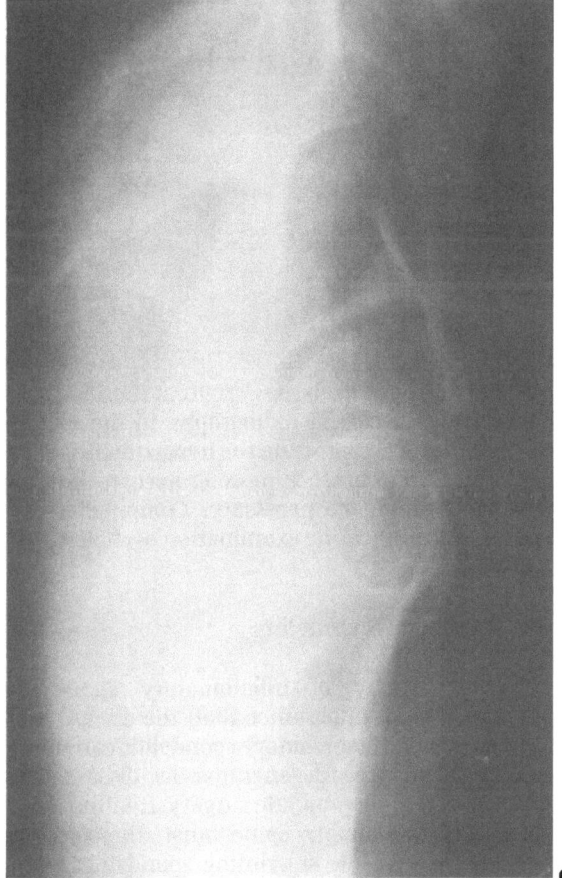

Fig. 4.17a–c. Additional views of the pelvis are available. Among the most useful are the inlet (a) and reverse inlet (b) described by Pennal, and the lateral (c), which allows assessment of congruence of the acetabulum and femoral head.

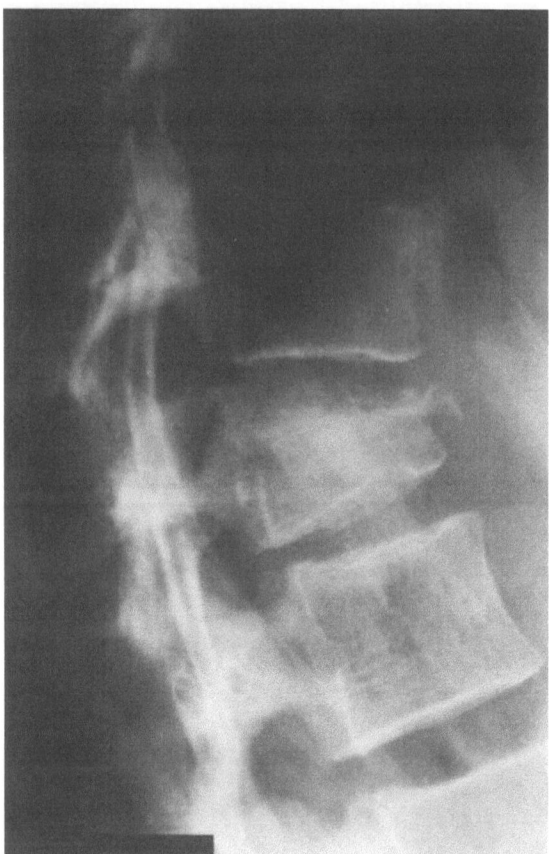

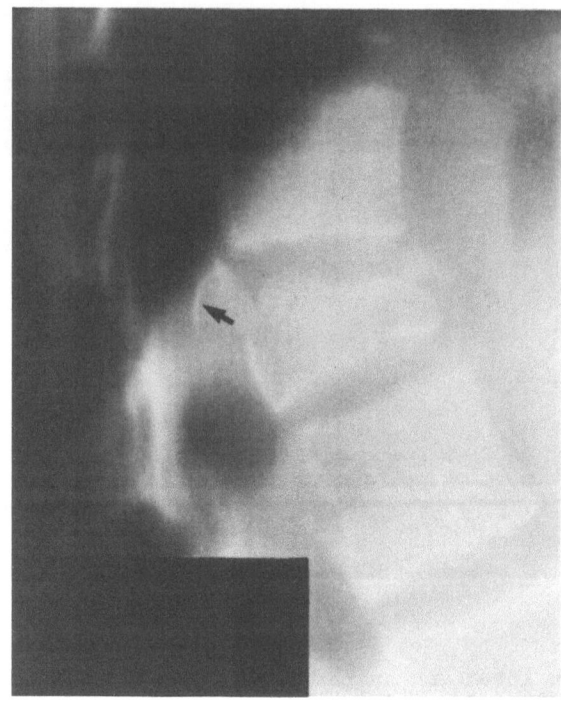

Fig. 4.18a,b. Tomograms decrease the information recorded on a film but do so disproportionately to emphasize a particular plane. They do not demonstrate things not recorded on standard radiographs but are able to give that illusion by removing unwanted information. Note the retropulsed bone fragment (*arrow*).

at the level above the lysis. Certain authorities have suggested that careful radiography in the oblique projection will demonstrate the hypertrophic callus, but in everyday practice more esoteric techniques will be found to be necessary. Computed tomographic scanning is the examination of choice.

Inflammatory Spondylitis

The radiography of inflammatory spondylitis assumes greater importance than the disease itself merits because inflammatory spondylitis can mimic the clinical picture of degenerative disc disease exactly and lead to inappropriate surgery. Routine radiography of the lumbar spine must, therefore, be adequate to exclude ankylosing spondylitis and a frontal film of the sacro-iliac joints must be included. It is most conveniently obtained at the same time and on the same film as the inclined frontal projection of L5. The routine radiography of the lumbar spine must demonstrate the dorsi-lumbar junction adequately in order to exclude Romanus lesions (Fig. 4.20) because they are the hallmark of idiopathic inflammatory spondylitis (e.g. Reiter's syndrome and ankylosing spondylitis).

That inflammatory spondylitis involves the ligaments and capsules as well as the bones is well known, but it is worth repeating here that routine radiographic assessment of the cervical spine in a patient with inflammatory spondylitis must include a flexion film (Fig. 4.4). Otherwise, ligamentous involvement might not be demonstrated.

Facet Injuries

The facets, particularly in the cervical spine, are so aligned as to make their demonstration uncertain on routine radiography. As frontal films of the cervical facets require 45° of angulation, there is a tendency to make do, perhaps unwisely, with lateral films of the structures. Because both facets are superimposed on a lateral film confusion can arise.

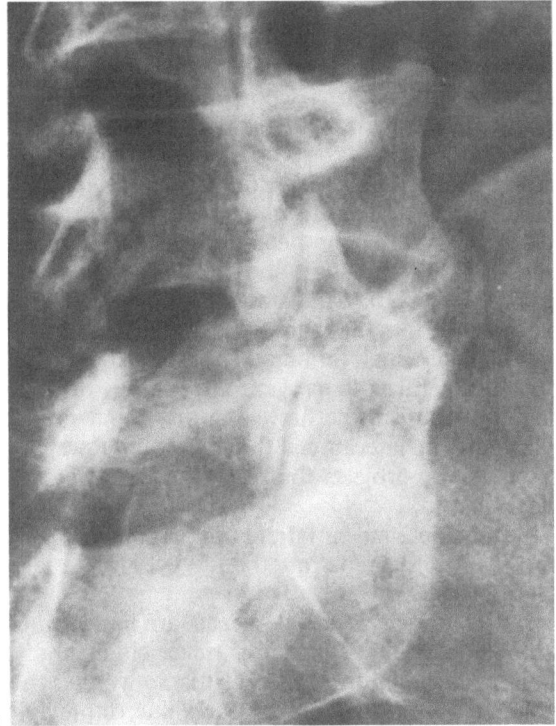

a

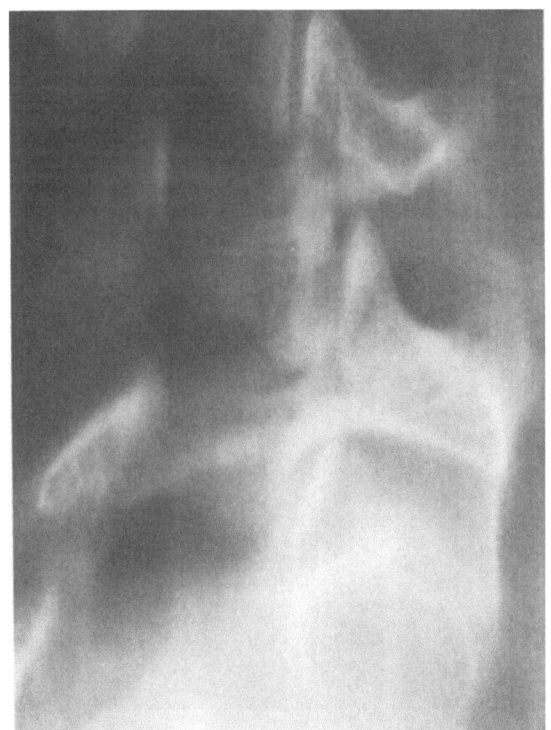

b

Fig. 4.19a–d. Defects in the pars interarticularis are not always easy to see even on oblique films. Sixty-degree oblique tomography is the examination of choice to demonstrate the pars interarticularis and its defects. (Reprinted with permission from *Orthopaedic Radiology*, ed. W. M. Park and S.P.F. Hughes. Blackwell Scientific, Oxford, 1987.)

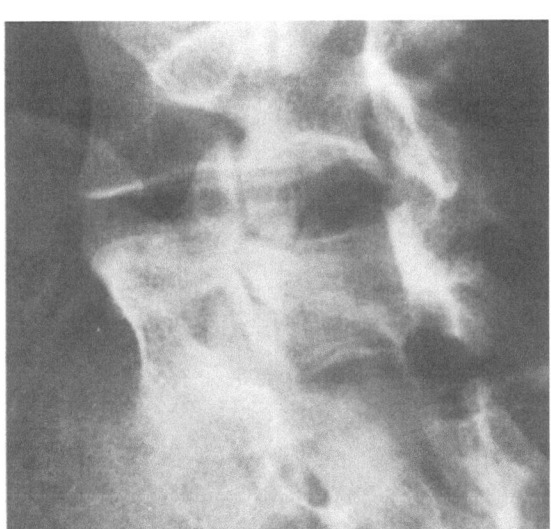

c

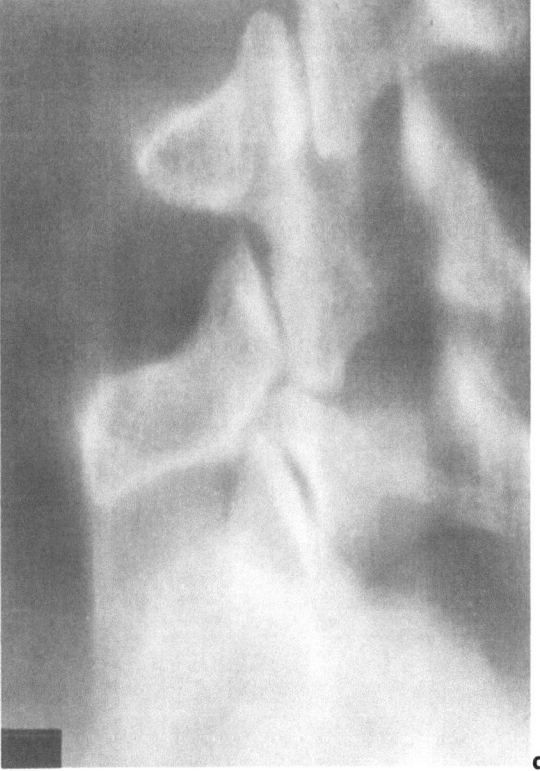

d

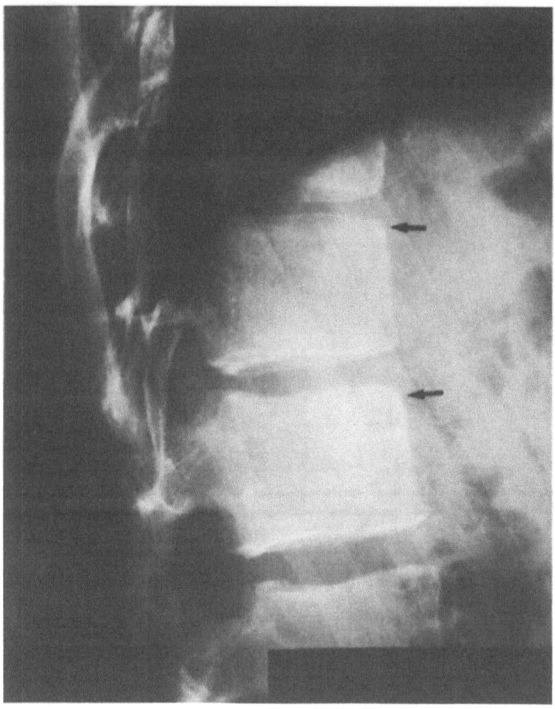

Fig. 4.20. The Romanus lesion of the vertebral body is best seen at the thoraco-lumbar junction and consists of an erosion with reactive sclerosis. It is the erosion of the corners more than infilling of the centres of the vertebrae that gives rise to the squaring of the vertebrae seen in ankylosing spondylitis.

It is natural to focus on a normal-appearing structure and if a normal facet is superimposed on an abnormal facet the abnormal one may not catch the attention of the reviewer. Assessment of facet injuries is best performed by slightly oblique projections, 10–15° being the best. It must be remembered that the obliquity should be obtained by angulation, not rotation, unless the whole patient is rotated as a log. Rotation of the head and not of the whole patient may well reduce and make invisible a facet injury (Fig.4.10). The amount of head rotation between the film that shows the dislocation and the film that does not is minimal. The aim of the shallow oblique lateral is to project one column of facets slightly behind the other column without greatly distorting the laterality of the projection. Reversing the obliquity projects the second column of facets into view.

Stereoscopy and/or lateral tomography are often necessary to demonstrate the full extent of a facet injury (Fig. 4.21).

In the lumbar region the facets are best seen on a 60° oblique film – which is never obtained as a routine in the injured patient. It is no wonder that lesions of the facets, quite clearly due to previous injury (Fig. 4.22), are all known as "normal variants".

Facets in the thoracic spine are often ignored. Whether they should be or not is a different matter.

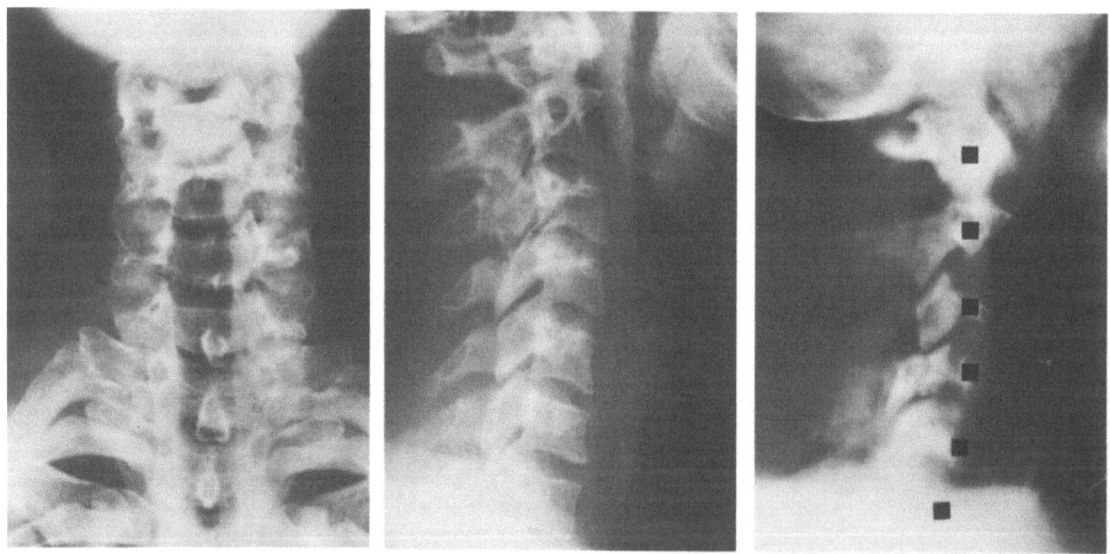

a, b   c

Fig. 4.21a–c. Only stereoscopy and tomography allow demonstration of one set of lateral masses whilst maintaining a lateral projection.

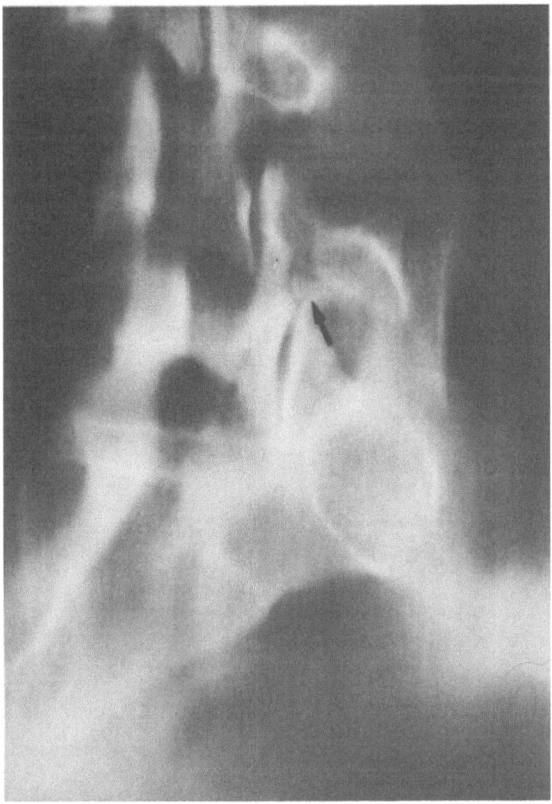

Fig. 4.22. It is difficult to believe that small fragments from facets are not the result of trauma, even though they are usually called "normal variants".

Scoliosis

No condition challenges radiography as much as does scoliosis – not so much because there is lateral angulation of the spine but because rotation accompanies the angulation. The radiographic projection of rotated angles is treacherous and can lead to impressive errors in interpretation. If an angled structure is rotated on its longitudinal axis (e.g. a patient with a scoliosis is turned) the radiographic projection of that angle can increase from its true measurement to 180°. The angle cannot be made more acute than it truly is by rotating the patient. The true measurement of the severity of the "curve" is obtained on a radiograph which is the frontal projection of the apical vertebra. This is most easily performed by rotating the tube 90° from the lateral of the apical vertebra which is obtained by using a beam parallel to the plane of the ribs at the level of the apex. Such a lateral film will frequently show

that the spine affected by "kypho-scoliosis" is, in fact, *lordotic* (Fig. 4.23). It is apparent that the easiest way to "correct" scoliosis radiographically is to rotate the patient. If radiographs are used to monitor the effect of surgery, rotation of the patient cannot be ignored (Fig. 4.23).

Rotation of an angle in another plane is a concern. If a scoliotic patient bends forwards, the radiographic projection of the angle can decrease from what it truly is to 0°, and the simplest way of making a scoliosis "worse" is to have the patient bend forward. In practice, forward flexion of the patient is not a significant cause of error in scoliosis radiography but rotation is .

Each unit has its own method of demonstrating flexibility in association with scoliosis, most using some variation of lateral bending; it must be remembered that prevention of rotation is an essential component of lateral bending radiography.

Acetabular Injuries

Radiography of the injured acetabulum must permit assessment of the posterior and anterior margins of the acetabulum and demonstrate the integrity of its roof. The anterior and posterior margins of the acetabulum and their supporting structures can most conveniently be seen on oblique films (30° internally and 30° externally). It is difficult for an injured patient to turn on to the injured side and the obliquity is best managed by angling the incident beam. Angulation which, in effect, causes internal rotation of the pelvis shows the posterior rim of the acetabulum and the anterior part of the supporting structures (Fig. 4.24a,b). The oblique view that causes, in effect, external rotation shows the anterior rim of the acetabulum and the posterior supporting structures (Fig. 4.24c,d). The lateral film demonstrates the roof of the acetabulum and is a convenient method of demonstrating the extent of acetabular roof injuries and the presence of marginal displacement of the femoral head from its normal location. It is the only projection which demonstrates acetabular involvement by vertical splits of the iliac crest (Fig. 4.24e,f).

Radiographic Signs of Bone and Joint Disorder

The cardinal signs of bone and joint disorder are not all visible in disorders of the spine. Those that are, are described below.

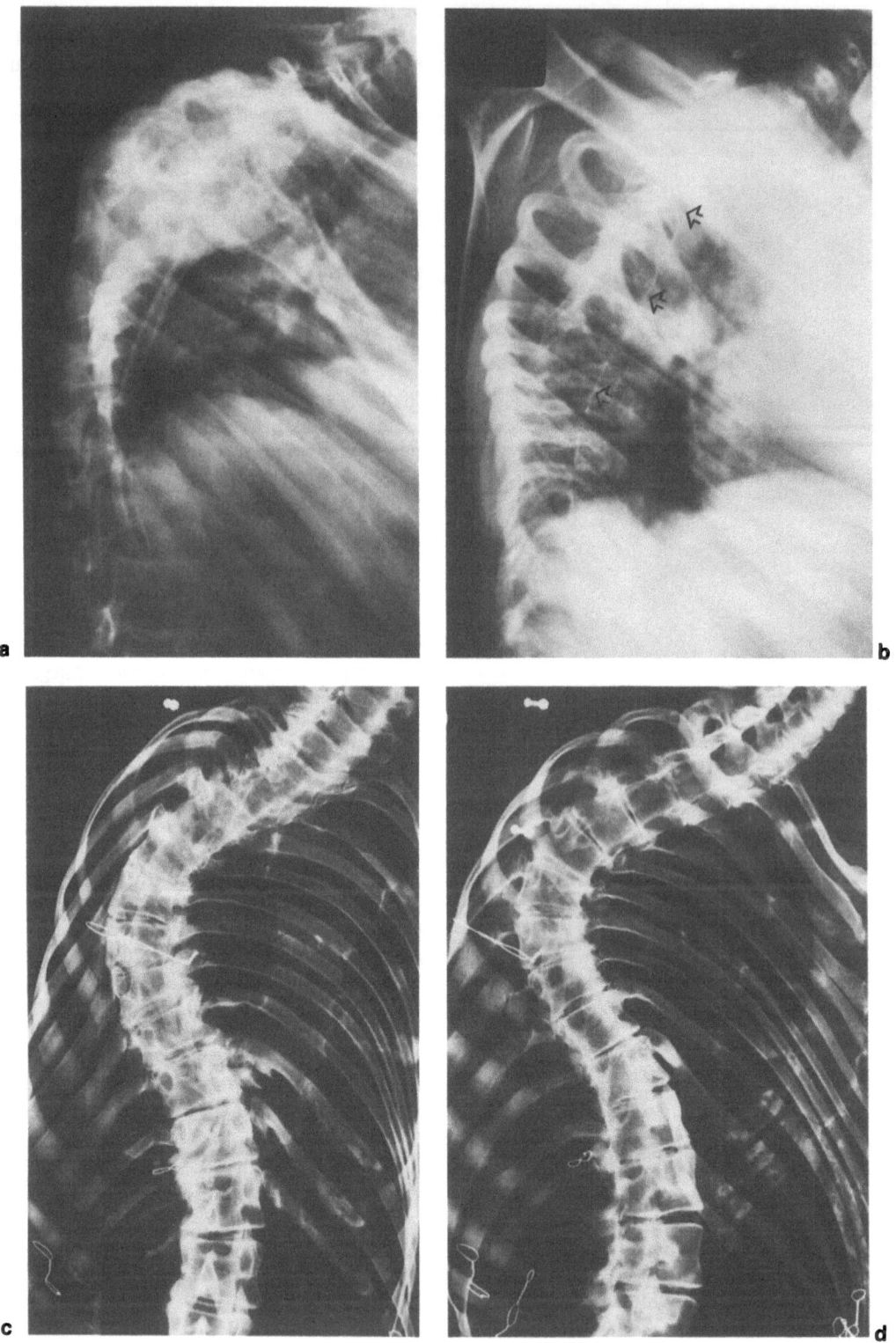

Fig. 4.23a–d. The lateral film of the patient with a scoliosis (a) appears to show a kyphosis whereas the lateral film of the spine (b) shows that there is, in fact, a lordosis. The frontal film of the patient with scoliosis (c) shows considerably less deformity than is shown on a frontal film of the spine (d).

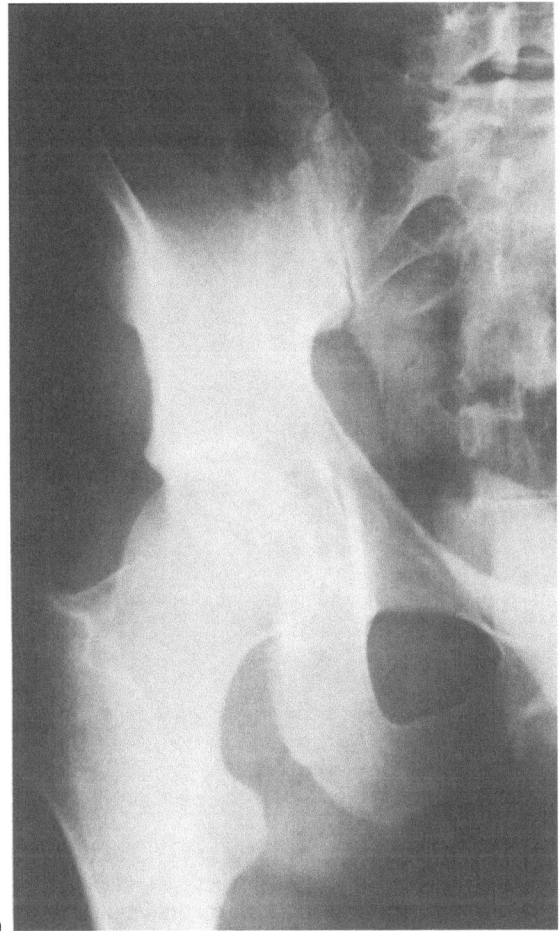

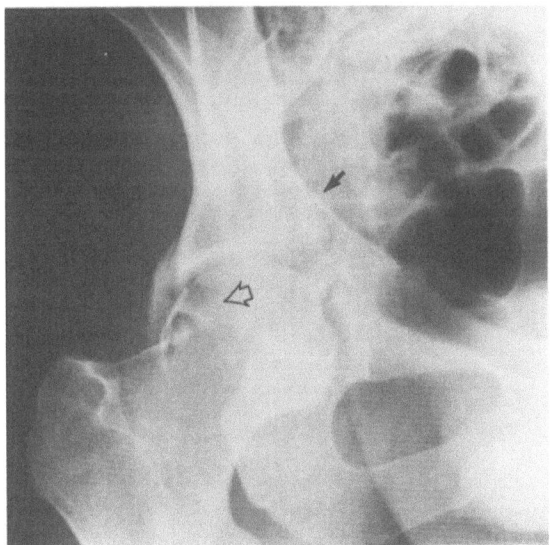

Fig. 4.24a–f. Radiographs of three patients. Internal rotation (b) shows the posterior margin of the acetabulum (*open arrow*) and the ilio-pubic bar (*closed arrow*) which are poorly seen on the frontal film (a). The external rotation view (d) shows the anterior margin of the acetabulum (*closed arrow*) and the ilio-ischial bone bar (*open arrow*). Compare this with the frontal film (c). The lateral film of the acetabulum (f) shows fracture lines and acetabular distortions not visible on frontal view (e) (next page).

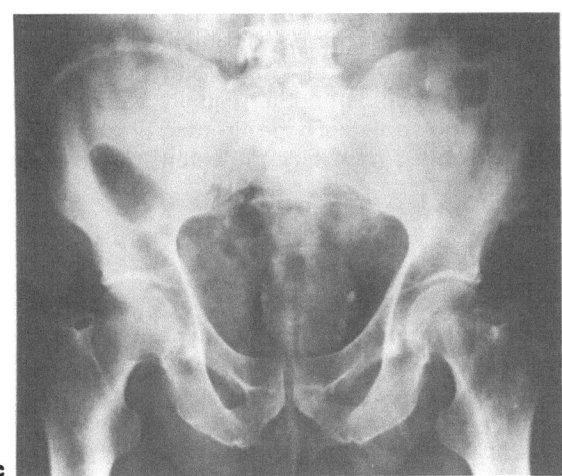

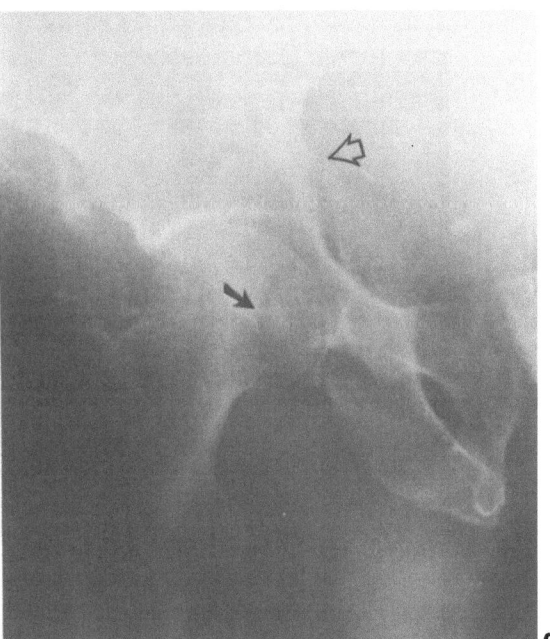

Fig. 4.24 *continued overleaf*

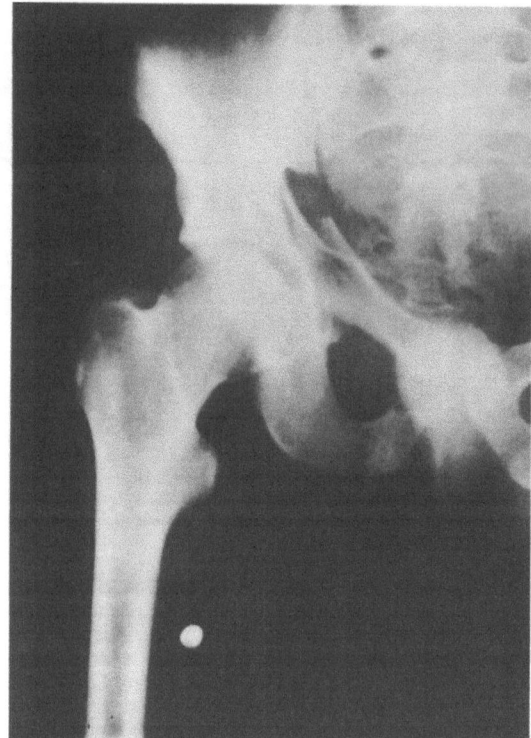
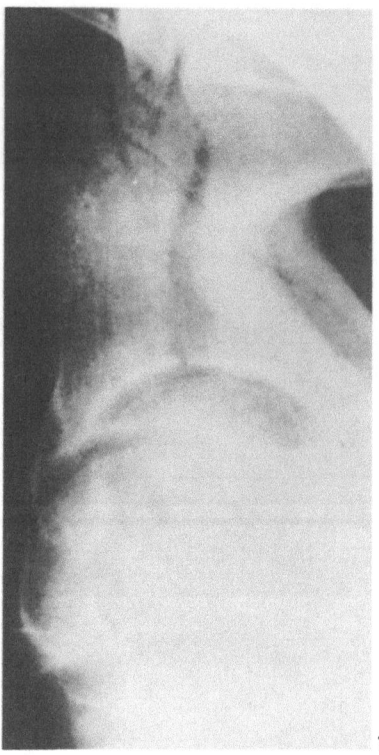

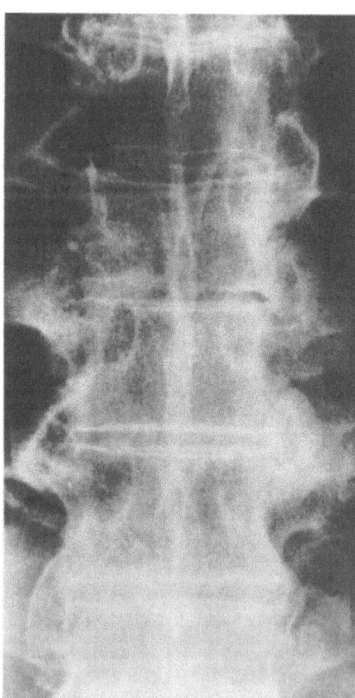

Fig. 4.25. Pedicle loss is another example of disappearance of cortical bone indicating bone disorder.

Loss of Cortical Integrity

Preservation of subperiosteal cortical bone is the sign of bone health, and its loss, the sign of bone disease (Figs. 4.1, 4.16). In the spine it may be difficult to see cortical bone clearly, but pedicle loss (Fig. 4.25) is an example of cortical bone loss. Loss of vertebral corners is another equally valuable but less well known sign of bone disorder. Precise radiography is often necessary to demonstrate cortical integrity.

Fracture

Radiographic demonstration of a fracture line requires that the X-ray beam be parallel to the fracture, so, as most fractures of the spine are in a plane not amenable to radiographic parallelism, the majority of fractures of the spine are not seen on radiographs. The advent of computed tomographic scanning has shown just how true that statement is. It may be necessary, therefore, to predict the presence of a fracture from another observation. The subject of spinal injuries is covered in Chap. 20, but it is worth mentioning here the significance of a displaced joint. If both sides of a joint are seen and the

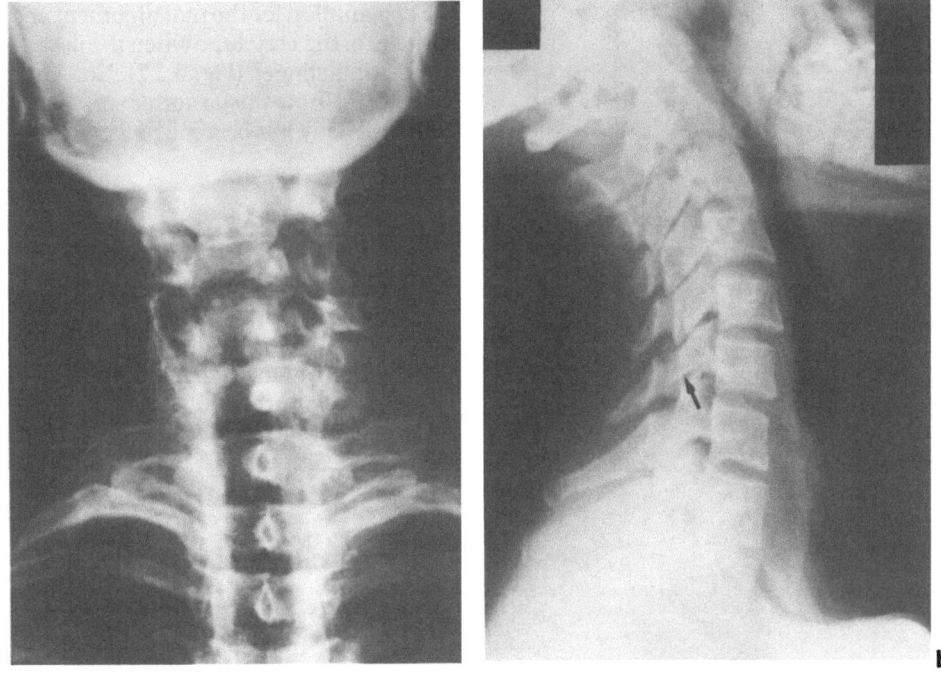

Fig. 4.26. The rotated facet (C6 left) is smaller, denser and more clearly defined than are the other facets (Fielding's sign).

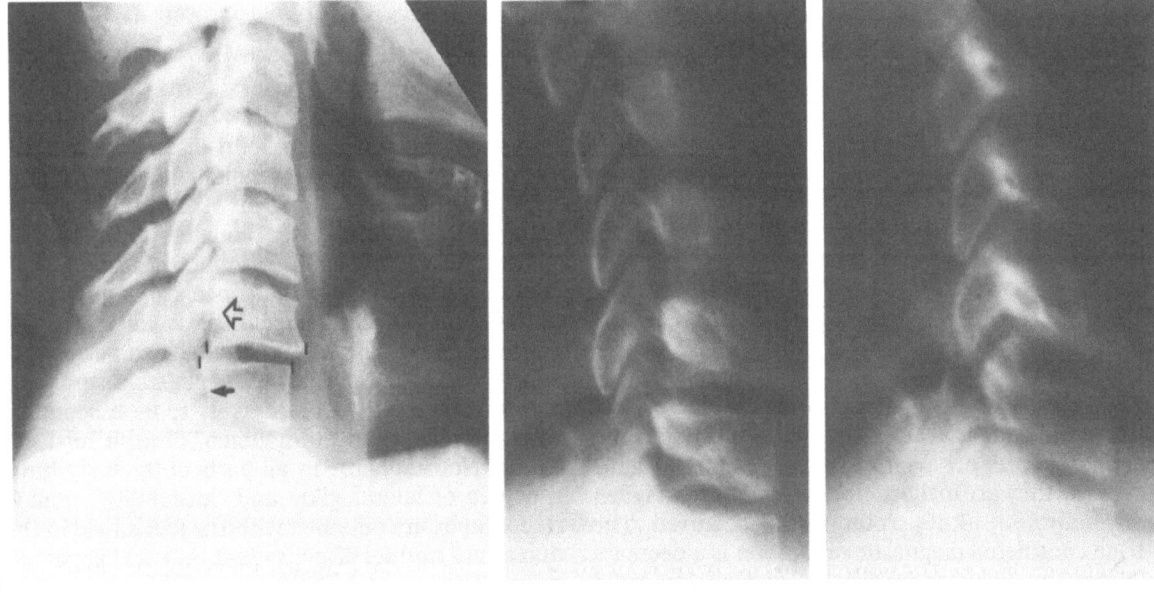

Fig. 4.27a–c. When an oval such as a vertebral body is rotated, its radiographic projection will change in size. This explains the apparent discrepancy in the antero-posterior depths of C6 and C7 on the lateral radiograph. Notice that the posterior surface of C7 is sharp (*closed arrow*) while that of the rotated C6 is indistinct (*open arrow*). The rotation occurred because one lateral mass was broken.

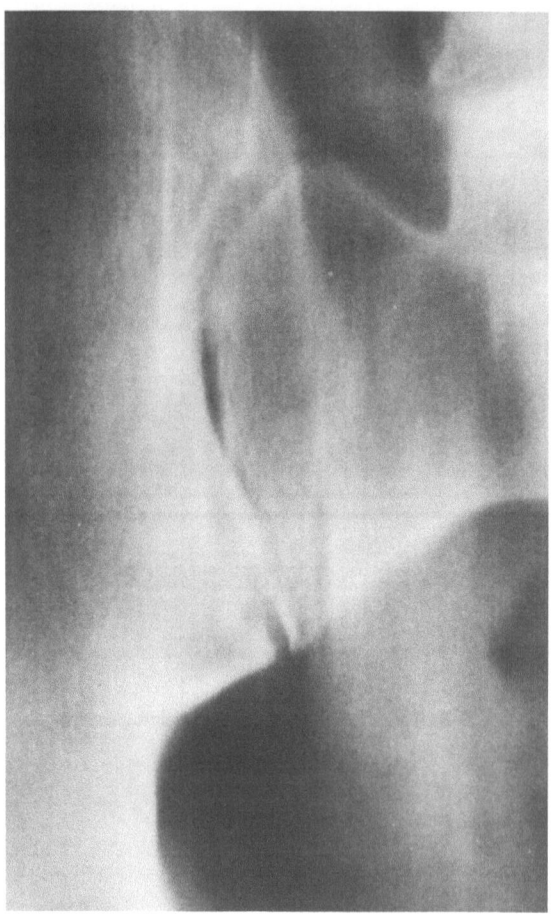

Fig. 4.28. Tomography may be necessary to show the loss of subchondral cortical bone that is the first sign of joint disease. It is illustrated here in a sacro-iliac joint.

joint lies in an abnormal place, there must be a fracture. This principle is of most value in assessing facet injuries and fractures of C1/C2.

Rotation

Rotation of bone will alter its radiographic projection if the bone is oval or rectangular in shape. The cervical facets are seen obliquely on frontal films because they are inclined normally; if a facet is seen distinctly (Fig. 4.26), rotation has occurred. The triad considered diagnostic of rotation is a decrease in size, an increase in density, and an increased sharpness of outline. Clearly if a structure is normally small, dense and sharp and becomes large, lucent and indistinct it, too, is rotated. The increase in the radiographic size of a rotated oval is obviously

the explanation for the malalignment of the anterior surfaces of the vertebrae when the posterior surfaces are less malaligned (Fig. 4.27). Note in the example in Fig. 4.27 how the posterior surface of the rotated vertebral body has become indistinct.

Repair

With very few exceptions, sclerotic bone is repaired bone and it is a sign of bone health. This is of some significance when one is attempting to biopsy the vertebrae. By and large, attempts to biopsy sclerotic vertebrae are unrewarding, both because it is technically difficult and because the sclerotic area is often the healthiest.

Loss of Subchondral Cortex

The cardinal manifestations of joint disease are rarely visible in the vertebral column and are usually difficult to appreciate in the sacro-iliac joints. Preservation of subchondral cortical integrity is difficult to establish both in the spine and in the sacro-iliac joints and it is usual to rely on evidence of repair to indicate that the joint is abnormal. Meticulous radiography will, however, permit demonstration of subchondral cortical loss in the sacro-iliac joints (Fig. 4.28) and attempts should be made to demonstrate it.

Malalignment

The only cardinal sign of joint disease that is frequently seen in the spine is malalignment.

Dislocations and other forms of malalignment will be covered in subsequent chapters, but there is virtue in discussing subluxation at this time. In the acutely injured patient the concept of subluxation as a partial dislocation has little validity and less practical value. The slightly malaligned vertebra is as likely to be normal as it is to be abnormal and if it is abnormal it is more likely to be a spontaneously reduced dislocation than a "little bit" of dislocation. Normal joints in all parts of the body have a degree of lateral glide and "instability", and if radiographs are obtained with the joints held in the maximum normal displacement they will appear to show subluxation. It is the view of this author that the term subluxation should be used to indicate, at least in the acutely injured, this entity of a joint being held at the extreme of its normal motion by a force external to that joint. Such a concept will

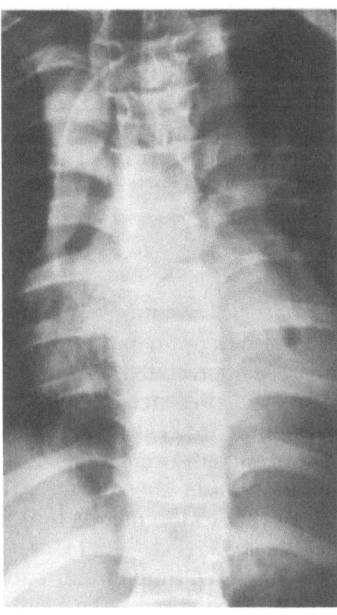

Fig. 4.29. A "little bit" of dislocation is much more likely to be spontaneous reduction of a total dislocation, as in this patient, than it is to be a "subluxation".

make one look elsewhere for the cause. C1/C2 rotational subluxation demonstrated by the cardinal signs of bone rotation described above (Fig. 4.2) is a normal movement and indicates muscle spasm consequent on a lesion somewhere else.

If subluxation were reserved for normal movement, dislocation would describe all degrees of abnormal movement. In the acutely injured spine this is not a bad principle as even the slightest amount of excessive displacement is usually associated with severe soft tissue damage and spinal instability (Fig. 4.29). The normal disc will allow 2–3 mm of antero-posterior gliding and 1 mm of lateral gliding. This degree of displacement should not be considered pathological but is, in fact, subluxation caused by muscle spasm and/or an injury to other supporting structures such as the facets. It is incorrect to assume that a facet injury associated with subluxation is unstable or is more important than a facet injury alone. On the other hand, a facet injury associated with a "little bit of dislocation" of the vertebral bodies greater than 2–3 mm indicates a major injury.

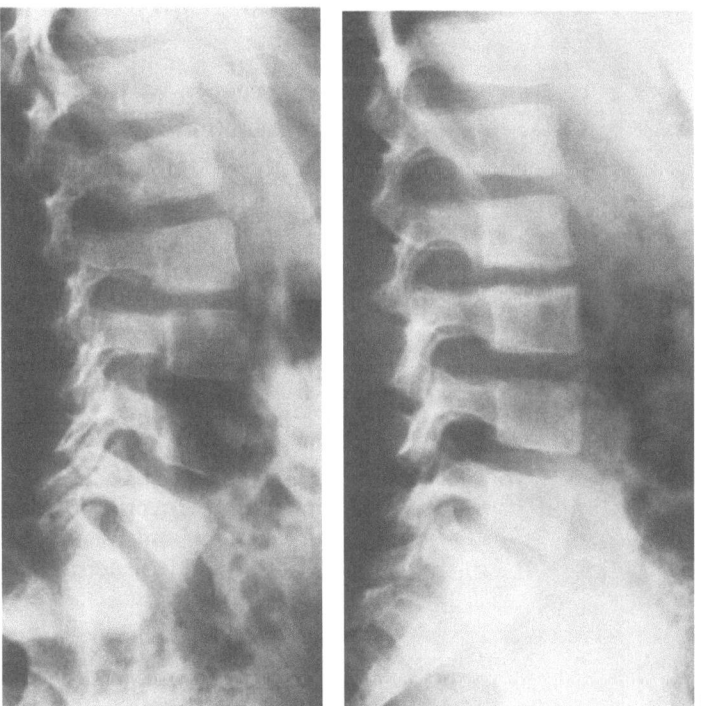

a   **b**

Fig.4.30a,b. Hyperlordosis is a common but little-known sign of paravertebral muscle spasm in the young. In **a** it should draw attention to the abnormally narrowed L2/3 disc space, allowing a diagnosis of discitis rather than waiting until the disease is more advanced (**b**).

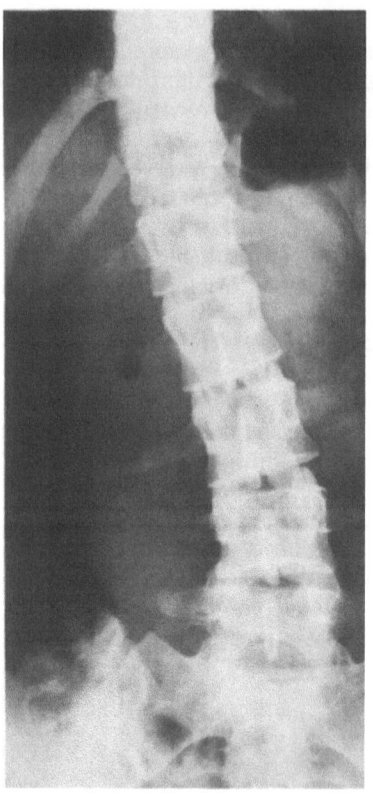

Fig. 4.31. Paravertebral muscle spasm can be severe enough to topple the patient off balance, invariably leading to a diagnosis of mental derangement. Notice that there is no rotation and that this is not, therefore, a structural scoliosis.

Spasm

Hyperlordosis is a common manifestation of paravertebral muscle spasm in the young but its significance is rarely appreciated on radiographs. It is a good sign of the presence of significant spinal disease and it should make one search carefully for the early signs of such disorders (Fig. 4.30).

Paravertebral muscle spasm can cause severe scoliosis of the spine to the degree that the patient will topple sideways (Fig. 4.31). As it is not infrequently present without much back pain the patient is usually considered to be mentally disturbed and a primary lesion in the spine may be overlooked (Fig. 4.31).

Errors in Diagnosis "Caused" by Radiography

Errors Due to an Inadequate or Incomplete Examination

Inadequate and incomplete examinations have been fully covered in the preceding material and here it need only be repeated that such examinations cannot be considered "normal", "negative", "no significant abnormality" or "grossly normal", but must be repeated and improved. The commonest cause of an error in radiological interpretation is, without doubt, an incorrect radiographic study. Certain examinations are accepted as being complete by definition, even though they are not and those, too, have been fully covered in the preceding material. It is worth emphasizing that errors may be caused by underpenetrated films, particularly of the pelvis. Underpenetrated films are treacherous.

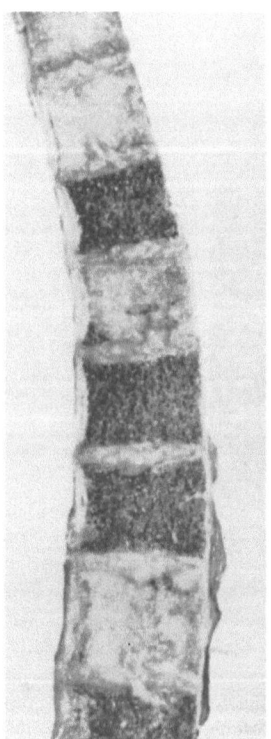 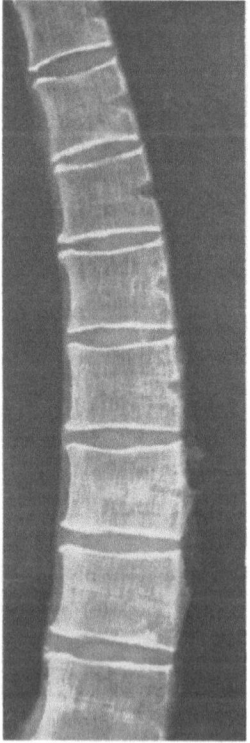

a   b

Fig. 4.32a,b. The dissected specimen (a) and the radiograph of that specimen (b) illustrate that extensive vertebral infiltration can occur without the radiographs being abnormal. (Reprinted with permission from Lodvic (1971).)

Errors Due to the Inherent Deficiencies of Radiography

All of us who practice diagnostic radiology gradually forget the inherent deficiencies of our techniques and the errors that those deficiencies cause. The prime deficiency of bone radiography is its inability to demonstrate medullary bone destruction. Lodvic (1971) has studied this deficiency thoroughly and his original work is to be recommended. A single illustration from his text demonstrates that radiography of the spine, even of a dissected specimen, cannot exclude extensive infiltration (Fig. 4.32). All of us who report radiographs of the spine should keep this illustration at the front of our memory.

Bone continuity cannot be verified radiographically. Any of the standard criteria used to define bone continuity can be mimicked by overlap and the diagnosis of continuity relies on a failure to demonstrate discontinuity. A single film demonstrating continuity is, therefore, unacceptable. Even a number of oblique projections may fail to demonstrate a pseudarthrosis if one is present. The radiological diagnosis of bone continuity must always be suspect.

Finally, it must be remembered that a radiograph does not demonstrate dynamic processes but only a stage in those processes. "Chip" fractures are a case in point. Virtually all chip fractures in the spine occur at the insertion of ligaments and/or capsules and not tendons, and are therefore due to disruption rather than traction and indicate movement. The combination of disruption and movement is, by definition, dislocation, and chip fractures of the spine must be considered to be part of a dislocation until that is disproved.

References

Lodvic GS (1971) The bones and joints. In: Hodes PJ (ed) An atlas of tumor pathology. Year Book Medical Publishers, Chicago.

5 Myelography

J. V. Occleshaw

Introduction 77
Myelographic Techniques 77
Radiographic Technique and Normal Myelographic Appearances 78
    Lumbar Segments 78
    Dorsal Segments 79
    Cervical Segments 80
Post-Myelographic Care 81
Pathological Appearances 81
    Spinal Compression 81
    Disc Herniations and Spondylosis 84
    Traumatic Nerve Root Avulsion 87
References 88

Introduction

The first myelographic studies performed in the 1920s employed air as the contrast agent, which was exchanged with the cerebrospinal fluid by lumbar puncture. Air ascended to the level of spinal cord compression and this was demonstrated on radiographs. In 1931 Arnell and Lindström injected the irritant iodinated water-soluble contrast agent Abrodil into the lower spinal canal after the administration of spinal anaesthesia, and demonstrated lumbar disc herniations with this positive contrast agent. The necessity for spinal anaesthesia restricted this type of myelography to the lumbar region and the technique enjoyed very limited application outside the Scandinavian countries.

The development of the oily positive contrast agent Pantopaque in 1942 provided a contrast agent that was heavier than the cerebrospinal fluid and could readily be manipulated within the spinal canal by gravity; at the same time it was so radiopaque that it was readily visualized at fluoroscopy and on radiographs. Pantopaque was widely accepted as an agent for myelography at all levels within the spine, but was not the ideal myelographic contrast agent. It could produce a form of chemical meningitis which on occasions led to adhesive arachnoiditis with serious consequences to the patient.

In the last ten years, non-ionic water-soluble contrast agents have been developed, starting with Metrizamide (Amipaque) and followed by Iopamidol (Niopam) and Iohexol (Omnipaque), which are suitable as myelographic agents for use at all levels within the spinal subarachnoid space. These agents have greatly increased both the short-term and long-term safety of myelography and have also enabled the spinal cord and nerve roots to be more readily visualized than with Pantopaque, which has a high radiographic density.

The methods of myelography to be described and illustrated in this chapter relate mainly to water-soluble contrast myelography, which has universally displaced Pantopaque myelography in recent years.

Myelographic Techniques

Water-soluble contrast agents injected into the subarachnoid space mix freely with the cerebrospinal fluid to produce a column of opacified cerebrospinal fluid with a higher specific gravity than the non-opacified adjacent fluid. Tilting the patient will allow the opacified fluid to run up or down the spinal canal under the influence of gravity, but at the same time will encourage further dilution of the contrast and result in a reduction of its radiographic density. Before starting a myelographic examination some idea as to the level of the lesion must be known so that the contrast medium

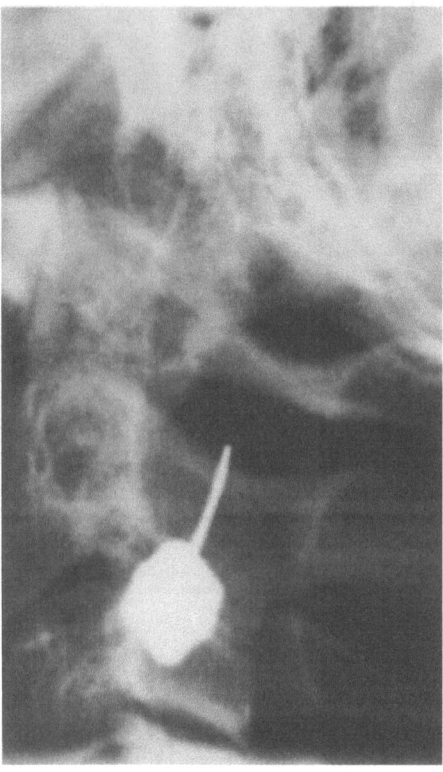

Fig. 5.1 Lateral radiograph showing the lumbar puncture needle inserted for lateral approach to the cervical subarachnoid space between the first and second cervical vertebrae.

15 ml of contrast in a concentration of 300 mg iodine per ml and careful manipulation of the patient to avoid overdilution.

Two methods are in common use for examination of the cervical segments of the spinal canal. In the first method a larger amount of contrast (up to 20 ml) at a concentration of 300 mg iodine per ml is slowly injected by lumbar puncture to avoid over-dilution, and under fluoroscopic control the patient is slowly tilted cranially with the head extended to trap the contrast in the cervical canal. The patient is levelled out when contrast is seen entering the cervical region during fluoroscopy. The second method, first employed by Amundsen and Skalpe (1975), is to introduce the contrast into the cervical canal by direct puncture of the spine laterally between the first and second cervical vertebrae. The patient is placed in the prone position, and again extension of the head is important to avoid contrast ascending into the basal cisterns. This method of spinal puncture is most readily performed under fluoroscopic control for both infiltration of local anaesthetic agent and the introduction of the spinal puncture needle (Fig. 5.1). The chief advantage of the cervical puncture technique is that smaller amounts of contrast agent are required: the exam-ination can readily be performed using 8–12 ml of contrast in the concentration range 200–250 mg iodine per ml.

can be introduced into the spinal canal as near to the lesion as possible, thus avoiding excess dilution. Manipulation of the patient must be carefully con-trolled by the examining radiologist. Ideally contrast injections should be made under screening control, firstly to ensure that all the injected contrast is enter-ing the subarachnoid space and secondly to avoid injecting more contrast agent than is really required for each examination.

For examination of the lumbar region and lower half of the dorsal region, contrast is usually injected by lumbar puncture and slow injection of the con-trast prevents overdilution. The volume and con-centration of the contrast vary with the size of the patient and the anatomy of the lumbar subarach-noid space. Most lumbar examinations are carried out with 10–15 ml of contrast agent in a concentra-tion of 200–300 mg iodine per ml. In children and some very thin adults it is occasionally possible to reduce the concentration of the contrast to the near-isotonic level of 180 mg iodine per ml. Dorsal spine examinations usually require the slow injection of

Radiographic Technique and Normal Myelographic Appearances

Lumbar Segments

After the introduction of the myelographic contrast agent the patient is placed in the prone position with the caudal end of the table slightly depressed to con-fine the contrast to the lumbar canal and the upper sacral area. Routine antero-posterior, lateral and 25°–30° oblique radiographs are then obtained. Films taken in the oblique projections are essential to demonstrate the nerve roots as they pass out to the intervertebral foramina. The normal appear-ances of the lumbar region are illustrated in Fig. 5.2. Nerve roots can be seen outlined by the contrast as they descend the spinal canal and pass laterally to their respective intervertebral foramina. The lower segments of the nerve roots are visualized by the opacified cerebrospinal fluid in the arachnoid sleeve that accompanies each nerve root. Lateral films

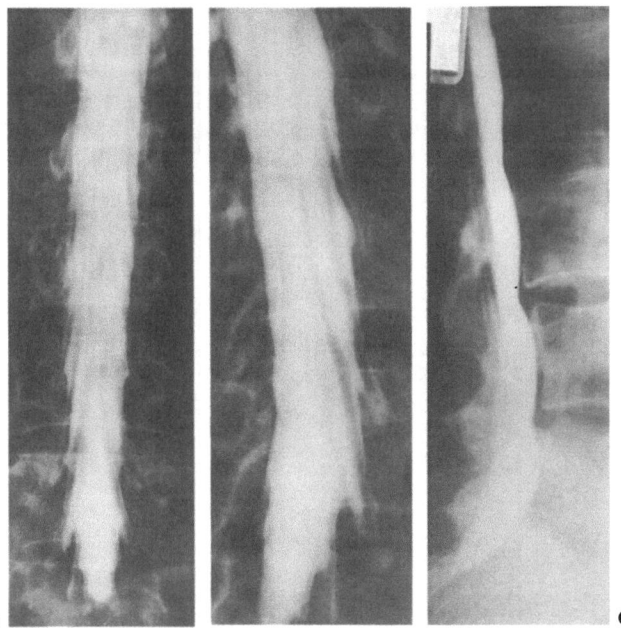

Fig. 5.2a–c. Normal appearance in the lumbar spine in the antero-posterior (a) oblique (b) and lateral (c) projections. The nerve roots are readily visualized by the contrast that has entered the nerve root sleeve.

taken with the patient standing in attitudes of flexion and extension are occasionally necessary when subluxation of the spine is suspected.

Tilting the patient slightly head-down will allow the contrast to ascend into the upper lumbar segments, and again lateral and antero-posterior films are obtained. Oblique films are of little value as the upper lumbar nerve root sleeves are very short so detail of the upper nerve roots is not obtained. Antero-posterior films with the patient in the lateral decubitus positions, though, will on occasion provide some detail of the lateral nerve root sheaths in the upper lumbar segments.

Dorsal Segments

After examination of the lumbar segments the patient is placed in the lateral decubitus position with the shoulders and head slightly elevated with pillows. Slow tilting into the 10°–20° head-down attitude will allow contrast to ascend slowly into the lower dorsal segments, while the elevation of the head and shoulders prevents the contrast from reaching the cervical level. Lateral films can be taken to cover the lower and mid-dorsal segment. Antero-posterior films with the patient supine clearly outline the lower spinal cord (Fig. 5.3).

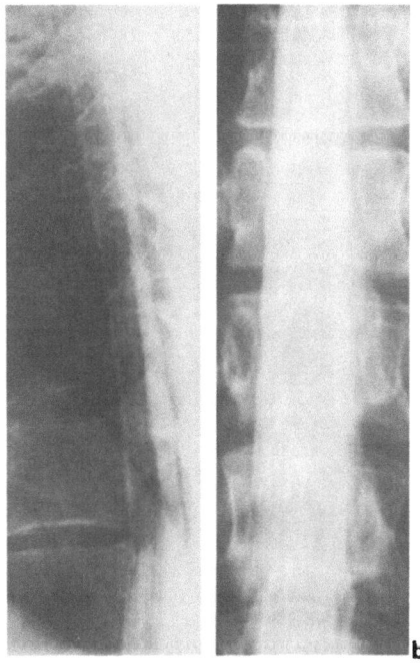

Fig. 5.3. a Spinal cord outlined by contrast in the lower dorsal spine as seen in the lateral projection. **b** Antero-posterior film showing the conus of the spinal cord and the lower dorsal segment.

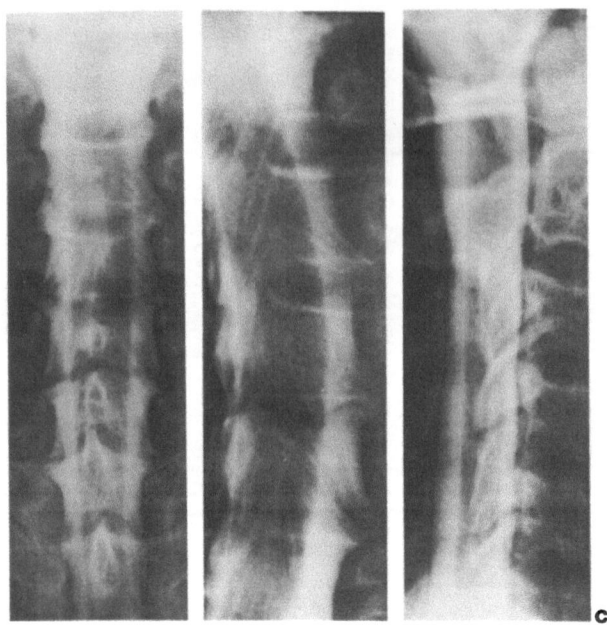

a, b

c

Fig. 5.4a–c. Normal appearances of the cervical segments of the spine in the antero-posterior (a) oblique (b) and lateral (c) projections.

Cervical Segments

If the contrast has been introduced by lumbar puncture, then provided there is a normal degree of dorsal kyphosis, the contrast will pass readily to the cervical region by depressing the head of the table while the patient is lying prone. In the presence of excessive dorsal kyphosis the contrast can be manipulated into the cervical spine with the patient lying in lateral decubitus position with the lower arm held behind. On tilting the head of the table down the contrast can be observed running into the cervical canal; the patient is then turned into the prone position with head extended and the table returned to the horizontal. Antero-posterior, 25°–30° oblique and lateral films should be obtained. These show the spinal cord surrounded by contrast and the nerve roots are also visualized crossing the lateral subarachnoid space to the intervertebral foramina (Fig. 5.4). Tomography carried out in the lateral projection can also be of value, especially for the demonstration of small cervical disc herniations compressing the spinal cord.

The position of the cerebellar tonsils is of great importance in cases of both "full-blown" and occult Chiari malformations. After placing the patient carefully in the supine position, lateral films of the cranio-cervical junction will demonstrate or exclude

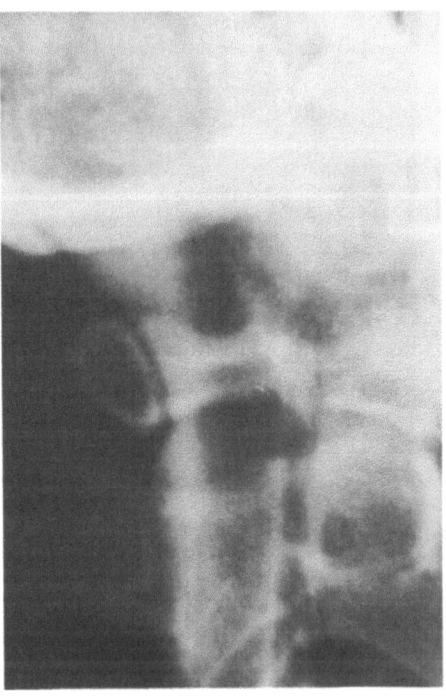

Fig. 5.5. Lateral appearances of the cranio-cervical junction in the supine position when the posterior subarachnoid space at this level is clearly visualized and free from herniation of the cerebellar tonsil.

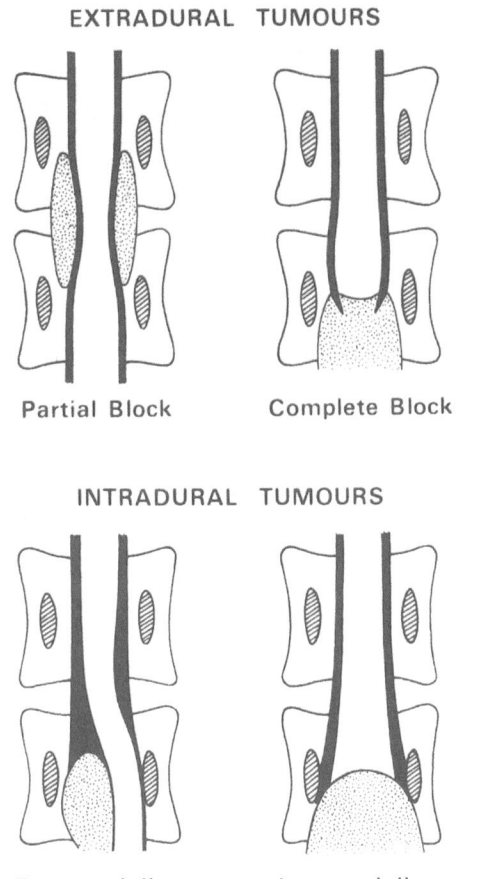

EXTRADURAL TUMOURS

Partial Block   Complete Block

INTRADURAL TUMOURS

Extramedullary   Intramedullary

Fig. 5.6. Schematic representation of the myelographic appearances in spinal compression from extradural and intradural tumours.

excreted in the urine in 24–36 hours, the greater part of the process occurring in the first 8 hours. Absorption occurs mostly via small Pacchionian granulations in the spinal nerve root sleeves, but there is evidence from computed tomographic studies that some contrast penetrates the spinal cord and the brain tissues (Drayer and Rosenbaum 1977).

Most patients experience some discomfort following myelography with non-ionic contrast agents, the most common effect being headache of a mild degree. On occasions this may be severe enough to require analgesics and, if accompanied by vomiting, anti-emetic drugs. Great care should be taken not to administer neuroleptic drugs to patients following myelography as the interaction of these drugs with certain contrast agents is well recognized (Hindmarsh et al. 1975). Encouraging patients to drink a large amount of fluid after myelography will significantly reduce the incidence and severity of post-myelography headache (Eldevik et al. 1978). Other complications following myelography and their treatment are to be found in Ansell (1986).

Pathological Appearances

The chief indications for myelography in orthopaedic practice are the investigation of patients with suspected spinal cord or nerve root compression and include spinal tumours, inflammatory spinal disease, degenerative disc disease, spondylosis and spinal trauma.

cervical herniation of the cerebellar tonsils. The normal appearances of the cranio-cervical junction are shown in Fig. 5.5.

Spinal Compression

The traditional neurosurgical division of spinal compression is into three types depending upon the anatomical site of the lesion:

Extradural compression
Intradural compression
    Extramedullary
    Intramedullary

Post-Myelographic Care

At the end of the examination the patient is returned to the ward either in the sitting position or lying in bed with the head and shoulders elevated. This is necessary to confine the contrast to the spinal canal and allow absorption to take place as quickly as possible. Studies on the dynamics of contrast absorption have shown that for all practical purposes the contrast will have been completely absorbed and

As the myelographic features are specific to the site of the pathological process producing the spinal compression, it is very convenient to classify the myelographic appearances in a similar way. The myelographic features of each type of lesion are illustrated in Fig. 5.6

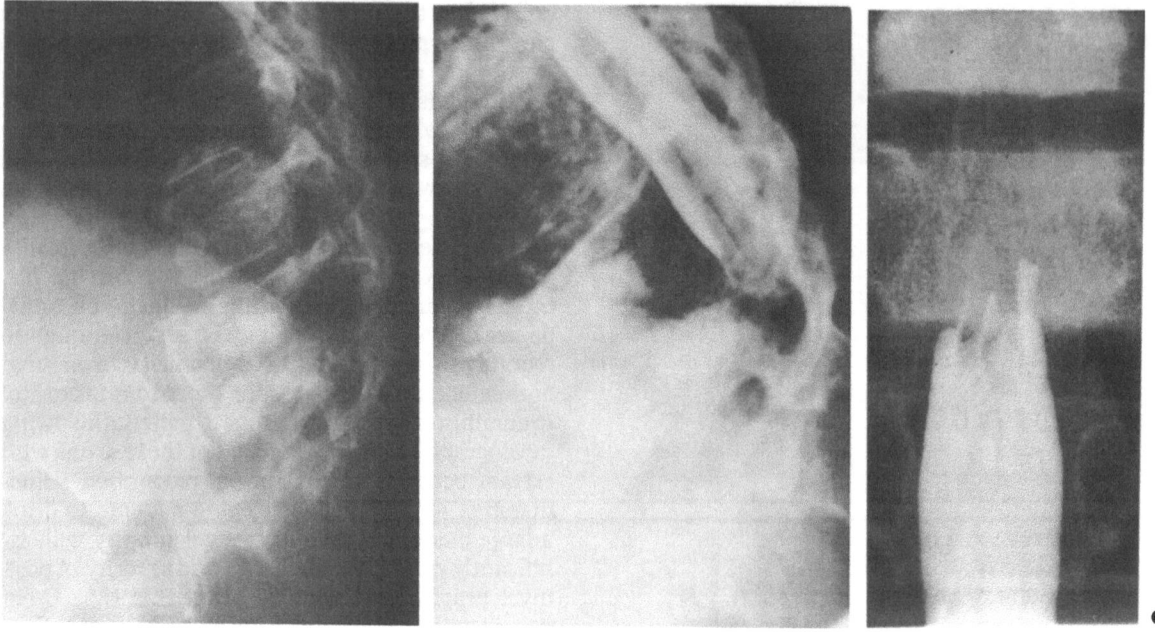

Fig. 5.7. a Tuberculous disease of the dorsal spine with marked dorsal kyphosis. b Complete extradural block as seen on descending myelography in the lateral projection. c Extradural block from lymphomatous deposits in the dorsal spine with intraspinal spread. Note the "bundle of twigs" appearances.

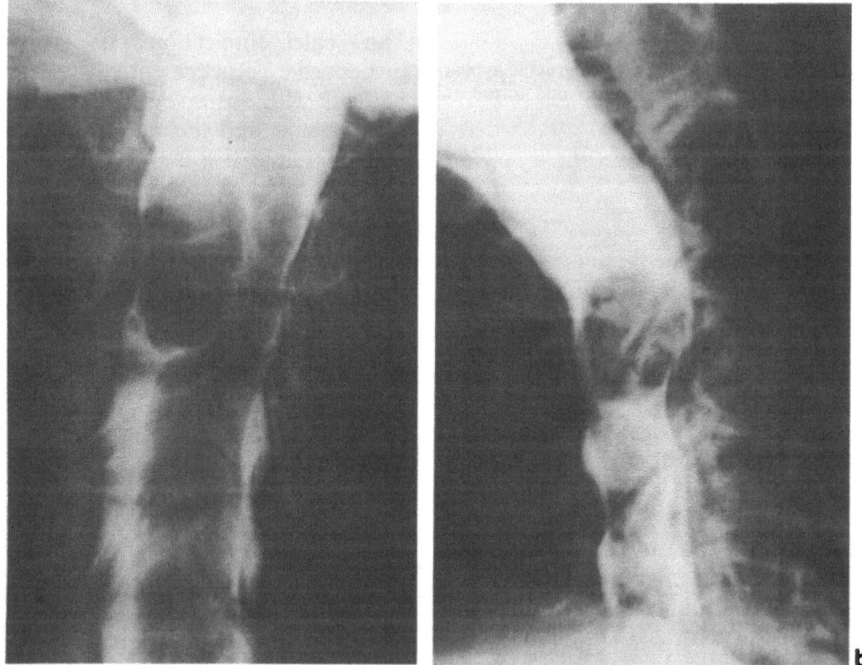

Fig. 5.8a,b. Cervical meningioma compressing and displacing the spinal cord laterally and producing the classical changes to the subarachnoid spaces as seen in the antero-posterior projection. Contrast has completely outlined the tumour in the antero-posterior (a) and lateral (b) projections.

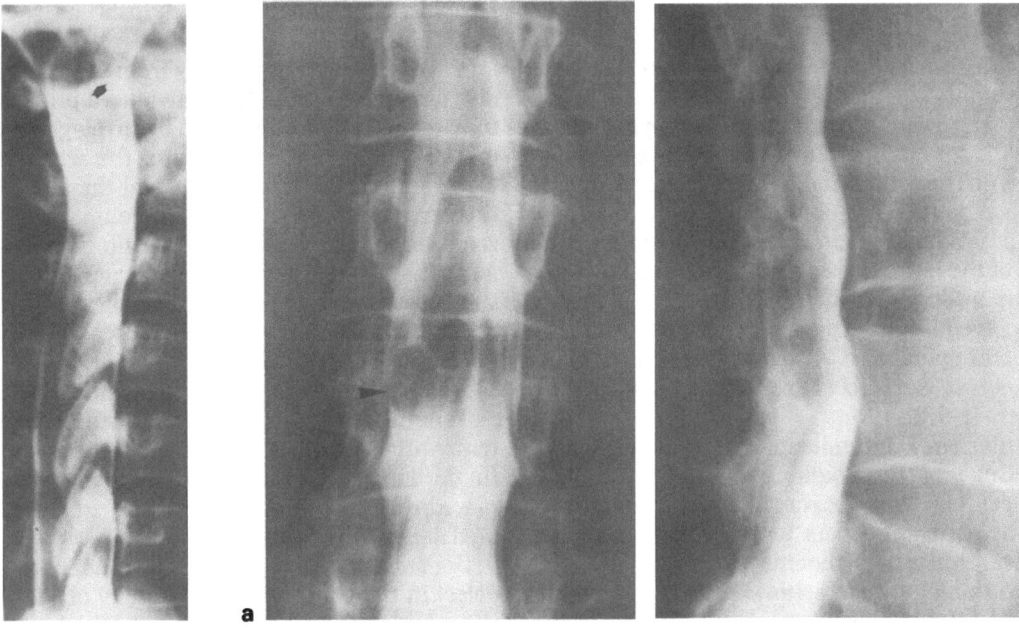

Fig. 5.9 (*left*). Syringomyelia, with contrast outlining the expanded cervical cord. Note the herniated tonsils producing a posterior filling defect down to the level of the arch of the first cervical vertebra (*arrow*).

Fig. 5.10a,b (*centre and right*). Spinal dysraphism with tethered spinal cord and fibrolipomatous tumour within the spinal cord and with extramedullary extension (*arrowhead*). Antero-posterior (**a**) and lateral (**b**) radiographs.

Extradural Compression

Extradural compression usually results from primary or secondary bone tumours, osteomyelitis or septic arthritis, or spinal trauma (fracture and/or dislocation). The spinal cord is partially or completely surrounded by tumour or abscess etc., so that the myelographic contrast is prevented from flowing freely along the spinal canal. This produces a partial or complete "myelographic block". Careful examination of the contrast immediately adjacent to the obstruction will often show a tapering of the contrast in the subarachnoid space and displacement of the spinal cord due to the encroachment on the spinal canal. The appearances of dorsal cord compression due to the extradural compression in Pott's disease of the dorsal spine are illustrated in Fig. 5.7a,b. Figure 5.7c shows the typical tapering block of extradural compression in a case of lymphomatous deposits in the dorsal spine with intraspinal spread. The tapering encirclement of the spinal cord and nerve roots by the tumour tissue produces an appearance resembling a "bundle of twigs".

Intradural Extramedullary Compression

Intradural extramedullary tumours are commonly either neurofibromas arising from the nerve roots within the dural compartment or meningiomas arising from the spinal dura. The myelographic appearances of these lesions are quite specific. The tumour displaces the spinal cord to one side, the subarachnoid space being widened on the side of the lesion just below the upper or lower pole of the tumour while the space on the opposite side is narrowed due to the displacement of the spinal cord. The rounded upper or lower pole of the tumour can be clearly identified and if the spinal block is not complete then contrast may pass around the tumour, outlining it completely. Fig. 5.8 shows the myelographic appearances of a neurofibroma of the third cervical nerve root in the antero-posterior and lateral projections.

Intradural Intramedullary Compression

Intramedullary tumours are either gliomas or ependymomas arising in the ependymal lining of the central canal of the spinal cord. Gliomas of the cord may produce a cystic cavity or syrinx within the spinal cord, but a fluid-filled syrinx within the spinal cord is more commonly encountered in syringomyelia. Any solid or cystic space-occupying lesion within the spinal cord may produce a myelographic block, with the contrast adjacent to the block outlining the expanded spinal cord. If no myelographic block is produced then contrast will outline the whole of the expanded segment of the spinal cord. Figure 5.9 illustrates the appearances in a case of syringomyelia with expansion of the cervical segment of the spinal cord. Also noted is the downward herniation of the cerebellar tonsils as described by Gardner (1965).

Occasionally intramedullary tumours may extend out of the spinal cord and have both intramedullary and extramedullary components. This phenomenon occurs with some gliomas and also with intraspinal lipomas in cases of spinal dysraphism. Figure 5.10 shows the appearances in a case of spinal dysraphism, with tethering of the spinal cord and a lipomatous tumour arising in the tethered lower spinal cord with extramedullary extension.

Disc Herniations and Spondylosis

Lumbar disc herniations vary from massive central disc prolapse to small laterally placed prolapse and may readily be demonstrated by myelography. The reduced radiographic density of the water-soluble myelographic contrast agents and the ability to fill the nerve root sleeves enable the course of the nerve roots to be followed out to the intervertebral exit foramina. Quoted accuracy for water-soluble contrast myelography in the diagnosis of the disc herniations varies from 93.8% to 96% (Occleshaw 1979; Cook and Wise 1979).

Massive central disc herniations produce a classical extradural type of compression of the spinal contents with a complete or partial myelographic block. In the lateral projection the contrast is seen displaced well away from the disc space by the herniated disc material (Fig. 5.11).

Centerolateral disc herniations produce a filling defect in the contrast agent laterally at the level of the intervertebral disc, and as a result of nerve root compression, filling of the nerve root sleeve with contrast is impaired or absent. These features are more readily seen in the oblique projection when the nerve roots are visualized in profile (Fig. 5.12a)

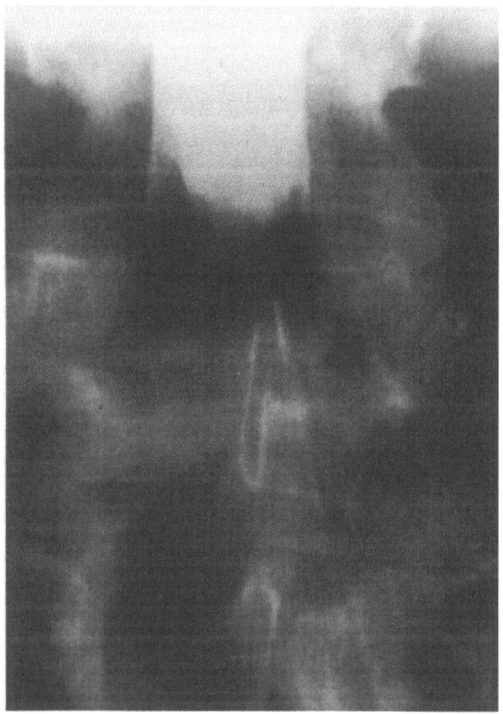 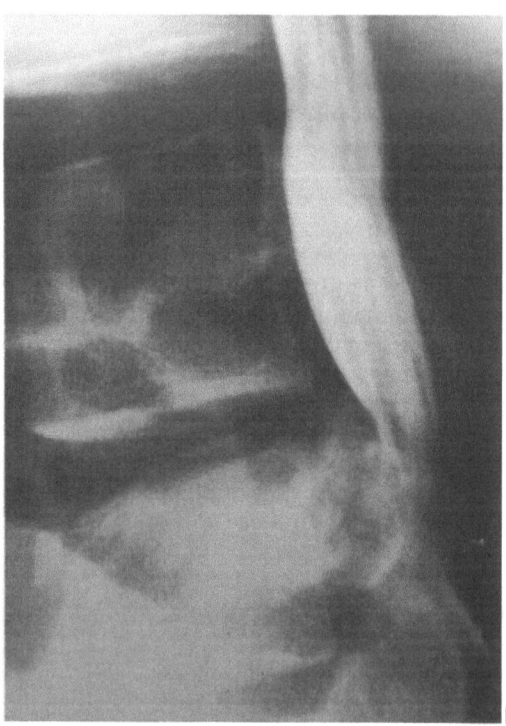

Fig. 5.11a,b. Massive central disc herniation following spinal trauma. Antero-posterior (a) and lateral (b) radiographs show complete myelographic block and marked posterior displacement of the subarachnoid space due to the herniated disc material.

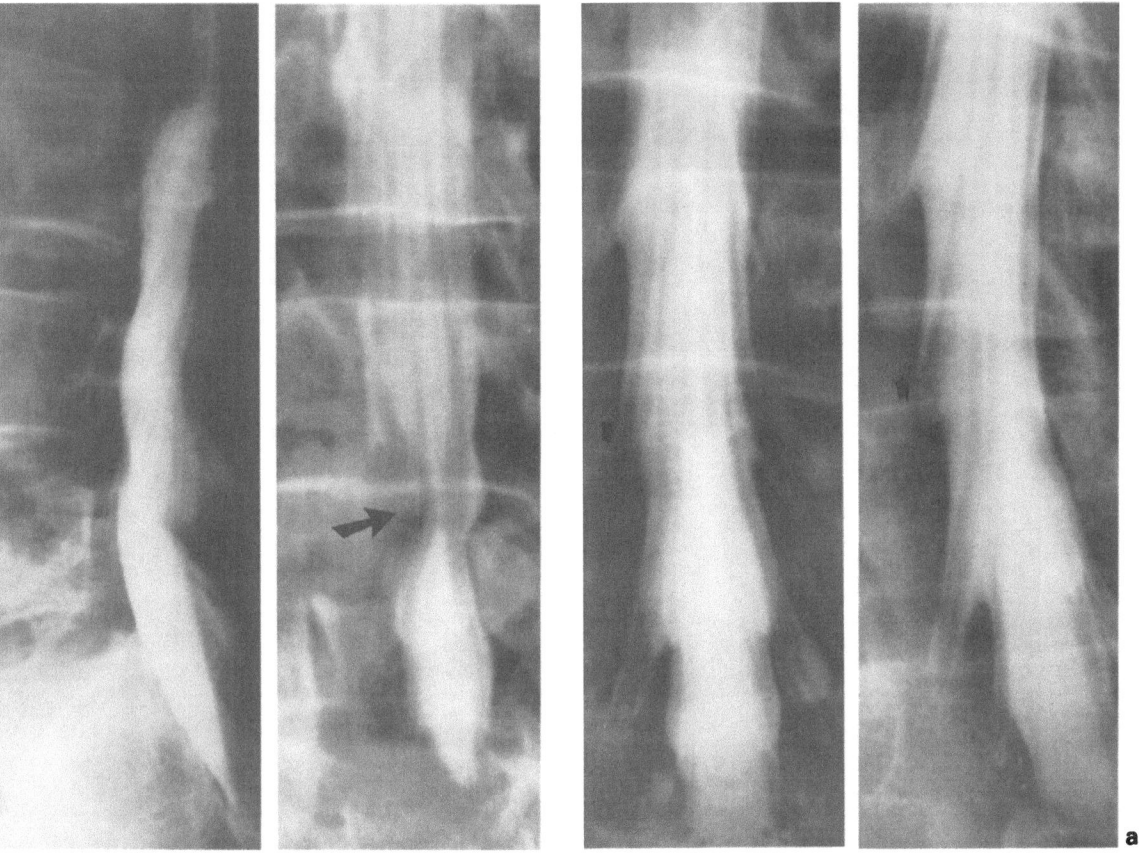

a, b   a, b

Fig. 5.12a,b. Centerolateral disc herniation. **a** Lateral radiograph showing small displacement of the contrast away from the posterior aspect of the disc. **b** Oblique projection showing a large laterally placed filling defect (*arrow*) and non-filling of the nerve root sleeve due to root compression.

Fig. 5.13a,b. Small lateral disc herniation showing nerve root sleeve "cut off" in the antero-posterior (a) and oblique (b) projections (*arrow*).

and are often accompanied by a moderate-sized anterior filling defect at the level of the offending disc in the lateral projection (Fig. 5.12b). Small lateral disc herniations adjacent to the intervertebral foramina may only reveal their presence by non-filling of the nerve root sleeve with contrast laterally, at the level of the offending disc, due to root compression (Fig. 5.13). Compression of the nerve root may cause the nerve to swell and appear larger than normal. This feature was described by Ecoiffier (1960) as the "signe du tromblon". However, this radiographic feature is rather non-specific and can occur as a result of other forms of root compression such as arachnoiditis, or from an osteophyte in osteoarthritic spondylosis.

Dorsal disc herniations are readily demonstrated when the patient is placed in the lateral decubitus position with the head slightly depressed to allow the contrast to pass to the dorsal segment. Massive dorsal disc herniations may produce a typical complete "extradural" block, while smaller lesions are completely outlined by the contrast at the level of the disc space and tomography may assist in demonstrating the full extent of the lesion. Figure 5.14 shows the degree of spinal cord compression and displacement resulting from a herniated dorsal disc.

Lumbar spondylosis may, as a result of ligamentous thickening, herniation of degenerate disc material and osteophyte formation, produce widespread compression of the spinal contents. Anterior filling defects are seen at the levels of the intervertebral discs in the lateral projection together with diffuse posterior defects from the posterior ligaments. Severe forms of this condition may cause the contrast to be broken up into a "step-ladder" type

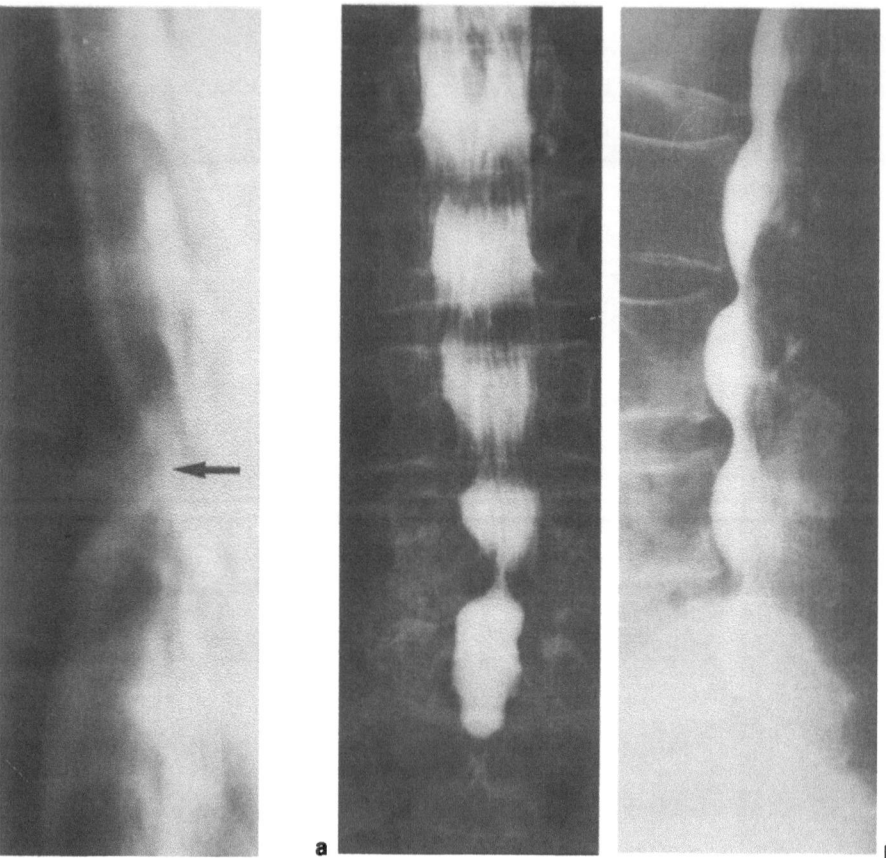

Fig. 5.14 (*left*). Dorsal disc herniation, showing herniated disc material indenting and displacing the dorsal spinal cord on tomography (*arrow*).

Fig. 5.15a,b (*centre and right*). Lumbar spondylosis. **a** In the lateral film there are anterior encroachments in the contrast at all lumbar disc levels and diffuse posterior indentations due to ligamentous thickening. **b** On the antero-posterior film the contrast is broken up into the typical "step-ladder" appearance of spinal stenosis. Note the lateral filling defects at the L4/5 and L5/S1 levels due to herniated disc material.

of appearance and produce the syndrome of spinal stenosis (Fig. 5.15). Osteophytes and herniated disc material produce multi-level lateral filling defects as seen in the antero-posterior and oblique projections.

Cervical disc herniations produce similar myelographic appearances to the herniations at lumbar or dorsal levels. Lateral filling defects from herniated disc material may be seen in the lateral aspect of the cervical canal (Fig. 5.16a–c), and non-filling or amputation of the nerve root sleeve may also be noted. Compression of the spinal cord in the antero-posterior axis may cause the lateral axis of the cord to increase and produce an apparent or "pseudo" expansion of the cord as seen in the antero-posterior radiographs. Often large central cervical disc herni-

ations may follow cervical trauma and can be seen displacing the cervical cord posteriorly (Fig. 5.16d).

Cervical spondylosis produces similar changes to those already described with lumbar spondylosis. Anterior indentations due to osteophytes are frequently seen in the lateral films with varying degrees of cord deformity or compression (Fig. 5.17a). Nerve root compression may be seen as simple "non-filling" of a nerve root sleeve or as a lateral filling defect in the contrast at nerve root level (Fig. 5.17b). Gross cervical spondylosis shows widespread cord compression due to the anterior indentations from herniated disc material and osteophytes, together with posterior indentations due to thickening of the posterior ligaments.

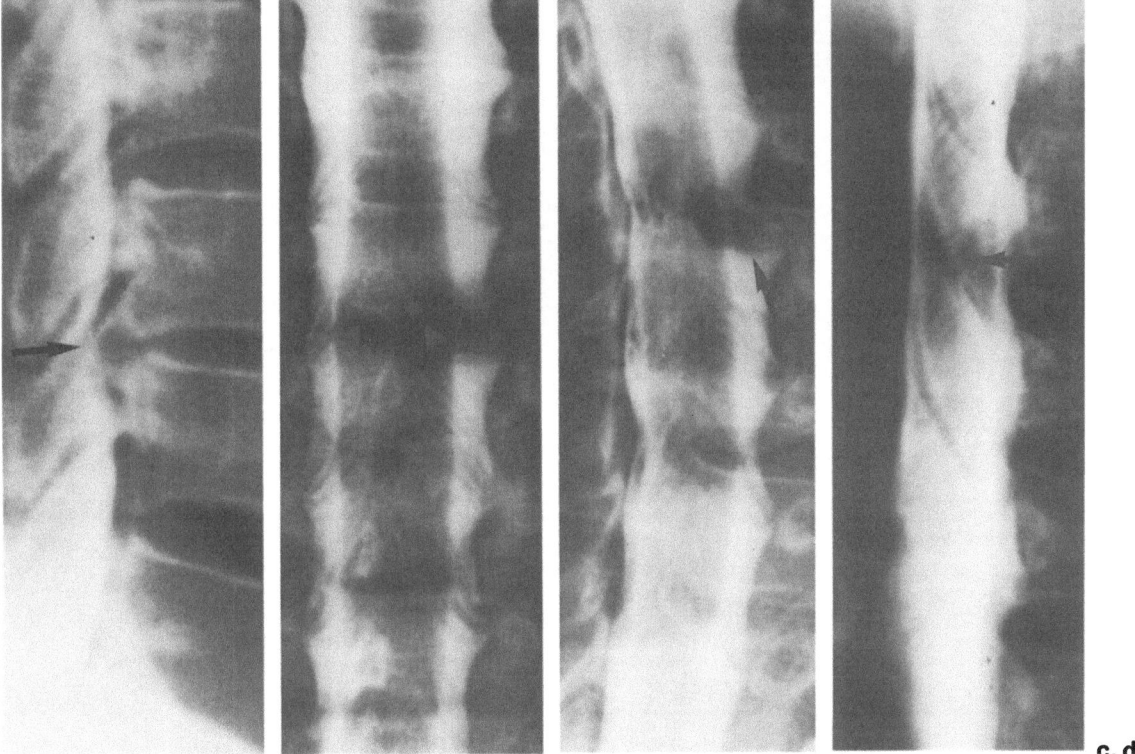

a, b   **c, d**

Fig. 5.16a–d. Cervical disc herniations. a Lateral film showing a herniated disc projecting posteriorly (*arrow*) b and c Antero-posterior and oblique projections showing the lateral filling defect and non-filling of the nerve root sleeve due to root compression (*arrow*). Note that there is some increase in the transverse diameter of the spinal cord at the level of the lesion (pseudo-expansion of the cord). d Massive central disc herniation following acute trauma. Tomography demonstrates the herniated disc compressing and deforming the spinal cord (*arrow*).

Traumatic Nerve Root Avulsion

Avulsion of the brachial plexus may follow trauma to the upper limb. In the early days following such an injury it is important to know whether the nerves have been completely avulsed, and myelography can provide valuable prognostic information. Complete avulsion is invariably accompanied by avulsion of the subarachnoid sleeves of the roots, and on myelography contrast is seen passing into diverticula-like cavities outside the inter-vertebral foramina (Fig. 5.18). Patients with signs of brachial plexus lesions not showing such appearances may in time show some evidence of nerve root recovery.

Despite the advances of newer imaging techniques in diagnostic radiology, the development of the new non-ionic contrast media for myelography, which has resulted in greater patient tolerance of the procedure, has helped myelography to maintain its position as a valuable method of investigating patients with spinal disease in present-day orthopaedic practice.

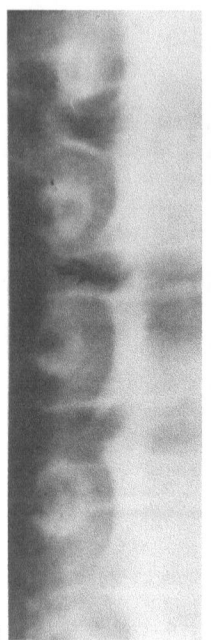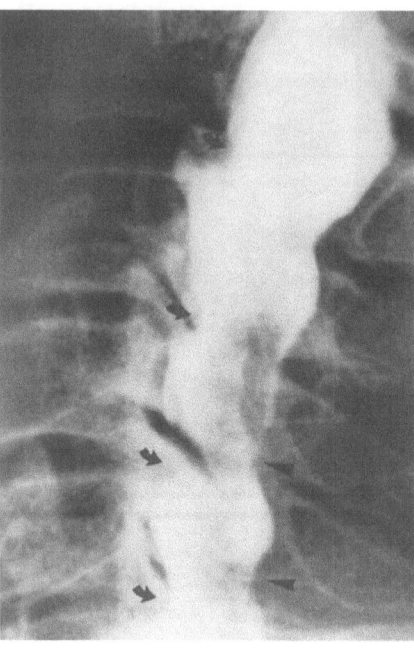

a, b

Fig. 5.17a,b. Cervical spondylosis. a Non-filling of the nerve root due to root compression from a small laterally placed osteophyte (*arrow*). b Gross spondylosis with anterior encroachment on the spinal canal at each disc level due to osteophyte and/or herniated disc material (*arrows*). Posterior indentations are seen in the contrast due to ligamentous thickening (*arrowheads*).

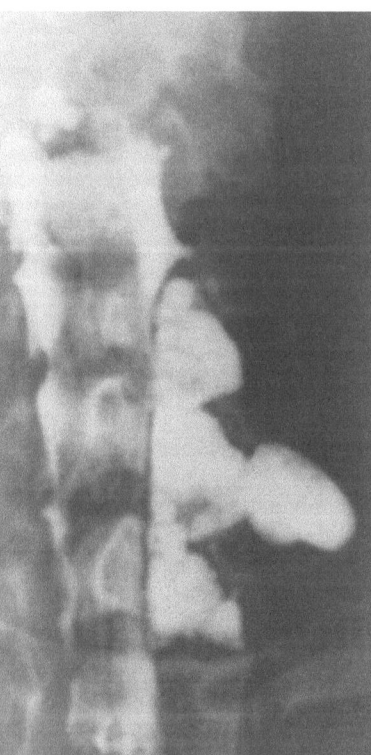

Fig. 5.18. Complete avulsion of the brachial plexus following traction injury to the arm. Myelographic contrast is seen escaping from the nerve root sleeves into "diverticula-like" cavities.

References

Amundsen P, Skalpe IO (1975) Cervical myelography with a water soluble contrast medium (metrizamide). Neuroradiology 8:209–212

Ansell G (1986) Complications in diagnostic radiology, 2nd edn. Blackwell Scientific Publications, Oxford

Arnell S, Lindstrom F (1931) Myelography with Skiodan (Abrodil). Acta Radiol 12:287–288

Cook PL, Wise KA (1979) A correlation of the surgical and radiculographic findings in lumbar disc herniation. Clin Radiol 30:671–682

Drayer BP, Rosenbaum AE (1977) Amipaque brain penetrance. Its correlation with adverse reactions and value radiodiagnostically. Acta Radiol [Suppl] 355:280–293

Ecoiffier J (1960) La radiculographie lombaire dans la sciatique. Masson et Cie, Paris

Eldevik OP, Nakken KO, Haughton VM (1978) The effects of dehydration on the side effects of metrizamide myelography. Radiology 129:715–716

Gardner WJ (1965) Hydrodynamic mechanisms of syringomyelia: its relationship to myelocele. J Neurol Neurosurg Psychiatr 28:247–259

Hindmarsh T, Grepe A, Widen L (1975) Metrizamide-phenothiazine interaction. Report of a case with seizures following myelography. Acta Radiol [Diagn] (Stockh) 16:129–134

Occleshaw JV (1979) Metrizamide myelography in the lumbar region. In: Grainger RG, Lamb JT (eds) Myelographic techniques with metrizamide. Nyegaard (UK) Ltd, pp 37–51

6 Epidurography

I. Emery and G. Hamilton

Relevance to Orthopaedic Surgery 89
Indications and Contraindications 89
Results 89
References 93

Epidurography is an established method of investigating the lumbar spinal canal and nerve roots (Luyendijk and van Voorthuisen 1966). The present authors' experience and technique are fully described elsewhere (Emery and Hamilton 1980; Hamilton 1983).

Relevance to Orthopaedic Surgery

Epidurography is of particular interest and value to orthopaedic surgeons for three reasons. First, it is a technically straightforward investigation requiring standard radiographic screening facilities, readily available and in most medical centres. Second, in an expanding speciality which may have limited in-patient facilities, it has particular value as it can be carried out as an out-patient or day case investigation. Third, it is possible to combine epidurography with the injection of a steroid, if desired, thereby combining a diagnostic and therapeutic procedure.

Indications and Contraindications

The technique may be used for the routine investigation of problems arising in the extradural space: lumbar disc prolapse and spinal stenosis. Contraindications are clinical evidence of any intradural lesion, or previous surgical exploration of the lumbar spinal canal.

Results

The accuracy of epidurography as a technique is demonstrated in Fig. 6.1. In the absence of the side-effects that may follow radiculography (Baker et al. 1978) the examination can be extended to include dynamic studies such as flexion and extension views (Fig. 6.2), lateral flexion views and stress views.

The presence of a lumbar disc prolapse is readily apparent, usually on both the antero-posterior and lateral views (Fig. 6.3). To obtain results as illustrated it is important that the basic aspects of the investigative technique described below are strictly adhered to.

The patient must be lying prone and as symmetrically as possible over a foam wedge on the screening table and the needle must be inserted in the mid-line, otherwise the distribution of the contrast medium may be uneven due to factors other than the presence of any pathological features. A non-ionic low-osmolality contrast is essential; we usually use Iohexol 180 mg iodine per ml. This satisfies the requirements of low viscosity with optimal radiodensity. Up to 20 ml of contrast may be injected but overfilling should be avoided as some detail may be obscured. A lumbar approach using the space between the fourth and fifth spinous processes is recommended. The sacral route is not used because diagnostic filling of the lower lumbar canal cannot reliably be achieved; neither will an injection above L4/L5 as contrast tends to flow cranially. Since most disc protrusions occur at the lower two lumbar discs the approach recommended is that which gives the most consistent and satisfactory results.

In patients with spinal stenosis a very accurate outline of the extent of encroachment on the lumbar

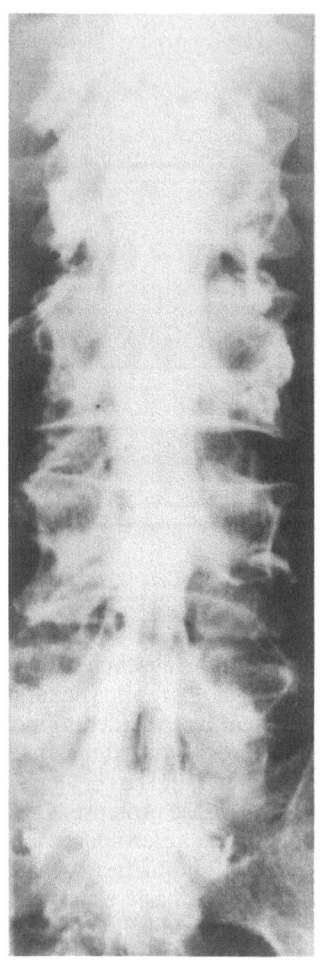

Fig. 6.1. a Normal appearance on antero-posterior view showing lumbar nerve roots and outline of lumbar canal. **b** Normal appearance on lateral view showing close outline of posterior longitudinal ligament and disc surfaces and true (A-P) diameter of spinal canal. **c** Normal appearance on oblique views (*below, centre and right*) showing lumbar nerve roots.

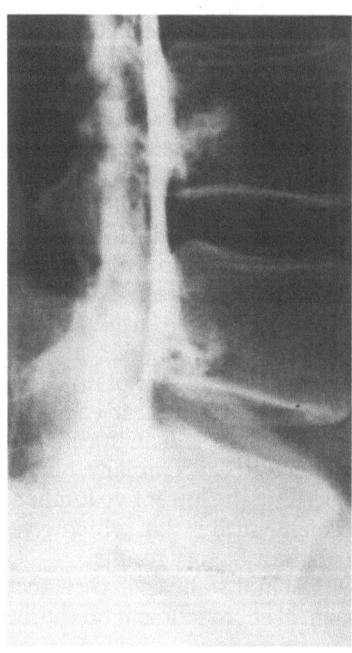

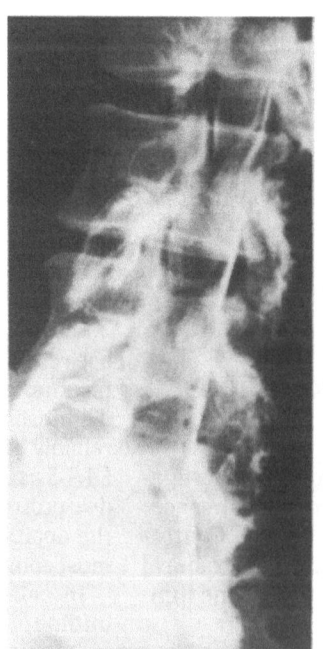

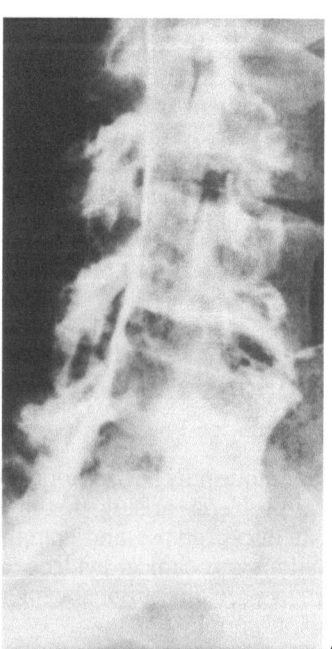

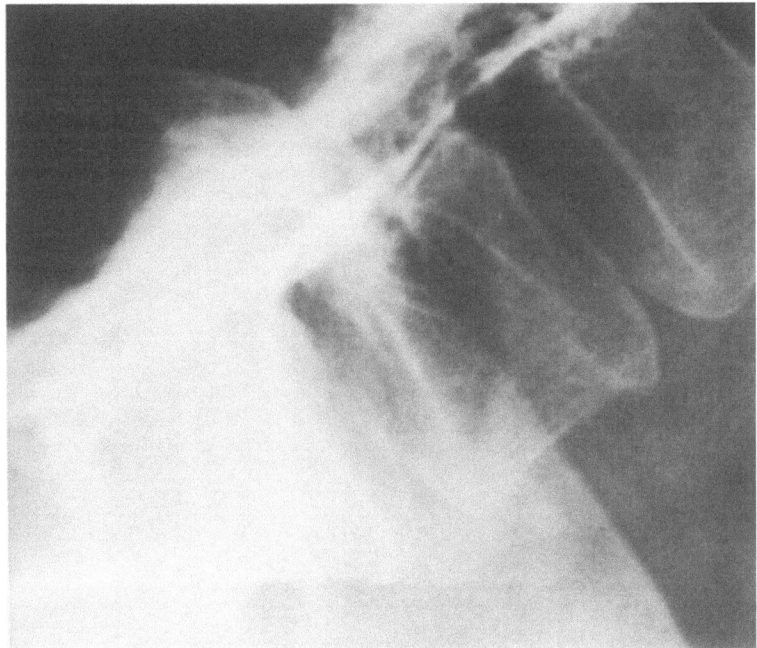

Fig. 6.2a,b. Normal appearance on lateral view during flexion (a) and extension (b).

Fig. 6.3 (*below*). a Antero-posterior view showing lack of filling at the L5/S1 level
due to a disc prolapse. b Lateral view showing L5/S1 disc protrusion in same patient.

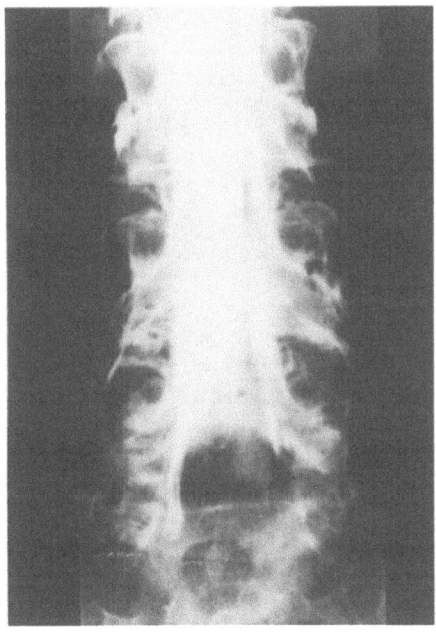
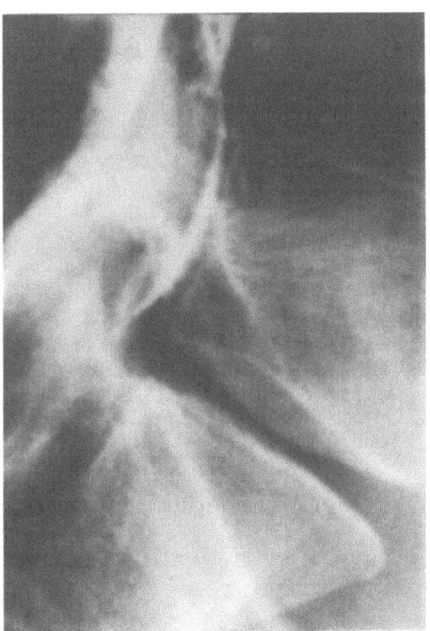

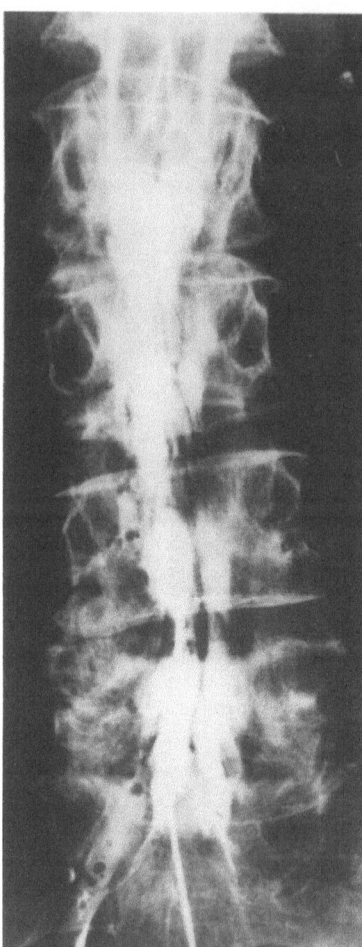

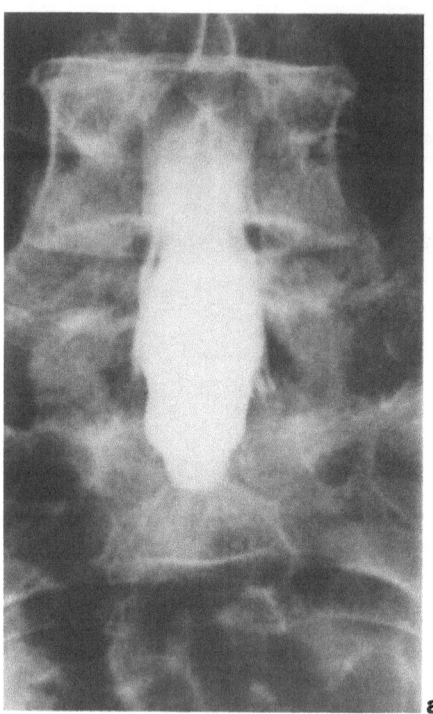

Fig. 6.4. Antero-posterior view showing severe spinal stenosis.

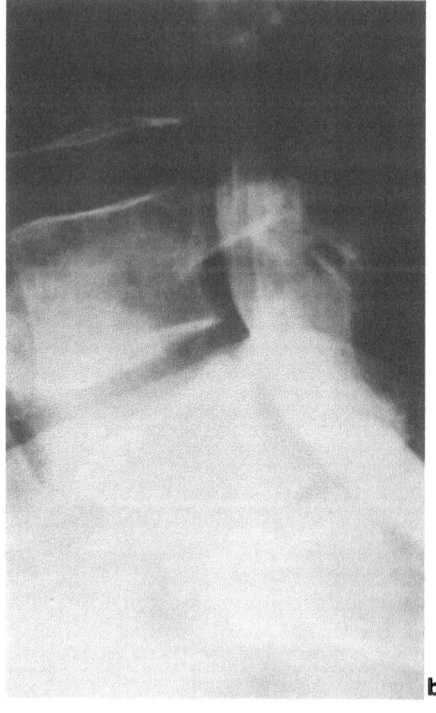

Fig. 6.5. a Antero-posterior view of radiculogram. Note the limited extent to which the roots are often outlined. **b** Lateral view of radiculogram on same patient. Compare with Fig. 6.6.

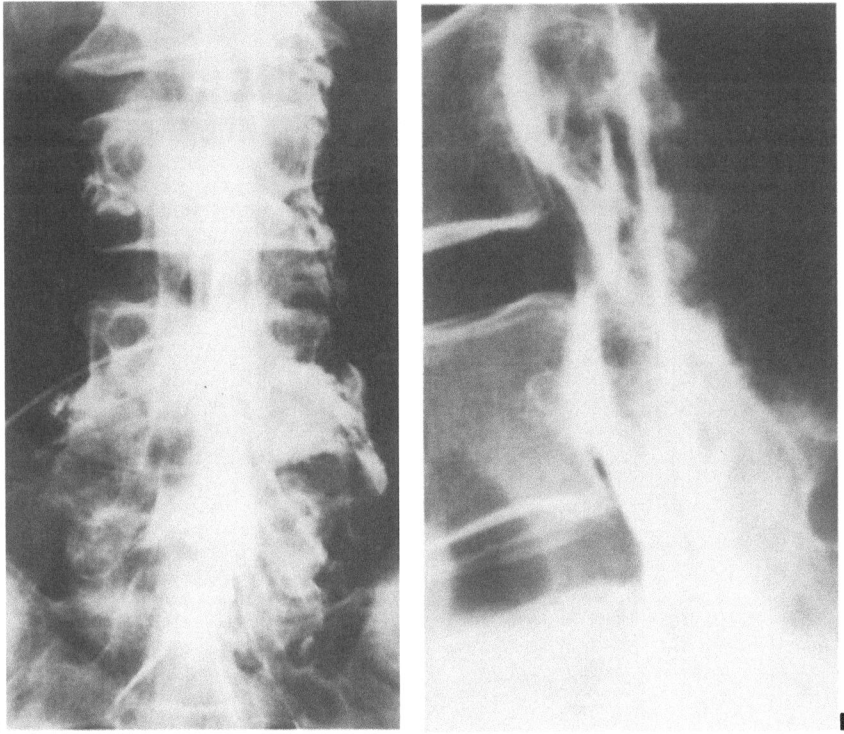

Fig. 6.6. Antero-posterior (a) and lateral (b) views of epidurogram on same patient shown in Fig. 6.5.

canal is obtained (Fig. 6.4), which is of importance in planning the extent of any proposed surgical decompression.

A comparison with radiculography (Chap. 5; Figs. 6.5, 6.6) demonstrates how accurate and informative epidurography can be, as the contrast is seen closely applied to the structures of most importance to the orthopaedic surgeon – the lumbar disc surfaces and the nerve roots to a level beyond the intervertebral foramina.

It is our experience that if a lumbar disc protrusion is not seen on routine views, it cannot be visualized by dynamic studies such as upright flexion, extension or even stress views. The latter are carried out with the patient holding weights from extended arms during flexion and extension. Any alteration that does occur during extension and flexion is negligible. We therefore conclude that any changes seen on flexion and extension during radiculography are probably due to the closer application of the outlined dural sac to a largely unaltered disc protrusion.

The authors have attempted the technique of introducing contrast through a catheter inserted via the sacral hiatus, as described by Hatten (1980). It was found to be difficult to direct the catheter and pain may be caused due to stimulation of nerve roots by the catheter.

References

Baker RA, Hillman BJ, McLennan JE, Strand RD, Kaufman SM (1978) Sequelae of metrizamide myelography in 200 examinations. AJR 130:499–502

Emery I, Hamilton G (1980) Epidurography using metrizamide: an out-patient examination. Clin Radiol 31:643–649

Hamilton G (1983) Metrizamide epidurography. J R Soc Med 76:126–130

Hatten HP (1980) Lumbar epidurography with metrizamide. Radiology 137:129–136

Luyendijk W, van Voorthuisen AE (1966) Contrast examination of the spinal epidural space. Acta Radiol [Diagn] (Stockh) 5:1051–1066

7 Angiography of the Axial Skeleton

G. Forbes

Introduction 95
Arteriography 95
  Clinical Indications 95
  Anatomy 97
  Technique 98
  Therapeutic Embolization 99
  Radiographic Findings 99
Epidural Venography 102
  Technique 103
  Radiographic Findings 103
References 105

Introduction

Angiography of the spine has a small but often criti-cal place in the evaluation of some spinal lesions. Clinical angiography of the axial spine can be divided into two different types: arteriography of the spinal cord and venography of the epidural venous plexus. Arteriography is generally used to evaluate the small, select group of patients with known or suspected arteriovenous malformations of the spine, spinal cord or supporting tissues, and is occasionally used to investigate a highly vascular spinal tumour. Epidural venography has been used predominantly as a secondary, or less commonly as a primary, examination for lumbar disc protrusion, although lately it has been replaced in this role by the less invasive techniques of computed tomography and magnetic resonance imaging. Because the clinical problems and clinical roles of angiography and venography are quite different, these examinations will be discussed separately. The clinical indications, vascular anatomy and pathophysiology, as well as the technique, need to be fully understood for proper utilization of these examinations in clinical practice.

Arteriography

Clinical Indications

The main indications for spinal arteriography are to establish the presence of an arteriovenous malfor-mation (AVM) in the cord (suggested by myelogra-phy) or in the paraspinal tissues (indicated by computed tomographic scanning) and to define in detail the arteriovenous anatomy of such a lesion or occasionally of a known highly vascular tumour.

Arteriography is not used to evaluate ischaemic or vascular occlusion in the spinal cord because of the limits of resolution of small vessels, nor as a screen for vascular lesions because of the complexity of the examination. However, once an AVM or highly vascular lesion has been detected or strongly suggested by myelography, selective spinal arterio-graphy is essential as the only means of defining with accuracy the vascular anatomy of the lesion and surrounding territory. Other non-invasive tests, such as plain films, computed tomography and, more recently, magnetic resonance imaging, can

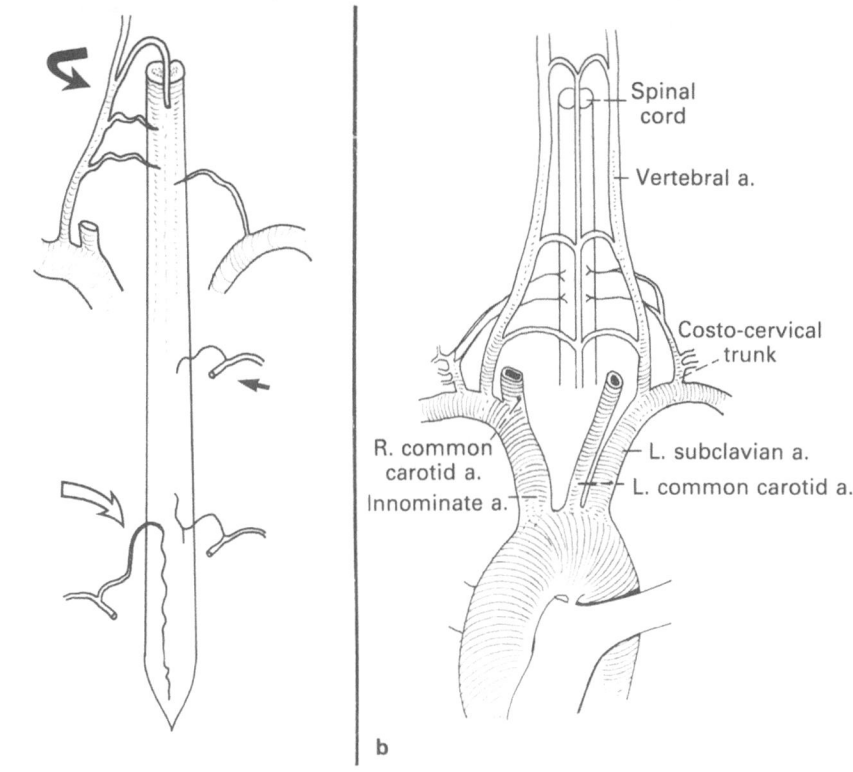

Fig. 7.1a,b. Spinal cord arterial supply. **a** Segments of spinal cord are supplied by different groups of arteries, including the artery of Adamkiewicz (*open arrow*), thoracic intercostal arteries (*straight black arrow*) and anterior spinal and cervical medullary arteries (*curved black arrow*). See text. **b** In the cervical region, vertebral arteries and thyrocostal cervical trunk vessels both supply spinal cord extending from the medulla to a watershed zone in the upper thoracic level. (By permission of the Mayo Foundation.)

demonstrate spinal AVMs, but myelography, properly carried out, remains the most reliable screening method.

Patients with vascular lesions of the spine requiring arteriography may have progressive locomotor disability and loss of bowel or bladder control; in acute presentations there will probably be associated haemorrhage, pain and sudden neurological deficit. In a series of 60 patients (Aminoff and Logue 1974) the presenting symptoms were of acute onset in 20%. In patients with a progressive history, the mean interval between the first symptom and the greatest persistent gait disorder was 5.7 years. In another series (Houdart et al. 1966) 11 of 15 adult patients had their first symptoms before age 12. The differences between acute and chronic presentations are likely to depend on the type of vascular malformation. Some authors believe that the symptoms of parenchymal angiomas are more frequently of sudden onset whilst dural lesions may have a more chronic and progressive course (Symon et al. 1984).

If a myelogram demonstrates serpiginous defects suspicious of an AVM, then arteriography is indicated. Rarely, other causes of serpiginous defects, such as the enlarged spinal nerves of Dejerine–Sottas syndrome or dilated veins beneath total blockage of the spinal canal, mimic an AVM. These disorders can usually be differentiated from a true AVM. A complete myelographic block in the thoracic region usually indicates tumour, but such a block occasionally occurs with an AVM following previous haemorrhage (Symon et al. 1984).

The extensive vascular supply to the spine may result in the failure of the first attempt at demonstrating a suspected AVM. The question then arises as to how aggressive one should be in continuing the search. It is usually accepted that an end-point has been reached when satisfactory negative examinations of all standard arterial supplies to the spinal cord have been accomplished. These include all thoraco-lumbar intercostal, both subclavian and vertebral, and both iliac arteries.

Although this examination is sometimes accomplished in one session, two are often necessary. On occasion an AVM may be found on a third or fourth study – an encouragement to a more aggressive approach. Although demonstrating the spinal artery of Adamkiewicz is important, this cannot be used as an end-point, since dural-based malformations usually arise some distance from the anterior spinal artery supply and often well above the level indicated by a clinical deficit. Location of the myelographic filling defects is of only limited value, since they more frequently represent only the dilated draining venous channels and may be far removed from the source of the arteriovenous connection.

Anatomy

For purposes of arteriography, the vascular supply to the spinal cord can be considered in two segments: the cervical and the thoraco-lumbar (Fig. 7.1). Branches from both vertebral arteries and from costo-cervical trunk vessels supply the cervical cord. Access to this system is obtained through catheterization of the subclavian arteries. Branches from the intercostal arteries arising along the length of the aorta supply the thoraco-lumbar cord and conus. Along the length of the cord, direct-feeding arteries are arranged in two separate systems: an anterior and a posterior chain. The anterior arterial chain extends along the anterior surface within the anterior median sulcus and thus lies in the mid-line when viewed from an antero-posterior direction. The posterior arterial chain consists of two channels running along the postero-lateral surface of the cord and, therefore, offset slightly from the mid-line when viewed from an antero-posterior perspective. Both the anterior and the posterior chains are supplied by radicular arteries arising from the paired intercostal arteries in the thoraco-lumbar region, the costo-cervical and vertebral arteries in the cervical region, and, in the case of the anterior chain, the junction of two anterior spinal branches from the upper vertebral arteries.

A major source of supply to the anterior chain in the thoraco-lumbar region is the artery of Adamkiewicz, sometimes referred to as the anterior spinal artery. This artery usually arises from an intercostal vessel between T8 and L2, first ascending and then descending, forming a sharp characteristic hairpin loop before entering the anterior median sulcus. Djindjian (1969) found it to arise on the left between T9 and T12 in 75% of cases. Inadvertent interruption of this arterial supply as a result of orthopaedic or aortic surgery involving the intercostal arteries can result in catastrophic spinal ischaemia. The supply to the smaller posterior lateral chains is more sporadic, arising from various intercostal vessels along the length of the cord. A common origin of blood supply to dural malformations and to the spinal cord from the same segmental artery is occasionally found (Doppman et al. 1971). Extensive anastomotic channels connect segments of the anterior and posterior chains along the cord.

The intercostal arteries can be identified by midstream aortography, but visualization of the smaller radicular arteries, the anterior spinal artery of Adamkiewicz and the arterial chains requires selective injections into the intercostal arteries together with a magnification–subtraction technique of high quality. Demonstration of the anterior spinal artery by digital vascular imaging has been recorded (Yeates et al. 1985), but meticulous technique with filming of high quality remains the method of choice for complete demonstration of these small vessels.

Veins directly draining the spinal cord are not customarily visualized, even with selective arteriography, unless they are pathologically enlarged.

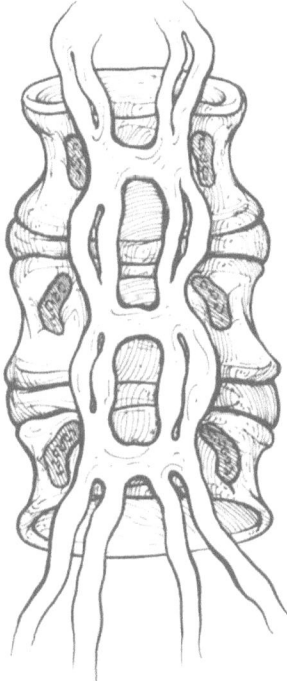

Fig. 7.2. Epidural venous plexus. The schematic diagram demonstrates the hexagonal appearance of the large anterior internal vertebral veins when viewed from an antero-posterior perspective. (By permission of the Mayo Foundation.)

Small radicular veins exit the cord on both sides to join intervertebral veins running longitudinally within the epidural venous plexus. The epidural venous plexus consists of paired anterior internal vertebral veins running longitudinally within the spinal canal and paired anterior lateral veins outside the canal in the paravertebral gutters (Fig. 7.2). Lateral intervertebral veins connect these two systems through branches, called "suprapedicular" and "infrapedicular", passing just above and below each bony pedicle. Cross-connections between the anterior internal vertebral veins as they course between the pedicles complete a lattice that appears as a series of hexagons when viewed from an antero-posterior perspective. A smaller chain of posterior longitudinal veins connects around the dural sac. This entire system can be opacified from retrograde catheterization of the ascending lumbar or iliac veins. The paravertebral system communicates with the caval system in multiple locations that allow access by catheters for epidural venography.

Technique

Arteriography of the spinal cord requires an experienced radiological team using sophisticated equipment in order to produce the highly detailed vascular studies necessary for proper diagnostic evaluation.

In practice, angiography of the spinal cord can be divided into investigation of the cervical region and of the thoraco-lumbar region. Both regions can be approached through any one of several peripheral vessels, although the femoral artery has become the most widely used. The Seldinger technique is used, employing a catheter specifically chosen for the selective catheterization required. If a thoraco-lumbar myelogram reveals the serpiginous vessels indicative of an AVM, selective catheterization of all the lumbar radicular and thoracic intercostal arteries is necessary to determine the full extent of the blood supply to the lesion, regardless of the level of the myelographic filling defect or the clinically indicated deficit. For cervical studies, selective catheterization of both vertebral arteries and opacification of the thyro-cervical and costo-cervical trunks are required. Direct catheterization of the latter carries a high risk and is usually unnecessary unless the vessels are enlarged, in which case selective injections may be indicated, though injection into the subclavian arteries just proximal to the origins of these small vessels can provide satisfactory demonstration. Two to five ml of a non-sodium meglumine contrast medium are usually sufficient for the individual thoracic and lumbar

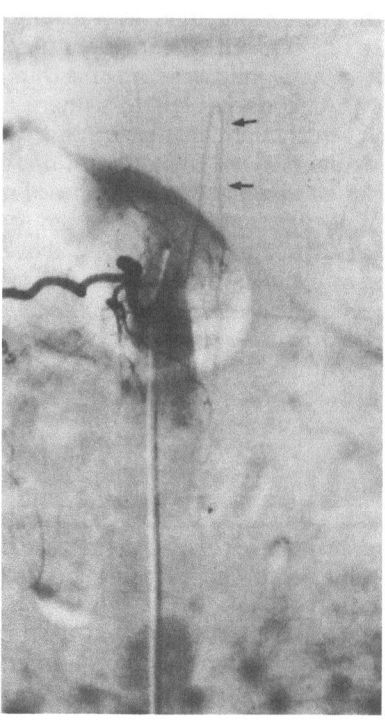

Fig. 7.3. Anterior spinal artery of Adamkiewicz. Selective injection into the intercostal artery that gives rise to the artery of Adamkiewicz demonstrates the superior course and hairpin curve (*arrows*) characteristic of this vessel.

arteries. Depending on the size of the arteries, injections of 7–12 ml for the proximal subclavian and 5–8 ml for selected vertebral arteries may be required.

Subtraction films are obtained for each arterial injection. The intercostal artery that supplies the artery of Adamkiewicz is identified, and a film series is obtained (Fig. 7.3). If the first angiogram does not demonstrate the AVM and selective catheterization of the intercostals is incomplete, a second angiogram can be undertaken in 24–48 hours. When the AVM is detected, serial filming in both antero-posterior and lateral planes is carried out with delayed films up to 20 seconds after injection. In the presence of a known vascular tumour, injection of bilateral regional intercostal arteries may be sufficient.

Normal post-angiographic care includes short bed rest, observation of vital signs, and monitoring of peripheral pulses below the areas of catheterization. Ischaemic symptoms can occur during or after catheterization of the spinal arteries, although they are not common if the angiographer is experienced.

Most studies of neuroangiographic risks and complications include cerebral examinations or combined cerebral and spinal examinations, making it difficult to provide definitive statistical conclusions about untoward effects of various stages of spinal arteriography. Transverse myelitis has been observed after selective bronchial arteriography (Feigelson and Ravin 1965), and cord lesions, including paraplegia, have been reported after aortography (McAfee 1957; Anthony 1958; Grossman and Kirtley 1958; Killen and Foster 1960, 1966; Efsen 1966). Djindjian (1969) observed no permanent complications in 180 spinal arteriographic studies, although eight patients had "medullary epilepsy". Complete spinal cord angiography performed by an experienced angiographer should carry a risk of less than 5% for minor reversible neurological change, depending on the age and condition of the patient.

Therapeutic Embolization

If therapeutic embolization of an AVM or tumour is performed, it is undertaken in a separate session and is directed towards occluding the component leading to the abnormal arteriovenous shunting while preserving the normal blood flow to the spinal cord.

The techniques for therapeutic embolization of spinal cord lesions have evolved during the past decade (Djindjian 1975; Russell and Berenstein 1984). Generally, a sheath placed in the femoral artery with the Seldinger technique is used to introduce into the feeding artery a thin-walled embolization catheter with a small tapered tip. Occlusive material in the form of a finely powdered particulate and liquid slurry or a liquid polymerizing glue is passed either directly through the catheter or through a smaller coaxial balloon-catheter system towards the lesion. The procedure is performed under fluoroscopic control with digital or film recording to monitor the process. Continuous evoked-potential recordings are made throughout the procedure, in addition to clinical testing of the mildly sedated patient, in order to identify any adverse neurological changes. If improvement occurs as a result of the embolization, signs can be identified in some patients within the first few weeks. Post-embolization care is similar to that after angiography, with increased emphasis on physical therapy and home care training.

The goals of therapeutic embolization angiography are to occlude abnormal arteriovenous shunting as close to the capillary level as possible, to decrease the venous pressure, and to preserve arterial supply to the remaining normal tissue. The procedure may be carried out as an adjunct to planned surgical resection or as the sole means of treatment if the risks of surgical removal are considered too high.

Radiographic Findings

Arteriovenous Malformation

An AVM is usually identified as a result of its draining veins (Fig. 7.4), which become enlarged and tortuous (serpiginous) within the confined space of the spinal canal giving rise to filling defects at myelography. Defects due to enlarged feeding arteries are seen only later if the lesion has progressed.

Because the vascular system is more or less continuous along the length of the spinal cord and the myelographic defects are usually caused by draining veins, there is often poor correlation between the level of the myelographic abnormality and the location of the primary pathological condition, i.e. the arteriovenous shunt. Thus the AVM may be found a substantial distance away from the myelographic defect (Fig. 7.5). At angiography small lesions are sometimes first detected as the result of early filling of a vein. A characteristic tuft of small vessels together with a persistent vascular stain is usually found in slightly larger lesions. As the malformation expands, classic changes of enlarged, tortuous feeding arteries from one or more levels and associated rapid venous shunting appear. Doppman and colleagues (1971) have indicated that the luminal diameter of arterial feeders supplying a spinal AVM may, in many instances, decrease by as much as 50% just inside the spinal canal, this site representing the point of dural penetration. In some cases, however, the lesion is large but the shunt remains small, and filling of the enlarged veins corresponding to specific myelographic defects may then only be found on delayed filming.

It is important to identify the presence or absence of supply by the anterior spinal artery of Adamkiewicz. Successful treatment through either surgery or embolization of a lesion deriving its supply from the anterior spinal artery must take into account the potential effects of closure of the arterial supply to a significant segment of the lower thoracic cord and conus. Most such lesions are predominantly anterior to the cord and are considered intra-axial (Fig. 7.6). Dural-based lesions derive their blood supply predominantly from extra-axial vessels, such as small meningeal perforating branches from intercostal arteries, and are found most

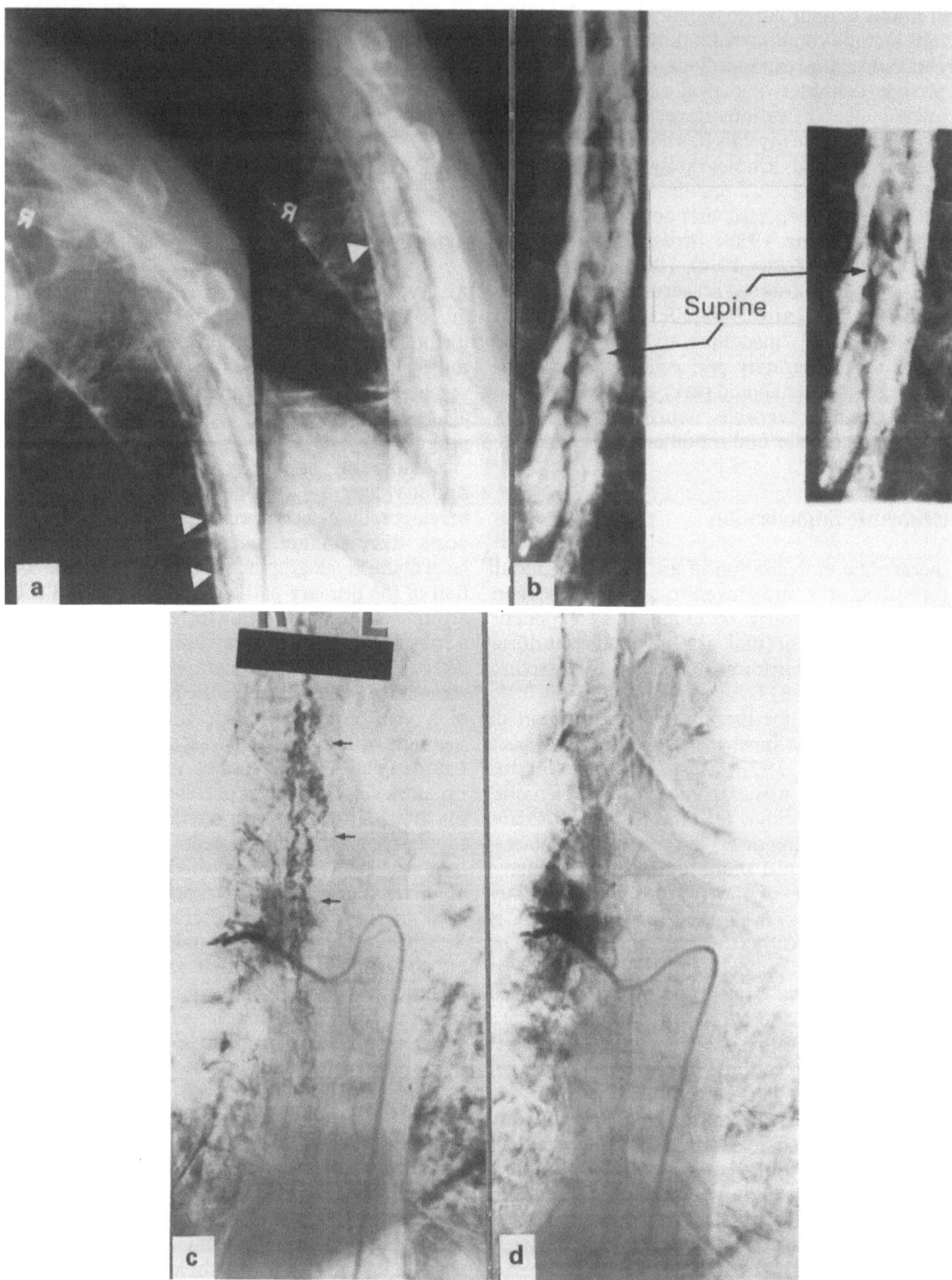

Fig. 7.4a–d. Myelography of arteriovenous malformation. **a** Irregular serpiginous vessels (*arrowheads*) are seen coursing along the length of the cord in a myelogram made using water-soluble contrast material. Markings may be subtle and poorly seen, particularly if high concentrations of contrast material and supine filming are not used. **b** A supine study with iophendylate in the same patient shows the irregular vascular markings (*arrows*) to better advantage. **c** A selective spinal arteriogram in this patient demonstrates extensive abnormal vascular channels of a thoracic arteriovenous malformation (*arrows*) that produced myelographic filling defects. **d** There is lack of filling of abnormal vessels after therapeutic embolization.

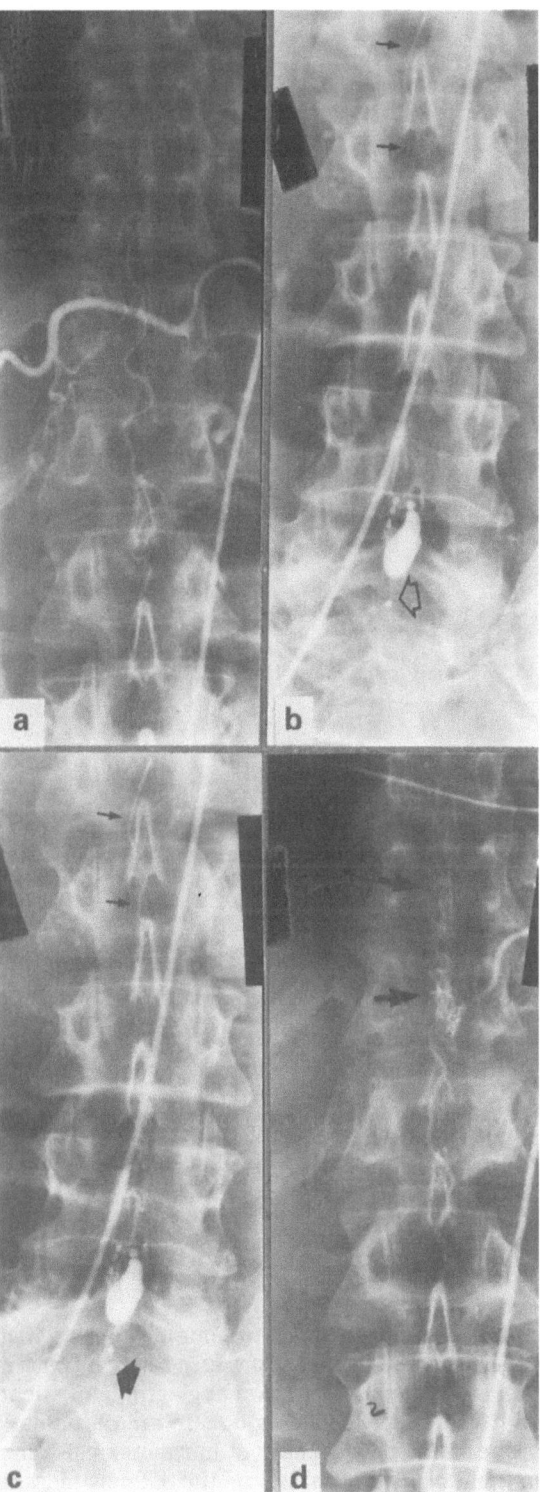

frequently postero-lateral to the cord (Fig. 7.7). The terms "intramedullary" and "extramedullary" can be confusing, since many extramedullary lesions can invaginate the cord and others can be mixed in character. The nature of the arterial supply relative to the cord largely dictates concerns of risks to the cord and potential recurrence after occlusion or resection. Evidence of a predominantly dural supply to a malformation does not eliminate the risk of cord ischaemia after treatment. Doppman and colleagues (1985) recently demonstrated that small arterial feeders to the posterior spinal chain may arise from extra-axial vessels supplying a dural malformation.

Tumour

Occasionally, spinal angiography is used to evaluate a vascular spinal tumour, although this may not be a standard procedure unless surgical resection is

Fig. 7.5a–d. Distant arteriovenous malformation. The patient had bilateral lower leg paresis and slight loss of bladder tone suggestive of a conus lesion. **a** No arteriovenous malformation was found with full thoracic and lumbar intercostal arteriography; however, the artery of Adamkiewicz was slightly larger than normal. **b** Another injection into this vessel with filming over the lumbar region showed a slow but persistently abnormal arterial course 20 seconds later (*small arrows*). Note the single droplet of residual iophendylate in a cul-de-sac (*open arrowhead*). **c** Further delayed filming at 40 seconds demonstrated a tiny arteriovenous shunt (*small arrows*) in the cul-de-sac. Note the arteriovenous malformation adjacent to the residual droplet of iophendylate (*filled arrowhead*). **d** Additional delayed filming over the low thoracic region finally demonstrated abnormally enlarged draining veins at conus level 60 seconds after intercostal injection (*arrows*).

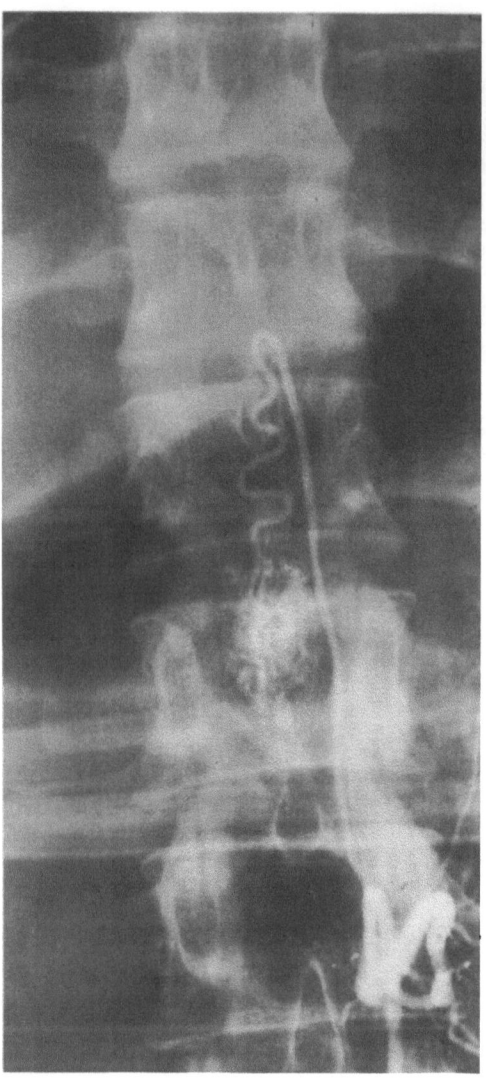

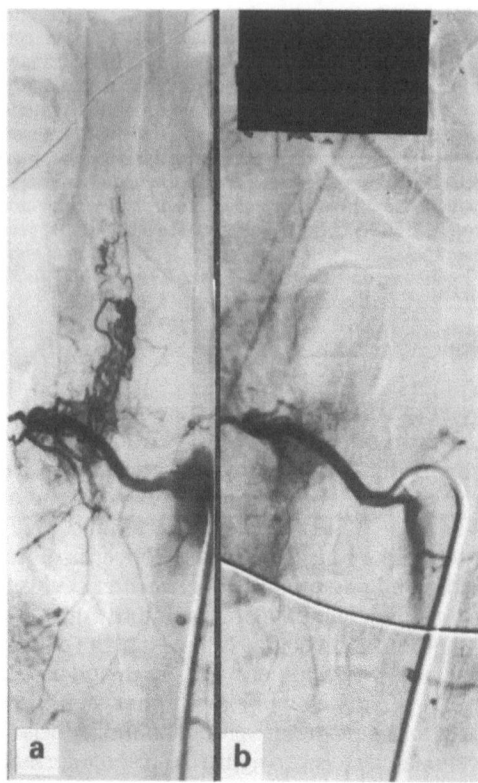

Fig. 7.7a,b. Dural-based arteriovenous malformation. a Dural vessels arising from the thoracic intercostal artery supply an arteriovenous malformation. When a lesion is this large it may be judged partially intramedullary at surgical exploration. The anterior spinal artery arises from another intercostal vessel distant from this site and is normal. b The malformation was successfully embolized, with subsequent improvement in the patient's leg weakness.

Fig. 7.6. Intramedullary parenchymal arteriovenous malformation. The lesion is supplied by an enlarged artery of Adamkiewicz arising from a low thoracic intercostal artery. This lesion involves the conus and also is intimately associated with the normal vascular supply to normal cord tissue.

contemplated. Any spinal tumour may be vascular, but haemangioblastomas produce a specific pattern that is well demonstrated on angiography. Patients with von Hippel–Lindau's disease are particularly prone to the development of haemangioblastomas in multiple sites, including the kidney, adrenal gland, pancreas, orbit and cerebellum, as well as the spinal cord. These lesions sometimes are found incidentally during angiography in these patients (Di Chiro and Doppman 1969; Herdt et al. 1972) (Fig. 7.8). Their angiographic appearance is charac-

teristic regardless of their site of origin. The lesion is well demarcated, highly vascular, and produces a persistent stain or blush. Cystic components are common. Arterial supply is usually from intra-axial vessels supplying the cerebellar or spinal cord parenchyma. The tumours are frequently multiple, and may be found along the length of the spinal cord. Most are intramedullary in the posterior aspect of the cord (Fig. 7.8).

Epidural Venography

Epidural venography has been used for the evaluation of protruded discs, primarily in the low lumbar

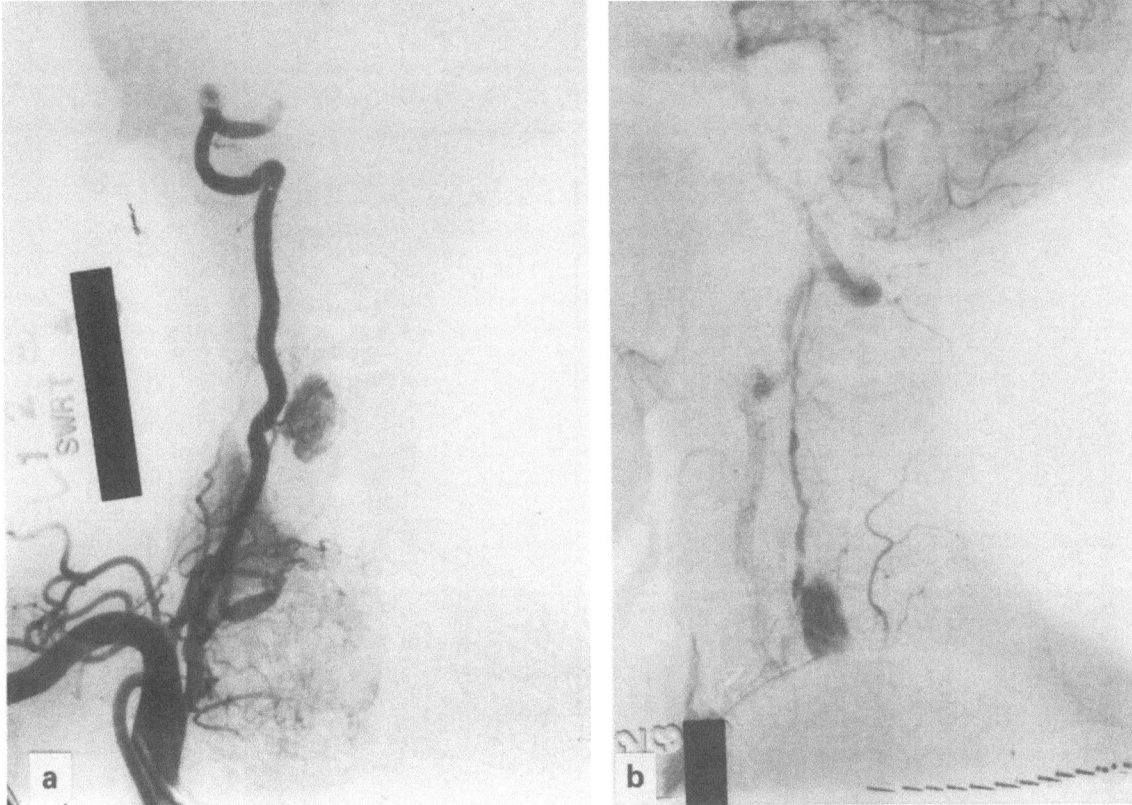

Fig. 7.8a,b. Haemangioblastoma. This large intramedullary cervical tumour, which is highly vascular, is supplied from multiple perforating branches from the vertebral artery (a) and anterior drainage into a large medullary spinal vein (b).

region and usually as a complementary procedure when myelographic results are negative or indeterminate (Bücheler and Janson 1973; LePage 1974; Gershater and Holgate 1976). The technique has largely been replaced by computed tomography – which is less invasive, less expensive and easier to accomplish – and more recently by magnetic resonance imaging. Today, epidural venography is only of value when direct visualization of the epidural venous plexus is considered essential.

Technique

A small, specially curved 5F catheter is introduced by the Seldinger technique into the femoral vein with selective catheterization of a presacral and ascending lumbar vein. Two or three injections of contrast medium with abdominal compression and Valsalva manoeuvres result in opacification of all or most of the vertebral plexus at the low lumbar levels. Although requiring angiographic expertise, the procedure is relatively quick, well tolerated and, because only a superficial vein is used, normally does not require hospitalization. A history of phlebitis or previous pelvic or lumbar surgery may preclude the examination.

Radiographic Findings

As a disc herniates into the spinal canal, it compresses and occludes one or more of the anterior internal vertebral veins. An important distinction to remember in angiography is that arteries are displaced but seldom occluded by masses, whereas veins are frequently occluded before being displaced by similar

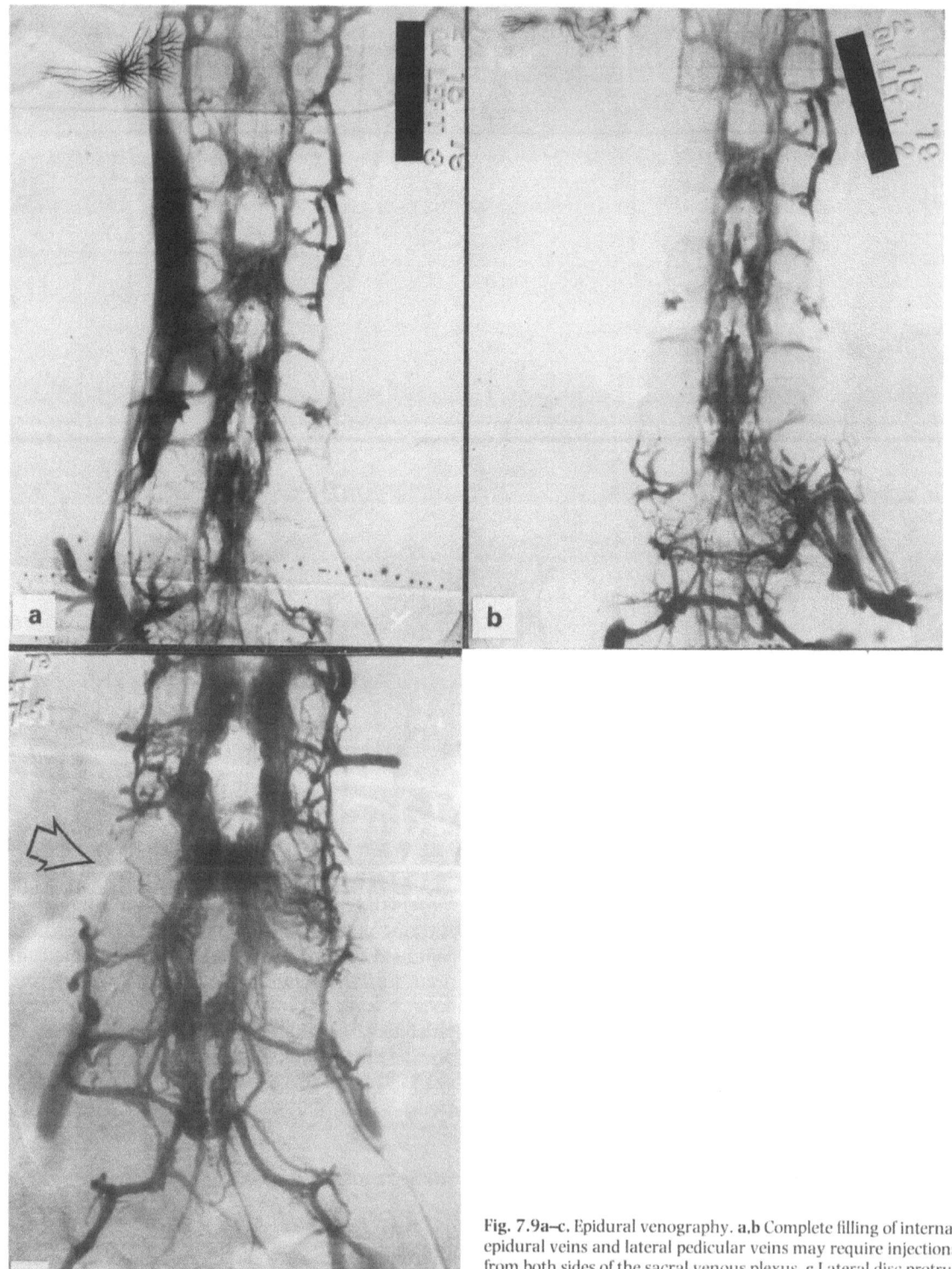

Fig. 7.9a–c. Epidural venography. **a,b** Complete filling of internal epidural veins and lateral pedicular veins may require injections from both sides of the sacral venous plexus. **c** Lateral disc protrusion prevents filling of the pedicular vein (*open arrow*) even though venous plexus above and below this site is opacified.

masses. To ensure that a vein is truly obstructed and not simply failing to opacify, all the adjacent veins must be carefully inspected (Fig. 7.9).

A lateral disc protrusion tends to obstruct both the medial and the lateral anterior internal vertebral veins at the interspace level. If a fragment is extruded into the neural canal, the pedicular (foraminal) veins may be compressed and occluded. Non-visualization of the pedicular veins alone, however, without associated anterior internal vertebral vein abnormalities may be a flow phenomenon. Other findings include collateral venous channels and dilated veins adjacent to the obstruction.

References

Aminoff MJ, Logue V (1974) The prognosis of patients with spinal vascular malformations. Brain 97:211–218

Anthony JE Jr (1958) Complications of aortography. Arch Surg 76:28–34

Bücheler E, Janson R (1973) Combined catheter venography of the lumbar venous system and the inferior vena cava. Br J Radiol 46:655–661

Di Chiro G, Doppman JL (1969) Differential angiographic features of haemangioblastomas and arteriovenous malformations of the spinal cord. Radiology 93:25–30

Djindjian R (1969) Arteriography of the spinal cord. AJR 107:461–478

Djindjian R (1975) Embolization of angiomas of the spinal cord. Surg Neurol 4:411–420

Doppman JL, Di Chiro G, Ommaya AK (1971) Percutaneous embolization of spinal cord arteriovenous malformations. J Neurosurg 34:48–55

Doppman JL, Di Chiro G, Oldfield EH (1985) Origin of spinal arteriovenous malformation and normal cord vasculature from a common segmental artery: angiographic and therapeutic considerations. Radiology 154:687–689

Efsen F (1966) Spinal cord lesion as a complication of abdominal aortography: report of four cases. Acta Radiol [Diagn] (Stockh) 4:47–61

Feigelson HH, Ravin HA (1965) Transverse myelitis following selective bronchial arteriography. Radiology 85:663–665

Gershater R, Holgate RC (1976) Lumbar epidural venography in the diagnosis of disc herniations. AJR 126:992–1002

Grossman LA, Kirtley JA (1958) Paraplegia after translumbar aortography. JAMA 166:1035–1037

Herdt JR, Shimkin PM, Ommaya AK, Di Chiro G (1972) Angiography of vascular intraspinal tumors. AJR 115:165–170

Houdart R, Djindjian R, Hurth M (1966) Vascular malformation of the spinal cord. The anatomic and therapeutic significance of arteriography. J Neurosurg 24:583–594

Killen DA, Foster JH (1960) Spinal cord injury as a complication of aortography. Ann Surg 152:211–230

Killen DA, Foster JH (1966) Spinal cord injury as a complication of contrast angiography. Surgery 59:969–981

LePage JR (1974) Transfemoral ascending lumbar catheterization of the epidural veins: exposition and technique. Radiology 111:337–339

McAfee JG (1957) A survey of complications of abdominal aortography. Radiology 68:825–838

Russell EJ, Berenstein A (1984) Neurologic applications of interventional radiology. Neurol Clin 2:873–902

Symon L, Kuyama H, Kendall B (1984) Dural arteriovenous malformations of the spine: clinical features and surgical results in 55 cases. Neurosurg 60:238–247

Yeates A, Drayer B, Heinz ER, Osborne D (1985) Intra-arterial digital subtraction angiography of the spinal cord. Radiology 155:387–390

8 Discography

J.T. Patton

History 107
Technique 109
    Mid-Line Approach 109
    Oblique Extra-Thecal Approaches 110
Radiological Appearances 110
    Normal Disc 110
    Disc Degeneration 111
    Disc Prolapse 112
Cervical Discography 112
    Technique 112
    Appearances 112
The Choice of Discography 113
    Indications for Discography 113
    Advantages of Discography 114
    Disadvantages of Discography 114
Current Status of Discography 114
References 114

History

Discography was first described by Lindblöm in 1948 in these words "Diagnostic disk puncture with injection of opaque medium demonstrates disk ruptures and protrusions and tells if the patient's symptoms originate from the punctured disk. The method seems to be of great practical value".

In the 40 years since then opinions have been fairly sharply divided about its practical use. Enthusiasts have regarded it as an essential investigation prior to disc surgery; others have been violently opposed on the grounds of (theoretical) damage to a normal disc consequent upon injection of a contrast medium of high osmolality (Gardner et al. 1952). In the days of myelography with iodized oil, workers such as Collis and Gardner (1962) "preferred lumbar discography rather than myelography in the routine radiological investigation of intervertebral disc disease".

With the advent of safer, water-soluble contrast agents the major objections to myelography have disappeared and there has been less incentive to perform discography. Nevertheless, the traditional investigation of disc disease by myelography, whatever the contrast agent, depends upon morphological changes in the disc causing distortion of the theca or root pockets. Other features such as instability at a particular level may or may not help in the assessment (Fig. 8.1), but unless there is thecal or root compression, myelography is unlikely to be of diagnostic help. Discography was the first investigation to give evidence of qualitative change in the disc; definite signs of degenerative disc disease were clearly evident on discography whether or not there was herniation or other morphological changes. In addition to the radiological appearances, other evidence was forthcoming from the response of the patient to any pain produced by the injection. A response similar to the patient's symptoms was regarded as further confirmation of a discogenic cause for symptoms (Collis and Gardner 1962). This type of observation forms part of what is nowadays known as Provocational Radiology (Park 1980).

In 1968, Wiley et al., in a series embracing 1092 patients at 2517 disc levels, established criteria for discography which remain true today. The point

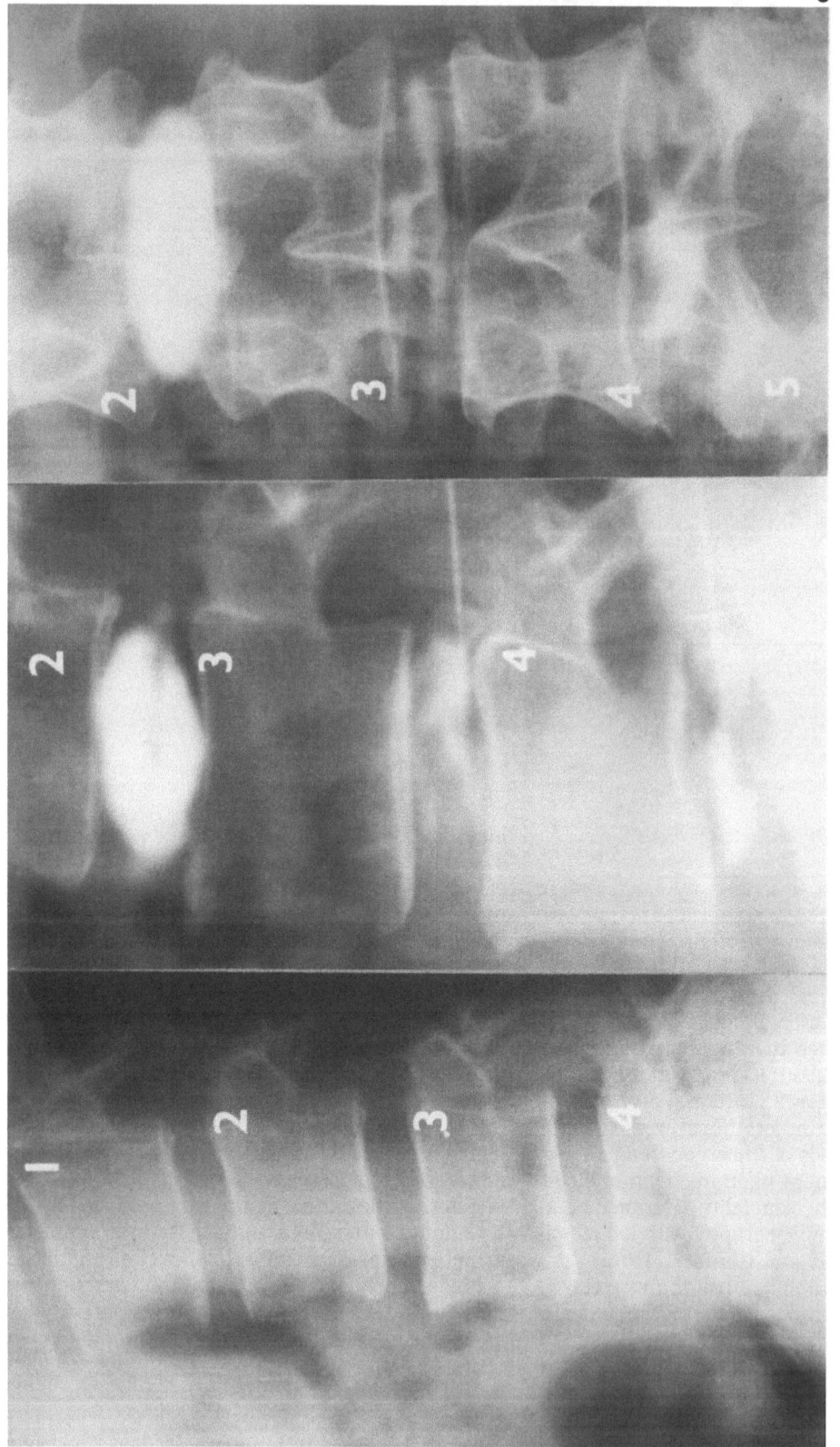

Fig. 8.1. a Hypermobility at L2/3 on flexion raised suspicion of disc disease at this level. **b,c** Subsequent discography revealed degenerative disc disease with bulging annulus at level below, where traction spurs are also present. The L2/3 nucleus is normal but of higher capacity and the disc space is wider than normal. These features are felt to indicate an "overworked" disc compensating for reduced movement at level below; hence the hypermobility on the flexion view.

was made that "where a diagnosis of disc herniation is made clinically, a myelogram/radiculogram rather than a discogram is advised if radiological confirmation is desired. Although myelography is highly accurate in disc herniation, if the prolapse is unusually far lateral, if the subarachnoid sac is short or narrow or if the sac is not applied closely to the back of the L5/S1 disc space, the herniation may not be visualized. In these cases discography is a valuable secondary procedure". Wiley et al. went to on to say that the chief value of discography is in the investigation of the patient with symptoms arising from disc degeneration without herniation and pointed out that in this group myelography is valueless.

The procedure also, of course, establishes whether symptoms are arising from more than one level, essential knowledge if spinal fusion is contemplated.

Technique

Early workers (Collis and Gardner 1962) devised a frame upon which the patient was placed in a flexed, prone position with the extremities fastened to the frame to prevent movement. Today most investigators simply place the patient on the X-ray table in the left lateral-decubitus position and the skin is surgically prepared and draped.

Mild sedation is useful to enhance muscle relaxation but deep sedation would interfere with the patient's response to injection.

There are three alternative approaches to the disc, one trans-thecal the others extra-thecal. By far the easiest method (used by the author) is the mid-line trans-thecal approach which has the advantage of enabling a specimen of CSF to be obtained *en route*.

Mid-line Approach

A 21-G needle is introduced through the interspinous ligament and, providing the patient is kept truly lateral and the needle horizontal, the only variable is cranial or caudal angulation of the needle which is checked by fluoroscopy with a standard under-couch X-ray tube. Once the needle has entered the dura, the direction of the tip cannot be altered so it is important to align the needle accurately with the disc space before entering the theca. If not, the needle must be withdrawn from the theca and re-directed. Cerebrospinal fluid may be collected while crossing the subarachnoid space

and providing the needle is introduced very slowly, free nerve roots are automatically displaced. If there is root entrapment, the advancing needle will cause sudden and severe referred pain and, therefore, it is essential that the spinal needle is advanced very slowly with great care.

When the resistance of the posterior annulus is encountered (and this is 2–3 mm posterior to where the beginner might expect) the stilette is removed and a 26-G needle 1.5 cm longer than its fellow is inserted through the spinal needle into the nucleus pulposus. In the normal disc the process so far is quite painless. Sometimes the patient experiences pain when the needle comes in contact with the annulus. This is variable in severity but is not as great as root irritation from which it obviously has to be distinguished. Such annular sensitivity is commonly encountered in what otherwise appears to be a normal disc and it has been suggested that this may result from overlap of segmental distribution from adjacent discs (Edgar and Nundy 1966, Wyke 1980). In annular sensitivity, the degree of pain response is variable but the patient is usually able to tolerate the insertion of the 26-G needle which would not be the case in nerve root entrapment.

The contrast medium of choice is meglumine iothalamate. The author uses Conray 130 but more dilute concentrations may be used. Injection is made using a 1-ml tuberculin syringe as the injection pressure required in an intact nucleus is high. The normal lumbar nucleus pulposus will accept up to about 1.0–1.2 ml of contrast medium, but usually 0.5 ml is sufficient to demonstrate normality. There is a theoretical possibility that excessively high pressure within the nucleus can create a plane of cleavage and induce degenerative change (Park 1980) and overfilling of a disc simply to improve the appearance of the radiographic record is to be avoided.

Jayson et al. (1973) investigated the bursting pressures required to rupture the annulus in cadaveric specimens and Quinnell and Stockdale (1980a) showed that by using a pressure transducer attached to a side tube, characteristic tracings would alert the operator to faulty injections around the nucleus. This technique arose from the discovery that the morphology of the nucleus is frequently complex and that quite commonly the needle tip is not within the cavity of the nucleus. The authors therefore recommended a needle with several additional side-holes near the tip (Quinnell and Stockdale 1980b).

In grossly degenerate discs, there is no feeling of rebound on releasing the plunger of the syringe and the sensation is little different from an intramuscular injection. The disc will easily accept 2 ml and

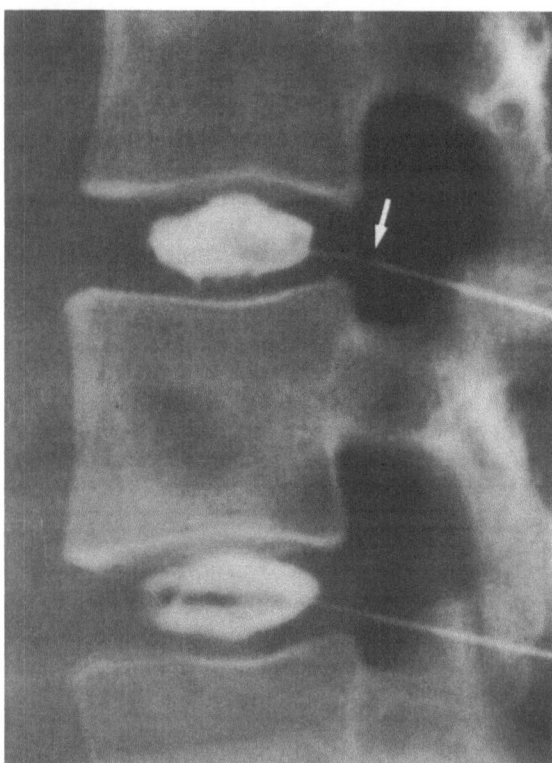

Fig. 8.2. Lumbar discogram. Note the bilocular nature of the nucleus pulposus and the position of the tip of the spinal needle (*arrow*) against the posterior annulus.

more of contrast medium which spreads throughout the disc space and is not confined to the area of the original nucleus.

Injection of the normal disc is usually painless but injection of the degenerate disc is painful, the degree of pain depending upon the integrity or otherwise of the annulus. If there is a prolapsed nucleus or a fissure in the annulus allowing escape of the contrast medium into the epidural space this will be more painful than if the contrast is contained within an intact, albeit bulging, annulus.

Symptom reproduction is variable and for detailed analysis the reader is referred to the work of Park (1980), Simmons and Segil (1975), Gardner et al. (1952) and Butt (1966).

Oblique Extra-Thecal Approaches

The postero-lateral and lateral oblique approaches enable the disc to be injected without crossing the subarachnoid space, the former through the extra-dural space of the spinal canal and the latter from a more lateral position between the transverse processes. Both methods eliminate the necessity of multiple perforations of the dura and are essential if it is intended to proceed to chemonucleolysis. They do, of course, preclude CSF sampling.

If the approach is to be made through the canal, the needle is inserted about 4 cm from the mid-line and advanced at an angle of 15° to the sagittal plane. The more lateral approach is made with the needle inserted about a hand's breadth (8–10 cm) from the mid-line and directed at an angle of between 45° to 60° depending upon the size of the patient. In both approaches the position of the needle tip is constantly monitored fluoroscopically.

In the lateral oblique approach, the L3/4 and L4/5 discs can frequently be entered through the same skin puncture (Park 1980) but entry into the lumbo-sacral disc can be difficult, particularly when the lumbo-sacral junction is set deeply within the pelvis.

The author usually leaves the needles in position when proceeding to subsequent levels. In this way, further saline injections may be made to compare pain responses and, if appropriate, steroid may be injected at certain levels as a therapeutic test immediately prior to removal of the needles.

In the author's experience, the theoretical objections to multiple dural puncture have not been encountered. In particular, post-operative headache has not been a feature which it still is post-myelography even with the non-ionic and low osmolar contrast agents. However, the approach has the serious disadvantage that it cannot be used in chemonucleolysis and anyone intending to commence discography may feel it preferrable to develop skill in the extra-thecal approaches.

Radiological Appearances

Normal Disc

The contrast medium is contained within the nucleus pulposus which in the upper four lumbar discs shows a bilocular appearance (Fig. 8.2). This feature is less common at the lumbo-sacral level where the nucleus frequently shows a simple discoid appearance; its variability is probably related, at least to some extent, to any degree of sacralization which may be present.

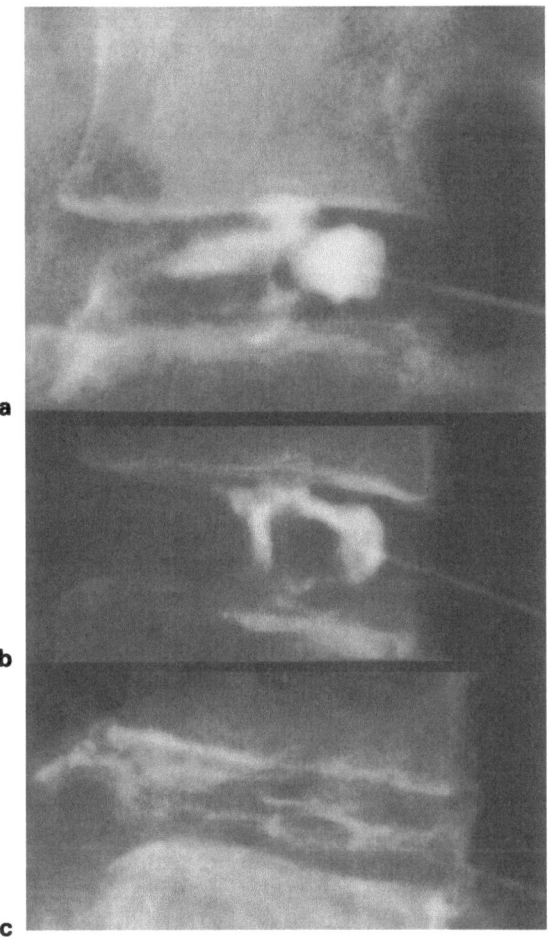

Fig. 8.3a–c. Lumbar discogram. Three levels in the patient shown in Fig. 8.2. **a** Schmorl's nodes superiorly and inferiorly at L3/4. **b** Partial filling of normal nucleus at L4/5. **c** Long-standing degenerative disease at lumbo-sacral level.

In the lateral projection, contrast medium does not normally extend into the anterior third or posterior fifth of the disc space (Fig. 8.2) nor extend lateral to the pedicles on the anterior view. It is interesting that the bilocular nature of the nucleus has been confirmed in magnetic resonance imaging.

Disc Degeneration

In long-standing disease, the disc space is probably already reduced, contrast medium diffuses quickly throughout the disc and the injection pressure is much reduced (Fig. 8.3). At an earlier stage, where the disc space may not yet be reduced, there is fre-

quently a fissured or "louvred" appearance, the contrast medium again dispersing throughout the region of both nucleus and annulus (Fig. 8.4).

Once the integrity of the nucleus is lost, the injection is accompanied by pain, usually quite severe, which persists after the injection is completed.

Distinction between normality and established degenerative change presents little problem. Difficulty may arise in recognizing early degenerative change and in determining whether or not the radiological appearances represent true herniation of nuclear material or simply extravasation through a fissure.

Early Changes – Annular Fissuring

The significance of fissuring of the posterior annulus without nuclear prolapse, especially in the adolescent and young adult, was emphasized by Brad-

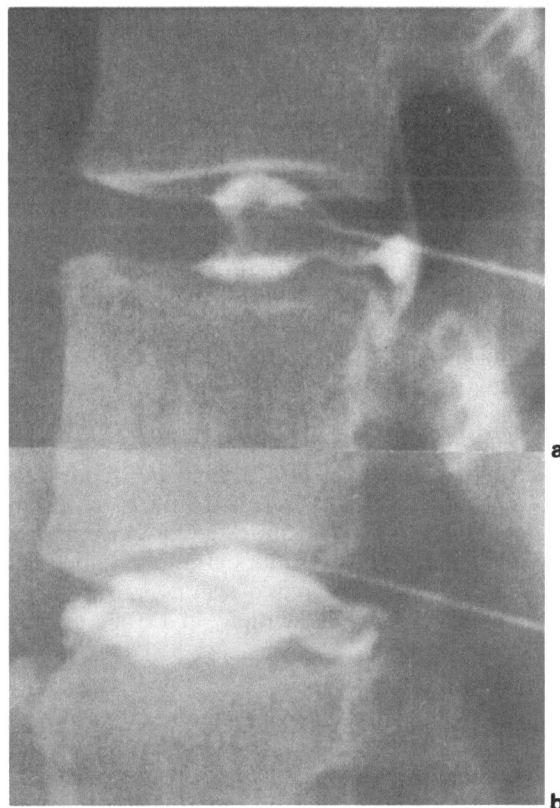

Fig. 8.4a,b. Lumbar discogram of the same patient shown in Fig. 8.2, to illustrate degenerative disc disease at an earlier stage. Two levels are illustrated. **a** Posterior annular fissure (AP view showed this to be lateral to the needle track). **b** The posterior annulus with a "louvred" appearance and bulging.

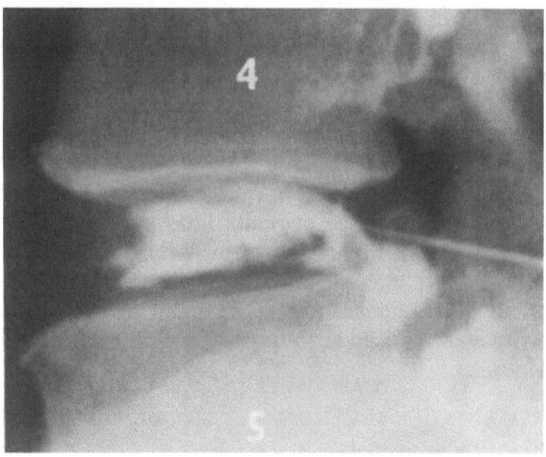

Fig. 8.5. Degenerative disease with disc prolapse. There is residual lipiodol above and below.

and does not diffuse as it does when extravasated through a fissure. While discography will demonstrate lesions of this nature, obviously they also will be well and more simply shown on myelography and certainly the trans-thecal approach to the disc is not advisable because of the risk of encountering trapped roots within a compressed cauda equina.

Intra-osseous (Schmorl's Nodes)

Defects of the vertebral end-plate from direct herniation of disc material into bone or as a result of damage to the growth plate in the latter years of growth (Hilton et al. 1976) will be confirmed on discography when contrast material will be seen to outline the herniated disc material (Fig. 8.3a).

ford and Garcia (1971). In this group the clinical picture is very suggestive of acute disc herniation but the absence of signs of root entrapment may inhibit the clinician from seeking an invasive investigation such as myelography or discography. The absence of morphological change makes myelography of no value, but discography shows a characteristic appearance in this condition (Park et al. 1979). The typical discographic appearance is of a normal or near-normal nucleus showing extravasation of contrast medium posteriorly through the fissure where it collects locally to produce a collar-stud appearance subsequently diffusing in the epidural space. In the example shown in Fig. 8.4a the diffusing contrast has outlined the posteriorly displaced dura raising the suspicion that there may already be some herniation of nucleus. The point is made by Park et al. (1979) that such fissures are rarely discernible at operation and in suspected cases, discography is an essential pre-operative investigation. Those authors also found good correlation between the areas of symptomatic pain and those provoked by discography in 12 of a series of 14 patients.

Disc Prolapse

Trans-annular

This may present as a localized bulge of the annulus (Fig. 8.4b) or as a sequestrated fragment (Fig. 8.5). In the latter, the contrast medium remains localized

Cervical Discography

In the author's experience, this examination has failed to fulfill earlier expectations and is nowadays rarely practised in the UK. Degenerative disc disease in the cervical spine is so common as to be almost universal in the elderly and in the symptomatic age group the demonstration of a degenerative disc is frequently offset by similar disease at adjacent levels. The provocational value is also limited since pain reproduction is usually poorly localized and frequently indistinguishable from pain at other levels.

Technique

An antero-lateral approach is made, under screen control, with a 21-G needle advanced under local anaesthetic between the carotid sheath and trachea (Smith and Nichols 1957). When the disc is reached, a 26-G needle is inserted through the outer needle about 0.75 cm into the disc space and 0.2–0.5 ml contrast medium injected.

Appearances

In the normal disc, an ovoid nucleus pulposus is outlined (Fig. 8.6); with continued pressure contrast medium will be seen to pass laterally into the neuro-central joints (Fig. 8.6). This always occurs in degenerative disc disease and usually occurs in the normal adult disc; in the young adult or juvenile

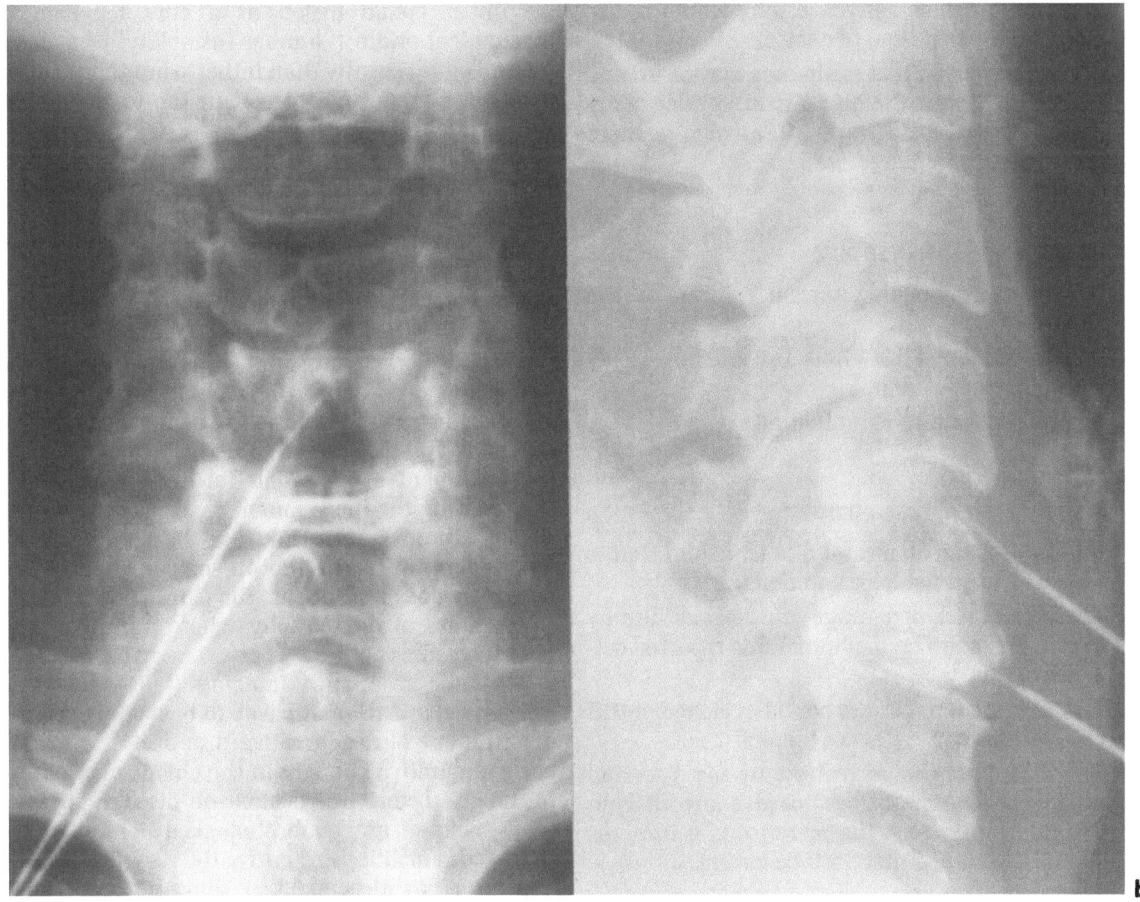

Fig. 8.6. Cervical discography. At C4/5 there is filling of the nucleus with lateral extension into the neuro-central joints without evidence of degenerative disease. At C5/6 the needle tip is not in the nucleus and contrast medium is shown surrounding the nucleus and again extending into the neuro-central joints.

such filling is accompanied by a distinct "give" of the syringe piston as though a passage (? false passage) has been opened by the pressure of the injection. This finding re-opens the old argument as to whether the neuro-central joints are true, genetically determined structures or simply adventitious arising from wear and tear after skeletal maturity (Payne and Spillane 1957).

The Choice of Discography

Indications for Discography

1. Where there is strong evidence of disc disease and this usually only after negative or equivocal myelography. It has no place in the diagnosis of back pain of unknown cause. Disc disease may include:
   a Suspected prolapse with negative myelography.
   b Degenerative disc disease.
   c Rupture of the annulus without prolapse.
2. As a preliminary to surgical treatment should the findings so indicate. It has no place in conservative management.
3. To determine the normality of the discs at levels adjacent to that of intended surgery.
4. Post-discectomy syndrome.

Contra-Indications to Discography

1. Clinical suspicion of a large disc protrusion where compression might be exacerbated. In

these circumstances myelography would be the standard investigation of choice.

2. Clinical suspicion that symptoms may be arising elsewhere than in the disc. Again, myelography and computed tomography (CT) would be more appropriate procedures.

Advantages of Discography

1. Demonstration of the normal as well as the abnormal disc.
2. Demonstration of the whole disc and not simply a posterior protrusion.
3. It is a very accurate examination.

Disadvantages of Discography

1. Injection of the abnormal disc is painful, but is an intrinsic part of the examination.
2. Theoretical risk of damage to a normal disc by needle and contrast medium. Little reported evidence of this.
3. Risk of infection. Little reported evidence of this or of serious consequences thereof.
4. The technique demonstrates only the disc, and unlike myelography, does not give any alternative information e.g. the presence of a tumour, should the clinical diagnosis be wrong.

Current Status of Discography

Opinions are still divided upon the value of provocational radiography. Whilst it is always encouraging to receive a definite, unprompted statement from the patient that the pain induced is identical to or very similar to the symptoms, in practice such information, in the author's experience, is rarely forthcoming. Much more commonly the patient will state that the pain is "similar to the symptoms but not quite the same".

In the cervical spine where, in the middle-aged, multiple level disease is common, symptom reproduction or something similar may occur at several levels, sometimes at variance with other clinical evidence of the probable level in question. As a result of this failure to distinguish between multiple level disease, whether by the patient response or radiological appearances, cervical discography is now rarely used as a preliminary to cervical fusion.

Lumbar spinal fusion as a cure for pain of mechanical origin ("lumbar instability") has been less in vogue recently than hitherto but there now is evidence of renewed interest in the technique. In those patients where myelography, with or without CT scanning, has proved unrewarding and yet there is still good clinical evidence of disc disease there is no doubt that discography can be of great help prior to fusion or discectomy, particularly in cases where the lumbo-sacral angle is acute with the theca sloping sharply away from the lumbo-sacral spine.

The indications for discography as presented by the earlier workers must now be re-appraised in the light of more recent imaging techniques. Current CT scanners have the resolution to demonstrate herniated disc material directly and to give evidence of encroachment of disc material upon epidural fat surrounding the theca and nerve roots as they pass through the foramina. However, the technique once again depends upon morphological change and obviously does not include the extra provocational information of discography where multiple levels are involved.

Magnetic resonance imaging (MRI), however, has proved in a dramatic way to be a very accurate determinant of degenerative disc disease showing early qualitative changes in the chemical structure of the disc before it is evident on discography and long before any morphological change has occurred. Facilities are currently very limited and expensive but it seems likely that as MRI becomes more widely available it must inevitably play an important part in the assessment of disc disease. Whilst it seems likely that MRI could eventually replace discography in the early diagnosis of degenerative disc disease, by its very nature it, too, cannot give the "provocational" information of discography.

Discography therefore, still has an important role in the pre-operative assessment of patients, particularly those without root involvement or where the surgeon wishes to avoid exploration of the disc.

References

Bradford DS, Garcia A (1971) Lumbar intervertebral disc herniations in children and adolescents. Orthop Clin North Am 2:583–592

Butt WP (1966) Discography – some interesting cases. J Can Assoc Radiol 17:167–175

Cloward RB, Buzaid LL (1952) Discography; technique, indications and evaluation of normal and abnormal intervertebral disc. AJR 68:552–564

Collis JS, Gardner WJ (1962) Lumbar discography – an analysis of 1000 cases. J Neurosurg 19:452–461

Edgar MA, Nundy S (1966) Innervation of the spinal dura mater. J Neurol Neurosurg Psychiatry 29:530–534

Erlacher PR (1952) Nucleography. J Bone Joint Surg [Br] 34:204–210

Gardner WJ, Wise RE, Hughes CR, O'Connell FB, Weiford EC (1952) The X-ray visualization of the intervertebral disc with a consideration of the morbidity of disc puncture. Arch Surg 64:355–364

Hilton RC, Ball J, Benn RT (1976) Vertebral end-plate lesions (Schmorl's nodes) in the dorsolumbar spine. Ann Rheum Dis 35:127–132

Jayson MIV, Herbert CM, Barks JS (1973) Intervertebral discs nuclear morphology and bursting pressures. Ann Rheum Dis 32:308–315

Keck C (1960) Discography, technique and interpretation. Arch Surg 80:580–585

Lindblöm K (1948) Diagnostic puncture of intervertebral discs in sciatica. Acta Orthop Scand 17:231–239

Massie WK, Stevens DB (1967) A critical evaluation of discography. J Bone Joint Surg [Am] 49:1243–1244

McCulloch JA, Waddell G (1978) Lateral lumbar discography. Br J Radiol 51:498–502

Park WM (1980) Radiological investigation of the intervertebral disc. In: Jayson MIV (ed) The lumbar spine and back pain, 2nd edn. Pitman Medical, Tunbridge Wells, pp 185–230

Park WM, McCall IW, O'Brien JP, Webb JK (1979) Fissuring of the posterior annulus fibrosus in the lumbar spine. Br J Radiol 52:382–387

Payne EE, Spillane JD (1957) Cervical spine: anatomico-pathological study of 70 specimens (using special techniques) with particular reference to the problem of cervical spondylosis. Brain 80:571–596

Powell MC, Wilson M, Szpryt P, Symonds EM, Worthington BS (1986) Prevalence of lumbar disc degeneration observed by magnetic resonance in symptomless women. Lancet II:1366–1367

Quinnel RC, Stockdale HR (1980a) Pressure standardised lumbar discography. Br J Radiol 53:1031–1036

Quinnel RC, Stockdale HR (1980b) An investigation of artefacts in lumbar discography. Br J Radiol 53:831–839

Simmons EH, Segil CM (1975) An evaluation of discography in the localisation of symptomatic levels in discogenic disease of the spine. Clin Orthop 108:57–69

Smith GW, Nichols P (1957) The technique of cervical discography. Radiology 68:718–720

Wiley JJ, MacNab I, Wortzman G (1968) Lumbar discography and its clinical applications. Can J Surg 11:280–289

Wyke B (1980) The neurology of low back pain. In: Jayson MIV (ed) The lumbar spine and back pain. Pitman Medical, Tunbridge Wells, pp 265–339

9 Facet Arthrography

I.W. McCall

Introduction 117
Technique 119
Clinical Studies 120
Conclusion 122
References 122

Introduction

Interest in the role of the posterior intervertebral joints as a source of back pain has undergone a revival in the last decade, but the original ideas date back to the early part of the century. The earliest writers implicated the facet joints as a cause of sciatica either in the form of a neuralgia from vertebral arthritis chiefly involving the articular facets (Putti 1927) or by creating nerve root pressure (Ghormley 1933). It was Badgley (1941) who suggested that irritation of the capsule of the lumbar facets could produce referred pain through the dermatome of the lumbar nerve roots by passage of the stimuli from the facets through the posterior primary ramus.

The concept of pain referral had already been defined by Kellgren (1939), who found that when the connective tissues in the posterior elements were stimulated, pain was perceived at a distance from the stimulus in patterns which he called sclerotomes. These differed from the dermatomes in both distribution and precision. Similar concepts were proposed by other authors, although the specificity of the pattern was not supported by some (Sinclair et al. 1948; Hockaday and Whitty 1967).

Experimental work using methylene blue (Hirsch et al. 1963) identified nerve endings in the facet capsule similar in nature to the annulus of the disc. These authors also injected hypertonic saline into the facets and disc area, which showed the latter to be more sensitive than the former and also that the pain referral from the facet was into the buttock and thigh. Injection into the posterior ligamentous structures did not give evidence of back pain. Mooney and Robertson (1976) rekindled interest in

the facets and showed that radiographically controlled injections of hypertonic saline into the joint produced referral pain in the low back, lateral or posterior thigh and sometimes the calf. There was no clear pattern to the referred pain and greater quantities of saline produced greater pain distribution.

Provocation studies, using radiographic control to allow precise positioning of small quantities of hypertonic saline, have shown that there is a significant overlap of pain referral from the facet joints as far apart as L1/2 and L4/5, but generally the more caudal the site of the injection, the more caudal was the referred pain. Furthermore, very similar pain patterns resulted from intracapsular injections and from those made into the pericapsular tissue. Pain referral from the joints did not cross the mid-line (Fig. 9.1) (McCall et al. 1979).

Anatomical studies of the posterior articular structures have revealed a profuse innervation which has considerable overlap of nerve supply. The posterior primary ramus at each segmental level forms the main nerve supply to the whole of the posterior elements. There is an ascending branch from each posterior primary ramus which passes to the facet of the segment above. The medial branch supplies the facet at the same level and also sends branches to multifidus, the interspinous ligaments and to the superior aspect of the facet below (Paris 1983). It is, therefore, not surprising that a significant overlap of the areas of pain referral exists when at least three different neurological segments are innervating each joint.

A second important anatomical factor with regard to facet arthrography is the juxtaposition of the nerve root and the dorsal root ganglion to the facet joint, its capsule and especially the ligamentum

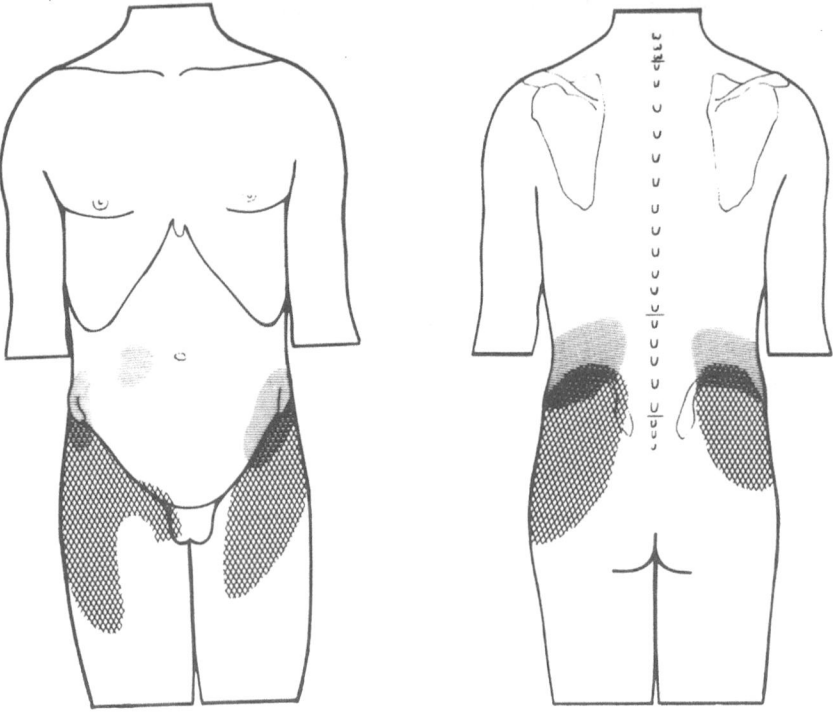

Fig. 9.1. The normal distribution of referred pain from the L1/2 (*hatched areas*) and L4/5 (*cross-hatched areas*) facet joints.

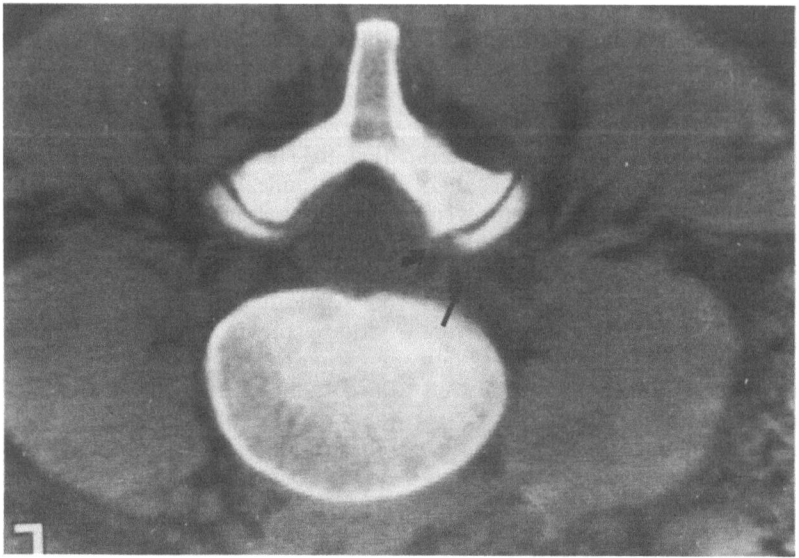

Fig. 9.2. Computed tomography. The ligamentum flavum (*short curved arrow*) is clearly demonstrated forming the anterior facet capsule. The nerve roots are shown within the foramen (*long straight arrow*) and are in close juxtaposition with the joint capsule.

flavum, which is extensively innervated (Fig. 9.2).

It is clear from this introduction that if facet arthrography is to be a precise diagnostic test, it has to be performed with a high degree of technical accuracy.

Technique

The injection is performed as an out-patient procedure without premedication. The patient is placed prone on an X-ray table; if the table top can rotate, this is an additional help. The patient is rotated until the articular surfaces of the facets to be injected are seen as a parallel line. The amount of rotation required will depend on the alignment of the facets. The lower lumbar facets tend to be more coronal in alignment and, therefore, a greater degree of rotation will be required. A small intradermal injection of local anaesthetic is made directly over the joint. A 22 gauge 3-inch spinal needle is inserted into the skin and passed perpendicularly downwards into the joint (Fig. 9.3).

At the L5/S1 level, where considerable rotation will have been necessary to see the joint lines, the posterior edge of the iliac crest may overlie the joint in some cases. In this situation the needle will encounter the bone of the crest if inserted perpendicularly and it must, therefore, be inserted nearer the mid-line and angled outwards down to the joint. The bone on either side of the joint may be struck, but usually the needle passes easily into the joint and a recognizable "give" will occur on perforation of the capsule. If there is a degree of degenerative disease, the passage of the needle through the capsule may not be felt. If the X-ray screen showed the needle against the joint, a small test injection of contrast will define the position of the tip. In patients with substantial osteoarthritis it may be impossible to perform the examination.

Once the needle is placed satisfactorily, contrast medium is injected to confirm the intra-articular position. The characteristics of the facet joint are similar to those of other diarthodial joints. The posterior aspect of the joint is covered by a fibrous layer holding the articular surfaces together while the capsule on the inner side is provided by the ligamentum flavum to which the synovium which lines the whole joint is relatively loosely attached (Fig. 9.2).

The anatomical extent of the facet capsule can be demonstrated by the injection of 1 ml of contrast medium, which identifies a large recess at either

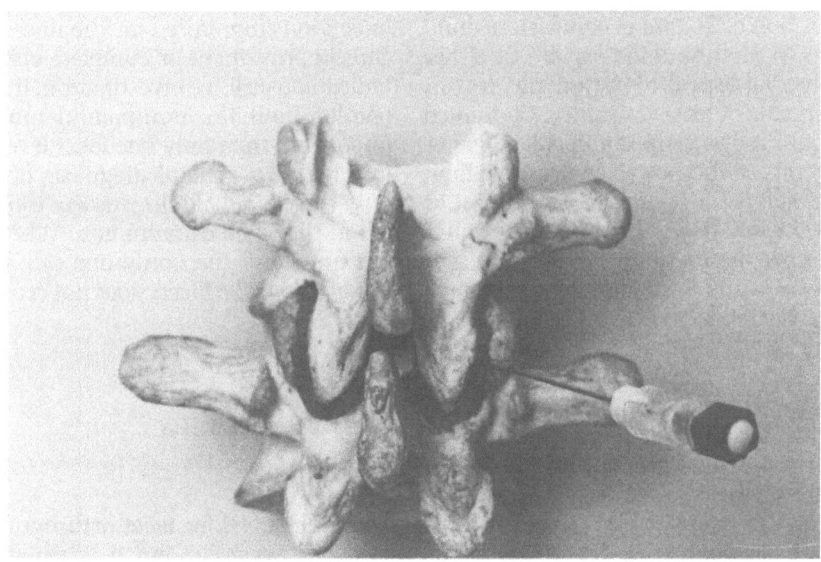

Fig. 9.3. Facet arthrography. The needle penetrates the joint capsule and contrast is injected into the joint. The amount of rotation required is dependent on the plane of the joints.

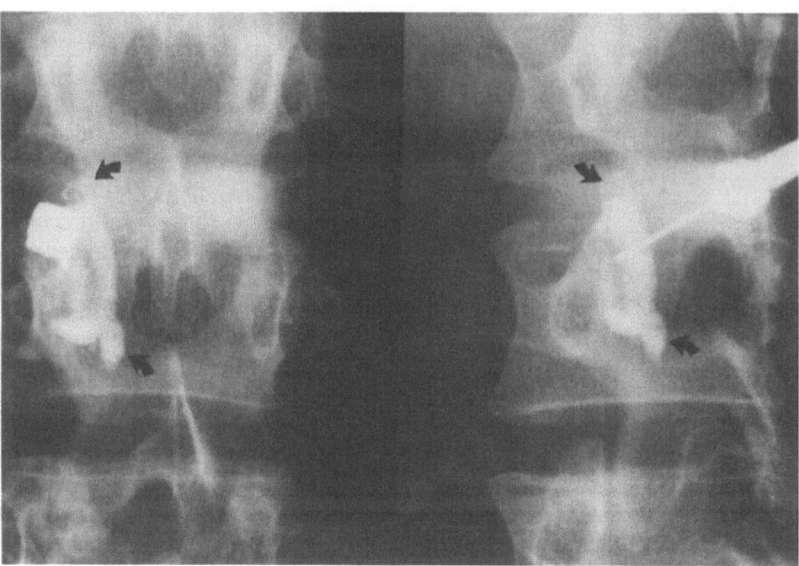

Fig. 9.4. Contrast outlines the extent of the facet capsule. The synovial recesses are identified at each pole of the joint (*arrows*).

extremity of the joint (Fig. 9.4). The inferior recess is always substantially larger than its superior counterpart. Diverticula have been demonstrated both superiorly and inferiorly and infrequently a meniscoid structure inserted between the facets near their superior portions has been noticed (Dory 1981). The injection of 2–3 ml of contrast medium frequently leads to rupture of the capsule at either the lateral or medial aspect of the inferior recess, which are the points of least resistance. Computed tomographic scanning performed immediately after injection of 2–3 ml of fluid showed contrast medium passing into the soft tissues posterior to the joint or into the epidural space (Dory 1981). The capsular capacity of the upper lumbar facets is less than that of the lower facets, with L5/S1 joint being the most capacious (McCall et al. 1979).

In view of the fact that extravasation may occur, the amount of contrast medium and local anaesthetic injected should be kept low. Between 0.1 and 0.2 ml of contrast is all that is usually required to confirm the intra-articular position of the needle. Full anatomical delineation of the facet is of no diagnostic assistance. Any pain that is produced at this point is recorded and compared with the patient's symptoms. The small quantity of contrast used is often insufficient to provoke a significant symptomatic response. Local anaesthetic (0.4 ml of 0.5% bupivacaine (Marcaine)) is then injected and after a short delay the needle is removed. The type of local anaesthetic is not fundamentally important. Some

authors use 1% or 2% lignocaine. The amount of lignocaine injected is kept constant at 0.4 ml and there is a theoretical advantage in injecting local anaesthetic of the higher percentage strength when only a small quantity is used.

The response of the patient's symptom to the injection is monitored for the next 4 hours. Significant improvement or complete obliteration of pain indicates a positive investigation. If separation of the painful from the non-painful motor segments is important, then only one facet level per day can be injected. If a general diagnosis of facet syndrome only is required, all three lower levels may be injected at the same examination. When the symptoms are unilateral then only one side need be injected as pain from the facets does not cross the mid-line.

Clinical Studies

The indications for facet arthrography are difficult to define precisely, but it is usually performed in patients who have low back pain, with or without leg pain, with no specific dermatomal sensory loss or motor weakness and in whom a disc prolapse and/or nerve root compression has been excluded. Relief of pain on a temporary basis has to be judged as a successful response to the injection and has been considered diagnostic of facet-originated pain. The accuracy of the examination is still unclear as it has usually been assessed in uncontrolled studies using broad patient groups.

This line of approach was initiated by Mooney and Robertson (1976) who studied 100 patients by injecting a mixture of local anaesthetic and steroids totalling between 3 and 6 ml into the facet joints at the lower three lumbar levels. Sixty-two patients obtained initial relief of their symptoms; 20 of these continued with complete relief at 6 months and a further 32 had partial longer-term relief of pain. Carrera (1980), applying the same principle, used between 2 and 4 ml of local anaesthetic and steroid mixture and reported initial relief of pain in 13 out of 20 patients with persistence of relief in 6. In a further report by the same author (Carrera and Williams 1984) 66% of 93 patients had initial relief with 25% recording persistent benefit. Similar percentages of around 50%–60% of patients experiencing initial relief have been reported by other authors (Destouet et al. 1982; Schroeder 1984). While these results would seem to suggest a high incidence of facet-induced pain in patients with non-dermatomal-type back and leg pain, there has been a notable lack of placebo controls and variability of symptoms has been considerable.

Proper assessment of the value of facet arthrography would be enhanced if subsequent longer-term treatment methods correlated with a positive arthrographic test. Unfortunately, assessment of the value of the technique has been bedevilled by a lack of a suitable standard against which it may be correlated. Longer-term treatment has centred predominantly around methods of denervation of the joints. Shealy (1975) used a system of soft tissue destruction by radiofrequency thermal effect and obtained instant relief in a number of patients. Other authors have also reported a satisfactory response with this method (Ignezi and Cummings 1980; Rashbaum 1983). Denervation may also be achieved by direct visualization via a surgical approach, freezing the nerve using a cryoprobe, or by the injection of phenol in the region of the nerves. The complex innervation of the facet joints makes complete denervation by these approaches almost impossible. Some reduction in the level of innervation may, however, decrease the excitatory threshold and thus lead to a temporary response.

The alternative treatment is immobilization of the motor segment by fusion. Unfortunately, while providing relief of pain in many cases, it also stabilizes the disc, thus severely limiting the treatment's specificity for judging the efficacy of facet arthrography.

Steroid injections alone have also been used. The form of injection must be seen purely as a therapeutic procedure in which the diagnostic component lies in the result of therapy. Eighty per cent of patients treated in one study had improvement of their symptoms for at least 3 days (Theron et al. 1983). Fairbank and colleagues (1981) have used an alternative approach by attempting to define the clinical features of the facet syndrome more precisely. These authors investigated a series of patients who had suffered their first significant and persistent attack of back or leg pain. The facet injections were performed under radiographic control as described above at the site of greatest tenderness. A randomly assigned control injection was also performed at a different level to exclude the non-specific effect of needle puncture and local anaesthetic. The patients were divided into two groups according to whether they experienced complete pain relief (a good response) or no relief (no response) after intra-articular injection of local anaesthetic. Statistically significant differing clinical features were identified between the two groups. The 54% of patients who responded to facet injections were found to have had a more acute onset of pain, often with a twisting or bending injury. They had less leg pain and the straight-leg-raising test produced back pain only. The pain was increased by sitting with forward flexion. Those who failed to respond to the injection had a more insidious onset of pain which was also made worse by standing. Straight-leg-raising in this group caused leg pain. Pain in extension was not found to discriminate between the two groups.

Support for some of these findings has been provided by other authors. Jackson and Craven (1984) also found pain and tenderness on hyperextension to be a poor predictor of success of facet injections. Schroeder (1984) found the results of injections were better when the history of pain was short. On the other hand, Lippitt (1984) in an uncontrolled retrospective survey which found a 42% response in 99 patients, suggested that symptoms of back and buttock pain were worse in the morning and with inactivity and that pain was exacerbated in hyperextension.

The specificity of facet arthrography as a diagnostic test is, in part, dependent on limiting the quantity of fluid injected into the joint. The capacity of the facet joint is limited and extravasation of local anaesthetic into the epidural space or surrounding soft tissues of the posterior elements will occur if excessive quantities of fluid are injected (Destouet et al. 1982). This fact has been stressed by Fairbank and others (1981), and Raymond and Dumas (1984), in a small study, suggested that the positive response to facet arthrography is substantially reduced from levels previously quoted by other authors if the total amount of local anaesthetic and contrast

122

medium is restricted to no more than 1 ml. These authors produced pain relief in only 1 patient out of 13 with uncomplicated chronic back pain using these limited quantities. Review of our own data on injections using small quantities of local anaesthetic indicates that in the chronic back pain group, rather than the acute group assessed by Fairbank and colleagues (1981), positive results from facet arthrography occurred in 25% of patients (I.W. McCall unpublished work, presented to the Society for Back Pain Research, Nottingham, March 1986).

The discrepancy in the results of these different series requires explanation. Many patients with chronic back pain have involvement of the whole motor segment with derangement of the disc associated with osteoarthritis of the facet joints, deformation of the spinal ligaments and muscle spasm. All of these features may be involved in pain production. It is, therefore, less likely that anaesthetizing only one part of the segment will relieve all symptoms. In some cases, however, osteoarthritis of the facet joints occurs without related disc damage (Lewin 1964), and capsular trauma or stress may be the main pathological process in others. In these cases, facet arthrography with small quantities of local anaesthetic will be diagnostic. The higher response in the younger age group with acute onset often associated with trauma (described by Fairbank and co-authors 1981) suggests that these cases may be due to trauma of the soft tissue of the joint. The lower incidence of response in chronic pain reflects the reduced number of patients with symptoms limited to the facets. When larger quantities of the local anaesthetic and steroid "cocktail" are injected, a larger area of tissue is anaesthetized, probably including the posterior primary ramus and possibly also the nerve root and sinu-vertebral nerve through epidural leakage. The patients responding may, therefore, include those with other pain sources in the motor segment.

Conclusion

Facet arthrography with small quantities of local anaesthetic provides a means of diagnosing those patients with a pain source localized to the facet. As yet there is no specific and completely reliable method of long-term conservative treatment to confirm the diagnosis. Intrafacetal and pericapsular injections of larger quantities of a local anaesthetic and steroids act as a vague method of pain localization and often provide temporary pain relief which, on occasion, may persist.

References

Badgley CE (1941) The articular facets in relationship to low back pain and sciatic radiation. J Bone Joint Surg [Am] 23:481–496

Carrera GF (1980) Lumbar facet joint injection in low back pain and sciatica: preliminary results. Radiology 137:665–667

Carrera GF, Williams AL (1984) Current concepts in evaluation of the lumbar facet joints. CRC Crit Rev Diagn Imaging 21:85–104

Destouet JM, Gilula LA, Murphy WA, Monsees B (1982) Lumbar facet joint injection: indication, technique, clinical correlation and preliminary results. Radiology 145:321–325

Dory MA (1981) Arthrography of the lumbar facet joints. Radiology 140:23–27

Fairbank JCT, Park WM, McCall IW, O'Brien JP (1981) Apophyseal injection of local anaesthetic as a diagnostic aid in primary low back pain syndromes. Spine 6:598–605

Ghormley RK (1933) Low back pain with special reference to the articular facets with presentation of an operative procedure. JAMA, 101:1773–1777

Hirsch C, Ingelmark BE, Miller M (1963) The anatomical basis for low back pain: studies on the presence of sensory nerve endings in ligamentous, capsular and intervertebral structures in the human lumbar spine. Acta Orthop Scand 33:1–17

Hockaday JM, Whitty CWN (1967) Patterns of referred pain in the normal subject. Brain 90:481–496

Ignezi RJ, Cummings TW (1980) A statistical analysis of percutaneous radiofrequency lesions in the treatment of chronic low back pain and sciatica. Pain 8:181–187

Jackson RP, Craven SD (1984) Facet joint injections in mechanical low back pain: a prospective statistical study. Orthop Trans 8:428

Kellgren JH (1939) On the distribution of pain arising from deep somatic structures with charts of segmental pain areas. Clin Sci 4:35–46

Lewin T (1964) Osteo-arthritis in the lumbar synovial joints. A morphological study. Acta Orthop Scand [Suppl] 73:1–112

Lippit AB (1984) The facet joint and its role in spine pain: management with facet joint injection. Spine 9:746–750

McCall IW, Park WM, O'Brien JP (1979) Induced pain referral from posterior lumbar elements in normal subjects. Spine 4:441–446

Mooney V, Robertson J (1976) The facet syndrome. Clin Orthop 115:149–156

Paris SV (1983) Anatomy as related to function and pain. Orthop Clin North Am 14:475–489

Putti V (1927) New conceptions in the pathogenesis of sciatic pain. Lancet II:53–60

Rashbaum RF (1983) Radiofrequency facet denervation: a treatment alternative in refractory low back pain with or without leg pain. Orthop Clin North Am 14:569–575

Raymond J, Dumas JM (1984) Intra-articular facet block: diagnostic test or therapeutic procedure. Radiology 151:333–336

Shealy CN (1975) Percutaneous radiofrequency denervation of spinal facets: treatment for chronic back pain and sciatica. J Neurosurg 43:448–451

Schroeder WF (1984) Facet arthropathy: diagnosis and treatment. Orthop Trans 8:439–440

Sinclair DC, Feindel WH, Weddell G, Falconer MA (1948) The intervertebral ligaments as a source of segmental pain. J Bone Joint Surg [Br] 30:515–521

Theron J, Blais M, Casasco A et al. (1983) Therapeutic radiology of the lumbar spine. Disc chemonucleolysis infiltration and coagulation of posterior articulations. J Neuroradiol 10:209–230

10 Computed Tomography

W. St. C. Forbes

Technical Aspects 123
    Advantages 123
    Disadvantages 124
CT Methods 124
    General 124
    Use of Intravenous Contrast Media 124
Clinical Applications 124
    Spine 124
    CT in Musculoskeletal Tumours 135
    Musculoskeletal Infection 139
    Joint Disease 140
    Miscellaneous Uses 141
    Quantitative Bone Mineral Analysis 141
Future Developments 142
Conclusion 142
References 142

Technical Aspects

Modern computed tomography (CT) scanners employ collimated fan beams directed only at the layer under investigation. The transmitted radiation is detected by arrays of scintillation or ionization detectors. The rotate/rotate principle is employed. In the third-generation scanner a rotating X-ray tube and rotating detector array is used; the fourth-generation scanner uses a fixed ring of detectors with the X-ray source within the ring.

Advantages

The technical developments of modern CT scanners have resulted in shorter scan times, improved collimation leading to thin sections (1 mm or less), faster data acquisition, shorter reconstruction times per section, a high repetition rate of scanning due to improvements in X-ray tube technology, improved spatial resolution and an extended dynamic range (-1000 to $+4000$ Hounsfield Units (HU)). These developments have had a significant impact on patient handling and have resulted in improved diagnostic capability in the musculo-skeletal system. The advantages of third and fourth generation CT scanners are:

1. The scout projection radiographic facility ("scannogram") enables accurate anatomical registration and reproducibility of the sections with important implications for examinations of the spine (Fig. 10.1).
2. Easier patient positioning permits transaxial, direct coronal and direct sagittal scanning.
3. The data obtained in the thin contiguous sections allow reconstruction in additional planes (coronal, sagittal, oblique), and with developments in soft-ware enables 3-dimensional reconstructions (3DCT) of bony structures.
4. Rapid sequence scanning of up to 30 sections in rapid sequence permits dynamic scanning and can provide information about the blood supply to normal or abnormal vascular structures.
5. The introduction of predetermined scanning protocols, with standardization of technique, lessens the likelihood of operator error.
6. CT guided biopsy techniques can be introduced.

Assessment of bone detail has been improved by the spatial resolution of modern rotate/rotate scanners with picture element (pixel) size as low as 0.5 mm × 0.5 mm. Furthermore, density discrimination of 1 part in 1000 may be obtained allowing visualization of some of the contents of the spinal canal. Use of a limited field of view, bone filters and the extended dynamic range of modern scanners provides very detailed information which has resulted in improved diagnosis of musculoskeletal disorders.

Disadvantages

Tissue Characterization

Despite its ability to discriminate among small differences in density, simple analysis of attenuation values does not permit precise histological characterization except when calcium (high density), or fat (low density), is present.

Partial Volume Effects

The tissue contained within the small volume (voxel) examined, is unlikely to be homogeneous in composition. The measured Hounsfield unit (HU), is an average of the different components of the tissue within a voxel. This "partial volume effect" becomes especially important when normal and pathological processes interface within a section. The boundaries of the abnormality, therefore, may be difficult to define with accuracy.

Radiation Dose

An average skin dose of 1 rad may be obtained on some systems. All modern CT scanners allow the operator to adjust the dose level and image quality. Contiguous and overlapping sections result in higher doses than non-contiguous sections. High resolution sections carry a higher dose penalty. Multi-planar reconstructions should be used in preference to direct scanning in planes other than the transaxial to reduce the radiation dose.

Movement

Any movement will produce artefacts which degrade the image quality even with the short scanning times of modern scanners.

Reproducibility

Precise positioning and accurate reproducibility of thin sections presents significant problems despite the scout-view facility. Careful external marking and a precise numbering code are helpful with follow-up examinations.

CT Methods

General

Thin sections in the transaxial plane as determined from the "scannogram" are used for imaging a defined area where detailed information is required. Multi-planar reconstructions can be obtained allowing more accurate visualization of the area being studied. Thick sections, usually 10 mm, with wider spacing, are used to sample a larger anatomical area, for example in the assessment of lymph node spread, diffuse skeletal metastases or intrapulmonary metastases.

Use of Intravenous Contrast Media

Administration of iodinated contrast media into the vascular system will raise the attenuation value of blood by 20–30 HU per mg/ml at 120 kVp. A rapid series of scans can be obtained using the dynamic scanning facility following a large bolus injection of contrast medium (Angio CT). The technique of dynamic sequential scanning requires a rapid series of scans at the same level. In dynamic incremental scanning, scans are performed at contiguous levels during a slower infusion (Isherwood et al. 1987).

Clinical Applications

Spine

Two methods of examination are applied to the investigation of Low Back Pain Syndrome and sciatica.

1. The more widely used method employs a series of angled sections parallel to the intervertebral disc (as determined from the scout view) starting through the lower part of the pedicle of the vertebra

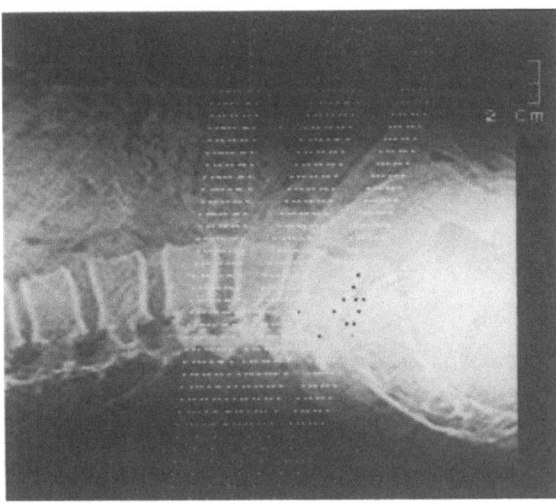

Fig. 10.1. Reconstructed digital radiograph ("scannogram"). The sections are obtained parallel to the vertebral end plates.

above and ending at the upper one third of the adjacent vertebral body (Buirski 1987, Fig. 10.1). This method excludes any distortion of normal anatomical structures but has the disadvantage that the whole area of the spine may not be covered, and free disc fragments may be missed.

2. A series of contiguous sections from the midpoint of the pedicle of L3 to the upper part of S1 without adjusting the gantry. This involves additional sections but has the advantage of providing a more comprehensive examination and allowing multi-planar reconstruction. Opinion regarding the value of reconstructed images is divided. Most radiologists rely on their assessment of transaxial sections only, resorting to reconstructed sagittal or coronal sections in difficult cases, or for accurate preoperative assessment of a longitudinal dimension.

Unenhanced transaxial sections are used in the assessment of prolapsed intervertebral discs, spinal stenosis, and facet joint disease. The more complex cases, e.g. spinal tumour, trauma, inflammatory masses may require the use of intra-thecal or intravenous contrast and reconstructions.

CT Myelography (CTM). Non-ionic water-soluble contrast agents achieve a uniform concentration in the cerebrospinal fluid, thereby increasing the sensitivity of CT to resolve the contents of the spinal canal. Either a low-dose technique using isotonic contrast media to enhance the contrast resolution

of the thecal sac using CT only or a high-dose technique combining conventional myelography with CT for anatomical localization, may be used.

Lumbar Disc Disease

The normal intervertebral disc exhibits homogeneous high density (80–110 HU). This is greater than the adjacent thecal sac or epidural fat which defines the posterior margin of the disc (Fig. 10.2). High resolution CT is a more accurate method for detecting the presence of a prolapsed intervertebral disc (Teplick and Haskin 1983). The herniated disc is seen as a smooth focal protrusion of the disc margin, continuous with the posterior annulus, lying beneath the posterior longitudinal ligament and displacing the epidural fat (Fig. 10.3, Williams et al. 1980). With large prolapses the epidural fat in the anterior and lateral portions of the canal and exit foramen will be replaced by the disc material.

A detection rate of 92% is achieved whereas myelography is positive in 80%–90%. Myelographic false-negative results are caused by lumbo-sacral and lateral disc protrusions. These cases may be successfully examined by CT. False-positive CT results are caused by the bulging annulus and the "pseudodisc" due to rotation or spondylolisthesis (Fig. 10.4). A false-negative CT usually results from interpretive errors or inadequate technique.

Compression of the thecal sac is seen in all but the most lateral disc prolapse and nerve root displacement can often be seen in the lateral recess (Fig. 10.3c). Prolapsed cervical discs are more difficult to identify. CT will detect a lateral disc protrusion in which myelography is normal with the disc material lying outside the canal either in the exit foramen or beyond it (Williams et al. 1982b). In some cases the lateral protrusion may be indistinguishable from a swollen root ganglion. Other atypical CT features of a prolapsed disc may be produced by calcification within a protruded nucleus pulposus (Fig. 10.3d, Teplick and Haskin 1983). This may simulate a posterior osteophyte especially when it arises close to the annulus. Atypical features may also be produced by a large isodense disc fragment if it completely fills the canal. Large extensions of protruded discs above or below the interspace and loose disc fragments are readily detected on CT providing the technique includes multiple contiguous sections above and below the interspace. Loose fragments may not be detected at myelography. A bulging annulus may be indistinguishable from a central disc protrusion (Fig. 10.5).

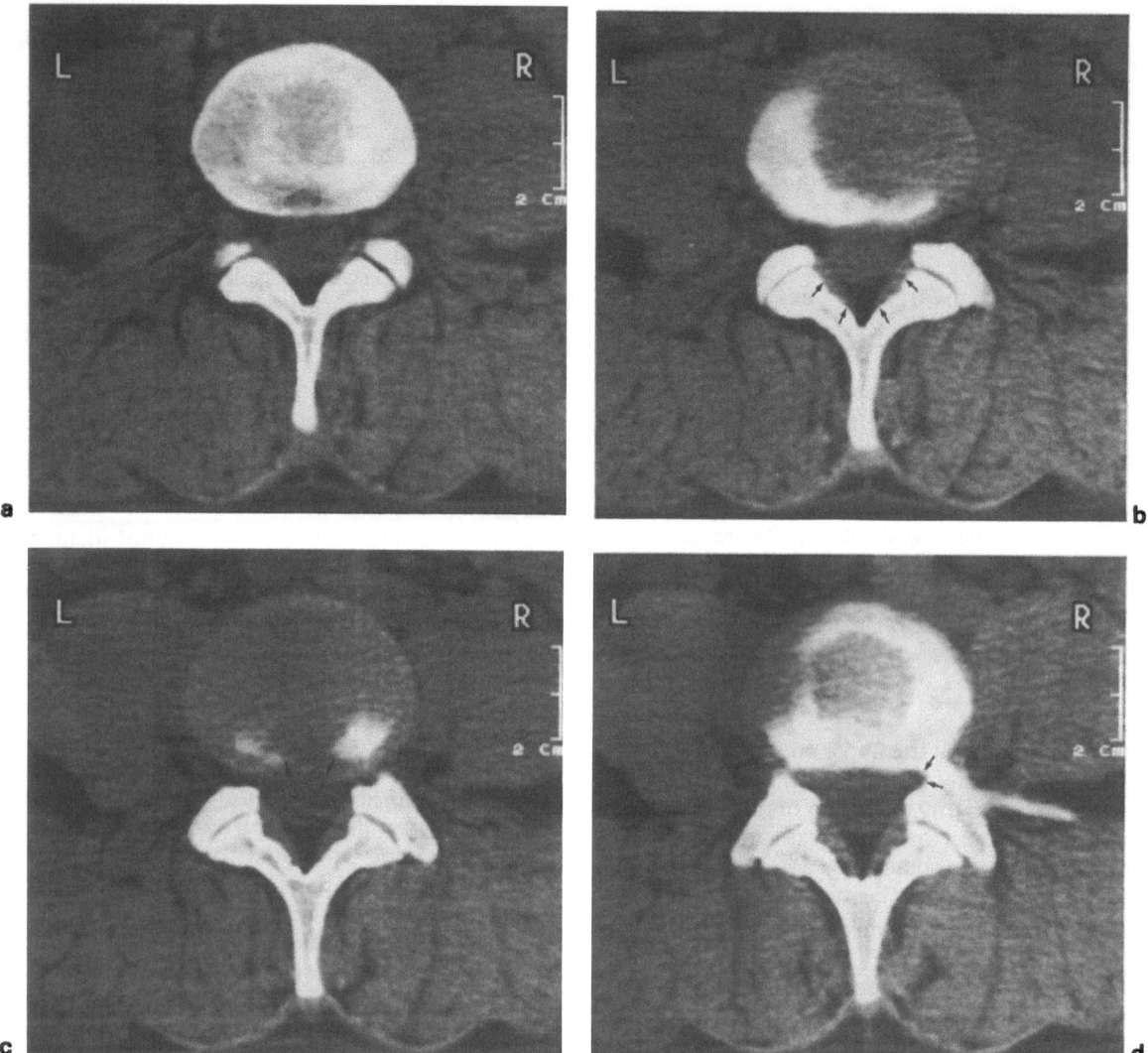

Fig. 10.2a–d. Normal anatomy. a Lower part of vertebral body. Nerve root ganglia in the neural exit foramina (*arrow*). b Lower end plate. Ligamenta flava form the posterior margins of the spinal canal (*arrows*). c Intervertebral disc. The disc annulus is seen anterior to the theca (*arrows*). d Upper end plate showing the lateral recesses of the bony spinal canal (*arrows*).

Myelography is not indicated in those cases where CT is unequivocally normal or abnormal, unless the clinical findings are inconsistent with the CT findings, but is indicated if CT is equivocal (Teplick and Haskin 1983).

CT has an additional advantage in the management of back pain syndrome of detecting unusual causes of root pain. Tumours of the nerve roots or root ganglia which do not compress the theca or root sheath will be missed on conventional myelography (Fig. 10.6a).

Bulging Annulus

The outward bulging of the intact degenerative disc margin beyond the adjacent vertebral body margin is readily identified on CT. The bulging annulus is usually symmetrical and most develop a convex posterior margin (Fig. 10.5). Asymmetrical bulging may be seen in patients with scoliosis. Bulging annuli frequently contain calcification and/or gas. CT, however, underestimates the severity of the degenerative change within the nucleus and

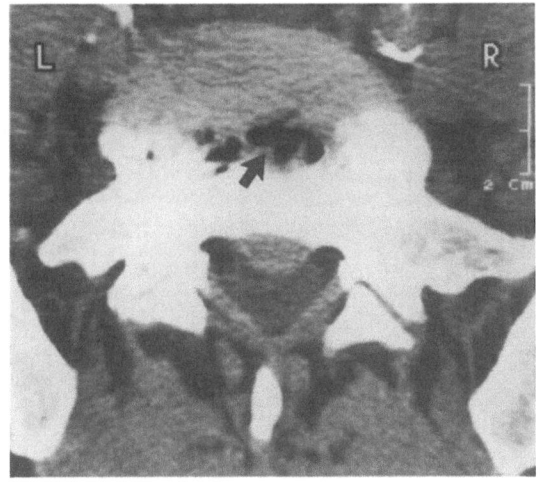

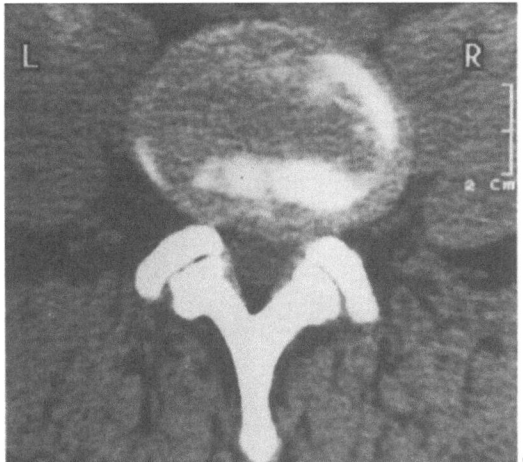

Fig. 10.3a–e. Prolapsed intervertebral disc. a Central posterior protrusion. The anterior epidural fat is obliterated. Note vacuum phenomenon in the nucleus (*arrow*). b Postero-lateral protrusion. The prolapsed disc material extends into the neural exit foramen. c Lateral. Recurrent disc protrusion. Disc material in the lateral recess. d Postero-lateral protrusion L2/3. Myelo CT. Small disc impression on the opacified theca extending into the lateral recess. e Calcified postero-lateral prolapsed disc L5/S1.

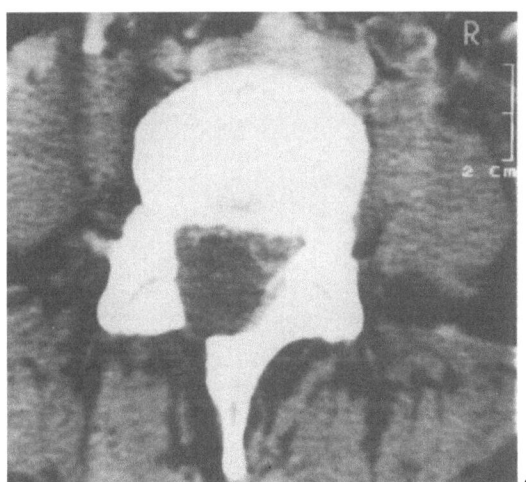

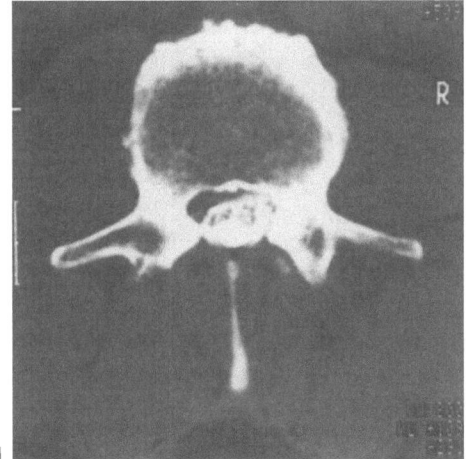

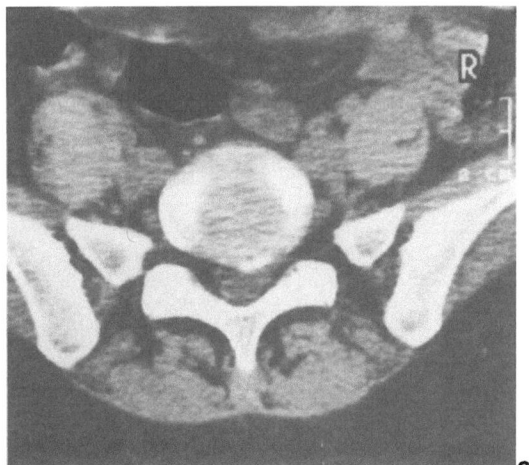

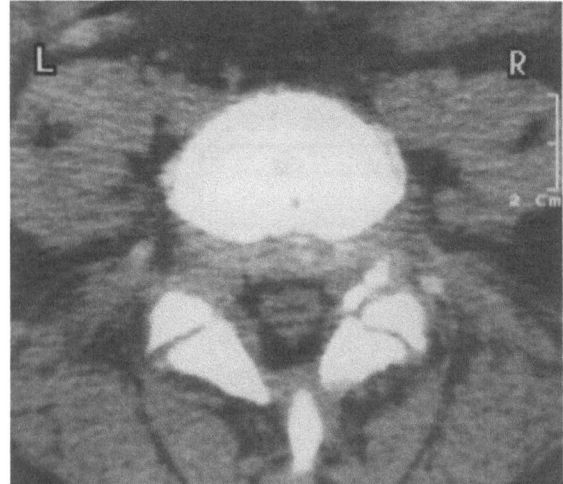

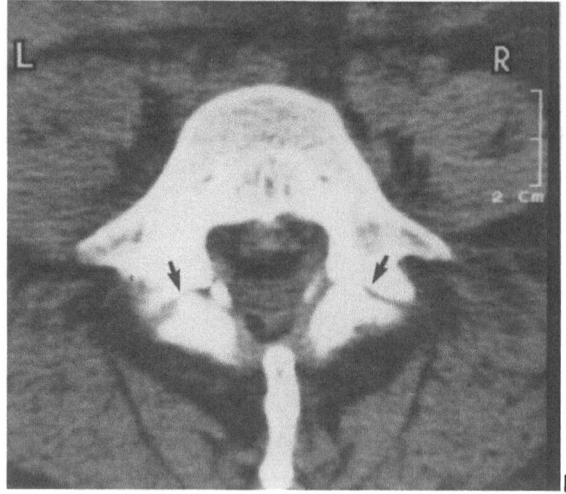

Fig. 10.4a,b (*above, left and right*). Spondylolisthesis L5/S1. a "Pseudodisc" due to uncovered intervertebral cartilage. b Defect in the pars interarticularis (*arrow*).

Fig. 10.5 (*left*). Bulging annulus L4/5. The disc margin extends beyond the vertebral end plate.

Fig. 10.6a,b (*below, left and right*). Neurofibroma L1/2. The tumour of the nerve root ganglion is shown as a well-defined mass of reduced attenuation within and extending outside the exit foramen (*arrow*). (Normal radiculogram.)

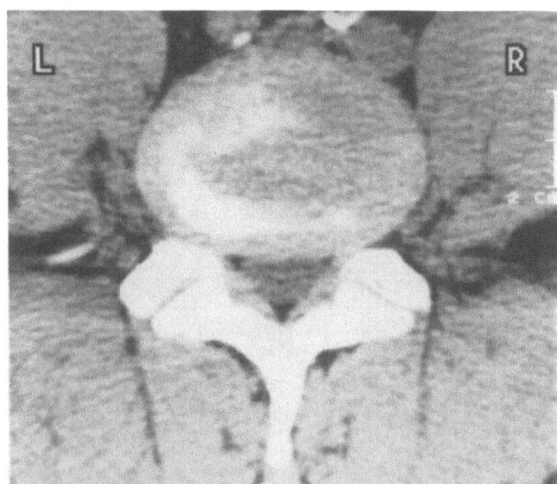

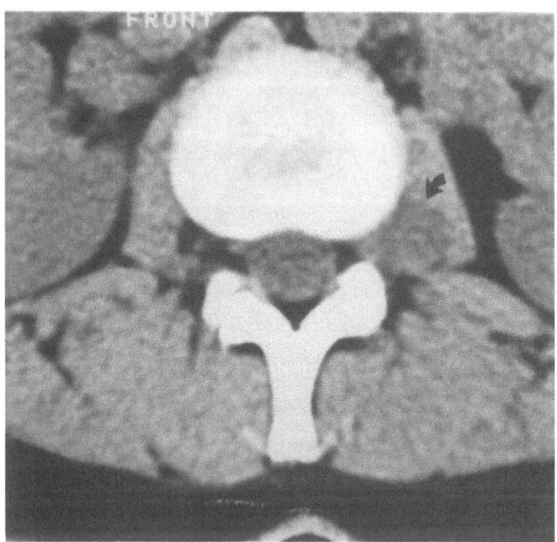

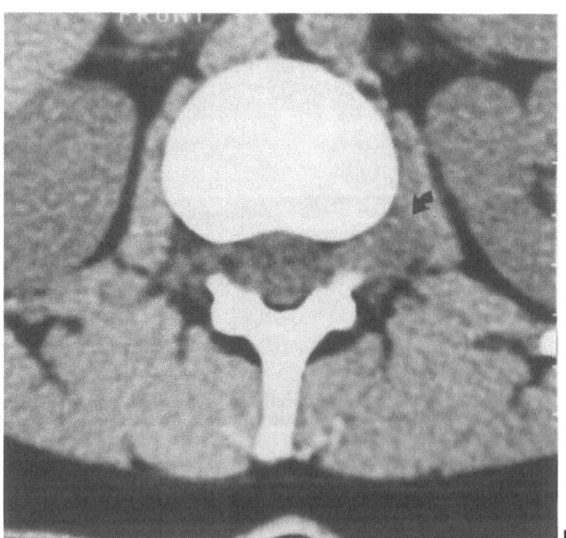

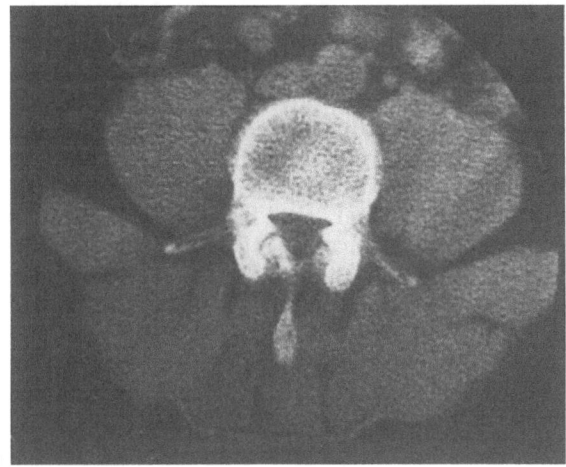

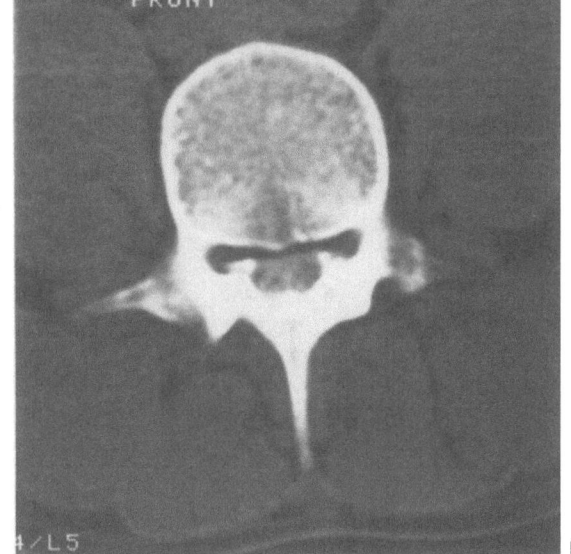

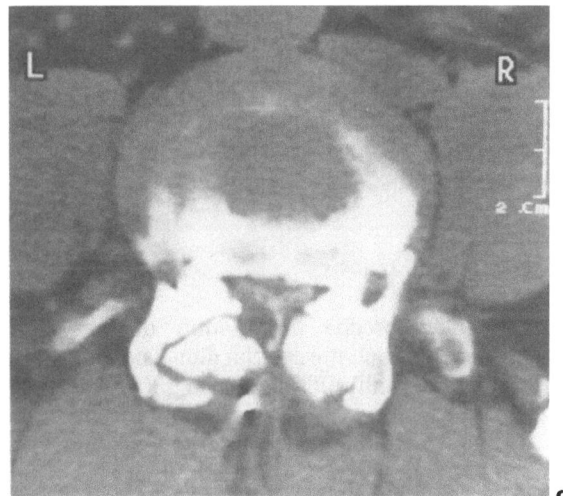

Fig. 10.7a–c (*above, left and right, and centre of page*). Congenital spinal canal stenosis. a Plain CT. Note short pedicles, hypertrophied facet joints, narrowed lateral recesses. b CTM. Severe narrowing of the sagittal and transverse diameter of the canal. c CTM. Congenital stenosis at L4/5 with severe degenerative disease in the facet joints. Previous laminectomy.

Fig. 10.8a,b (*below, left and right*). Acquired canal stenosis. a Lumbar. Grossly hypertrophied facet joints and "trefoil" canal. b Cervical CTM. Severe cord compression secondary to hypertrophied facet joints.

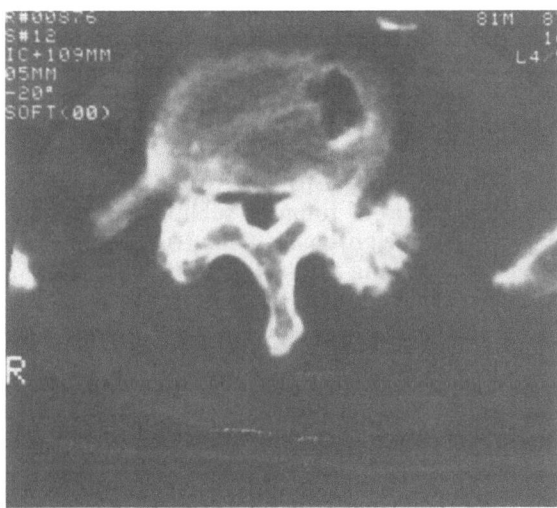

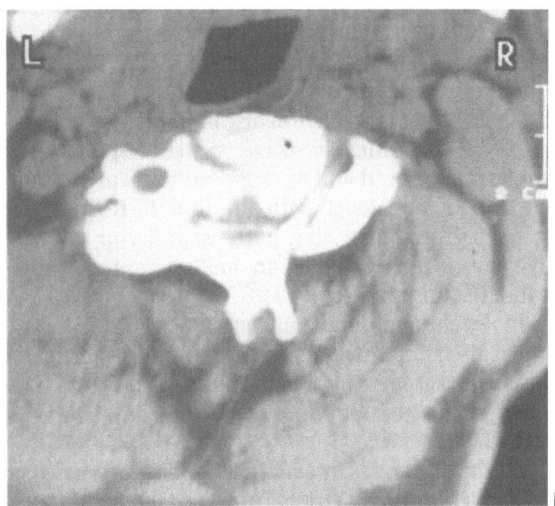

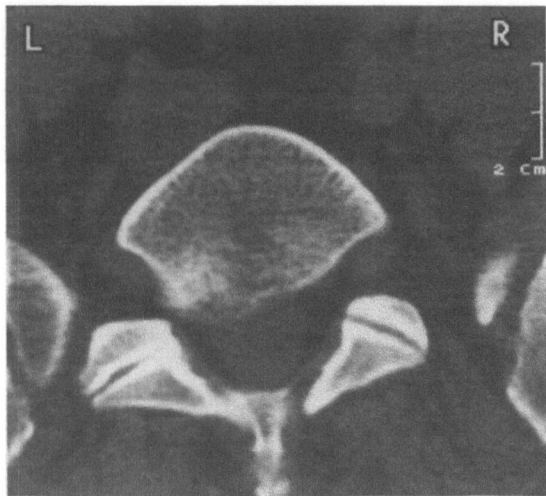

Fig. 10.9. Neural foraminal stenosis. Severe unilateral stenosis due to large postero-lateral marginal osteophyte.

annulus (Williams et al. 1982a). Above L5/S1, diffusely bulging annuli deform the anterior theca symmetrically and displace the epidural fat antero-laterally.

Spinal Canal Stenosis

CT provides precise information of the canal diameters of which the sagittal dimension is critical (11.5 mm is small) (Ullrich et al. 1980). The cross-sectional area can be measured; values less than 1.45 cm² are abnormal. Measurements must be made with the plane of the section parallel to the end plates. Information on the shape of the canal is provided. Subjective assessment of the dimensions and shape of the canal, however, are probably as accurate as direct measurement.

The appearances of the soft tissue structures, particularly the intervertebral disc and ligamenta flava, must be examined as these structures affect the shape of the canal and its cross-sectional area. Comparison of one level with another is helpful. An important ancillary sign is the scarcity or absence of epidural fat which is an indicator of a "tight" canal (Helms and Vogler 1982).

In developmental canal stenosis, both the central and sub-articular canals are stenosed (Fig. 10.7). The pedicles are short and enlarged, and the articular pillars and laminae may be massive (Dorwart et al. 1983).

Acquired canal stenosis due to marginal vertebral osteophytes and hypertrophy of the facet joints leads

to severe narrowing of the central and sub-articular canals (Fig. 10.8). The stenosis in these cases usually extends into the exit foramina (Fig. 10.9). Ligamentous hypertrophy and bulging disc annuli often accompany these osseous changes, and produce further narrowing of the canals with nerve root compression in the exit foramina and lateral recesses. The central canal in these cases assumes a "trefoil" appearance (Fig. 10.8a).

Less commonly, the soft tissue degenerative changes of a bulging annulus and hypertrophied ligaments produce the stenotic canal without stenosis of the bony spinal canal (Helms and Vogler 1982). Calcification may be seen within the hypertrophied ligaments.

Spondylolysis and Spondylolisthesis

The intervertebral cartilage that extends from the posterior edge of the forwardly displaced L5 body to the posterior edge of S1 gives rise to the "pseudodisc" appearance which is characteristic of spondylolisthesis (Fig. 10.4).

Canal stenosis occurs in spondylolysis without spondylolisthesis due to thickening of the pars interarticularis by masses of fibrocartilage which bridge the defect and encroach on the sub-articular canal (Heithoff 1982).

Spinal Trauma

CT has a major role in the assessment of both acute and late stages (Chap. 20). In the acute stage, CT is used in the assessment of fractures of the vertebral bodies and appendages, particularly in those patients with neurological deficit (Post and Green 1983). Its importance lies in the detection of fractures and assessment of displacement of the fragments. The degree of stenosis caused by the displaced fragments can also be accurately assessed on the axial sections and the multi-planar reconstructions (Figs. 10.10, 10.11). Facet distraction, the effects of rotatory subluxation and the presence of foreign bodies (Fig. 10.12) are easily detected. Following surgical correction the position of the fragments and surgical implants, clearance of the loose fragments and detection of un-united fractures are readily assessed.

Sagittal reconstructions may be required to assess the degree of canal stenosis in the acute or late stages and to define accurately the position of loose fragments within the spinal canal. Sagittal reconstructions may detect horizontal fractures and

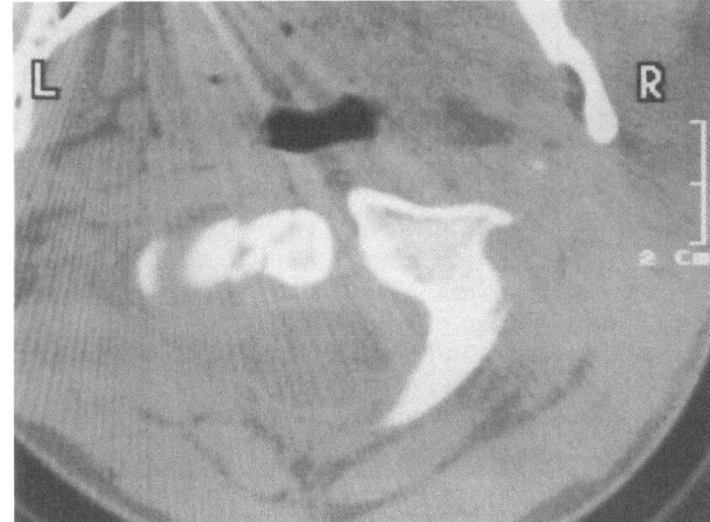

Fig. 10.10a–d. Fracture dislocation of C1 and C2. **a** Transaxial section. Oblique fracture through odontoid peg. **b** Coronal reconstruction. Odontoid peg. **c** Sagittal reconstruction. Odontoid peg. **d** Transaxial section. Oblique fractures through the vertebral body with displacement (*arrow*) and through the neural arch.

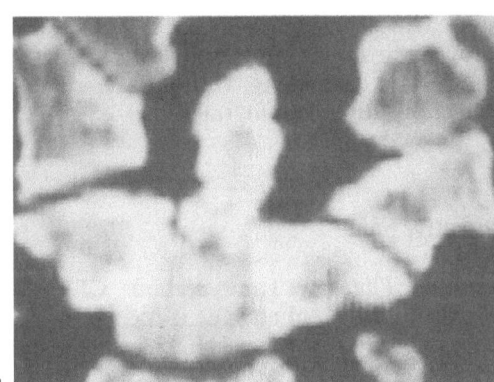

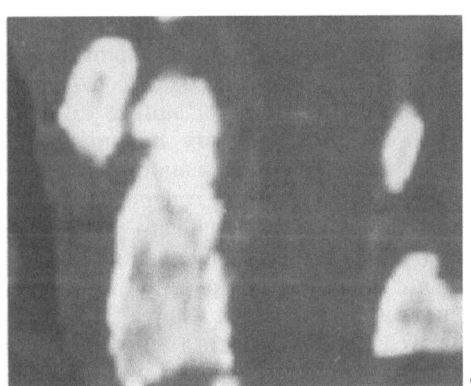

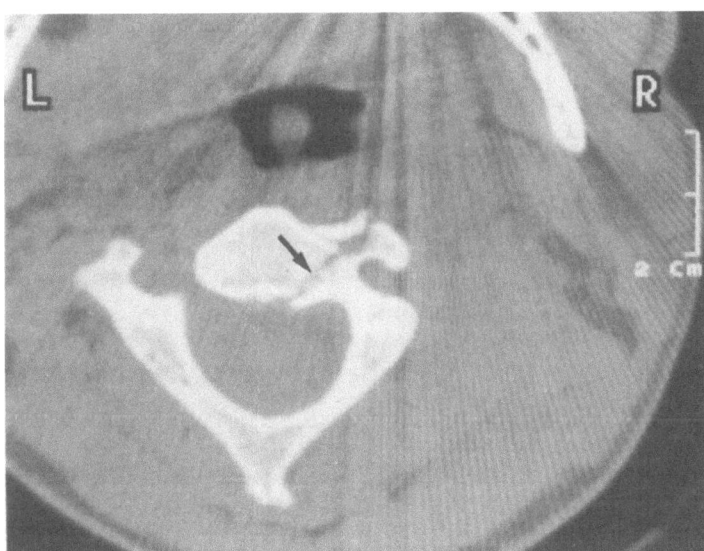

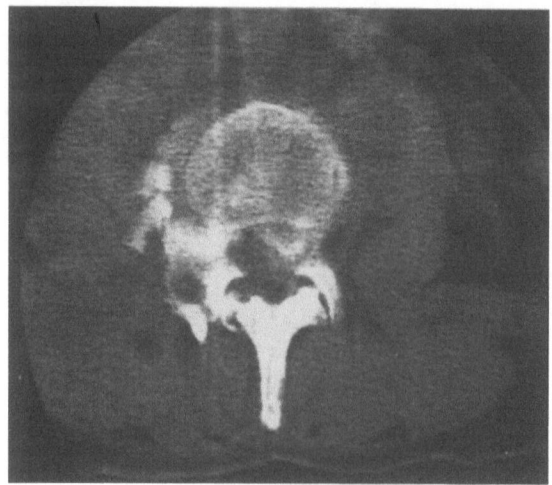 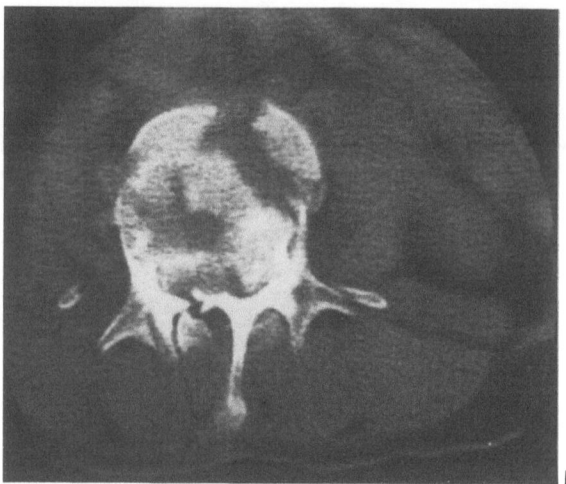

Fig. 10.11a,b. Fracture dislocation L2/3. **a** Comminuted fracture, widened facet joints. **b** Severe narrowing of spinal canal and disruption with displacement of the neural arch.

subluxations missed on axial sections (Faerber et al. 1979). Paraspinal haematomata, extra-spinal foreign bodies and CSF hygromas can be detected in the acute phase following trauma. Damage to neural tissue, such as intra-medullary haemorrhages, subarachnoid blood, epidural haematomata, herniated intravertebral discs, and cord oedema can also be detected in the early stages, whilst a post-traumatic syrinx (Fig. 10.13) or pseudomeningocoele may be identified as late complications. In these cases, diagnosis is enhanced using CTM, which shows delayed entry of contrast into the respective cavities.

CT provides a quick, easy, simple, comfortable and safe method of imaging, with lower radiation dose than conventional tomography.

Post-operative Spine

Post-operative Fibrosis. Thin section CT with intravenous contrast enhancement has an important role in identifying hypertrophic scar tissue and

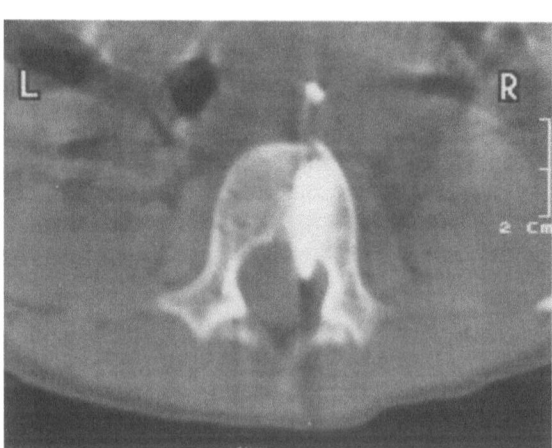 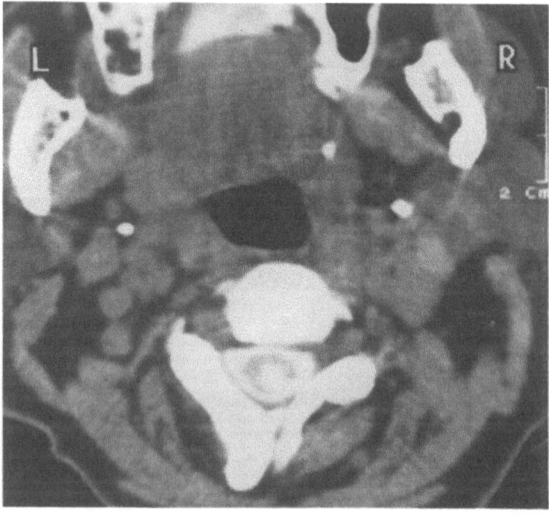

Fig. 10.12. Foreign body L1. Glass fragment impacted in vertebral body and spinal canal.

Fig. 10.13. Post-traumatic syrinx. CTM. Contrast-filled cavity within cervical spinal cord.

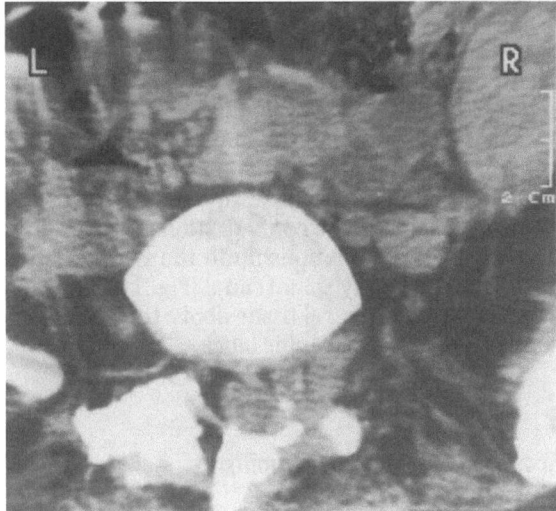

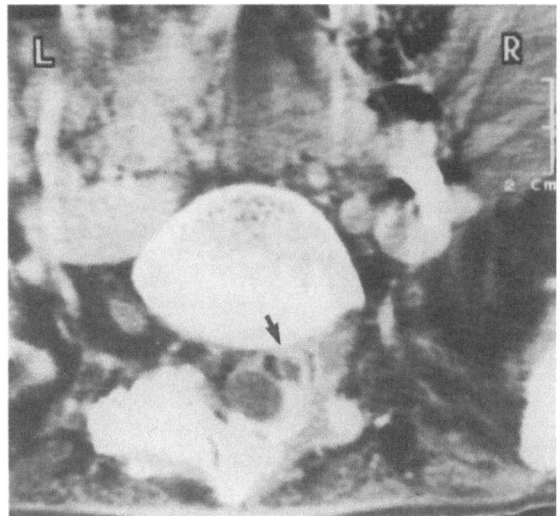

Fig. 10.14. Post-operative fibrosis. Previous laminectomy. a Pre-contrast. b Post-intravenous contrast. Scar tissue extending into exit foramen encasing the root ganglion. The epidural fat is obliterated and the theca displaced towards the scar. Enhanced fibrous strands anteriorly (*arrow*).

arachnoiditis and differentiating this condition from recurrent disc herniation (Schubiger and Valavanis 1982, Dixon and Bannon 1987). In the presence of scar tissue the thecal sac is retracted towards the soft tissue lesions which do not compress the thecal sac. The soft tissue lesion is contoured to the sac and does not compress it. Obliteration of the epidural fat by the scar tissue is a characteristic feature. The soft tissue scar does not arise from the annulus and will be seen separate from it. The density of the scar is less than 75 HU and enhances after a high dose of intravenous contrast (Fig. 10.14). CT occasionally may show concentric dural calcification and enhancing varices in severe post-operative arachnoiditis. The recurrent prolapsed intervertebral disc has a CT appearance similar to a primary herniated disc and will not enhance.

Other Post-operative Conditions. Assessment of the completeness of a laminectomy for canal stenosis

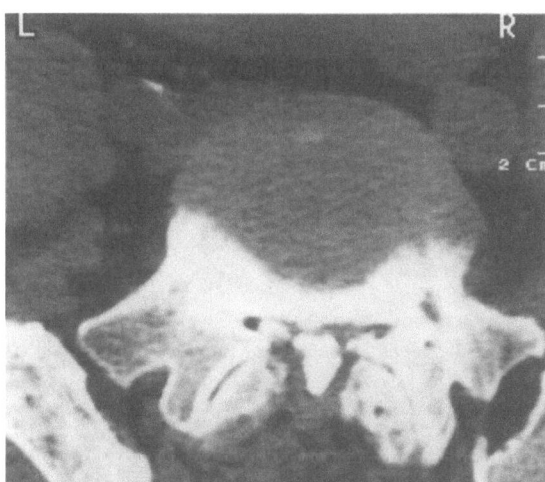

Fig. 10.15. Post-operative laminectomy for stenosis L4/5. The hypertrophied facets are unaffected by the laminectomy. Note the severe lateral recess stenosis.

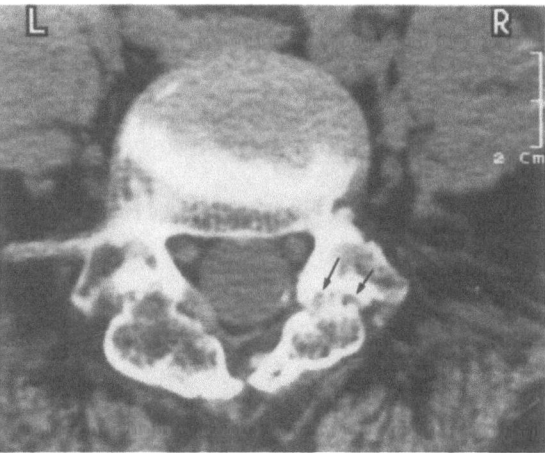

Fig. 10.16. Post-operative spinal fusion L4. Un-united inter-laminar graft (*arrow*). Normal spinal canal.

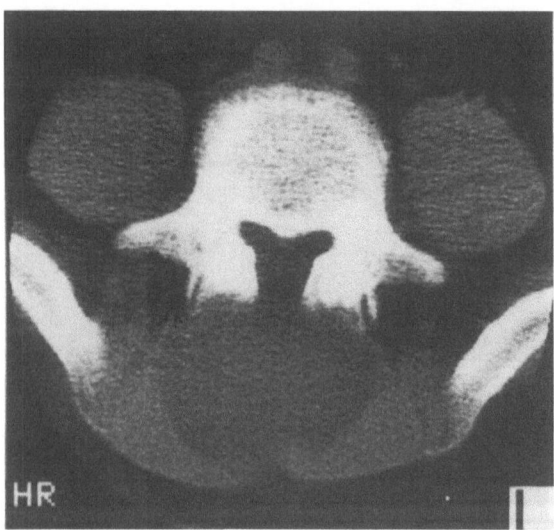

Fig. 10.17. Post-operative pseudomeningocoele. Large collection of CSF density herniating through the laminectomy defect. Note "trefoil" canal.

(Fig. 10.15), the capacity of the spinal canal, position and assessment of union of interlaminar and interbody (Fig. 10.16) spinal fusion are among the important post-operative indications for CT. The assessment of post-operative lateral recess or neural foraminal stenosis and the detection of the post-laminectomy pseudomeningocoele (Fig. 10.17), are important post-operative complications which can be detected by CT.

Intra-spinal Tumours

These uncommon causes of back pain are readily detected on CTM. Myelography is required for anatomical localization followed by high resolution CT with multi-planar reconstructions at the level of the spinal block, for detailed assessment. CT provides an accurate display of the configuration of the tumour (Fig. 10.18a), its relationship to the neural tissue, its effect on the bony spinal canal (Fig. 10.18b), and can visualize the neural tissue above the level of the conventional myelographic block.

Scoliosis and Spinal Dysraphism

Neither plain CT nor CTM have a role in the evaluation of idiopathic scoliosis. In congenital scoliosis myelography combined with CT has an important role in the detection of dysraphism which may not be evident on plain films. Diastematomyelia, lipoma and cord tethering may only be seen on the combined CT study (Fig. 10.19). Meningocoeles are readily detected on the conventional myelogram (Rothwell et al. 1988). An important advantage of CT in this condition is the evaluation of the spinal morphology in the axial plane with reconstructions providing additional information if required.

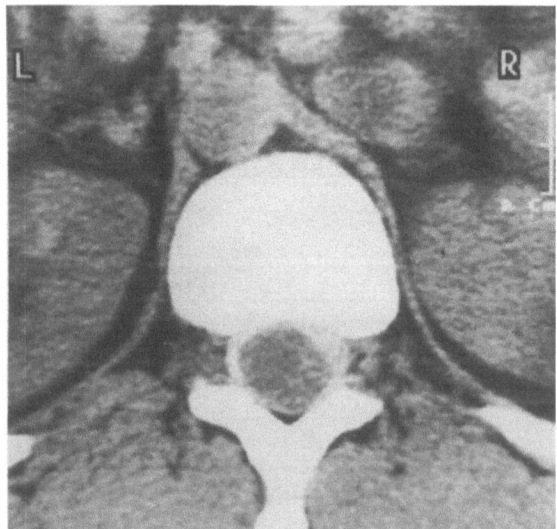
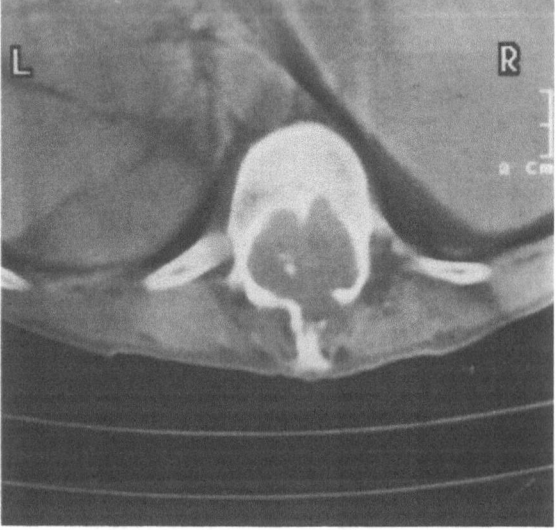

Fig. 10.18a,b. Intraspinal neurofibroma. **a** CTM. Expansion of conus. Note thin rim of opacified theca. Complete block shown on conventional myelogram. **b** CTM. Scalloped enlarged spinal canal. The theca is compressed and displaced anteriorly. Note calcification within low-density tumour.

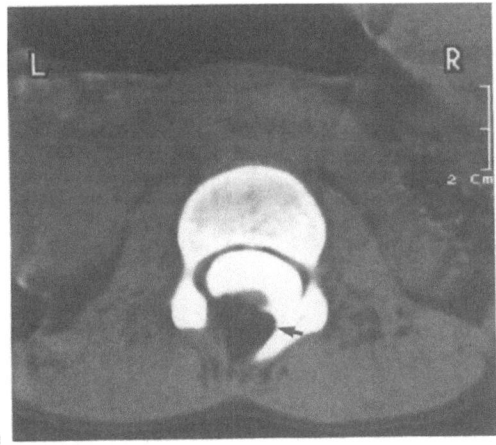 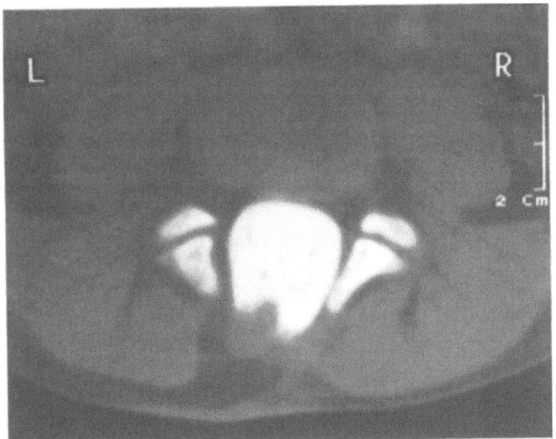

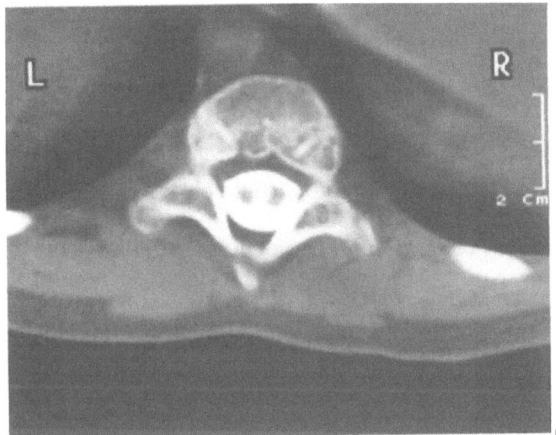

Fig. 10.19a–c. Spinal dysraphism; CTM showing spina bifida, enlarged thecal sac. **a** Lipoma shown as area of decreased density (*arrow*). **b** Cord tethering, posteriorly. **c** Diastematomyelia.

Discitis

Thin section CT may show destructive changes in the disc space extending into the adjacent end plates (Fig. 10.20), with no apparent extension of the disease into the spinal canal. A paraspinal abscess, if present, will be shown extending into or displacing the psoas muscles. CT, however, does not provide significantly more information than conventional X-ray examinations.

CT in Musculoskeletal Tumours

Diagnosis and Prognosis. CT has an important role in the diagnosis, treatment and prognosis of these tumours. The location, size, extent and the effects on normal adjacent structures are readily assessed. In malignant tumours, local and distant spread to lymph nodes, axial skeleton, liver and lungs may be detected. CT also has a role in the detection of recurrent disease.

Pre-operative Assessment. The quality of the adjacent bone can be assessed for the application of surgical devices and angio CT is used for identifying vessel encasement.

Soft Tissue Tumours

CT provides important information regarding the size, location and extent of soft tissue tumours (Genant et al. 1981). Solid tumours will be differentiated from cystic lesions. The attenuation characteristics of benign and malignant tumours with the exception of lipomata (Fig. 10.21), are non-specific. Benign tumours, however, show more homogeneous attenuation characteristics, are usually well-defined and encapsulated and displace adjacent structures. Malignant tumours, on the other hand, obliterate the fascial planes and infiltrate the adjacent muscle and subcutaneous adipose tissue (Fig. 10.22a). They usually show non-specific attenuation characteristics, often with calcification, and display irregular enhancement (Fig. 10.22b, DeSantos

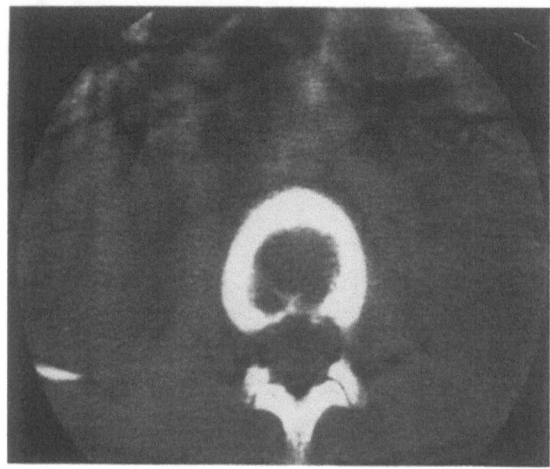

Fig. 10.20. Discitis. Large defect in sclerosed end-plate.

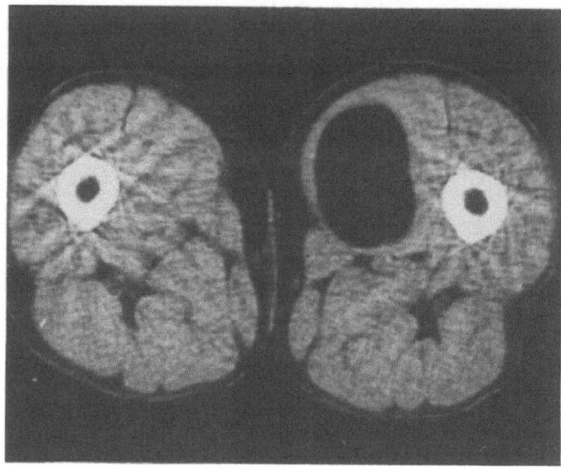

Fig. 10.21. Lipoma. Well-defined low density mass in antero-medial aspect of thigh.

et al. 1978). The tumour margins are frequently poorly-defined due to the partial volume effect and because of the inability to differentiate peri-tumoural oedema from tumour, and tumour from isodense normal soft tissue. Accurate assessment of the extent of the tumour, therefore, is not always possible. Despite this limitation, however, valuable

information regarding the extent and effect of the tumour on adjacent structures may be obtained.

The need for angiography has diminished due to the use of dynamic (angio) CT which displays the tumour blush and position of normal vessels in relation to the soft tissue tumour (Fig. 10.22c). CT has prognostic implications in its ability to detect local

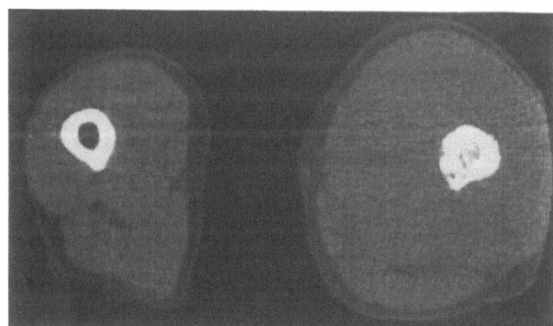

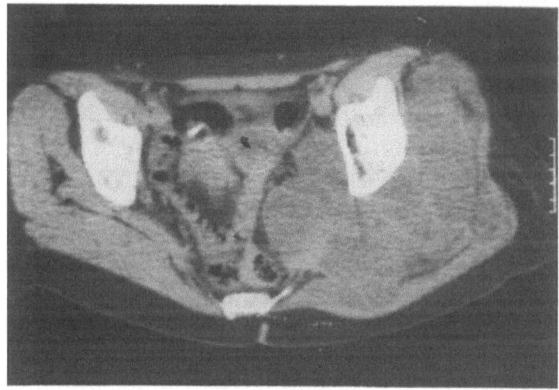

Fig. 10.22a–c. Soft tissue sarcoma. a Thigh. Uniformly enlarged thigh with loss of tissue planes. Note associated bony destruction. b Gluteal region – pre-contrast. Large mixed density mass with intraspinal extension. No bony involvement. c Same patient shown in b. Angio CT with multi-loculated, heterogeneous enhancement.

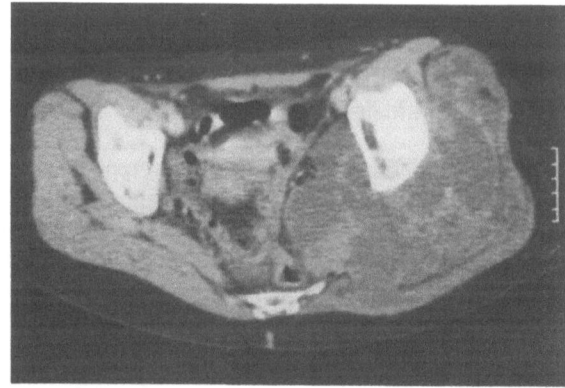

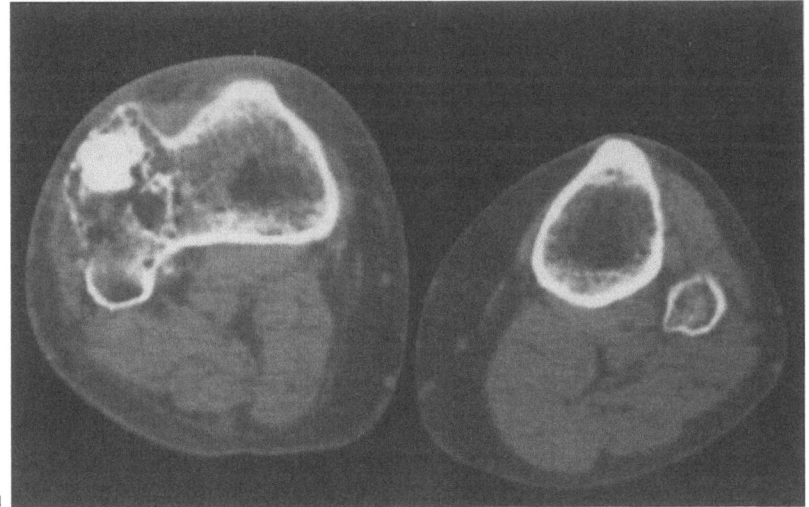

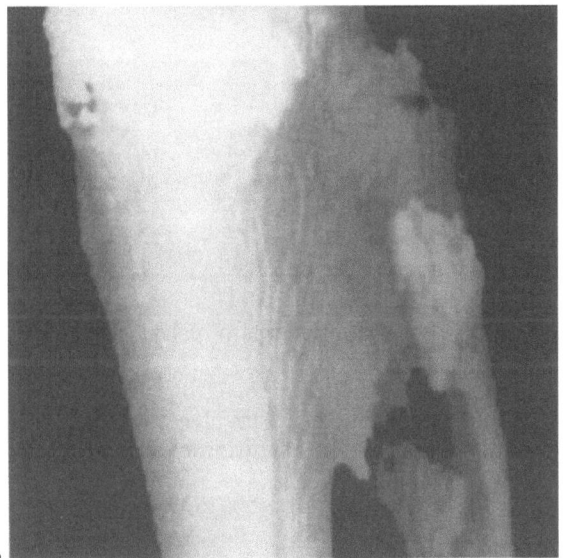
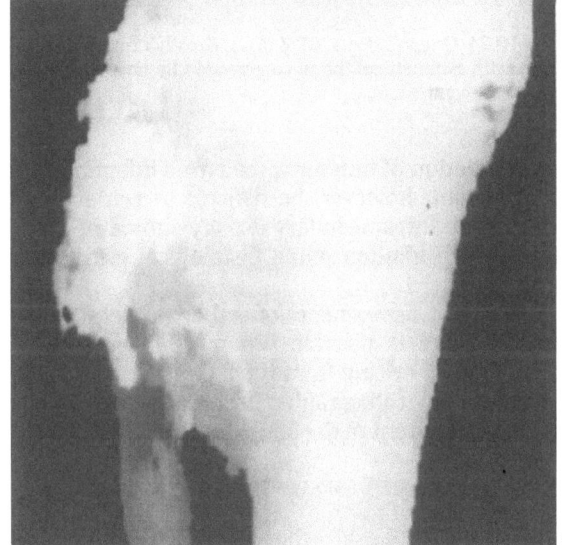

Fig. 10.23a–c. Chondroma. Transaxial section. Expansion of proximal tibia and calcification. **b,c** "3D" reconstructions showing extent of mass and displacement of fibula.

and distant metastases and in the detection of recurrent tumour, but its ability to detect small recurrences is limited in the presence of excess scar tissue.

Baseline CT scanning is necessary for monitoring purposes.

Skeletal Tumours

The typical characteristics of benign tumours are well demonstrated. The extent of the calcification and bony expansion of a chondroma of a long bone, and the spatial configuration of the bony mass and

its relationship to the long bone can be accurately assessed on 3DCT (Fig. 10.23).

The expansion of the cervical arch and the soft tissue component of an osteoblastoma is readily displayed together with its extension into the spinal canal (Fig. 10.24).

In osteosarcoma, the intramedullary and extra-osseous components can be distinguished (Fig. 10.25), although precise delincation of the margins of the extra-osseous soft tissue mass cannot be assessed with accuracy. CT will define the soft tissue mass outside the calcified or ossified portion of the tumour and beyond the cortical confines of long bones. The

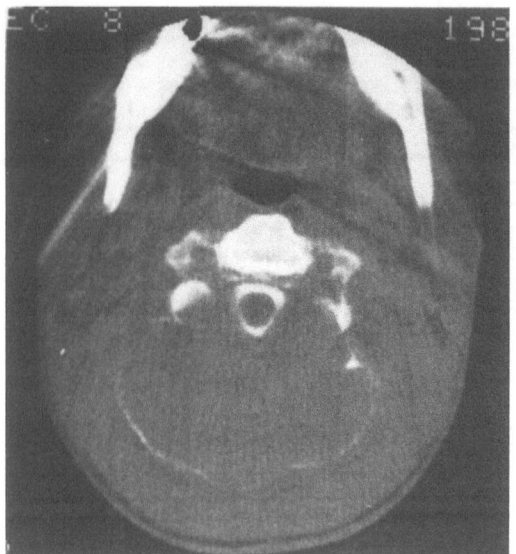

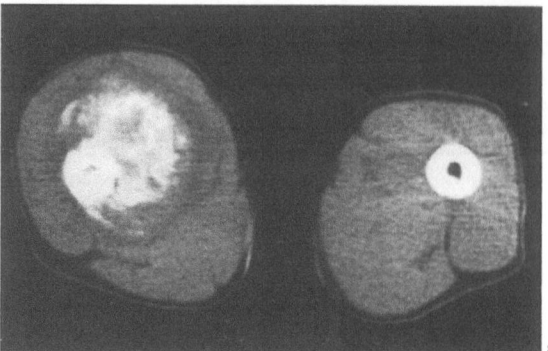

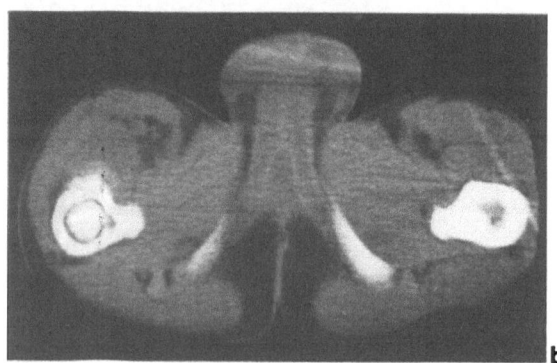

Fig. 10.24. Osteoblastoma, CTM of C3. Grossly expanded neural arch with symmetrical thecal compression by large intraspinal soft tissue component.

differentiation of tumour spread from inflammatory change can, however, be difficult to achieve and changes in intramedullary density should be interpreted with caution when histological evidence is lacking.

Accurate assessment of other skeletal bone malignancies is possible (Chap. 21), particularly those lesions arising from the axial skeleton where conventional radiographic techniques are inadequate. The extent of the bony destruction and asso-

Fig. 10.25a,b. Osteosarcoma of thigh. **a** Tumour extension into soft tissues. **b** Intramedullary extension.

ciated soft tissue components of pelvic lesions can be demonstrated (Fig. 10.26).

In spinal metastatic disease, CT has an important role in showing the extent of involvement of the posterior elements and the extension of any soft tissue

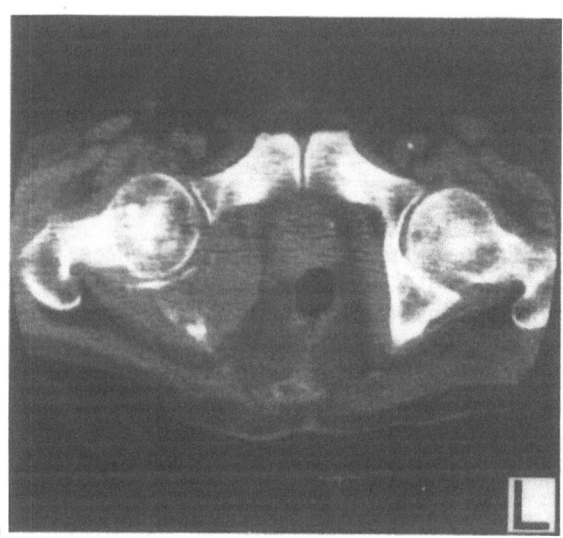

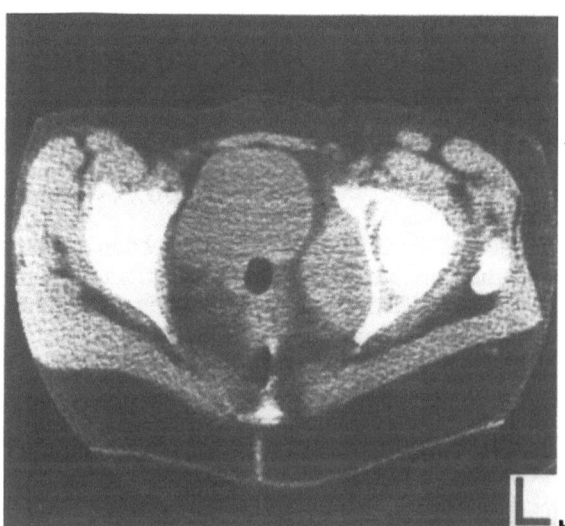

Fig. 10.26a,b. Metastases. **a** Destructive lesion in ischium. Large intra-pelvic soft tissue mass deforming the ischio-rectal fossa. **b** Displacement of bladder and cervix (outlined by air-containing tampon).

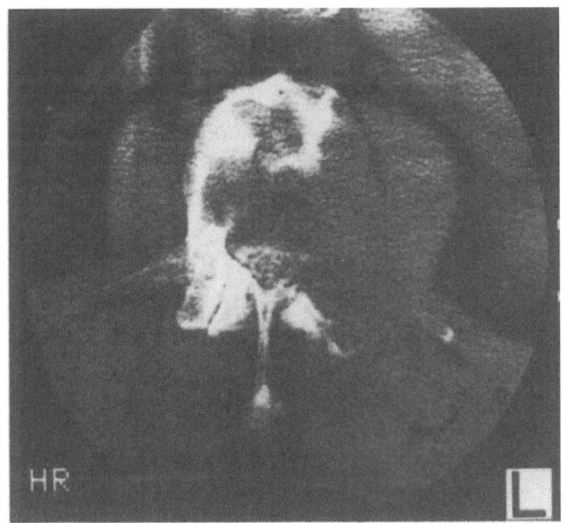

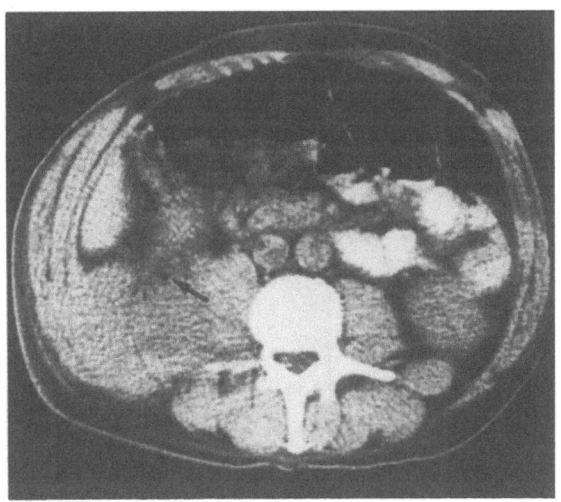

Fig. 10.28. Psoas abscess. Enlarged L Psoas major showing heterogeneous density and small gas loculus (*arrow*).

Fig. 10.27. Spinal myeloma. CTM. Destructive lesion in body and appendages. Thecal compression and para-spinal extension.

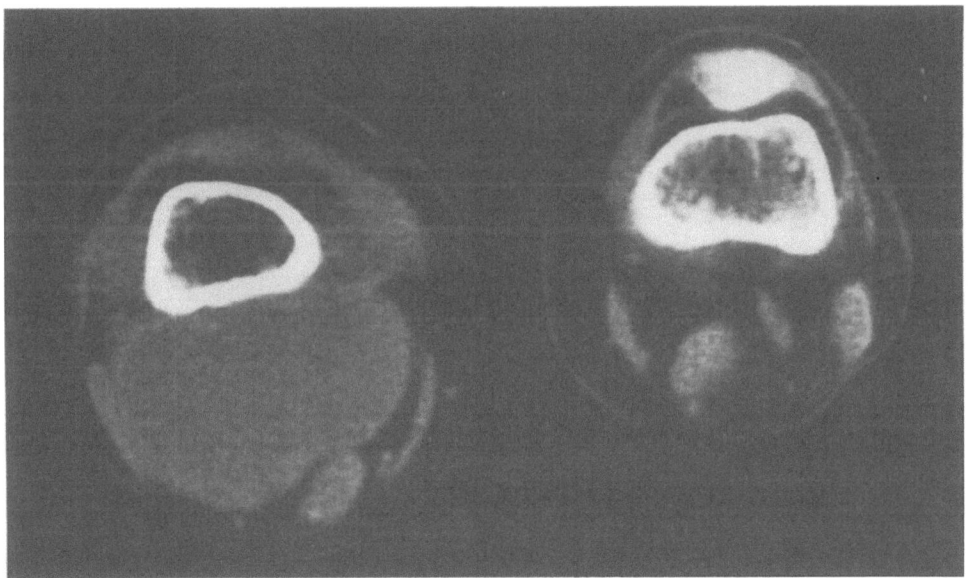

Fig. 10.29. Abscess in posterior thigh. Low density mass with rim of slightly increased density.

mass into the spinal canal (Chap. 22). In the presence of a block, CTM may be required to show the degree of cord compression (Fig. 10.27).

CT has a specific role in detecting degenerative disease in the costo-vertebral and apophyseal joints of the spine in those patients with malignant disease who demonstrate increased uptake of radionuclide where the conventional radiographic skeletal survey is negative (Best et al. 1979).

Musculoskeletal Infection

In spinal infection, CT complements conventional X-ray techniques but has a major role in diagnosing paraspinal infection and psoas abscess (Fig. 10.28). In the latter the psoas outline is enlarged, the psoas sheath distended and the abscess shows as decreased attenuation within the muscle. Rim enhancement may be shown.

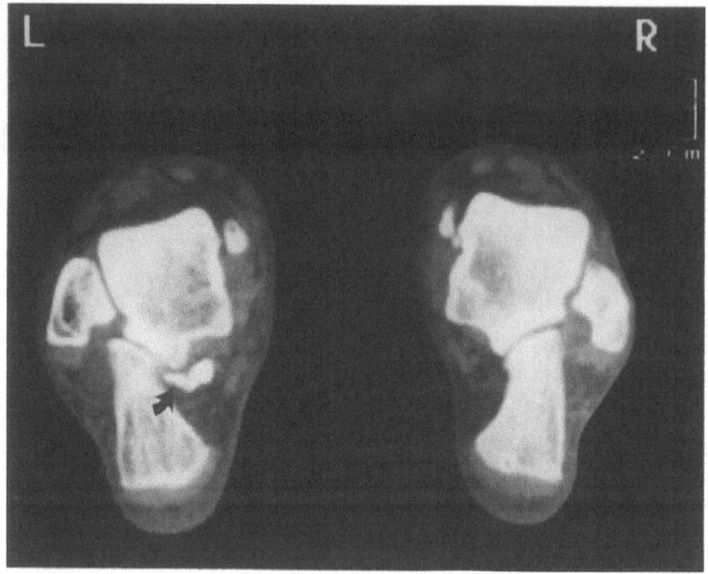

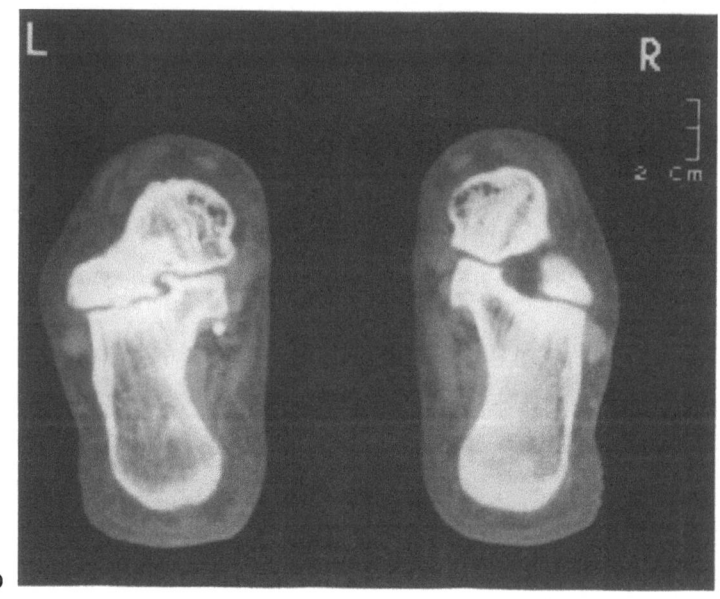

Fig. 10.30a,b. Sub-talar joints. **a** Un-united fracture of the sustentaculum tali (*arrow*). **b** Narrowed, irregular talo-tibial joint.

An abscess of the soft tissues of the limbs usually presents as a mass, of attenuation lower than normal soft tissue, and with a rim of slightly increased density which may enhance (Fig. 10.29). Differentiation from a soft tissue tumour is not always possible unless the clinical details are carefully considered.

Joint Disease

The hip joint is more easily studied than smaller and more complex joints which are more likely to be affected by the "partial volume effect". The use of thin sections to reduce the "partial volume effect" results in increased noise and difficulties in reproducibility. In certain situations, however, useful information can be obtained where conventional radiology has a limited role, e.g. the subtalar joints (Fig. 10.30).

In the pelvis, the hip and sacro-iliac joints are best examined by thin section CT. The femoral head, acetabulum and long axis of the femoral neck can then be demonstrated.

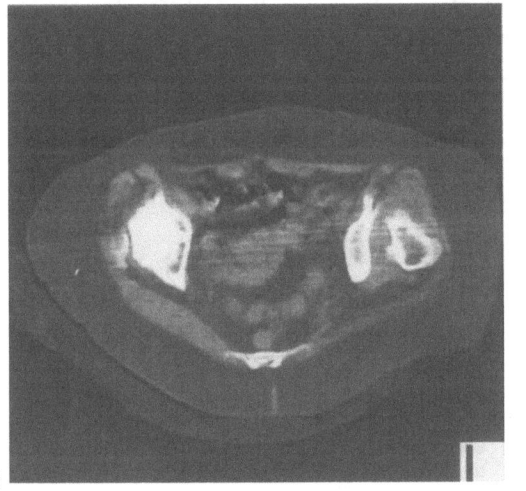 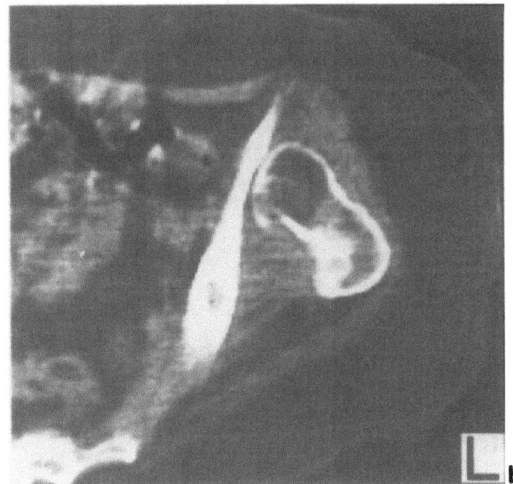

Fig. 10.31a,b. Acetabular dysplasia. a Shallow acetabulum. b False joint.

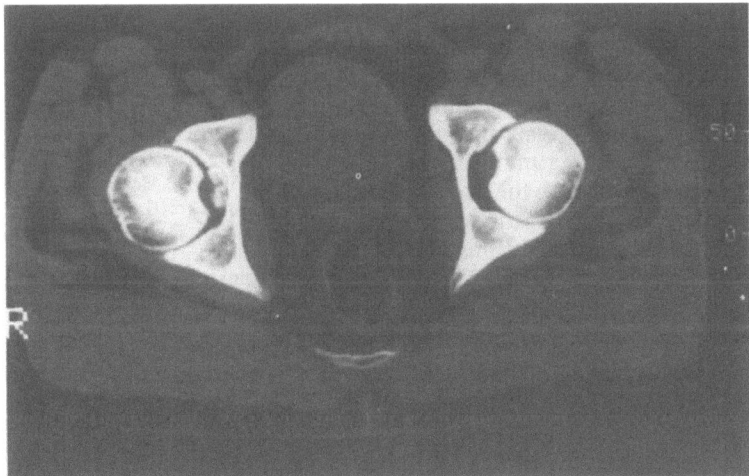

Fig. 10.32. Loose body in medial joint space, right hip.

Anteversion of the femoral neck (Hernandez et al. 1981), and the position, size and shape of the acetabulum are particularly well displayed in cross section, indicating a role for CT in the evaluation of acetabular dysplasia (Fig. 10.31), and in hip and shoulder joint trauma. Loose bodies in the hip joint are accurately located (Fig. 10.32).

Miscellaneous Uses

CT has been used in the pre-operative assessment of the adequacy of bone stock for total joint replacement (Genant et al. 1980). Plain CT (Pavlov et al. 1979) and CT combined with positive contrast arthrography have also been used in the evaluation of tears of the cruciate ligaments.

Quantitative Bone Mineral Analysis (see Chap. 19)

The ability of CT to measure the attenuation coefficients of each pixel provides a basis for accurate quantitative bone mineral analysis in trabecular and cortical bone (Genant and Boyd 1977, Pullan and Roberts 1978, Cann and Genant 1980). These measurements are independent of the overlying soft tissues. The attenuation values alone can be used as a measure of bone mineral content, but these values are subject to the "partial volume effect". Dual energy scanning, by separating high and low atomic matter elements, namely calcium and fat, can overcome some of these errors (Exner et al. 1979; Adams et al. 1982).

Future Developments

The technical aspects of modern CT systems are extremely complex and very sophisticated. Improvements in the soft-ware capabilities will continue to be made resulting in increased diagnostic capabilities. Recent developments include three-dimensional reconstruction, rotating and "walk-through" displays. Non-specific soft-tissue discrimination will remain the main disadvantage despite the excellent contrast resolution of the modern CT scanner.

The introduction of the newer generations of CT scanners has extended the indications for CT in the musculoskeletal system. The increased availability of CT will lead to a dramatic reduction in the incidence of invasive procedures such as angiography.

Conclusion

The indications for CT in musculoskeletal diagnosis are increasing in number and importance. With proper use of existing systems and up-grading of diagnostic procedures, CT can replace many conventional techniques and invasive procedures. The advantages of CT over conventional techniques – its 3-D imaging capabilities, excellent contrast resolution, accurate measurement of the attenuation coefficient and reduced exposure of the patient to radiation makes CT a powerful tool in musculoskeletal diagnosis. The impact of high resolution CT in the diagnosis of spinal disorders rivals the impact of the early generation of CT in neurological diagnosis.

References

Adams JE, Chen SZ, Adams PH, Isherwood I (1982) Measurement of trabecular bone mineral by dual energy computed tomography. J Comput Assist Tomogr 6:601–607

Best JJK, Forbes WStC, Adam NM, Isherwood I (1979) CT scanning and radioisotope bone scanning: a comparison. In: Gerhardt P, Van Raich G (eds) Total body computerized tomography. Georg Thieme Publishers, Stuttgart, pp 216–221

Buirski G (1987) The investigation of sciatica and low back pain syndromes: current trends. Clin Radiol 38:151–155

Cann CE, Genant HK (1980) Precise measurement of vertebral mineral content using computed tomography. J Comput Assist Tomogr 4:493–500

De Santos LA, Goldstein HM, Murray JA, Wallace S (1978) Computed tomography in the evaluation of musculo-skeletal neoplasms. Radiology 128:89–94

Dixon AK, Bannon RP (1987) Computed tomography of the post-operative lumbar spine: the need for, and optimal dose of, intravenous contrast medium. Br J Radiol 60:215–223

Dorwart RH, Vogler JB, Helms CA (1983) Spinal stenosis. Radiol Clin North Am 21:301–325

Exner GU, Prader A, Elsasser U, Ruegsegger P, Anliker M (1979) Bone densitometry using computed tomography. Part I: Selective determination of trabecular bone density and other bone mineral parameters. Normal values in children and adults. Br J Radiol 52:14–24

Faerber EN, Wolpert SM, Scott RM, Belkin SC, Carter SL (1979) Computed tomography of spinal fractures. J Comput Assist Tomogr 3:657–661

Genant HK, Boyd DP (1977) Quantitative bone mineral analysis using dual energy computed tomography. Invest Radiol 12:545–551

Genant HK, Cann CE, Chafetz NI, Helms CA (1981) Advances in computed tomography of the musculo-skeletal system. Radiol Clin North Am 19:645–674

Genant HK, Wilson JS, Bovill EG Jr, Brunelle FO, Murray WR, Rodrigo JJ (1980) CT of the musculo-skeletal system. J Bone J Surg 62A:1088–1101

Haughton VM, Williams AL (1982) Computed tomography of the spine. Mosby, St. Louis

Heithoff KB (1982) Pathogenesis and high resolution computed tomographic scanning of direct bony impingement syndromes of the lumbar spine. In: Genant HK, Chafetz N, Helms CA (eds), Computed tomography of the lumbar spine. San Francisco, University of California Press, pp 227–244

Helms CA, Vogler JB (1982) Computed tomography of spinal stenosis and arthroses. In: Genant HK, Chafetz N, Helms CA (eds), Computed tomography of the lumbar spine. San Francisco, University of California Press, pp 187–220

Hernandez RJ, Tachdjian MO, Poznanski AK, Dias LS (1981) CT determination of femoral torsion AJR 137:97–101

Isherwood I, Forbes WStC, Griffin J (1987) CT scanning – the body. In: Sutton D (ed), A textbook of radiology and imaging 4th edn. Churchill Livingstone, Edinburgh, pp 1691–1738

Pavlov H, Hirschy JC, Torg JS (1979) CT of the cruciate ligaments. Radiology 132:389–393

Post MJD, Green BA (1983) The use of CT in spinal trauma. Radiol Clin North Am 21:327–375

Pullan BR, Roberts TE (1978) Bone mineral measurement using an EMI scanner and standard methods: a comparative study. Br J Radiol 51:24–28

Rothwell I, Forbes WStC, Gupta SC (1988) Br J Radiol (in press)

Schubiger O, Valavanis A (1982) CT differentiation between recurrent disc herniation and post-operative scar formation: The value of contrast enhancement. Neuroradiology 22:251–254

Teplick JG, Haskin ME (1983) CT and lumbar disc herniation. Radiol Clin North Am 21:259–288

Ullrich CG, Binet EF, Sanecki MG, Kieffer SA (1980) Quantitative assessment of the lumbar spinal canal by computed tomography. Radiology 134:137–143

Williams AL, Haughton VM, Daniels DL, Thornton RS (1982a) CT diagnosis of lateral lumbar disc herniation. AJNR 3:211–213

Williams AL, Haughton VM, Meyer GA, Ho KC (1982b) Computed tomographic appearance of the bulging annulus. Radiology 142:403–408

Williams AL, Haughton VM, Syvertsen A (1980) Computed tomography in the diagnosis of herniated nucleus pulposus. Radiology 135:95–99

11 Digital Orthopaedic Radiography: Vascular and Non-vascular

W.D. Foley and C.R. Wilson

Introduction 145
Digital Subtraction Angiography 146
    Instrumentation 146
DSA Performance Parameters 147
    Spatial Resolution 147
    Contrast Sensitivity 147
Angiographic Techniques 148
Post-Processing 148
Quantitative DSA 149
Utilization of DSA in Clinical Orthopaedic Radiology 149
    Trauma 149
    Tumour 151
    Spinal Angiography 152
Digital Radiography 152
    Instrumentation 152
Specialized Orthopaedic Radiography 156
    Cast Radiography 156
    Scoliosis Radiography 156
    Dual Energy Radiography 156
    Digital Tomosynthesis 157
    Special Procedures 158
References 158

Introduction

The use of digital imaging techniques for static projection radiography is, at present, in a clinical evaluation phase (Stein 1976; Fraser et al. 1983; Tesic et al. 1983; Sonada et al. 1983). Further refinements in system architecture are possible, but have not yet been developed or tested in the laboratory or clinic. On the other hand, digital techniques for vascular imaging, using a digitized video signal, are well established and digital subtraction angiography (DSA) is now accepted as an integral component of a state-of-the-art angiographic system (Kruger and Reiderer 1984). DSA systems are characterized by rapid frame rate, enhanced on-line subtraction and instantaneous review on a television monitor. Post-processing techniques designed to improve anatomical registration and image quality as well as to remove motion artefacts have been developed and implemented (Foley et al. 1983). Relative to conventional film techniques a digital angiographic system has a limited field of view and inferior spatial resolution. Image contrast is somewhat poorer because of scattered radiation and veiling glare within the image intensifier. Thus, although it is relatively easy to digitize a video signal, image intensifiers with a larger field of view, when used for digital projection radiography, suffer from a relative loss of spatial resolution and contrast sensitivity in comparison with conventional film techniques. Other approaches to digital projection imaging are under development and promise improved performance over an image-intensifier-based system.

In this chapter, instrumentation and performance parameters of DSA and digital projection radiographic systems will be discussed and the clinical

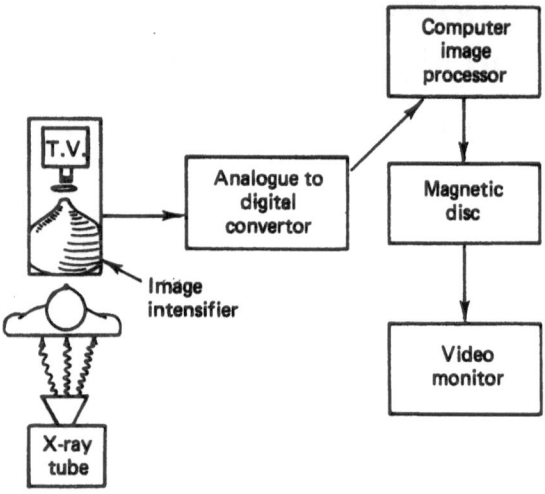

Fig. 11.1. Schematic block diagram of DSA system. The subtraction process is performed on-line in the computer with real time storage of images on the magnetic disc and display on the video monitor.

applications of DSA in orthopaedic imaging described. The role of static digital projection radiography is currently conjectural; implementation will depend on its diagnostic accuracy in relation to conventional film techniques, and upon the relative cost and logistics of such a system. If picture archiving and communication systems (PACS) (Capp et al. 1985) become an efficient cost-effective method of image display, transfer, storage and retrieval, it is likely that the majority of orthopaedic radiography performed in an institution with a PACS system will use digital imaging devices.

Digital Subtraction Angiography (DSA)

Instrumentation

In DSA, a video processor and digital disc are added to a fluoroscopic imaging chain to provide on-line viewing of subtraction angiographic images (Fig. 11.1). Early systems used video cameras with relatively high noise characteristics (signal-to-noise ratio of approximately 250 : 1 or less), employing frame averaging of an interlaced video format to provide an acceptable signal-to-noise ratio. Exposure times varied with patient thickness and

were typically 125—250 ms in duration. Such systems were sensitive to vascular motion which resulted in edge unsharpness during prolonged exposure times and were unable to record a sequence of rapid frame rate images. Adoption of high-performance video cameras with low noise characteristics (signal-to-noise ratio $\simeq 1000 : 1$) allowed single video frame pre-contrast and post-contrast images to be used for subtraction. In addition, a progressive rather than an interlaced video readout technique allowed the radiographic exposure to be separated in time from the video frame readout. At 30 cycles per second, video frame readout time is 33 ms. Thus, the use of progressive readout allowed exposure times shorter than 33 ms to be employed. The combination of high-performance video cameras and progressive target readout thus resulted in short exposure time and rapid frame rate capability – both important requirements for an intra-arterial angiographic technique.

Radiation dose and beam energy employed in a DSA system are comparable to those used in conventional film–screen angiographic units. In addition, basic angiographic techniques such as choice of frame rate, projection, field of view and exposure time have been adapted from film–screen angiographic systems to DSA units with little change. However, the concentration of the injected contrast bolus for intra-arterial DSA has been reduced compared with that employed for conventional film angiography because of the greater sensitivity of DSA. On-line storage of the digital image data is provided by memory storage in the image processor (for short-term storage) or digital disc (for short-term or medium-term storage). Image data stored in the video memory or on digital disc can be processed to improve image quality (by video frame averaging) or anatomical registration. The digital data can also be accessed for quantitative determinations including vessel diameter, cross-sectional area, volume flow rate and indices relating to capillary perfusion and myocardial contraction (Bursch and Heintzen 1985). Images are archived either on film or magnetic tape or both. Digital image storage allows the operator to review the image sequence on a video monitor, and to record on film and archive on magnetic tape only those images which are pertinent to the patient diagnosis. This has resulted in considerable savings in film cost over conventional angiography, an economic argument which in addition to the ease of use and on-line image display of DSA has resulted in a wide dissemination of this technology. It is likely that further developments in large-scale magnetic or optical storage media and image processing will occur with the utilization of DSA for cardiac angiography.

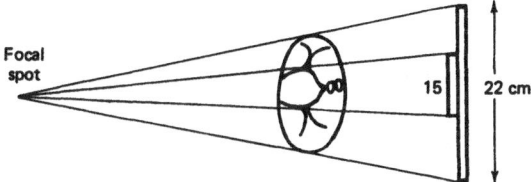

Fig. 11.2. Schematic diagram demonstrating the air gap magnification technique (outer radiation beam) and the use of electronic minification (inner radiation beam). Air gap magnification substantially reduces scattered radiation effects without the need for a radiographic grid. Thus, the dose efficiency (amount of input radiation required to form an image) is improved. Electronic minification further improves spatial resolution, though is more affected by focal spot penumbra.

DSA Performance Parameters

Spatial Resolution

The spatial resolution of an image system determines the "sharpness" of anatomical detail in the image. Traditionally, the clarity of small vessel display and of vessel margins is considered to reflect spatial resolution. The objective test of spatial resolution is provided by imaging of a bar phantom and the result expressed in line pairs/mm. With current 525-line video systems and the 512×512 matrix used, the primary determinant of DSA spatial resolution is the matrix, i.e. the number of picture elements into which each video frame is divided. The size each picture element represents in the object is determined by the field of view of the input phosphor of the intensifier, the magnification factor and the number of elements in the image matrix. Geometric magnification improves spatial resolution as, with increasing degrees of magnification, each pixel element in the image plane actually subtends a progressively smaller "pixel" in the object. Geometric magnification is achieved using the air gap principle, which reduces the amount of scattered radiation reaching the detector, thus reducing or eliminating the need for a radiographic grid. It is necessary, however, to use a small X-ray focal spot for geometric magnification to avoid edge unsharpness in the image due to the penumbra effect (Fig. 11.2). Since a microfocus X-ray tube tolerates less instantaneous heat loading than a larger focal spot, longer X-ray exposure must be used when the geometric magnification technique is employed.

Electronic minification decreases the intensifier field of view and for an identical matrix size, reduces pixel size in the object plane, thus improving resolution. However, this increases the radiation dose required to ensure equivalent photon statistics per pixel in comparison with images obtained with a larger intensifier field of view.

Spatial resolution can be maximized using a combination of geometric magnification, electronic minification and a small anode target size. The best spatial resolution achievable with a 512^2 image matrix and electronic minification to 11 cm diameter intensifier field of view is 2.5 line pairs/ mm. However, optimum spatial resolution may be achievable only by relatively long exposure times. When imaging pulsatile vessels, theoretical improvement in edge definition may be offset by motion unsharpness. A compromise solution is to use shorter exposure times with larger focal spot and some potential loss in edge resolution.

A 1024 matrix should, in theory, double the resolution of a digital vascular device. However, improvements in resolution are only in the range of 20%–30%. Continuing sources of image degradation, including scattered radiation within the intensifier and excessive electronic noise in the video camera, partially offset improvements expected from a doubling of the matrix size.

Contrast Sensitivity

Contrast sensitivity is the detection of a specific signal, in this case an opacified vessel as discriminated from the surrounding anatomical structure and background random electronic noise. The subtraction technique, by removing surrounding anatomy, isolates the opacified vessel making it more conspicuous. Vessel recognition depends upon the size of the signal provided by the opacified vessel, the combined noise due to photon statistics and electronic noise, and artefacts introduced by anatomical misregistrations in the subtracted image. The size of the perceived vessel signal is proportional to the arterial iodine concentration and inversely related to the energy of the X-ray beam. A higher arterial iodine concentration results in greater radiation absorption by the vessel and thus a stronger signal. This is the major reason for improved image quality with intra-arterial as compared with intravenous injections of contrast medium for DSA.

However, DSA systems have some limitation in dynamic range, (i.e. the range of signal intensities that can be faithfully recorded), and the contrast medium concentration used for conventional film angiography will exceed the dynamic range of the digital video recording system. Thus, it becomes necessary to reduce arterial iodine concentration relative to that which would be used for conventional film angiography of the same region. Angiographers may reduce the concentration of the injected contrast medium bolus using the same volume flow rate as for conventional film angiography. Alternatively they may use a similar contrast medium bolus concentration at a reduced volume flow rate, but the volume flow rate must be sufficient to produce adequate admixture of the injected contrast medium into the blood. Inadequate admixture may result in streaming with incomplete opacification of the vessel.

A lower beam energy also results in greater photon attenuation by the contrast-opacified vessels; however, lower beam energies also result in longer exposure times and reduced latitude or dynamic range in the image. As with the spatial resolution determinants of focal spot size and beam geometry, compromise is necessary. A beam energy sufficient to result in adequate contrast and dynamic range of the opacified vessels is chosen. In general, 70–75 kVp is used for angiography of the neck, thorax and extremities and 75–85 kVp employed for intracranial and abdominal vessel studies.

Quantum mottle is random variation in X-ray flux which is more noticeable at low X-ray exposures and results in "graininess" in the resultant image. Both quantum mottle and electronic noise in the receptor degrade DSA image quality by adding random noise to the images and decreasing contrast. In general, radiographic exposures for DSA sequences are similar to those for film–screen angiography and, if appropriately selected, result in acceptable quantum mottle. Electronic noise is primarily a reflection of the noise characteristics of the video camera, particularly its pre-amplifier. Additional noise is introduced by digitization of the continuous analog video signal. These latter sources of noise and their reduction are essentially an engineering problem. Experience has indicated that not only should the analog video signal contribute noise less than $\pm 1\%$ of the peak video signal, but in addition, the video signals should be accurately assigned to one of 1024 levels, i.e. a 10-bit depth in the analog-to-digital converters.

Angiographic Techniques

A convenient checklist for a radiologist performing angiography, whether conventional film–screen or DSA, is to consider:

1. Projection
2. Field of view
3. Frame rate
4. Exposure time
5. Contrast injection techniques

These factors determine how clearly the vascular pathology and regional vascular anatomy are displayed. The chosen projection should result in the least vessel overlap and a profile display of the vessel of interest. The chosen field of view should demonstrate regional vascular anatomy without extraneous content. The frame rate should be variable for the arterial, capillary and venous phases and be rapid enough to demonstrate dynamic events such as arteriovenous fistula. Short exposure times are required to "freeze frame" rapidly pulsating vessels such as the thoracic aorta, pulmonary arteries and coronary arteries. Longer exposure times are usually adequate for studies of the pelvis and extremities and for intracranial examinations. Contrast injection requires appropriate catheter placement and selection of contrast medium concentration and volume flow rate. In addition the radiologist should select beam energy, exposure factors and beam geometry to optimize spatial resolution and contrast sensitivity.

Post Processing

Digital image data can be retrieved from image memory or digital disc. The initial sequence of subtraction images can be processed to improve anatomical registration between the original (or an alternative) mask and subsequent images, and to increase DSA signal by averaging techniques. A convenient hierarchy of techniques is available and includes:

1. *Remask*. Selection of an alternative mask to improve anatomic registration.

2. *Integrated remask*. Video frame averaging improves the signal-to-noise ratio of the resultant image by the square root of the number of images that are integrated or averaged. The major perceived effect is a smoother image with less random fluctuations in the image. Both pre-contrast and post-contrast images can be integrated prior to subtraction, but integration may not be successful if patient motion occurs during the sequence of images that are to be integrated because it increases image unsharpness.

3. *Pixel shift*. This is an analytical technique employing submillimetre pixel shift in the X and Y dimensions in an attempt to reduce misregistration between the images. It is most commonly applied to reregister the craniofacial bones and the cervical spine as well as the extremities. Two techniques – translational or rotational – can be employed. Translational techniques involve motion in the X or Y plane only, while rotational pixel shift involves more complex manoeuvres. Translational pixel shift suffices for almost all clinical requirements.

4. *Temporal/energy subtraction*. This technique, also called "hybrid subtraction", uses dual energy exposure for each image. On-line viewing of the low beam energy exposures is used as in conventional temporal subtraction DSA already discussed. However, two image data sets are obtained for each composite low and high energy exposure. These image data sets may be combined with various degrees of weighting of the high-energy data set to result in soft tissue cancellation. Thus, pre-contrast images display bone with subtraction of surrounding soft tissue and post-contrast images display bone and iodinated vessels. A final temporal or mask mode subtraction is used to isolate the iodinated vessels. Soft tissue cancellation on the pre-contrast and post-contrast images also removes the misregistration artefacts resulting from soft tissue motion between pre-contrast and post-contrast exposures.

The hybrid subtraction technique has been found useful in the removal of the misregistration artefact resulting from swallowing during intravenous carotid arteriography and the peristaltic bowel motion artefact occurring during intravenous or intra-arterial aortorenal arteriography (Foley et al. 1983). The technique is not useful in intracranial or extremity imaging as these studies are not usually degraded by involuntary soft tissue motion. In thoracic imaging, rapid pulsatile vascular motion occurs between the low- and high-energy exposures resulting in unsharpness due to intrinsic motion and artefact in hybrid DSA images.

Quantitative DSA

An objective measurement of vessel diameter or cross-sectional area which is accurate and reproducible would be a significant advantage. It has been clearly demonstrated, using conventional film angiography, that intra-observer variation in subjective estimation of percentage stenosis is of the order of 10%–15%, while inter-observer variability

is of the order of 25%. This is a significant clinical limitation as angiographic estimation of percentage stenosis is considered the "gold standard" against which other, less invasive techniques are judged. Moreover, this estimate, in conjunction with clinical symptomatology, may determine whether operative or non-operative management is employed. Video densitometric techniques utilizing an edge detection algorithm in conjunction with background subtraction and linear smoothing have been employed in phantom and biological experiments (Jaques et al. 1985; Simons and Kruger 1985). These techniques have significant limitations, particularly in estimating percentage stenosis in small vessels with low iodine concentrations, because of low signal-to-noise ratio and limited resolution due to the matrix size. In addition, all techniques may be less accurate when stenoses are visualized "en face" rather than "in profile".

It is possible to estimate arterial volume flow rate by recording the appearance time of the leading edge of a contrast bolus as it progresses down the longitudinal axis of a vessel. The most accurate estimation is recorded when the leading edge of the bolus is registered on a pixel-by-pixel basis using rapid frame rate acquisition. The flow rate can then be separated into systolic and diastolic phases. Preliminary animal experiments have demonstrated good agreement between calculated and actual flow. For animal experiments, intravenous bolus injection of contrast material was employed (DF Smith et al. unpublished). Intra-arterial contrast injections with the catheter tip in close proximity to the measurement site may result in false estimation of the arterial flow above baseline values because of disruption of the flow introduced by the bolus.

Ultilization of DSA in Clinical Orthopaedic Radiology

In orthopaedic patients DSA can be used in the evaluation of trauma, bone and soft tissue sarcoma, spinal angiography and vascular interventional techniques.

Trauma

Extremity angiography in trauma patients is used to evaluate arterial occlusion, pseudoaneurysm and arteriovenous fistula (Smith et al. 1981). Patients

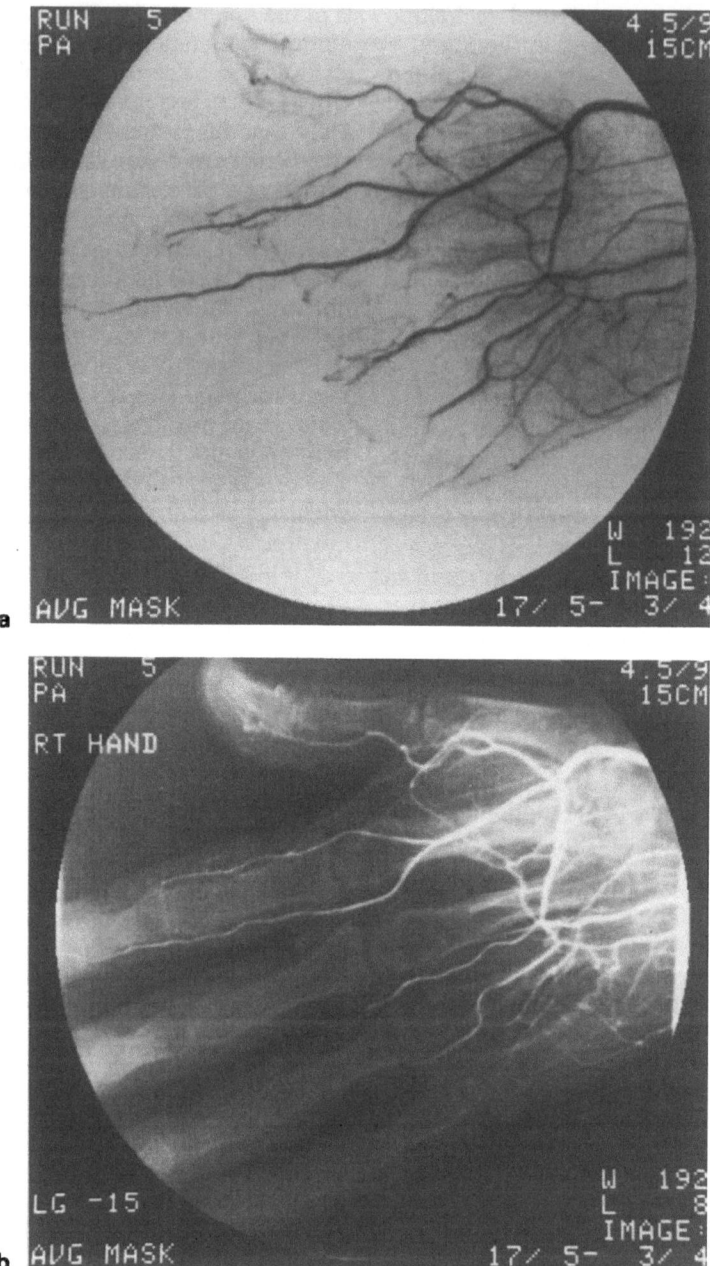

Fig. 11.3a,b. Intra-arterial DSA study of the right hand demonstrating thromboembolic obstruction of proper digital vessels to the index, ring and little fingers. Image quality reflects adequate intra-arterial iodine concentration, appropriate peak voltage, small field of view and adequate radiation dose. Note the use of the landmark feature (b) to detail skeletal reference landmarks in relation to the site of the vessel occlusion.

at risk include those with fracture or fracture dislocation involving the distal femur, knee and ankle regions. Reduced arterial inflow to the distal extremity may be a result of either arterial compression, intimal disruption and thrombus or arterial transection. Angiography may be performed prior to fracture reduction, particularly to detect the vessel that is displaced or injured by a bone or fracture fragment. Distal femoral fractures are more likely to result in this type of arterial injury. In this clinical setting, operative angiography may be used in preference to conventional angiographic approaches.

Careful manipulation of the fracture fragment can then be performed under direct vision with arterial repair to follow fixation of the fracture. In patients in whom direct arterial injury is not suspected, the distal extremity circulation may be re-assessed clinically following fracture reduction. Angiography should be performed in patients with persistent ischaemia to identify those who may benefit from either fasciotomy or from repair of an injured vessel segment.

DSA is most appropriate when used in the post-trauma patient for a unilateral intra-arterial study of the extremity (Goodman et al. 1984). The advantages of DSA over conventional film techniques are the rapidity of study with the ability to obtain multiple repeat projections easily. Bone subtraction is useful in clearly defining the more distal vasculature, particularly the pedal circulation. When ionic contrast material is used the studies are relatively pain-free as the contrast material is diluted to a 20%–30% concentration compared with the usual concentration of 60%. The most acceptable DSA studies in terms of clinical results are those performed using large field of view image intensifiers and the "landmark" feature (the electronic addition of a calculated percentage of the original mask image to the subtraction angiogram in order to provide the orthopaedic and vascular surgeon with skeletal reference landmarks). Angiographic studies performed following internal fixation of a fracture with metallic rods are less satisfactory as the site of vascular injury may be superimposed over the metallic device. In these circumstances multiple projections, best performed with a rotating X-ray tube detector gantry, are necessary.

As are lower extremity studies, unilateral upper extremity studies are usually performed using DSA techniques and intra-arterial catheter approaches. Adequate detail of the palmar arch, common digital and proper digital vessels is obtained, provided appropriate contrast medium concentrations (20%–30%) are used (Fig. 11.3). All DSA studies require patient cooperation to maintain the involved extremity motionless and so avoid anatomical misregistration.

Some radiologists advocate the use of intravenous DSA to evaluate suspected extremity trauma in cooperative haemodynamically stable patients (Gavant et al. 1986).

In certain patients with multiple sites of significant trauma a "pan-arteriogram" may be necessary. This could include studies of the brachiocephalic vessels, thoracic aorta, liver, spleen, kidneys and pelvis. In as much as patient cooperation will permit, these studies can be performed using DSA with intra-arterial catheter techniques. DSA studies of the thoracic aorta of quality sufficient to diagnose or exclude aortic disruption at a confidence level equivalent to that achievable with film angiography, can be obtained in the majority of patients using modern DSA equipment (Fig. 11.4). Rapid frame rate image acquisition in combination with selective remasking should be used. The most common indication for a post-traumatic pelvic arteriogram is evaluation for suspected arterial disruption and pseudoaneurysm in a patient with pelvic fracture and significant extraperitoneal bleeding. Transcatheter embolization techniques are effective in stopping arterial bleeding. However, patients may continue to bleed internally due to venous disruption.

In patients with suspected visceral abdominal trauma, contrast-enhanced computed tomography (CT) has superseded angiography as the investigation of choice (Federle 1983). Thus, in patients with multiple trauma, the sequence in which angiography and CT are performed will depend upon clinical factors, particularly the site at which the most significant injury is suspected. DSA is of value in these circumstances, as the total load of contrast medium is reduced compared with that which would have been used had conventional film techniques been employed. In general, DSA requires one-quarter to one-half of the total load of contrast medium used for conventional film angiography.

Tumour

Angiography may be employed as a vascular mapping procedure in patients scheduled for resection of bone and soft tissue tumours of the extremities (Paushter et al. 1983; Lee et al. 1986). Tumours in this category include: giant cell tumour, aneurysmal bone cyst involving sites such as the fibular head and femoral trochanter, and malignant fibrous histiocytoma. In these patients DSA is used to define the feeding vessels, and lesion vascularity and extent (Fig. 11.5). A relatively large field of view display format in conjunction with landmarking to display skeletal reference structures is appropriate. Transcatheter embolization of painful metastatic bone lesions in non-weightbearing areas of the long bones can be employed (Chuang et al. 1979). For embolization procedures DSA is useful in providing sequential studies during the procedure and in providing a "vascular road map" for selective placement of a catheter tip prior to coil release (Fig. 11.6) (Turski et al. 1982). Transcatheter arterial chemotherapy is also utilized at some institutions

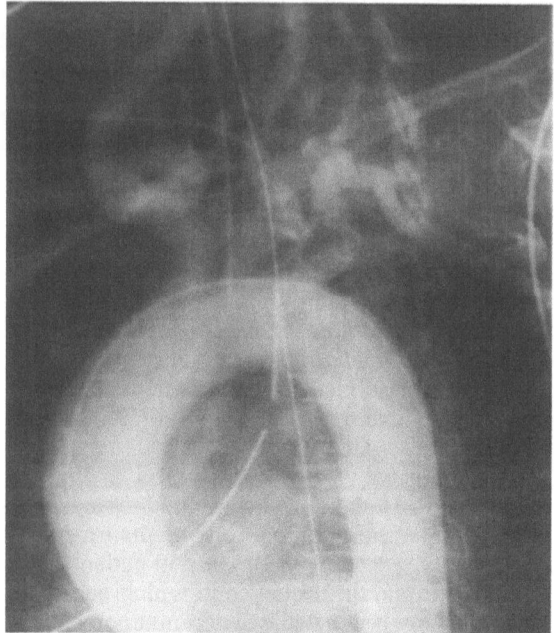
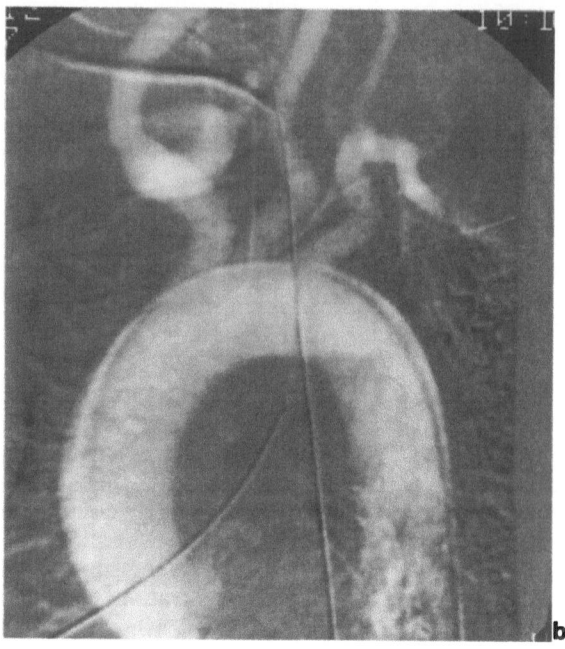

Fig. 11.4a,b. Intra-arterial film angiography (a) and DSA (b) in a patient with suspected thoracic aortic injury. Both studies are diagnostic and exclude the possibility of thoracic aortic tear. Intra-arterial DSA requires less contrast material and is a faster examination. The DSA technique is especially useful in patients who subsequently require contrast-enhanced CT to evaluate suspected abdominal injury.

in the treatment of bone sarcomas (Chuang and Wallace 1981). The therapy is given as part of a treatment protocol including radiation therapy and subsequent amputation. Selective catheter placement is facilitated by the "road map" feature of DSA.

Spinal Angiography

Spinal angiography is performed as a diagnostic procedure in those patients with suspected arteriovenous malformation involving the spinal cord and as a pre-therapy procedure in patients having spinal cord surgery for tumour or cyst or operative correction of scoliosis deformity (Yeates et al. 1985). Spinal angiography may be a time-consuming procedure requiring review of multiple images to identify the artery of Adamkiewicz and other spinal cord feeders. On-line review of DSA studies facilitates the procedure (Fig. 11.7). The artery of Adamkiewicz and other spinal-feeding arteries can be reliably identified on intra-arterial DSA studies. A significant advantage of intra-arterial DSA is the reduced concentration of contrast material required for selective lumbar, intercostal and vertebral artery injections. As with extremity angiography, patients must be motionless during the angiographic sequences to

avoid misregistration artefact. Bowel motion artefact can be reduced with concurrent intravenous glucagon and the use of central abdominal compression. Combined temporal/energy DSA may be of potential value in lumbar spinal angiography, though it would be anticipated that the hybrid subtraction technique could significantly reduce the contrast signal from a small spinal artery.

Digital Radiography

Instrumentation

The five major components of a radiographic system are:

1. Source
2. Detector
3. Processor
4. Display
5. Image storage and retrieval

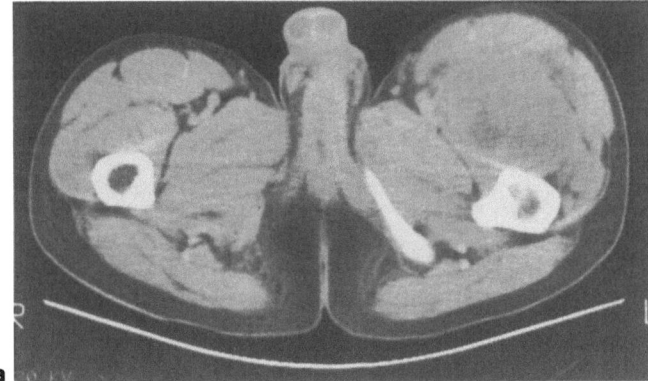

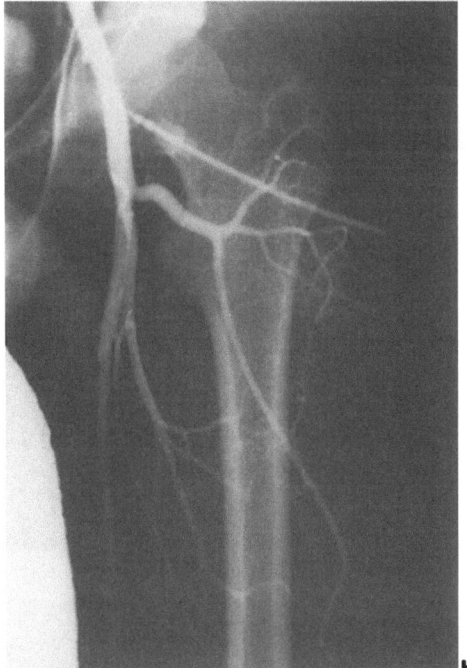

Conventional radiographic systems use a film–screen detector to receive the transmitted radiation image. A grid is interposed between the subject and receptor when imaging thick body parts to reduce the scattered radiation which decreases contrast. However, the interposed radiographic grid increases the radiation dose requirement. The exposed silver halide film is chemically developed and the resultant film image displayed on a light box illuminator using transmitted light. Ordinarily image processing is not performed because of the lack of suitable equipment. However, laser film digitizers and improved display terminals are being used in selected research sites to evaluate computerized image processing of film radiographs.

Digital radiographic systems offer many potential advantages related to improvements in image quality, contrast sensitivity, exposure latitude, interactive contrast enhancement through image processing and display windowing, and more efficient storage, retrieval and transmission of radiographic image data. Digital images may be displayed on film using a laser film writer or on a video monitor. Commercially available video monitors are 525 line systems. One thousand line systems are becoming available but both of these systems are inadequate for skeletal radiology. Two thousand line video monitors will probably be required for adequate definition of skeletal radiographs. Such systems would display a 2000 × 2000 matrix image covering a 20 cm × 20 cm field of view with a potential resolution of 5 line pairs/mm (0.1 mm pixel element). Prototype flicker-free 2000 line monitors have been developed. However, such systems are currently extremely expensive and appropriate clinical evaluations must be performed before they can be considered adequate display devices for

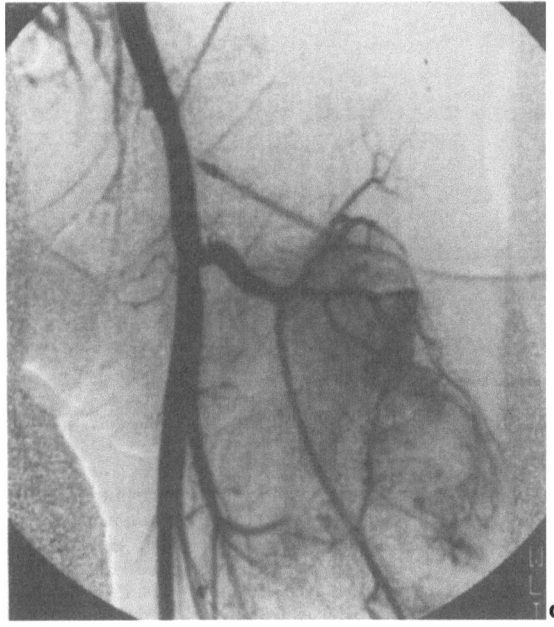

Fig. 11.5a–c. CT scan (a), conventional film angiography (b) and intra-arterial DSA (c) in a patient with malignant fibrous histiocytoma of the anterior left thigh. Note the improved display of abnormal capillary stain in the tumour mass provided by the DSA study. This reflects the improved contrast sensitivity of DSA compared with film angiography. CT scan demonstrates that the tumour is contiguous with bone. There is no periosteal reaction.

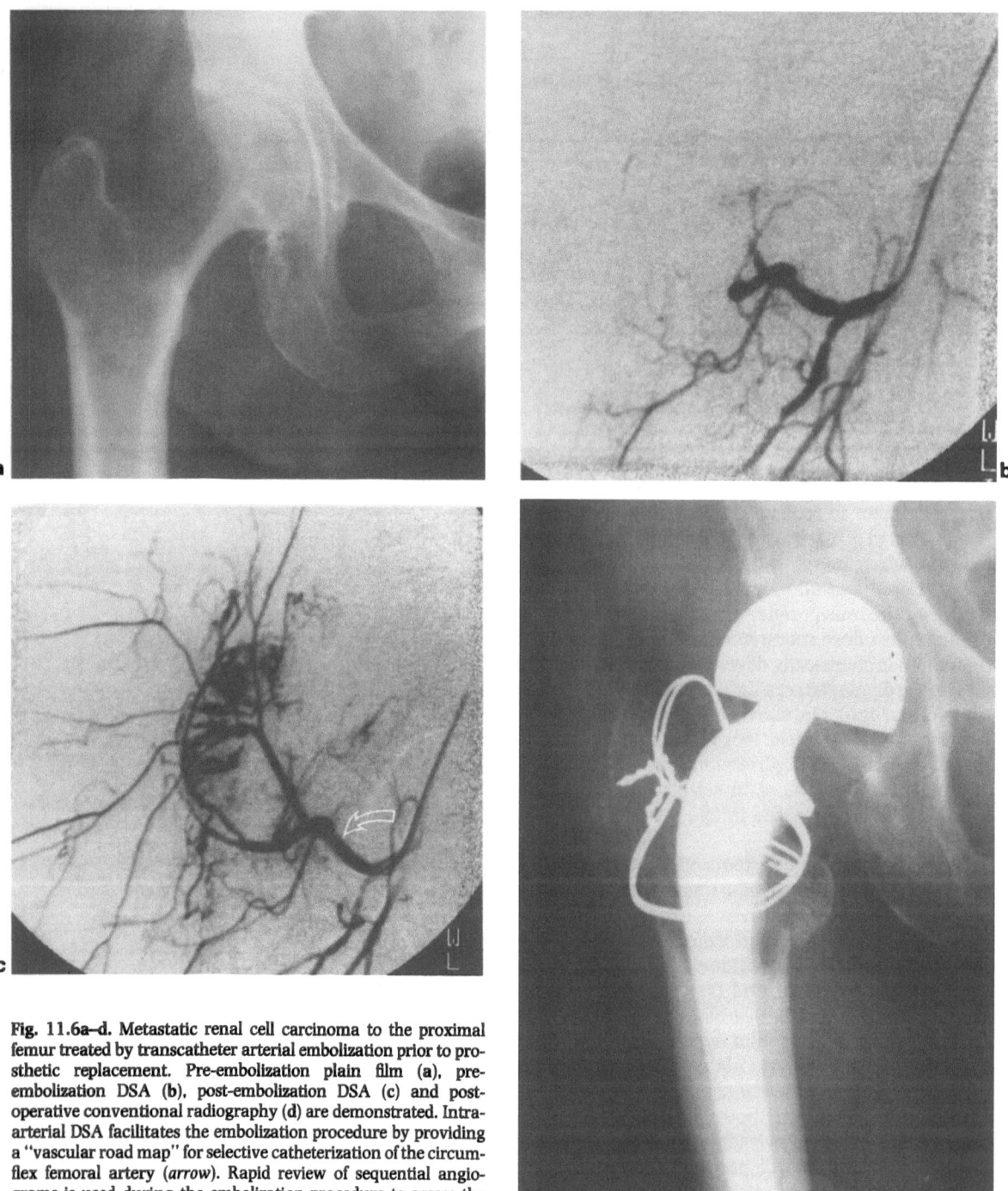

Fig. 11.6a–d. Metastatic renal cell carcinoma to the proximal femur treated by transcatheter arterial embolization prior to prosthetic replacement. Pre-embolization plain film (**a**), pre-embolization DSA (**b**), post-embolization DSA (**c**) and post-operative conventional radiography (**d**) are demonstrated. Intra-arterial DSA facilitates the embolization procedure by providing a "vascular road map" for selective catheterization of the circumflex femoral artery (*arrow*). Rapid review of sequential angiograms is used during the embolization procedure to assess the adequacy of vessel occlusion in the tumour bed.

orthopaedic images. Electronic storage, retrieval and transmission will depend upon the development and implementation of a PACS system. Interface standards for PACS networks have been developed by the American College of Radiology and National Electrical Manufacturers Association of the United States. However, further developments and standards are required in image storage methods and network transmission. Successful implementation of a PACS system would be a significant advance in view of the well-recognized logistic problems with the storage and retrieval of radiographic film, particularly film tracking and retrieval time.

Conventional film techniques use an area beam with a short total exposure time. Scattered radiation constitutes a significant component of the transmitted photon beam and degrades image contrast. Pencil beam and fan beam radiographic techniques markedly diminish the percentage of scattered radiation incident on the receptor and are more efficient in this regard than a radiographic grid with an area beam technique (Stein 1976; Tesic et al. 1983). However, there is increased total exposure time and susceptibility to motion distortion. Pencil beam and fan beam techniques can be used more efficiently with electronic detectors if the electronic receptor is more sensitive to input radiation than a film–screen device. Types of beam geometry and detector architecture used in digital radiography are outlined in Fig. 11.8. Total exposure times of 500 ms for abdominal and chest imaging appear feasible with new techniques in fan beam digital radiography. It should be understood that exposure time for any segment of the image is minimal and only a small percentage of the total exposure time. Such techniques should be free of image distortion due to either peristaltic bowel motion or cardiac wall motion. A moving fan beam technique could result in effective motion stopping with the added advantage of significant scatter reduction.

A significant advantage of image digitization is the capability for producing data with low noise and a wide dynamic range suitable for window-level analysis in a manner comparable to that employed on a CT scanner console. Interactive variation of window level at a video display console can result in significant improvement in perceived contrast. Other electronic manipulations include tonal reversal, and image processing techniques such as spatial filtering and histogram equalization (Sartoris and Sommer 1984; McAdams et al. 1986). Tonal reversal will change a white-on-black format to a black-on-white format. Spatial filters provide edge enhancement and improved perceived dynamic range. Though such techniques do not increase the information content within the image or improve

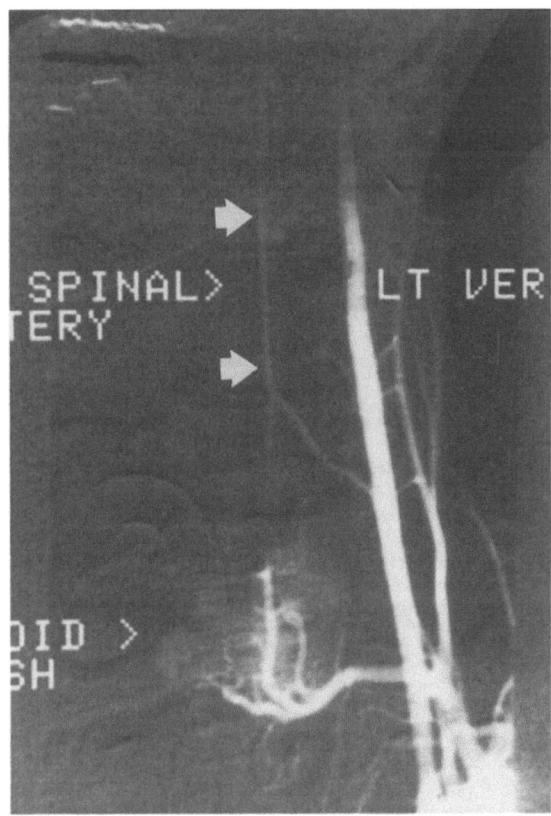

Fig. 11.7. Intra-arterial DSA in spinal angiography. This is an example of a left subclavian artery injection with opacification of the left vertebral artery, thyrocervical and ascending cervical artery. The anterior spinal artery (*filled arrows*) arises from a direct feeder off the left vertebral artery. Improved contrast sensitivity and the use of repeat "on-line" angiography make DSA a better method than conventional angiography in cooperative patients.

spatial resolution, they may make fine detail, both anatomical and pathological, more apparent to the observer (Fig. 11.9).

The spatial resolution of a conventional film–screen system is dependent on focal spot size, beam geometry and the characteristics of the detector. Slow detail screens and film are capable of 10 line pairs/mm resolution. Such resolution is usually only apparent with a magnifying lens. A reasonable goal for most skeletal radiography would be a 100 micron pixel corresponding to 5 line pairs/mm and a matrix size of 2000 × 2000 for a 20 cm × 20 cm field of view. The resolution required for adequate definition of the fine meshwork pattern of bony trabeculae is, as yet, unknown, as there have been

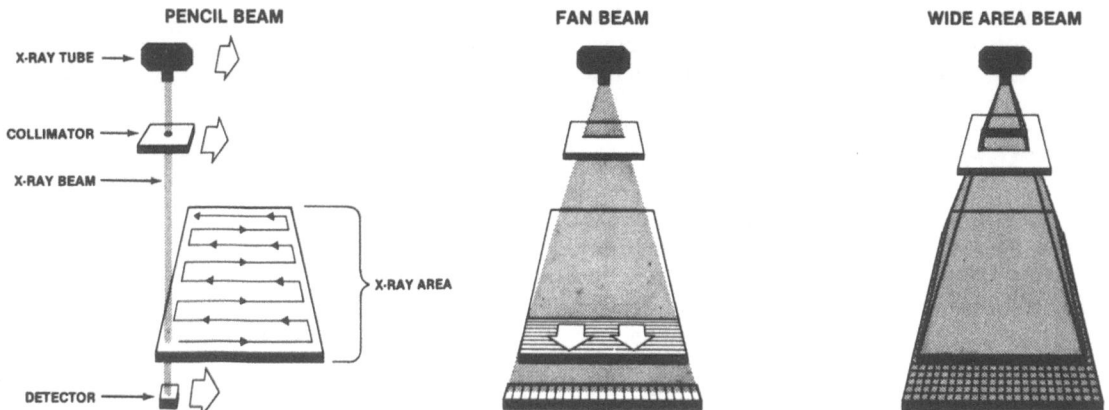

Fig. 11.8. Schematic diagram of different beam geometries which could be implemented for digital radiography. The pencil beam approach utilizes a narrow X-ray beam used in a raster scan fashion in conjunction with a single crystal photomultiplier detector. This system provides the lowest X-ray exposure and best scatter reduction, but is associated with the longest scan times and potential motion distortion. Wide area beam systems operate either by digital readout of a receptor plate (photostimulable phosphor, selenium plate) or require a large array of discrete electronic detectors, a prohibitively expensive proposition. Fan beam systems with acceptably short exposure times offer significant exposure and scattered radiation reduction. The receptor may be a phosphor/photodiode combination, an ionization chamber or a proximity focused image intensifier.

no comparative studies of observer performance analysing skeletal radiographs at different pixel sizes. Abnormalities which need to be clearly defined on digital radiographs of the skeleton include: hairline fractures, focal trabecular destruction, cortical erosions, early periosteal new bone formation, small soft tissue calcifications, pseudofractures and small osteophytes (Fig. 11.9). Improved image contrast at adequate levels of spatial resolution may actually make focal abnormalities of the types just mentioned more perceptible to an observer reviewing digital radiographic images on a video monitor.

Specialized Orthopaedic Radiography

Cast Radiography

Analysis of fracture healing or non-union by the radiography of extremities immobilized in plaster is often difficult. This is due to the limited exposure latitude of conventional film techniques. Improved latitude, as is possible with a digital device, does result in improved perception of cortical and cancellous bone.

Scoliosis Radiography

The potential advantage of digital techniques in scoliosis radiography is exposure reduction to the adolescent population in which this technique is most commonly used. In addition, quantitative determinations can be performed easily on digital image data, allowing precise determination of the scoliotic deformity and comparison with previous studies.

Dual Energy Radiography

Dual energy radiography may be implemented using a dual photon technique employing rapidly switching beam energy, tube current and the use of differential filtration to avoid spectral overlap. Another and perhaps preferable technique employs a dual energy receptor compartmentalized into two components, the input window being sensitive to relatively low energy and the back end of the receptor to higher energies. Dual energy techniques may be employed for bone mineral analysis and for selective cancellation of bone or soft tissue in projection radiography. By "removing" overlying soft

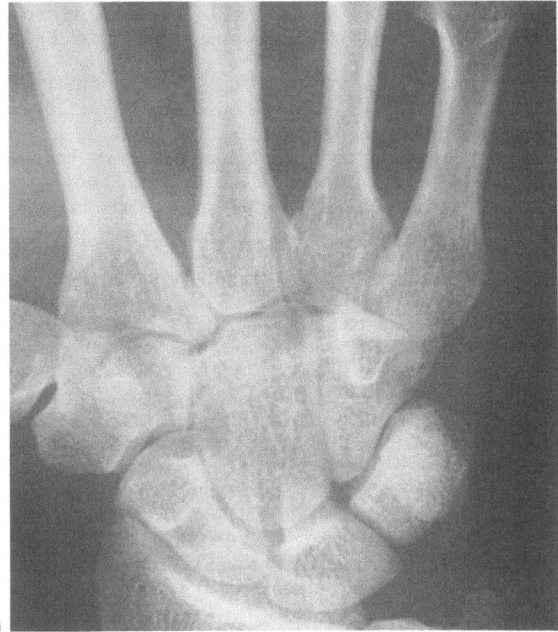

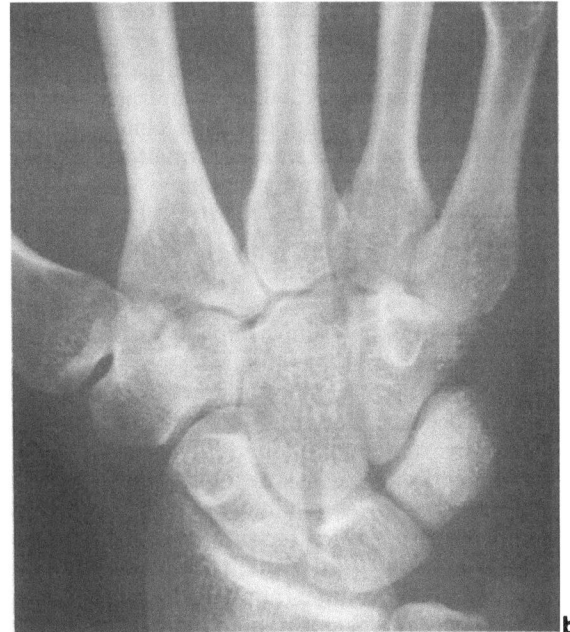

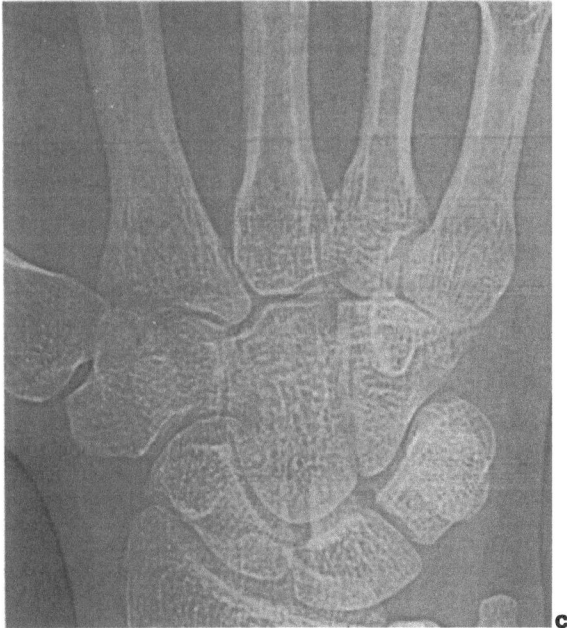

tissue, such techniques may improve the display of the thoracic spine and shoulder girdle in chest radiography, and of the lumbar spine and pelvic girdle in abdominal imaging (Brody et al. 1981). Dual image techniques involve image subtraction, which introduces electronic noise into the images. Thus the technique is best implemented with a detector extremely sensitive to input radiation.

Digital Tomosynthesis

In conventional tomography a thin object plane is selected by appropriate motion of the X-ray source and detector around a plane defined by the fulcrum of the central beam axis. Structures in the object above and below the desired image plane are removed by blurring. Repeated tomograms with different settings of the fulcrum height are needed to produce a contiguous sequence of predefined section planes within the object. Thus, conventional tomography entails a considerable radiation dose compared with a single projection radiograph. An alternative low-dose technique for coronal plane tomography using a digital image receptor is digital tomosynthesis (Maravilla et al. 1983; Friedenberg et al. 1985). With this technique, multiple contiguous object planes can be isolated by utilizing rapid digital readout during multiple exposures at different times during motion of the tube and detector.

Fig. 11.9a–c. Linear fracture at the base of the right fourth metacarpal bone. Conventional radiography (a) is compared with video display of digitized conventional film (b) and the edge-enhanced (computer processed) image (c). The digitized images b, c were acquired with a 0.2 mm pixel size (2.5 line pairs/mm). The original conventional radiograph was obtained using geometric magnification. The spatial resolution of a 2.5 line pairs/ mm digital image is not equivalent to conventional radiography. Image processing techniques result in improvements in perceived bony detail. Such techniques could be useful in digital orthopaedic radiography, provided there is adequate spatial resolution in the image data.

Digital tomosynthesis has been implemented with a planar electron tube (PET scope), video camera and analog-to-digital converter. Data are recorded in a manner analogous to the nonsubtraction mode of a DSA system. Multiple image planes can be obtained with one exposure. Reformations in other than the coronal plane are possible.

Special Procedures

Special imaging procedures such as arthrography, and interventional techniques such as biopsy, require fluoroscopic monitoring. Using a digital video processor, and time integration of video signals by a recursive filter, high-quality video images without significant motion lag can be obtained at far lower radiation doses than currently employed with conventional fluoroscopic systems (Jaffe et al. 1982). In addition, video images may be synthesized by integration and the electronic images photographed on a multiformat camera, thus reducing or eliminating the need for conventional spot radiographs.

References

Brody WR, Cassel DM, Sommer FG et al. (1981) Dual energy projection radiography: initial clinical experience. AJR 137:201–205

Bursch JH, Heintzen PH (1985) Parametric imaging. Radiol Clin North Am 23:321–323

Capp MP, Roehrig H, Selley GW et al. (1985) The digital radiology department of the future. Radiol Clin North Am 23:349–355

Chuang VP, Wallace S (1981) Arterial infusion and occlusion in cancer patients. Semin Roentgenol 16:13–25

Chuang VP, Wallace S, Swanson D et al. (1979) Arterial occlusion in the management of pain for metastatic renal carcinoma. Radiology 133:611–614

Federle MP (1983) Computed tomography of blunt abdominal trauma. Radiol Clin North Am 21:461–475

Foley WD, Keyes GS, Smith DF et al. (1983) Temporal energy "hybrid" subtraction and intravenous digital subtraction angiography. Radiology 148:265–271

Fraser RG, Breatnach E, Barnes GT (1983) Digital radiography of the chest: clinical experience with a prototype unit. Radiology 148:1–5

Friedenberg RM, Lightfoote JB, Wang SP, Smolin MF (1985) Digital tomography: description and preliminary clinical experience. AJR 144:639–643

Gavant ML, Gold RE, Fabian TC, Tonkin ILD (1986) Vascular trauma to the extremities and lower neck: initial assessment with intravenous digital subtraction angiography. Radiology 158:755–760

Goodman PC, Jeffrey RB Jr, Brant-Zawadzki M (1984) Digital subtraction angiography in extremity trauma. Radiology 153:61–64

Jaffe CC, Orphanoudakis SC, Ablow RC (1982) The effect of a television digital noise reduction device on fluoroscopic image quality and dose rate. Radiology 144:789–792

Jaques P, DiBianca F, Pizer S, Kohout F, Lifshitz L, Delany D (1985) Quantitative digital fluorography: computer versus human estimation of vascular stenoses. Invest Radiol 20:45–52

Kruger RA, Reiderer SJ (1984) Basic concepts of digital subtraction angiography. GK Hall Medical Publishers, Boston

Lee KR, Cox CG, Price HI, Johnson JA, Neff JR (1986) Intra-arterial digital subtraction arteriographic evaluation of extremity tumors: comparison with conventional arteriography. Radiology 158:255–258

Maravilla KR, Murray RC Jr, Horner S (1983) Digital tumor synthesis: technique for electronic reconstructive tomography. AJR 141:497–502

McAdams HP, Johnson GA, Suddarth SA, Ravin CE (1986) Histogram directed processing of digital chest images. Radiology 21:253–259

Paushter DM, Borkowski GP, Buonocore E, Belhobek GH, Marks KE (1983) Digital subtraction angiography for preoperative evaluation of extremity tumors. AJR 141:129–133

Sartoris DJ, Sommer FG (1984) Digital film processing: applications to the musculoskeletal system. Skeletal Radiology 11:274–281

Simons MA, Kruger RA (1985) Vessel diameter measurement using digital subtraction radiography. Invest Radiol 20:510–516

Smith PH, Lim WN, Ferris EJ, Casali RE (1981) Emergency arteriography in extremity trauma: assessment of indications. AJR 137:803–807

Sonada M, Takano M, Miyahara J, Kato H (1983) Computed radiography utilizing scanning laser stimulated luminescence. Radiology 148:833–838

Stein JA (1976) X-ray imaging with a scanning beam. Radiology 117:713–716

Tesic MM, Mattson RA, Barnes GT, Sones RA, Stickney JB (1983) Digital radiography of the chest: design features and considerations for a prototype unit. Radiology 148:259–264

Turski PA, Stieghorst MF, Strother CM, Crummy AB, Lieberman RP, Mistretta CA (1982) Digital subtraction angiography "road map". AJR 139:1233–1234

Yeates AE, Drayer BP, Heinz ER, Osborne D (1985) Intra-arterial digital subtraction angiography of the spinal cord. Radiology 155:387–390

12 Magnetic Resonance Imaging (MRI)

J.P.R. Jenkins and I. Isherwood

Introduction	159
Technical Aspects	159
Instrumentation	159
Image Acquisition	160
Safety	162
Normal Anatomy	163
Musculoskeletal System	163
Spine	164
Musculoskeletal Pathology	165
Tumours	165
Musculoskeletal Infection	166
Vascular Lesions	167
Trauma	167
Joint Disease	169
Muscle Disease	171
Spinal Pathology	171
Degenerative Disc Disease	171
Infection	171
Trauma	173
Congenital Anomalies	173
Tumours and Arteriovenous Malformations	173
Syringomyelia	175
Bone Marrow Disease	176
Magnetic Resonance Spectroscopy (MRS)	176
Present Research and Future Aspects	176
References	177

Introduction

Magnetic resonance imaging (MRI) is established as an important diagnostic technique, most clearly showing its clinical utility and efficacy in the central nervous system, spine and musculoskeletal system.

In the spine and musculoskeletal system MRI has particular advantages (Table 12.1), including a high soft tissue contrast resolution and discrimination, the ability to image in any plane, the absence of bone and some metal artefacts in the image and the use of non-ionizing radiation. Artefacts from respiration, cardiac motion and bowel peristalsis can degrade images of the spine when conventional scanning techniques are used but can be much reduced by the application of surface coils, cardiac gated or faster imaging sequences (*vide infra*). Disadvantages (Table 12.1) include high cost, limited availability, relatively long data-acquisition times, poor compact bone and calcium detail and claustrophobic effects.

Technical Aspects

Instrumentation

MRI systems require the following:

Magnet
Radiofrequency (rf) coils (transmitter/receiver)
Gradient coils
Computer, display unit and digital storage facilities

Table 12.1. The advantages and disadvantages of MRI

Advantages
   High intrinsic soft tissue contrast and discrimination
   Direct transverse, sagittal, coronal and oblique imaging
   Multisection imaging
   No bone or air artefacts
   Artefacts only from some metals
   No ionizing radiation used
   Demonstration of normal development and function
   No known biological hazard

Disadvantages
   Long scanning times
   Many protocol options
   Correct choice of rf pulse sequence parameters essential
   Poor bone and calcium detail (including periosteal reaction)
   Motion artefacts with scanning thorax and abdomen
   Relative difficulty in monitoring/maintaining ill patients
   Patients with pacemakers restricted
   Claustrophobia (2%–5% cases studied)
   High capital and revenue costs
   Limited availability
   ? Long-term side effects

Magnet

An essential component of an MRI system is a relatively stable and homogeneous static magnetic field. This is provided by one of three main types of magnet designs – permanent, resistive or superconducting. Each has its advantages and disadvantages (McFarland and Rosen 1986). The single most costly item for a magnetic resonance (MR) system is the magnet, and new and more compact designs are currently being developed.

The static main magnetic field strength for MRI ranges at present from 0.01 to 2.0 T[1]. There is no consensus as to the optimum field strength for MRI, although Hoult et al. (1986) proposed a medium field strength (0.5–1.0 T) as the best current compromise. If spectroscopy or imaging of nuclei other than protons is required, then a high field system is necessary. An MRI system usually operates at a fixed field strength, although some manufacturers are now producing "rampable" systems where the main magnetic field can be varied from 0.5 to 2.0 T.

[1]Field strength is measured in Tesla(T) (SI unit) or Gauss(G). 1 T = 10 000 G. The earth's magnetic field strength varies with position but is approximately 0.5 G or 0.05 mT.

Radiofrequency Coils

The basic radiofrequency (rf) coil surrounds the part of the patient to be examined and is used to transmit and receive rf signals to and from the patient. This produces the appropriate signal data from which digital images can be produced. Surface and close-coupled receiver coils are of smaller diameter, improve the signal-to-noise ratio and allow thinner sections to be obtained with consequent improvement in spatial resolution and soft tissue discrimination.

Gradient Coils

The main magnetic field is modified during scanning for short periods (typically a few milliseconds) by gradient magnetic fields. Gradient field strengths are usually only about 2% of the main field. By the use of such a gradient system, sections of tissue in any plane, as well as within the section, can be identified from the magnetized volume. There are three sets of gradient coils (called X, Y and Z) that are orientated in three orthogonal directions, and each can affect the main field. Two or more coils can be energized simultaneously to produce a gradient on the main field in any direction in space.

Computer, Display Unit and Digital Storage

These facilities are very similar to those employed in computed tomography (CT) and are required to collect and process the signal data to form images, which can then be displayed in digital form on a viewing console. Data acquisition times for conventional MRI are typically of the order of minutes, whereas image data reconstruction takes only seconds. Digital data can be stored as in CT on magnetic tape, optical or floppy disc, or a hard copy can be made.

Image Acquisition

The physical principles of MRI are discussed in greater detail elsewhere (Bradley et al. 1983, Wehrli et al. 1983, Jenkins and Isherwood 1987a,b). In outline, atomic nuclei with an odd number of protons and/or neutrons (e.g. proton (^{1}H), sodium (^{23}Na), phosphorus (^{31}P) and carbon (^{13}C)) possess an intrinsic spin, thus generating a magnetic moment. Nuclei of tissues placed within the main magnetic field tend to align along the direction of that field. Application of rf pulses can be used to induce resonance of particular sets of nuclei. The

Table 12.2. Main rf pulse sequences with their major signal intensity weighting

rf pulse sequence	Image weighting
Partial saturation recovery (PSR)	Proton density + T_1 Phase-contrast
Spin echo (SE)	
Short TR/short TE	T_1
Long TR/long TE	T_2
Long TR/short TE	Proton density
Inversion recovery (IR)	
Medium to long TI	T_1
Short TI ("STIR")	$T_1 + T_2$

required frequency of the rf pulse is determined by the strength of the magnetic field and the particular nucleus under investigation. Resonance refers to a change in the alignment, and thus energy level, of the nuclei in the main field. The energy absorbed during this transition (higher energy state) is subsequently released to the environment when the rf pulse is turned off as the nuclei relax back to equilibrium (lower energy state). The release of energy can be recorded as an electrical signal and provides the data from which digital images can be derived. Such an image is usually constructed using a mathematical process called two-dimensional Fourier transform (2DFT).

The proton, i.e. the hydrogen nucleus, is the one most suitable for conventional imaging. It is the most abundant in the human body and yields the strongest MR signal compared with other spinning nuclei. The protons which give rise to the MR signal are mainly those in water and lipids, with water protons in the majority. Protons which do not contribute significantly to the resultant MR signal include those in proteins, DNA and solid structures such as cortical bone.

The strength (amplitude) of the signal will depend not only on the number of measurable or mobile protons ("proton-" or "spin-density") in the tissues, but also on a variety of other parameters such as relaxation times, blood flow, chemical shift or phase-contrast effects, magnetic susceptibility, diffusion, perfusion and rf absorption. Two relaxation times are described, termed T_1 and T_2. The T_1 (otherwise known as "spin lattice" or "longitudinal") relaxation time is a term used to describe return of protons back to equilibrium following application and then removal of the rf pulse. T_2 (otherwise called "spin-spin" or "transverse") relaxation time is a term used

to describe the associated loss of coherence or phase between individual protons immediately following the rf pulse. Both time constants are exponential terms and are parameters that have the potential to characterize normal and pathological tissues (Jenkins et al. 1985, 1987c; Johnson et al. 1987; Isherwood et al. 1987; Prendergast et al. 1987).

A variety of rf pulse sequences can be used to generate an image. The most commonly used sequences are termed partial saturation recovery (PSR), inversion recovery (IR) and spin echo (SE). Different pulse sequences give different weighting in the received signal to the various tissue parameters (Table 12.2). A high signal intensity, using typical sequences, is observed from tissues with an increased proton density, short T_1 or a prolonged T_2. A low signal is produced by tissues with the opposite parameters (see Table 12.3). The MR signal related to flowing blood is a complex interplay of many factors, including blood velocity, direction of flow, flow profile (laminar or turbulent), pulse sequences employed and field gradients applied. Turbulent and fast flowing (arterial) blood produces little or no signal, whereas static or slow moving (venous) blood can give a high signal. Thus arteries and veins can be detected. Chemical shift effects occur because there is a change in the MR behaviour relating to differences in the chemical environment between protons attached to carbon in a lipid molecule and those bound to oxygen as in water. This difference can be exploited in chemical shift imaging to produce separate water and lipid or composite ("phase-contrast") images (see Fig. 12.12) (Bydder and Young 1985a; Paling et al. 1987).

For each rf pulse sequence there are a number of operator-dependent factors (called "machine"

Table 12.3. Signal intensity of musculoskeletal tissues on T_1W and T_2W sequences

High signal on T_1W and T_2W images
    Fat, marrow, haematoma/thrombus (varies with age), slow-flowing blood

Low signal on T_1W and T_2W images
    Cortical bone, air/gas, ligaments/tendons, fibrocartilage, calcification, turbulent/fast flowing blood

Intermediate signal on T_1W and T_2W images
    Muscle, nerves, spinal cord, hyaline (articular) cartilage, annulus fibrosis of disc

Low–intermediate signal on T_1W and high signal on T_2W images
    Cerebrospinal fluid, urine, nucleus pulposus of disc, most tumours, infection, cysts, effusions

parameters) *viz.* echo time (TE), inversion time (TI) and repetition time (TR), any one of which can be varied with dramatic alteration in image contrast. Typically, an rf pulse sequence, with its defined timing parameters, needs to be repeated 128 or 256 times, each with a new gradient increment, in order to produce an image on a 256×256 or a 512×512 matrix. Each gradient increment can be repeated, typically twice, to give two signal excitations, which are then averaged. The overall scanning time per sequence can be calculated by multiplying the TR of the sequence by the number of gradient increments and signal excitations used. A single section MR image, using typical sequences, can take 2–8 minutes to collect the data, together with a few seconds of data processing. Much of the time taken for data collection is non-productive and represents the time allowed for tissue relaxation processes to occur before re-excitation. Use can be made of this relaxation period by exciting protons in adjacent sections, thus obtaining sufficient data to image 4–16 contiguous sections in the same time taken to image one or two sections. Such multisection imaging significantly reduces the scanning time needed for a patient and allows the full extent of lesions to be determined.

Safety

No genetic or mutagenic effects have been demonstrated using presently available MRI instrumentation (Budinger 1981; Saunders and Smith 1984). Recommendations for magnetic field limitations in MRI are based on present guidelines issued by the Bureau of Radiological Health (BRH) (1982) and the National Radiological Protection Board (NRPB) (1983). There are three potential sources of hazard that exist relating to the different types of magnetic fields encountered in MRI.

Static Main Magnetic Field Effects

There is no evidence to suggest any biological risk for those exposed to MRI from the static main field. Of practical concern is the attractive force on ferromagnetic objects which increases with (field strength)[2] and inversely with (distance from the magnet)[3]. Loose ferromagnetic metal objects can thus become dangerous projectiles.

Most orthopaedic implants are non-ferromagnetic or demonstrate a weak magnetic effect. Some vascular clips are, however, ferromagnetic and may be displaced by the static field. Even if the clips or other implants are made from non-magnetic

material, cold cutting during manufacture or bending can induce significant ferromagnetism within stainless steel (New et al. 1983). The degree of risk can be reduced or eliminated by appropriate selection of alloys for implant manufacture (such as high nickel impregnated stainless steel alloys, tantalum or titanium). A further practical problem concerns cardiac pacemakers, two types of which contain reed switches activated by magnetic fields (either static or time-varying). Patients with pacemakers in situ should not be examined by MRI, and such individuals should not enter the 0.5 mT (5 G) stray field line.

It is important to stress that the main magnetic field is not confined to the bore of the magnet, but extends for a significant distance in all directions, increasing with magnetic field strength, unless magnet shielding is used.

Time Varying (Gradient) Magnetic Field Effects

Rapidly changing magnetic fields induce electric currents in tissues, since the body acts as a conductor. The magnitude of the effect is proportional to the rate of change of field. Saunders and Smith (1984) have pointed out that skin sensations and muscular contractions would be induced before ventricular fibrillation because of the higher densities in these tissues. The NRPB (1983) guidelines limit the induced current density in tissues to about a tenth of that required to induce fibrillation in the normal myocardium. It is uncertain, however, if this is the same for the electrically unstable abnormal myocardium. Bone healing is stimulated by the application of changing magnetic fields, although it will not occur with sinusoidal pulses that are used in MRI. Even so, the limit set would avoid this effect. Tooth pain and taste sensation have been reported due to movement of the patient's head through a changing magnetic field. This effect probably relates to tooth nerves sensing an induced electrical current and may indicate that patients should not be moved quickly when gradient fields are on.

Rapid gradient switching, especially during multislice acquisition or fast scanning techniques, produces mechanical noise as the rf coils move in response to changing fields. Manufacturers are working on improved designs to minimize this effect.

Radiofrequency Magnetic Field Effects

Most of the rf pulse power used to excite nuclei is dissipated as heat in tissue. The recommendations

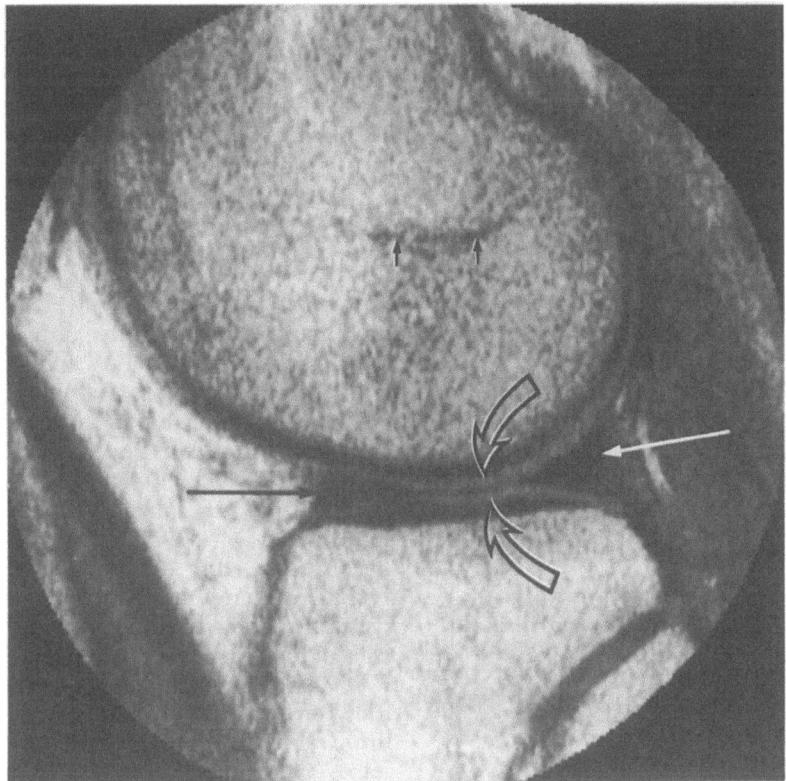

Fig. 12.1. Normal adult knee on sagittal (SE with TR/TE of 600/40) image. Menisci are shown as low signal (*long straight arrows*) with high signal from articular cartilage (*curved arrows*). A linear low signal in the femoral condyle (*small straight arrows*), in keeping with trabecular bone, marks the previous location of the epiphyseal growth plates.

on field limitations restrict exposure so as to avoid any significant rise in temperature of sensitive body tissues (particularly avascular structures such as the lens of the eye). Caution is required when examining patients with metallic implants, e.g. hip prostheses, where there is a possibility of heating within the implant (Davis et al. 1981).

Monitoring critically ill patients can be difficult within the "tunnel" of the magnet, but intubated patients can be scanned successfully using non-ferromagnetic equipment. Defibrillators function satisfactorily in the magnetic field but the monitoring electrocardiographic trace can be affected. Although no evidence exists to suggest that the embryo is sensitive to the magnetic and rf fields encountered in MRI, examinations in early pregnancy are restricted to certain research centres at the present time.

Normal Anatomy

The signal intensities of various musculoskeletal and spinal tissues calculated using conventional T_1- and T_2-weighted (T_1W and T_2W) sequences is given in Table 12.3. Similar variability in signal intensity is noted for tissues using the PSR sequence, except that the vertebral marrow appears as low signal (due to chemical shift effect from the phase difference between the lipid (fatty marrow) and water (haemopoietic marrow) proton species and both articular cartilage and intervertebral disc give high signal (see Fig. 12.12).

Musculoskeletal System

There is good delineation of the fascial planes, subcutaneous fat, vessels, nerves, ligaments, tendons

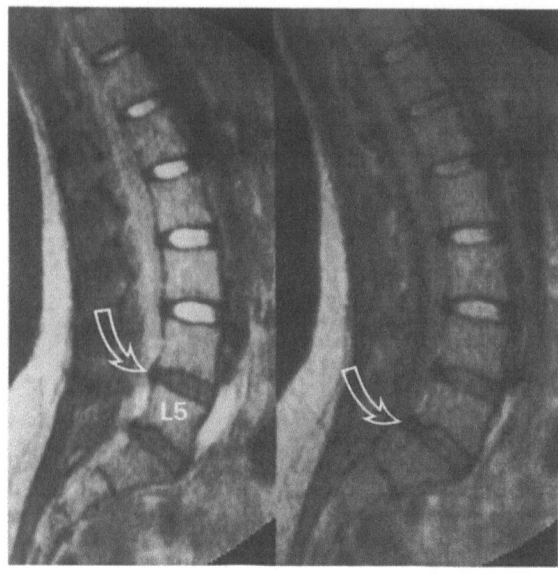

Fig. 12.2. Contiguous sagittal T_2W (SE 3000/80) images in a young adult showing degenerative and posteriorly herniated L4/5 and L5/S1 intervertebral discs (*curved arrows*). Using this sequence, the cerebrospinal fluid is of high signal. Note cleft of low signal within the nucleus pulposus of the normal hydrated discs above.

and muscles on both T_1W and PSR sequences. The capsule, ligaments, cartilages and menisci, as well as the articulating bone and growth plates, are well distinguished (Fig. 12.1). Multiplanar, including oblique, surface coil imaging, allows a complete assessment of most joints. Detailed normal MR anatomy of some major joints has been described, including the knee (Harms and Muschler 1986), hip (Littrup et al. 1985), ankle and foot (Beltran et al. 1986b), shoulder (Seegar et al. 1987), wrist (Weiss et al. 1986a) and temporomandibular joint (Westesson et al. 1987). Early studies reported poor visualization of neurovascular bundles in the extremities, but with improved spatial resolution achieved by localized surface coils, these can now be routinely imaged.

There is an age-related change in the relative proportions of fatty and haemopoietic marrow within cancellous bone. Young children have a more extensive distribution of haemopoietic marrow compared with adults (Kricun 1985). This is reflected in lower marrow signals on T_1W sequences in the appendicular skeleton and spine. With increasing age the haemopoietic marrow (long T_1) gradually

recedes from the appendicular skeleton, being replaced in part by fatty marrow (short T_1) (Littrup et al. 1985) and is demonstrated as a high signal on PSR and T_1W images.

Spine

The spinal cord, including the conus, cauda equina and nerve roots, can be directly and routinely demonstrated on both T_1W and PSR sequences (see Fig. 12.9). The surrounding cerebrospinal fluid (CSF) within the spinal canal has a low signal whilst epidural fat and veins have a high signal. On heavily T_2W images, a high signal is obtained from CSF (because of its long T_2), producing an "MR myelogram" effect (Fig. 12.2). High resolution surface coil imaging *in vivo* (on a 0.3 T permanent magnet system) has consistently shown dorsal and ventral rootlets coursing within the subarachnoid space on transverse sections (Flannigan et al. 1987). The longitudinal ligaments are of low signal (low proton density) and cannot be distinguished from adjacent cortical bone. Although compact bone gives no signal, the fatty and haemopoietic marrow content of cancellous bone in adults appears as high signal on T_1W and T_2W images and low signal on PSR images.

Although the use of surface coils for spinal imaging markedly reduces artefacts from respiratory and cardiac motion, significant flow artefacts from CSF can occur, particularly in the cervical spine. Improvement in image quality, without extending scanning time, has been achieved by a combination of CSF-gating and flow compensation sequences (using low rf pulse angles and even echo rephasing) (Rubin JB et al. 1987).

The two components of the intervertebral disc can be distinguished on moderate to heavily T_2W images, whereby the normal nucleus gives a high signal (long T_2) and the annulus a low signal (short T_2). On T_1W and PSR sequences there is no such separation, and the disc appears intermediate and high signal respectively. A thin line or cleft of reduced signal intensity within the nucleus pulposus on T_2W images is found consistently in subjects over the age of 30 years (Fig. 12.2). Although the exact histological correlation of this cleft is uncertain, it would appear to represent fibrous tissue secondary to fissuring as part of a normal ageing process. High resolution sections of cadaveric discs have demonstrated the characteristic laminated structure of the annulus observed in the young disc (Hickey et al. 1986).

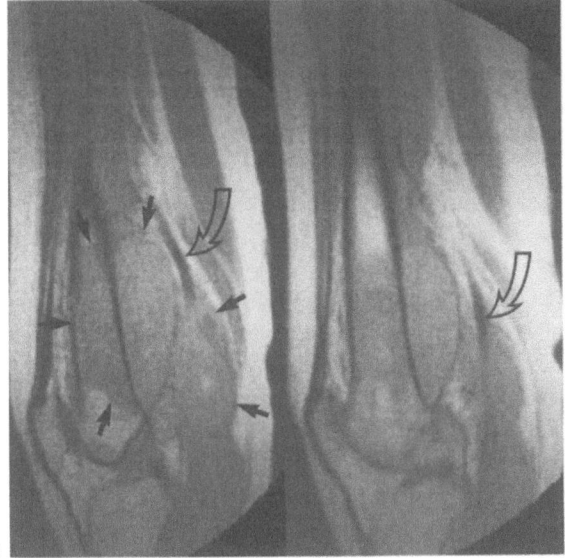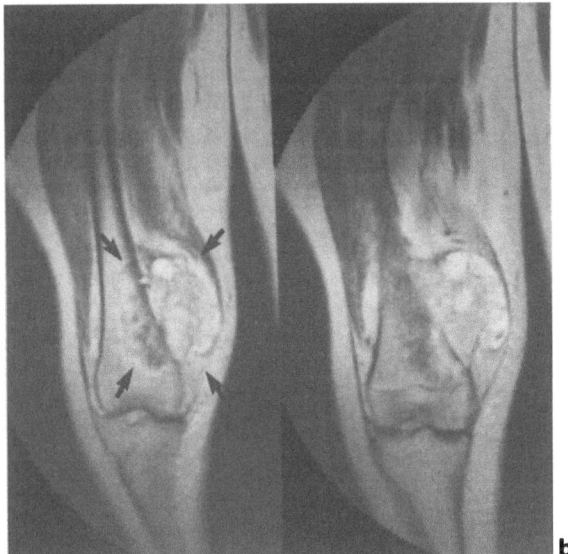

a   b

Fig. 12.3a,b. Osteosarcoma in distal femur on contiguous (a) sagittal T₁W (SE 1100/26) and (b) coronal T₂W (SE 2000/80) images. The extent of the tumour within bone and soft tissues (*straight arrows*) is clearly delineated. The popliteal artery (*curved open arrow*) is displaced but separate from the extra-osseous mass.

Musculoskeletal Pathology

Tumours

The improved contrast resolution, together with the multiplanar facility of MRI allows both the intra- and extraosseous extent of bone and soft tissue tumours to be more clearly and accurately defined compared with plain radiographs and CT (Fig. 12.3) (Zimmer et al. 1985; Weekes et al. 1985; Aisen et al. 1986; Totty et al. 1986; Petasnick et al. 1986; Boyko et al. 1987). Displacement or involvement of adjacent neurovascular structures by soft tissue tumours can also be accurately assessed (Petasnick et al. 1986). In primary bone tumours, MRI is superior to CT in demonstrating not only the intraosseous extent (including the presence or absence of skip lesions), but also in assessing the integrity of the growth plate, joint space and adjacent tissues.

Pettersson et al. (1987) examined 176 consecutive primary musculoskeletal tumours with a 0.15 T resistive system and observed that, in tumours confined to the bone, MRI was excellent for evaluation of the extent of the lesion, but not necessarily better than CT or radionuclide scanning. For soft tissue tumours and bone tumours with soft tissue extension, MRI was significantly better than any other

modality in delineating between tumour and muscle, fat, vessel, joint or bone. Cortical bone destruction, although demonstrated by MRI, is more easily shown on CT.

In general there are no specific characteristics that distinguish a malignant from a benign tumour on MRI and similar morphological criteria hold as for CT. Whether a lesion is well demarcated from or infiltrating adjacent tissues is not a reliable indicator of benignity or malignancy (Fig. 12.4). Malignant and benign tumours usually overlap in signal intensity. Most tumours, and indeed other soft tissue masses, have long T₁ and long T₂, appearing as low or high signal on T₁W or T₂W images respectively. Homogeneity in signal intensity is often seen with benign soft tissue tumours but some, particularly neurofibromas and haemangiomas, have heterogeneous signal intensity on T₂W images (Petasnick et al. 1986). Most malignant lesions exhibit homogeneous and heterogeneous signal intensity on T₁W and T₂W images respectively (Fig. 12.3). Although lipomas (short T₁, long T₂) have a characteristic MRI appearance, appearing as high signal on both T₁W and T₂W images, Petasnick et al. (1986) noted no differences in signal intensity in the majority (6 of 7) of benign and malignant fatty tumours. Similar signal intensity changes to fat have been noted in intramuscular haemorrhage and haematomas (Unger et al. 1986), and from

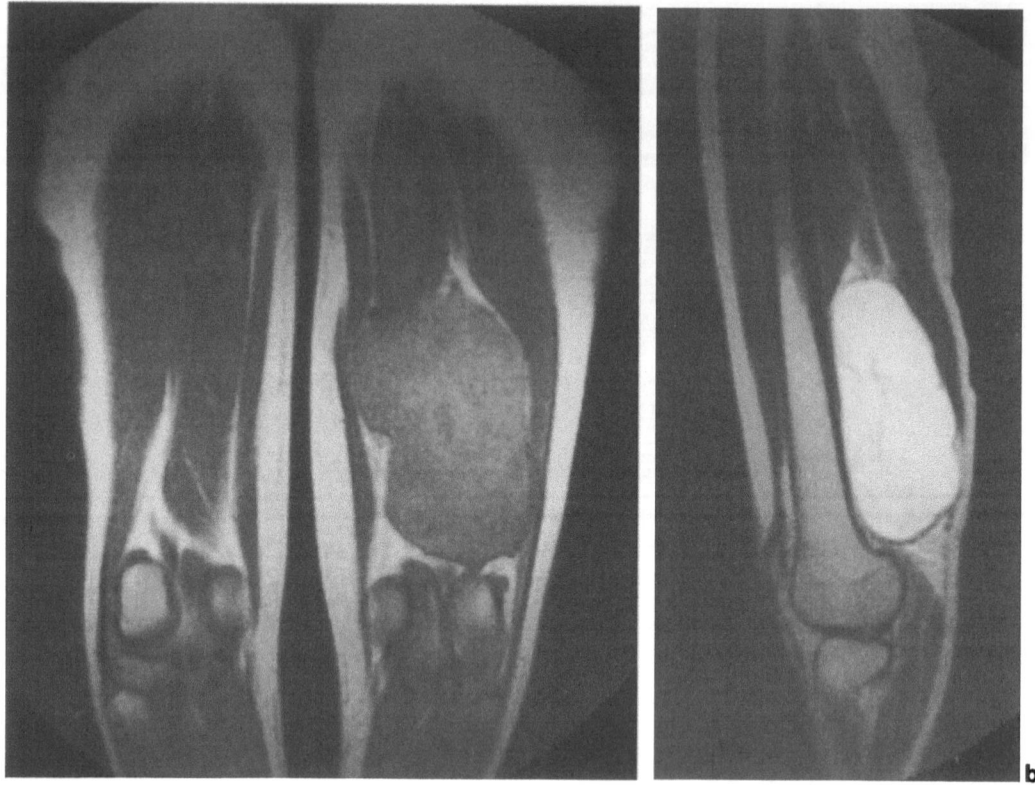

Fig. 12.4a,b. Liposarcoma on (a) coronal T_1W (SE 1000/26) and (b) sagittal T_2W (SE 2000/80) images. The tumour has a relatively homogeneous signal, different in intensity to that of surrounding fat. Note it is well marginated with a low intensity rim.

haemorrhage within tumour. Areas of necrosis and cystic change are characterized by prolonged T_1 and T_2 values, giving very low or high signals on T_1W or T_2W images respectively. Fluid levels containing blood of various ages may be observed in aneurysmal bone cysts. Both benign and malignant fibrous tumours have been noted to have low signal on all sequences, in keeping with a low proton density related to abundant collagen and marked acellularity within the tumour (Sundaram et al. 1987). Although MRI localizes abnormalities more clearly than other imaging modalities it is limited, at present, in determining specific pathology.

The advantages of MRI over CT are especially evident in the extremities, where there is less fat and muscle bulk. In the assessment of tumour recurrence in the post-operative patient, metallic surgical clips and prostheses produce only minimal localized artefact on MRI and diagnostic scans can be produced in the majority of cases (Weekes et al. 1985; Zimmer et al. 1985). Some metallic implants, however, are ferromagnetic or have ferromagnetism induced during manufacture (New et al. 1983), producing significant artefact.

CT or plain radiography remain superior in demonstrating calcification, periosteal reactions, fractures and gas formation. CT is the imaging method of choice in the assessment of pulmonary metastases, whilst radionuclide bone scanning is preferred in the identification of bone metastases. In MRI, as in CT, problems can arise in separating tumour from reactive or post-operative oedema, infection or acute haemorrhage (Brady et al. 1983; Beltran et al. 1987; Vanel et al. 1987). Chronic fibrosis due to scar tissue, however, has a low signal on T_2W sequences and, usually, can be differentiated from tumour.

Musculoskeletal Infection

In a preliminary study, Berquist et al. (1985) compared MRI with Indium-III-labelled leucocyte scans in patients with proven infection following surgery and trauma. Indium-III-labelled leucocyte scan was positive in all 12 cases of documented low-grade infection and MRI demonstrated bone and/or soft

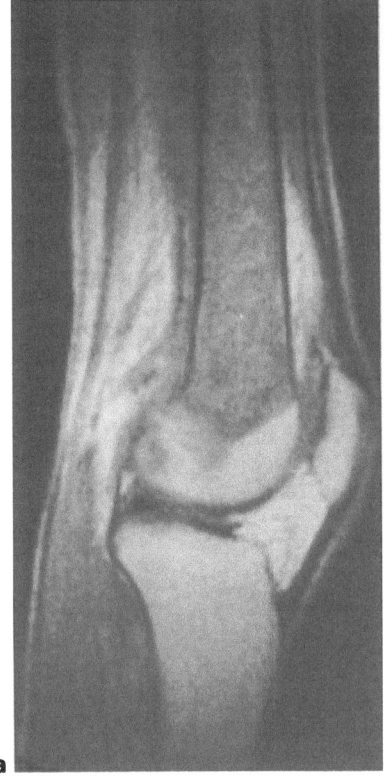

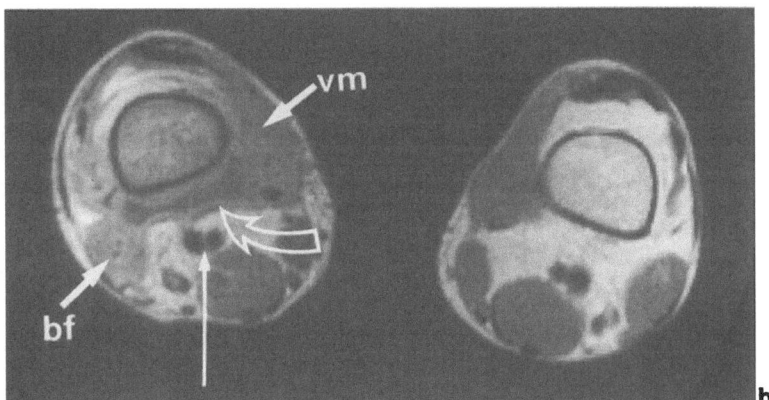

Fig. 12.5a,b. Osteomyelitis in a renal transplant patient involving the distal femoral shaft on (**a**) sagittal and (**b**) transverse intermediate T_1W (SE 1000/40) images. The extensive infiltration of the bone marrow is shown in (**a**). The adjacent soft tissue abscess (*open arrow*) postero-medial to the femoral shaft and anterior to the popliteal vessels (*long straight arrow*) is demonstrated in (**b**), together with involvement of the vastus medialis (*vm*) and biceps femoris (*bf*) muscles. (Reproduced from Sutton 1987, by kind permission.)

tissue changes in 11. In one patient, a localized artefact from a metal prosthesis prevented adequate evaluation of the bone–metal interface. MRI, however, more clearly localized the site of infection, i.e. medullary, cortical or adjacent soft tissues (Fig. 12.5). As with CT, difficulty was noted in differentiating fracture healing and post-surgical change from active infection.

In another group of 15 patients presenting with symptoms typical of an acute infection, Berquist et al. (1985) observed no differentiation between infection (in 12) or tumour (in 3). Both pathologies in the majority of cases produced lengthening of the relaxation times. Some cases of culture-proven osteomyelitis have also demonstrated low signal on both T_1W and T_2W images, making differentiation from fibrous dysplasia, bone infarction or benign sclerosis difficult (Modic et al. 1986a).

Vascular Lesions

Peripheral arteriovenous malformations and haemangiomas have been demonstrated by MRI with the full extent, size and location of the soft tissue components of the lesion more correctly represented, compared with contrast-enhanced CT (Fig. 12.6) (Cohen et al. 1986; Totty et al. 1986; Petasnick et al. 1986; Kaplan and Williams 1987). The exact feeding and draining vessels and associated phleboliths, however, have not consistently been shown by MRI.

Although angiography is required to demonstrate the feeding and draining vessels, and for performing pre-operative or therapeutic embolization, it cannot relate the full extent of the lesion to muscle groups and adjacent nerves so well, and is not without attendant risks.

Trauma

Haematomas in the acute stage (1–6 days) have similar signal intensity to skeletal muscle on T_1W images with a lower signal on T_2W images (Rubin JI et al. 1987). Subacute and chronic haematomas (up to 10 months duration) appear as areas of high signal with a low intensity rim on both T_1W and T_2W images (Fig. 12.7) (Unger et al. 1986). This lower signal on the T_2W images in acute haematomas can be difficult to visualize at low magnetic fields except when a modified PSR

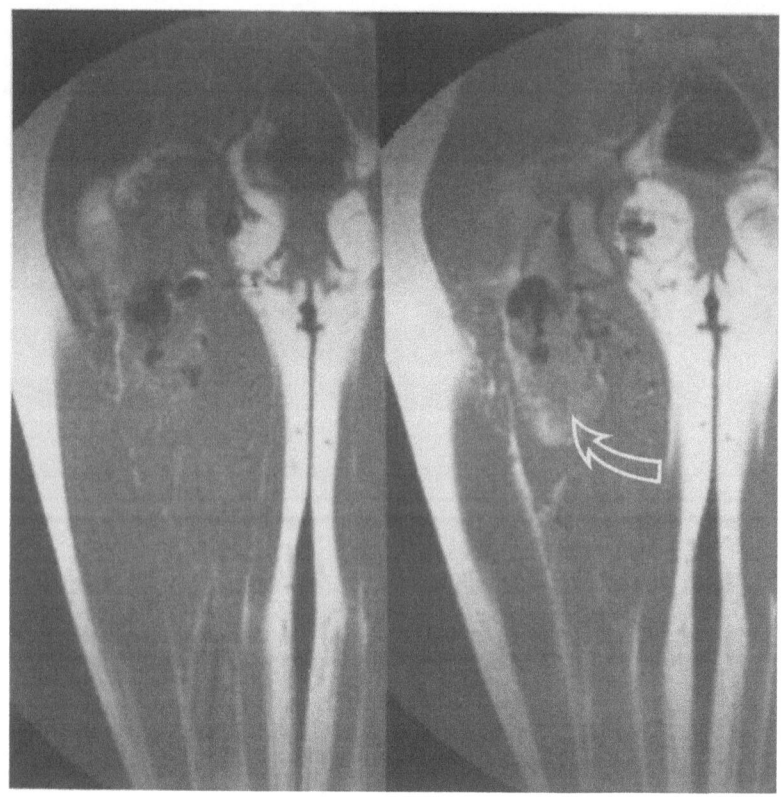

Fig. 12.6. Intramuscular haemangioma in the upper thigh on two contiguous coronal T_1W (SE 560/26) images. The vascular and soft tissue components (*arrowed*) are well demonstrated.

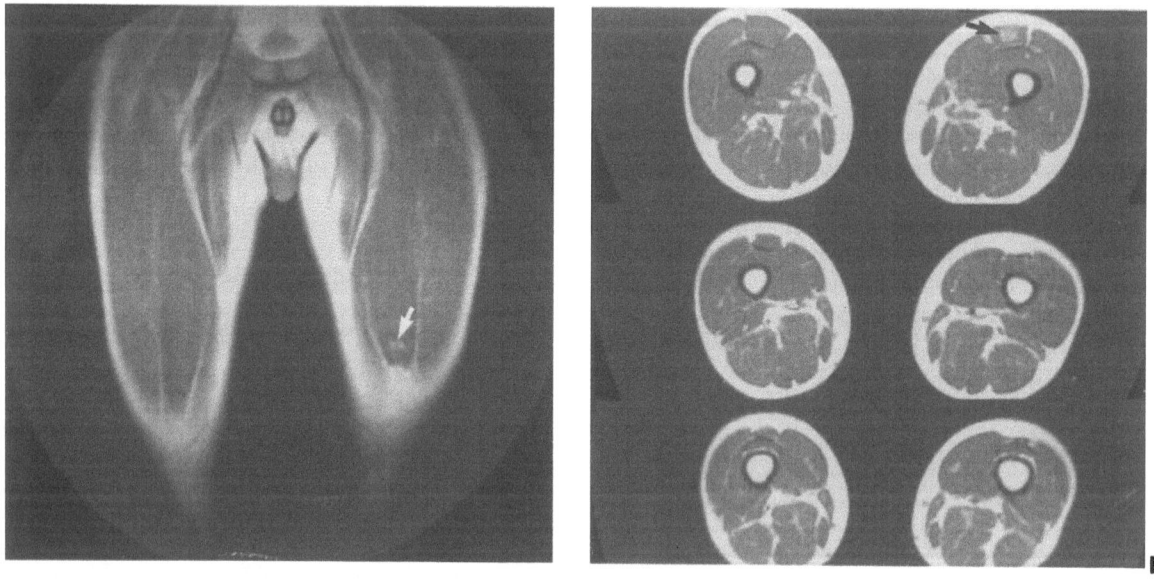

Fig. 12.7a,b. Ruptured rectus femoris tendon with associated intramuscular haematoma (*arrowed*) on (**a**) coronal T_1W (SE 1100/26) and (**b**) transverse intermediate T_1W (SE 1000/40) images.

sequence is used (Edelman et al. 1986; Unger et al. 1986; Rubin JI et al. 1987). The reduced signal intensity associated with haemorrhage is due, in the acute phase, to deoxyhaemoglobin and, in the subacute and chronic lesions, to the presence of haemosiderin (Gomori et al. 1985). The mechanism for the increased signal of subacute and chronic haematomas on T_1W images probably relates to increasing concentration of methaemoglobin which, being paramagnetic, produces T_1 shortening (Bradley and Schmidt 1985). Thus it would appear that haemorrhage and haematoma can be characterized using MRI.

In stress fractures extensive marrow and cortical abnormalities have been demonstrated (Stafford et al. 1986). The marrow changes are non-specific (long T_1/long T_2) and show similar change, as noted in other conditions, including malignancy. Similar non-specific changes in the bone marrow have been demonstrated in Sudeck's atrophy.

Joint Disease

Early studies of the knee were limited due to poor spatial resolution, which has been overcome by the use of surface coil imaging (Fig. 12.1) (Harms and Muschler 1986; Reicher et al. 1987; Hartzman et al. 1987). A wide variety of knee abnormalities have been depicted, including meniscal tears, ligamentous injuries, osteochondral loose bodies, bone ischaemia and pigmented villonodular synovitis (Reicher et al. 1987; Hartzman et al. 1987; Crues et al. 1987). Meniscal tears can be diagnosed if an abnormal linear high signal (probably representing joint fluid) within the low signal intensity meniscus extends to the surface margin, or if there is disruption to the meniscal surface (Crues et al. 1987). False-positive MRI results have been reported, mainly in the posterior horns (Reicher et al. 1987). In a study correlating MRI with histological review, focal non-linear areas of high signal without extension to the meniscal surface were due to myxoid degeneration (Stoller et al. 1987). The authors noted that these would not be evident at arthroscopy and they were considered to be precursors of frank tears. Thus the identification of such lesions may have prognostic significance in identifying patients at risk.

Precise localization of a ruptured patella tendon can be demonstrated by MRI, allowing operative repair, without exploration of the whole tendon (Reicher et al. 1987). Tendon rupture can be differentiated from partial tears or surrounding haemorrhage with continuity of the tendon, which may respond to more conservative treatment (Fig. 12.7). In the assessment of anterior cruciate ligament injuries, MRI is unable to differentiate midsubstance tears from avulsions (Reicher et al. 1987). MRI may be useful in patients suspected of anterior cruciate ligament tear, however, in the determination of concomitant meniscal tears, which occur in the majority. In three patients with posterior cruciate ligament injury, the MRI appearances corresponded with the findings on arthroscopy.

Disruption of the articular cartilage associated with osteochrondral loose bodies larger than 5 mm and low signal intensity subchondral defects can be detected. Joint effusions and synovial cysts can be shown, but haemorrhagic effusions can be difficult to differentiate from non-haemorrhagic fluid (Beltran et al. 1986a; Hartzman et al. 1987).

MRI has particular advantages compared with arthrography in that it is non-invasive, has a high soft-tissue contrast discrimination and requires no manipulation of an already painful joint. The potential of an intra-articular contrast agent for MRI remains to be explored (Hajek et al. 1987).

MRI is the most sensitive technique, superior to plain radiography, CT and radionuclide scanning, in the detection of bone ischaemia of the femoral head (Fig. 12.8) (Mitchell MD et al. 1986; Markisz et al. 1987). A chronological pattern of segmental MRI signal features may allow staging of bone ischaemia (Mitchell et al. 1987). Early bone ischaemia is characterized by retention of the normal fat signals throughout the lesion, except for a low signal rim; while advanced disease, including those with fractures, has a low signal throughout the lesion. This late effect is presumed due to replacement of fat by sclerosis and fibrosis. However, advanced disease, characterized by a large irregular region of reduced signal within the femoral head, may be difficult to differentiate from tumour or arthritis without appropriate clinical assessment.

The distribution of fatty (high signal) versus haemopoietic (low signal) marrow in the proximal femur with respect to age on T_1W images has been compared in patients with bone ischaemia of the femoral head and control subjects, using a 1.5 T system (Mitchell DG et al. 1986). An early conversion to fatty marrow was observed in the majority of patients with bone ischaemia (38 of 57 affected hips). This was presumed due to reduced vascularity in the proximal femur and may allow identification of patients at risk.

In addition to the early detection, staging and monitoring of bone ischaemia of the femoral head, MRI has been useful in selecting and monitoring

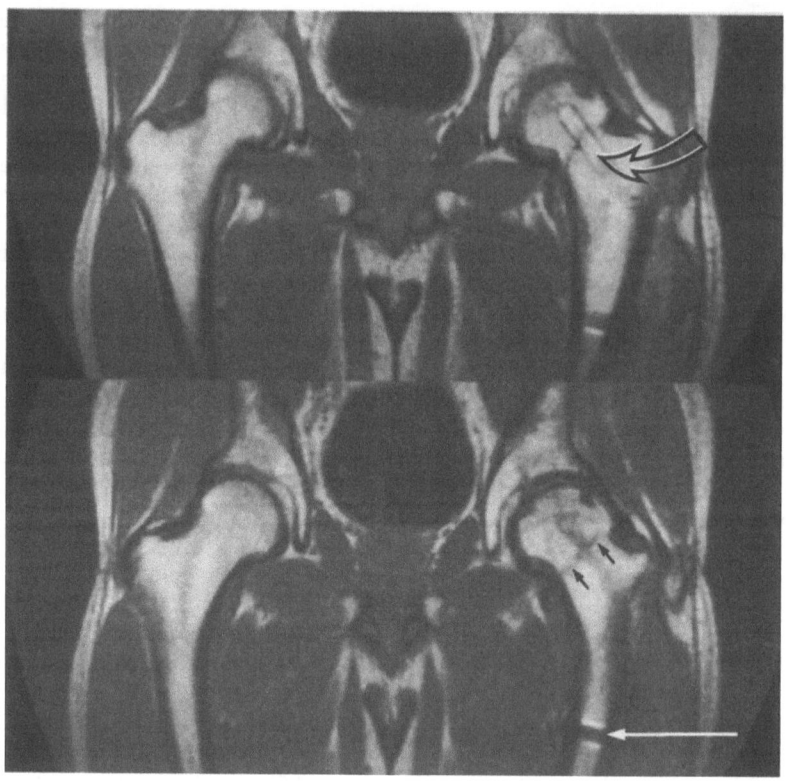

Fig. 12.8. Bone ischaemia of the left femoral head secondary to fracture of the femoral neck on two contiguous coronal T_1W (SE 600/26) images. Irregular area of reduced signal within the left femoral head, associated with distorted contour, is demonstrated, as is the site of the previous fracture (*small straight arrows*). Margins of a previous pin insertion (*curved arrow*) are outlined by low signal (trabecular bone) with a central area of high signal (fatty marrow). The low to high signal within the femoral shaft (*long straight arrow*) is due to a magnetic susceptibility effect produced by a retained surgical screw. Right hip shows a normal appearance for comparison.

treatment (Mitchell et al. 1987; Markisz et al. 1987). The tract from a core compression can be visualized separate from surrounding marrow, and signal intensity alterations in the marrow due to regression or progression of disease can be assessed on sequential studies. Bone ischaemia at sites other than the femoral head has been reported, including the humeral head, distal femur and proximal tibia, talus and carpal bones.

A variety of pathologies involving the bone marrow and soft tissues of the wrist have been observed using high field (1.0–1.5 T) systems with surface coil imaging (Weiss et al. 1986b; Middleton et al. 1987). Lesions studied included ganglions, rheumatoid arthritis, carpal fractures, osteochondritis of the lunate, carpal tunnel syndrome and tendon rupture. The soft tissue, cartilage and bone marrow abnormalities were better demonstrated on MRI compared with other imaging methods. In rheumatoid arthritis, synovial lesions including pannus formation and effusions could be detected, in addition to the subluxations and erosions observed on the plain radiographs. In one of three cases of osteochondritis of the lunate (Kienboch's disease) confirmed at surgery, radionuclide scanning was negative but MRI demonstrated altered signal within the bone in all cases. In patients with previous scaphoid fractures MRI may be helpful in predicting those at risk from pseudoarthrosis and non-union. MRI has also been found useful in detecting rupture of the distal radio-ulnar ligament, which previously has only been demonstrable on arthrography. Various abnormalities on MRI have been detected in the carpal tunnel syndrome, including segmental and diffuse swelling of the median nerve and thickening of the tendon sheath.

Recent reports have demonstrated the potential of high resolution surface coil imaging for the assessment of internal derangement of the temporomandibular joint (Katzberg et al. 1986; Westesson et al. 1987). Both sagittal and coronal imaging planes are required for complete assessment of the position of the meniscus. The soft tissue and osseous anatomy is well demonstrated, as are the margins between the meniscus and its attachment, which is an advantage of MRI over arthrography. Further refinements in MRI technology, to include assessment of joint movement, are to be expected.

Muscle Disease

The multiplanar facility, together with the high soft tissue contrast discrimination of MRI, provides a more effective technique compared with CT in the imaging of normal and diseased muscle (Fig. 12.7). No distinguishing features between the various primary and secondary muscle disorders on proton MRI have been reported, where muscle tends to be replaced by fat. Phosphorus-31 MR spectroscopy with high field (i.e. 1.5–2.0 T) systems, however, has significant advantages over imaging in characterizing normal and diseased energy metabolism in muscle with and without exercise in a non-invasive way (Radda et al. 1984; Bore 1985; Taylor et al. 1986; Heppenstall et al. 1986).

Spinal Pathology

It is in the assessment of spinal disorders that MR with surface coil imaging most clearly shows its clinical utility and efficacy. Several reports have demonstrated that MRI is superior to CT and myelography in the evaluation of disc degeneration, disc space infection, intramedullary masses and congenital anomalies of the spine. In rheumatoid arthritis, involvement of the cervico-medullary junction, erosive changes of the odontoid process and pannus formation are well demonstrated on T_1W images using extension and flexion views (Reynolds et al. 1987).

Degenerative Disc Disease

MRI is superior to all other imaging modalities, including discography, in the detection of degenerative disc disease (Modic et al. 1986b; Gibson et al. 1986a). The water content of the disc decreases with degeneration and age. This change is reflected on T_2W images by a reduction in the signal intensity from the nucleus pulposus with consequent loss of distinction between the nucleus pulposus and annulus fibrosis (Fig. 12.2). Although it is not possible on signal intensity changes alone to discriminate a degenerative from an ageing disc, the measurement of T_1 and T_2 values of the nucleus pulposus can achieve this separation (Jenkins et al. 1985). These measured parameters have been found to be highly significant indicators of degeneration. Degeneration appears to be a constant feature of herniated discs, but not all degenerative discs are herniated and so can be found in clinically asymptomatic, yet vulnerable, individuals.

In a study comparing surface coil MR with CT and myelography, Modic et al. (1986b) indicated that CT and MR were complementary techniques in the diagnosis of lumbar disc herniation and canal stenosis (Figs. 12.9, 12.10). Surface coil MR could be viewed as an alternative to myelography. Similar observations have been made in the cervical spine (Modic et al. 1986c), with improved accuracy in the diagnosis of disc disease, by using a combination of CSF gating and flow compensation techniques. Epidural fibrosis from post-operative scarring can be consistently differentiated from a recurrent disc prolapse by use of an intravenous paramagnetic contrast agent (Gadolinium-DTPA) (Jenkins et al. 1987d). Epidural fibrosis shows enhancement, whereas the disc does not demonstrate any signal intensity change immediately following Gadolinium-DTPA administration.

After chymopapain injection a gradual but marked reduction in the signal of the disc associated with narrowing of the interspace has been demonstrated (Gibson et al. 1986b). Transient end-plate changes, best shown on T_2W or STIR (see Table 12.2) images, consistent with a chemical discitis, were noted in approximately one third of cases.

Infection

MRI is more accurate in the detection of disc space infection and vertebral osteomyelitis compared with plain radiographs, CT and radionuclide scanning (Modic et al. 1985; Worthington et al. 1987). A characteristic diffuse increase in signal intensity on T_2W and STIR images of the whole disc and adjacent end-plates may be observed, together with an associated loss of the normal intranuclear cleft of the disc. The use of Gadolinium-DTPA increases conspicuity of disc and bone involvement, together with any soft tissue abscess formation (de Roos et al. 1986; Jenkins et al. 1987d). Worthington et al. (1987) have described the early changes (within three weeks) of disc-space infection in an animal model

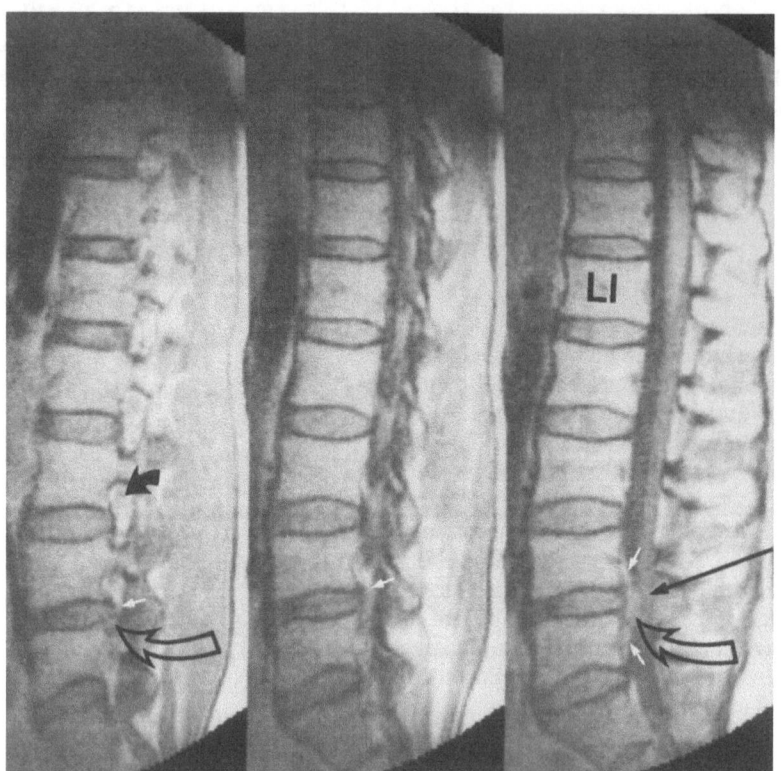

Fig. 12.9

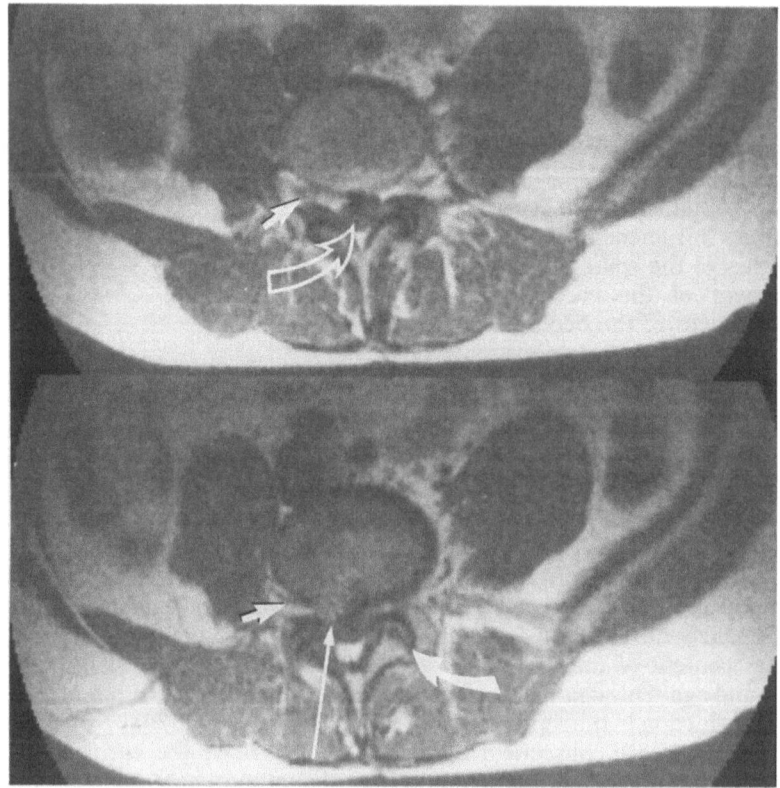

Fig. 12.10

Fig. 12.9. Postero-lateral prolapsed and partially fragmented L4/ 5 disc (*curved open arrows*) compressing spinal nerve roots (*long straight arrow*) on contiguous sagittal T_1W (SE 1000/26) images, from the right side to the mid-line. There is elevation of the epidural fat (*small straight arrows*) around the protruded disc. Exiting nerve roots (*small curved closed arrow*) are demonstrated within the epidural fat in the superior part of the lateral recesses. Note the conus of the spinal cord opposite T12/L1.

and demonstrated on STIR (Short Tau Inversion Recovery) images an initial reduction in signal from the infected disc associated with an increased signal from adjacent end-plates. The initial loss of signal from the disc is probably related to T_2 shortening from enzyme degradation. After three weeks the characteristic increase in signal of the disc is noted when repair and granulation tissue has formed. Following adequate antibiotic treatment, the disc and vertebral body changes slowly revert to normal, taking weeks and months respectively.

Similar signal intensity changes in the vertebral end-plates have been noted in metastatic disease, post-chymopapain injection and severe degenerative disc disease. Untreated disc-space infection and vertebral osteomyelitis of more than three weeks' duration, however, can be differentiated from these other conditions by the characteristic increased signal of the disc on both T_2W and STIR images, associated with typical enhancement following Gadolinium-DTPA, in the former case.

Trauma

MRI can demonstrate the extent of bony and soft tissue injury including spinal cord compression, cord swelling and haemorrhage, disc trauma and ligamentous injury more accurately than CT (McArdle et al. 1986; Tarr et al. 1987). Separation of stable from unstable fractures on MRI can be made on the basis of disruption of the posterior ligaments and elements. CT and plain radiographs nevertheless are superior to MRI in the detection of fractures, especially of the posterior neural arch and in assessing the number and origin of displaced fragments

Fig. 12.10. Postero-lateral herniated disc (*long straight arrow*) distorting the adjacent nerve root (*small straight arrow*) and thecal sac (*curved open arrow*) on oblique/transverse T_1W (SE 700/40) image. The posterior facet joints (*curved solid arrow*), including articular cartilage, are well demonstrated.

in comminuted injuries. Post-traumatic syringomyelia, myelomalacia and cord atrophy in patients with chronic trauma and cord injury can be more accurately assessed compared with CT myelography (Quencer et al. 1986).

Congenital Anomalies

Congenital anomalies, including Arnold-Chiari malformations, spinal dysraphism, meningocoeles, myelomeningocoeles, tethered cord and sacral lipomas can all be accurately delineated by T_1W and PSR sequences, without the need for more extensive invasive procedures (Fig. 12.11). Any associated hydrocephalus and syringomyelia can be defined. In diastematomyelia the duplicated cord can be demonstrated, as can the bony septum, but only if the latter contains fatty marrow. CT or plain radiographs are more accurate in demonstrating the presence of such a bony septum. Difficulties in achieving satisfactory sagittal sections in patients with severe scoliosis can be offset by using multisection coronal or oblique plane imaging.

Tumours and Arteriovenous Malformations

Most tumours produce a non-specific increase in T_1 and T_2 compared with normal spinal cord, and can be distinguished from surrounding CSF using moderately T_2W sequences. Vertebral body haemangiomas are an exception as they tend to have a short to intermediate T_1 and appear high signal on T_1W and T_2W images. Meningiomas and neurofibromas, which are the two most common intradural-extramedullary tumours, can be differentiated by signal intensity appearances in the majority. Meningiomas tend to have signal intensity characteristics similar to normal cord, whereas neurofibromas have increased signal on T_2W images. Intramedullary, intradural-extramedullary and extradural tumours can be differentiated with MRI providing more information than both myelography and CT (Di Chiro et al. 1985; Jenkins and Isherwood 1987a). The extent and location of tumours can be fully evaluated, particularly with the use of Gadolinium-DTPA (Fig. 12.12) where more lesions are demonstrated with increased conspicuity compared with non-enhanced MRI scans and other imaging methods (Bydder et al. 1985b; Jenkins et al. 1987d).

MRI can separate cystic from solid components of intramedullary tumours in the majority of cases

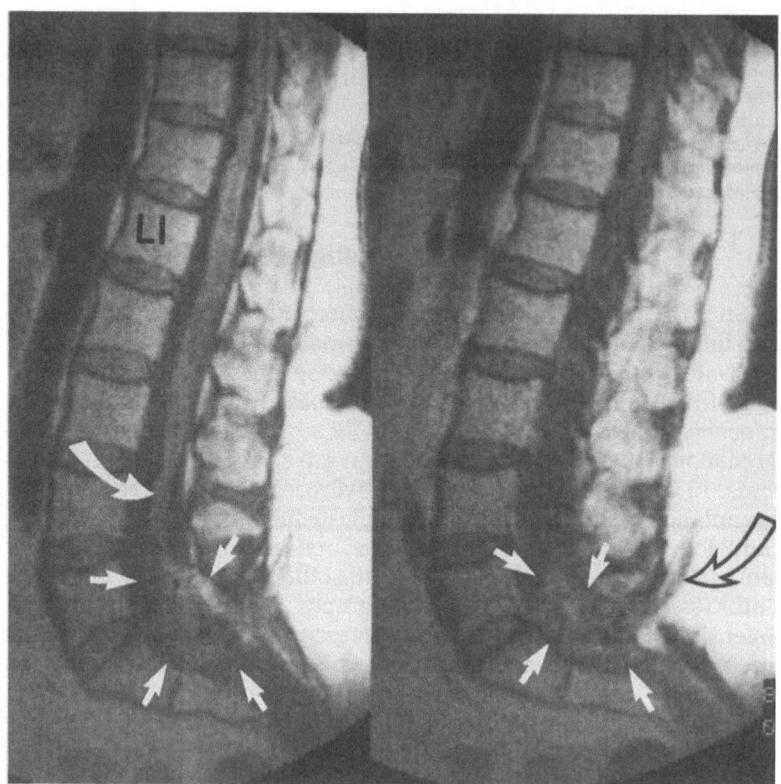

Fig. 12.11

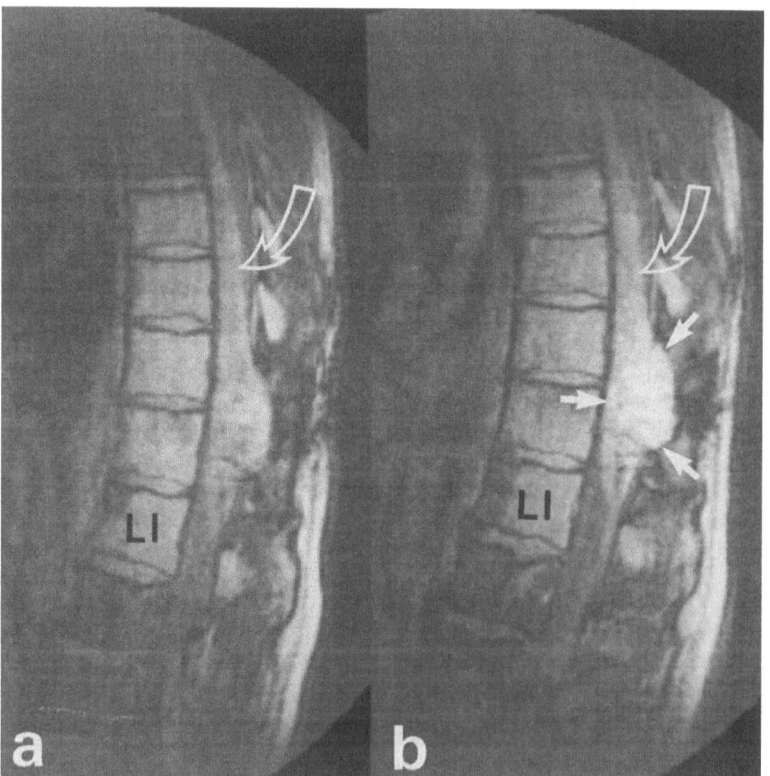

Fig. 12.12

Fig. 12.11. Spinal dysraphism, sacral meningocoele (*curved open arrow*) and subcutaneous lipoma, tethered cord (*curved solid arrow*) and intraspinal angiolipoma (*straight arrows*) on contiguous sagittal intermediate T_1W (SE 1000/40) images.

(Fig. 12.12). Ambiguities, however, can occur when cysts contain proteinaceous fluid, which can simulate solid components on MRI (Rubin et al. 1986; Goy et al. 1986). The accurate definition of the extent and components of an intramedullary tumour allows for improved surgical management. Extramedullary and intramedullary arteriovenous malformations can be differentiated from tumours and the full extent shown. Small lesions, however, are difficult to assess using current technology, as are the feeding and draining vessels. Thrombosis of an arteriovenous malformation following surgery or embolization can be demonstrated, indicating the potential value of MRI as a non-invasive method in the assessment of such cases (Di Chiro et al. 1985).

Syringomyelia

The extent and cavitation from syringomyelia, together with evaluation of an associated Chiari malformation, is readily assessed using T_1W or PSR sequences (Fig. 12.13). The cavity appears as low signal on both sequences. There are conflicting reports, however, concerning the accuracy of MRI in the detection of syrinx cavities within normal-sized or small cords, compared with CT myelography. MRI is generally considered to be superior to CT myelography but a lack of concordance has been noted in the normal-sized cord (Gillespie et al. 1987). In differentiating intramedullary tumours from syringomyelia, the appearance of distinct margins and uniform signal intensity equivalent to that of CSF correlated in the majority with syringomyelia (Williams et al. 1987). Difficulties

can occasionally occur in discriminating cystic tumours from syringomyelia, but improved specificity has been achieved using Gadolinium-DTPA. No enhancement was noted in cases of syringomyelia, whereas enhancement occurred early in tumour wall and later in tumoral cyst (Jenkins et al. 1987d). The MRI appearance of myelomalacia can be indistinguishable from cord cavitation (Gillespie et al. 1987).

In many cases of syringomyelia, a loss of signal within the syrinx cavity, termed CSF flow-void sign, using T_2W sequences, has been observed and is presumed to represent pulsatile flow in a cavity undergoing active expansion (Sherman et al. 1987). Indeed, the velocity and direction of CSF flow in volunteers and syringomyelia have been measured *in vivo* and shown to vary with different phases of the cardiac cycle (Ridgway et al. 1987; Turnbull et al. 1987). Absence of this flow-void sign has been noted in tumoral cysts – an observation which may help in their discrimination (Enzmann et al. 1987).

Fig. 12.12a,b. Recurrent intramedullary astrocytoma on sagittal PSR (TR/TE of 500/18) images, (a) before and (b) after intravenous Gadolinium-DTPA. The high signal from D9 to L1 vertebral bodies is due to fat replacement from previous radiotherapy and demarcates the field limits. There was early enhancement to the tumour (*straight arrows*) in (b) with late enhancement to a cystic expanded spinal cord above (*curved arrow*). The extent of the expanded cord is limited to the upper radiation portal and is in keeping with radiation necrosis. Note previous posterior laminectomy at tumour site.

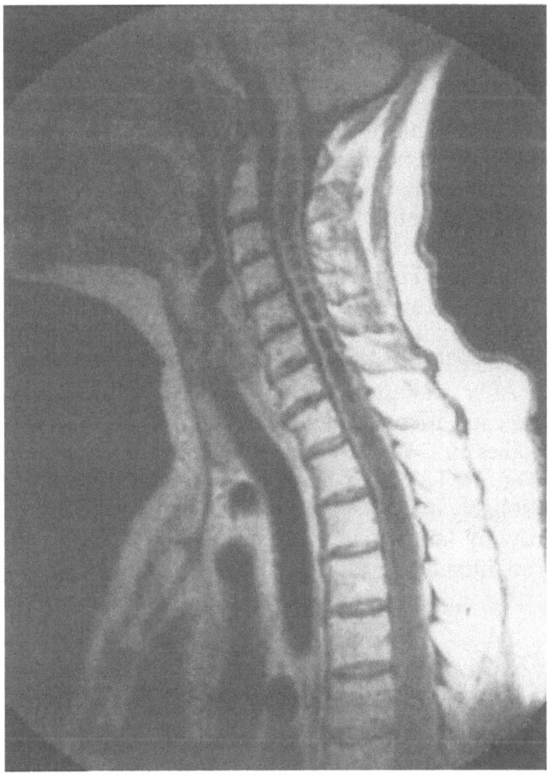

Fig. 12.13. Syringomyelia on a sagittal intermediate T_1W (SE 1000/40) image showing typical appearances, including haustrae within the syrinx cavity.

Table 12.4. Present and future aspects

Surface coil imaging
Oblique plane scanning
New pulse sequences/scanning techniques
Paramagnetic tracers
Tissue characterization
Blood flow imaging and measurements *in vivo*
Volume (3-dimensional) imaging
Other nuclei imaged (e.g. sodium ^{23}Na, carbon ^{13}C, fluorine ^{19}F)
Human (proton ^{1}H and phosphorus ^{31}P) spectroscopy *in vivo*

Bone Marrow Disease

MRI has a high sensitivitiy in the detection of bone marrow disease (Olson et al. 1986; Daffner et al. 1986; Pennock et al. 1986; Nyman et al. 1987). Chemical shift imaging (*vide supra*) is of value in more clearly demonstrating bone marrow abnormalities. Striking signal intensity changes on MRI within bone marrow and other organs have been detected in patients with transfusional haemosiderosis complicating thalassaemia major, where tissue deposits of haemosiderin develop after multiple blood transfusion (Brasch et al. 1984).

Measurements of relaxation times have been found useful in evaluation of acute lymphoma involving bone marrow and in monitoring response to treatment (Moore et al. 1986, Thomsen et al. 1987). Elevated T_1 values in the lumbar spine bone marrow were observed in patients with acute leukaemia. Following chemotherapy these returned to within the normal range in those patients who obtained a complete remission but remained elevated in those who did not.

After radiation therapy a well-defined homogeneous increase in signal intensity in vertebral bodies on T_1W and PSR images can be demonstrated (Fig. 12.12). This alteration in signal intensity is probably due to replacement of haemopoietic marrow by fatty tissue and effectively demarcates the radiation field.

Magnetic Resonance Spectroscopy (MRS)

In vivo, MRS is still at an inchoate stage but has considerable clinical potential, as indicated in several reviews (Radda et al. 1984; Evanochko et al. 1984; Bore 1985). The *in vivo* metabolic activity of tissues, including muscle and osseous structures and tumours, can be evaluated non-invasively (Nidecker et al. 1985; Taylor et al. 1986; Heppenstall et al. 1986; Ross et al. 1987). The energetics of human muscle have been investigated during and after fatiguing dynamic exercise and following injury. Changes in the Phosphorus-31 spectrum of human bone tumours in response to treatment have also been noted. A detailed review of MRS is outside the scope of this chapter.

Present Research and Future Aspects

Some of the future aspects presented in Table 12.4 are being evaluated at the present time, whereas others are at a developmental stage. Tissue characterization, i.e. the ability to discriminate quantitatively between normal and abnormal biological tissue and between different pathologies *in vivo*, can be achieved by a number of methods, including measurements of T_1 and T_2 relaxation times, the use of paramagnetic tracers or by chemical shift imaging. By using multiple point relaxation time data encouraging initial results have been achieved, not only in the intervertebral disc and vertebral body (*vide supra*), but in recurrent rectal carcinoma and prostatic disease (Jenkins et al. 1985; Johnson et al. 1987; Prendergast et al. 1987; Thomsen et al. 1987). Isherwood et al. (1987) have used T_1 and T_2 tissue maps of intervertebral discs and adjacent vertebral bodies before and after exercise and have shown redistribution of T_1 and T_2, indicating the effect of diurnal factors upon vertebral body relaxation times.

Refinements in surface coil technology, together with direct volume imaging, should permit thinner sections and higher spatial resolution. The use of faster scanning techniques, together with paramagnetic tracers, would be useful in the study of tissue perfusion.

Progress in MRI has been rapid over the last few years, and the diverse achievements that have already been demonstrated bear witness to its future role as a powerful diagnostic tool for musculoskeletal and spinal disease.

Acknowledgements. Financial support from the Medical Research Council, Cancer Research Campaign, British Heart Foundation, Department of Health and

Social Security, Picker International Ltd and Schering-AG, Berlin is gratefully acknowledged.

References

Aisen AM, Martel W, Braunstein EM, McMillin KI, Phillips WA, Kling TF (1986) MRI and CT evaluation of primary bone and soft tissue tumours. AJR 146:749–756

Beltran J, Noto AM, Herman LJ, Mosure JC, Burk JM, Christoforidis AJ (1986a) Joint effusions: MR imaging. Radiology 158:133–137

Beltran J, Noto AM, Mosure JC, Shamam OM, Weiss KL, Zuelzer WA (1986b) Ankle: surface coil MR imaging at 1.5 T. Radiology 161:203–209

Beltran J, Simon DC, Katz W, Weis LD (1987) Increased MR signal intensity in skeletal muscle adjacent to malignant tumours: pathologic correlation and clinical relevance. Radiology 162:251–255

Berquist TH, Brown ML, Fitzgerald RH, May GR (1985) Magnetic resonance imaging: application in musculoskeletal infection. Magn Reson Imaging 3:219–230

Bore PJ (1985) The role of magnetic resonance spectroscopy in clinical medicine. Magn Reson Imaging 3:407–413

Boyko OB, Cory DA, Cohen MD, Provisor A, Mirkin D, DeRosa GP (1987) MR imaging of osteogenic and Ewing's sarcoma. AJR 148:317–322

Bradley WG, Newton TH, Crooks LE (1983) Physical principles of nuclear magnetic resonance. In: Newton TH, Potts DG (eds) Modern neuroradiology: advanced imaging techniques. Clavadel Press, San Anselmo, pp 15–61

Bradley WG, Schmidt PG (1985) Effect of methemoglobin formation on the MR appearance of subarachnoid hemorrhage. Radiology 156:99–103

Brady TJ, Rosen BR, Pykett IL, McGuire MH, Mankin HJ, Rosenthal DI (1983) NMR imaging of leg tumours. Radiology 149:181–187

Brasch RC, Wesbey GE, Gooding CA, Koerper MA (1984) Magnetic resonance imaging of transfusional hemosiderosis complicating thalassaemia major. Radiology 150:767–771

Budinger TF (1981) Nuclear magnetic resonance (NMR) in vivo studies: known thresholds for health effects. J Comput Assist Tomogr 5:800–811

Bureau of Radiological Health (USA) (1982) Guidelines for evaluating electromagnetic risk for trials of clinical NMR systems. Department of Health and Human Services, Public Health Service, Food and Drug Administration, Rockville

Bydder GM, Young IR (1985a) Clinical use of the partial saturation and saturation recovery sequences in MR imaging. J Comput Assist Tomogr 9:1020–1032

Bydder GM, Brown J, Niendorf HP, Young IR (1985b) Enhancement of cervical intraspinal tumors in MR imaging with intravenous Gadolinium-DTPA. J Comput Assist Tomogr 9:847–851

Cohen JM, Weinreb JC, Redman HC (1986) Arteriovenous malformations of the extremities: MR imaging. Radiology 158:475–479

Crues JV, Mink J, Levy TL, Lotysch M, Stoller DW (1987) Meniscal tears of the knee: accuracy of MR imaging. Radiology 164:445–448

Daffner RH, Lupetin AR, Dash N, Deeb ZL, Sefczek RJ, Schapiro RL (1986) MRI in the detection of malignant infiltration of bone marrow. AJR 146:353–358

Davis PL, Crooks L, Arakawa M, McRee R, Kaufman L, Margulis AR (1981) Potential hazards in NMR imaging: heating effects of changing magnetic fields and RF fields on small metallic implants. AJR 137:857–860

de Roos A, van Meerten ELP, Bloem JL, Bluemm RG (1986) MRI of tuberculous spondylitis. AJR 147:79–82

Di Chiro G, Doppman JL, Dwyer AJ et al. (1985) Tumours and arteriovenous malformations of the spinal cord: assessment using MR. Radiology 156:689–697

Edelman RR, Johnson K, Buxton R, Shoukimas G, Rosen BR, Davis KR, Brady TJ (1986) MR of hemorrhage: a new approach. AJNR 7:751–756

Enzmann DR, O'Donohue J, Rubin JB, Shuer L, Cogen P, Silverberg G (1987) CSF pulsations within nonneoplastic spinal cord cysts. AJR 149:149–157

Evanochko WT, Ng TC, Glickson JD (1984) Application of in vivo NMR spectroscopy to cancer. Magn Reson Med 1:508–534

Flannigan BD, Lufkin RB, McGlade C et al. (1987) MR imaging of the cervical spine: neurovascular anatomy. AJR 148:785–790

Gibson MJ, Buckley J, Mawhinney R, Mulholland RC, Worthington BS (1986a) Magnetic resonance imaging and discography in the diagnosis of disc degeneration: a comparative study of 50 discs. J Bone Joint Surg [Br] 68:369–373

Gibson MJ, Buckley J, Mulholland RC, Worthington BS (1986b) The changes in the intervertebral disc after chemonucleolysis demonstrated by magnetic resonance imaging. J Bone Joint Surg [Br] 68:719–723

Gillespie JE, Jenkins JPR, Metcalfe RA, Isherwood I (1987) Magnetic resonance imaging in syringomyelia. Acta Radiol [Diagn] (Stockh) Supplementum 369:239–241

Gomori JM, Grossman RI, Goldberg HI, Zimmerman RA, Bilaniuk LT (1985) Intracranial hematomas: imaging by high field MR. Radiology 157:87–93

Goy AMC, Pinto RS, Raghavendra BN, Epstein FJ, Kricheff II (1986) Intramedullary spinal cord tumours: MR imaging, with emphasis on associated cysts. Radiology 161:381–386

Hajek PC, Barker LL, Sartoris DJ, Neumann CH, Resnick D (1987) MR arthrography: anatomic-pathologic investigation. Radiology 163:141–147

Harms SE, Muschler G (1986) Three-dimensional MR imaging of the knee using surface coils. J Comput Assist Tomogr 10:773–777

Hartzman S, Reicher MA, Bassett LW, Duckwiler GR, Mandelbaum B, Gold RH (1987) MR imaging of the knee. Part II: chronic disorders. Radiology 162:553–557

Heppenstall RB, Scott R, Sapega A, Park YS, Chance B (1986) A comparative study of the tolerance of skeletal muscle to ischemia: tourniquet application compared with acute compartment syndrome. J Bone Joint Surg [Am] 68:820–828

Hickey DS, Aspden RM, Hukins DWL, Jenkins JPR, Isherwood I (1986) Analysis of magnetic resonance images from normal and degenerate lumbar intervertebral discs. Spine 11:702–708

Hoult DI, Chen CN, Sank VJ (1986) The field dependence of NMR imaging. II: Arguments concerning an optimal field strength. Magn Reson Med 3:730–746

Isherwood I, Prendergast DJ, Hickey DS, Jenkins JPR (1987) Quantitative analysis of intervertebral disc structure. Acta Radiol [Diagn] (Stockh) Supplement 369:492–495

Jenkins JPR, Hickey DS, Zhu XP, Machin M, Isherwood I (1985) MR imaging of the intervertebral disc: a quantitative study. Br J Radiol 58:705–709

Jenkins JPR, Isherwood I (1987a) Magnetic resonance imaging – Technical aspects, CNS and spine. Chapter 64 In: Sutton D (ed) A textbook of radiology and imaging, 4th edition. Churchill Livingstone, Edinburgh, pp 1654–1690

Jenkins JPR, Isherwood I (1987b) Magnetic resonance imaging – The body. Chapter 68 In: Sutton D (ed) A textbook of radiology and imaging, 4th edition. Churchill Livingstone, Edinburgh, pp 1810–1849

Jenkins JPR, Braganza JM, Hickey DS, Isherwood I, Machin M (1987c) Quantitative tissue characterisation in pancreatic disease using magnetic resonance imaging. Br J Radiol 60:333–341

Jenkins JPR, Stack JP, Watson Y, Isherwood I (1987d) Magnetic resonance imaging of spinal lesions: the role of Gadolinium-DTPA. In: Proceedings of the Sixth Annual Meeting of the Society of Magnetic Resonance in Medicine (Society of Magnetic Resonance in Medicine, Berkeley) p 8

Johnson RJ, Jenkins JPR, Isherwood I, James RD, Schofield PF (1987) Quantitative magnetic resonance imaging in rectal carcinoma. Br J Radiol 60:761–764

Kaplan PA, Williams SM (1987) Mucocutaneous and peripheral soft-tissue hemangiomas: MR imaging. Radiology 163:163–166

Katzberg RW, Bessette RW, Tallents RH et al. (1986) Normal and abnormal temporomandibular joint: MR imaging with surface coil. Radiology 158:183–189

Kricun ME (1985) Red-yellow marrow conversion: its effect on the location of some solitary bone lesions. Skeletal Radiol 14:10–19

Littrup PJ, Aisen AM, Braunstein EM, Martel W (1985) Magnetic resonance imaging of femoral head development in roentgenographically normal patients. Skeletal Radiol 14:159–163

McArdle CB, Crofford MJ, Mirfakhraee M, Amparo EG, Calhoun JS (1986) Surface coil MR of spinal trauma: preliminary experience AJNR 7:885–893

McFarland EW, Rosen BR (1986) NMR instrumentation and hardware available at present and in the future. Cardiovasc Intervent Radiol 8:238–250

Markisz JA, Knowles RJR, Altchek DW, Shneider R, Whalen JP, Cahill PT (1987) Segmental patterns of avascular necrosis of the femoral heads: early detection with MR imaging. Radiology 162:717–720

Middleton WD, Kneeland JB, Kellman GM et al. (1987) MR imaging of the carpal tunnel: normal anatomy and preliminary findings in the carpal tunnel syndrome. AJR 148:307–316

Mitchell MD, Kundel HL, Steinberg ME, Kressel HY, Alavi A, Axel L (1986) Avascular necrosis of the hip: comparison of MR, CT and scintigraphy. AJR 147:67–71

Mitchell DG, Rao VM, Dalinka MK et al. (1986) Hematopoietic and fatty bone marrow distribution in the normal and ischemic hip: new observations with 1.5 T MR imaging. Radiology 161:199–202

Mitchell DG, Rao VM, Dalinka MK et al. (1987) Femoral head avascular necrosis: correlation of MR imaging, radiographic staging, radionuclide imaging, and clinical findings. Radiology 162:709–715

Modic MT, Feiglin DH, Piraino DW et al. (1985) Vertebral osteomyelitis: assessment using MR. Radiology 157:157–166

Modic MT, Pflanze W, Feiglin DHI, Belhobek G (1986a) Magnetic resonance imaging of musculoskeletal infections. Radiol Clin North Am 24:247–258

Modic MT, Masaryk TJ, Boumphrey F, Goormastic M, Bell G (1986b) Lumbar herniated disk disease and canal stenosis: prospective evaluation by surface coil MR, CT and myelography. AJR 147:757–765

Modic MT, Masaryk TJ, Mulopulos GP, Bundschuh C, Han JS, Bohlman H (1986c) Cervical radiculopathy: prospective evaluation with surface coil MR imaging, CT with metrizamide, and metrizamide myelography. Radiology 161:753–759

Moore SG, Gooding CA, Brasch RC et al. (1986) Bone marrow

in children with acute lymphocytic leukemia: MR relaxation times. Radiology 160:237–240

National Radiological Protection Board ad hoc Advisory Group on Nuclear Magnetic Resonance Clinical Imaging (1983) Revised guidelines on acceptable limits of exposure during nuclear magnetic resonance clinical imaging. Br J Radiol 56:974–977

New PFJ, Rosen BR, Brady TJ et al. (1983) Potential hazards and artifacts of ferromagnetic and non-ferromagnetic surgical and dental materials and devices in nuclear magnetic resonance imaging. Radiology 147:139–148

Nidecker AC, Müller S, Aue WP et al. (1985) Extremity bone tumours: evaluation by P-31 MR spectroscopy. Radiology 157:167–174

Nyman R, Rehn S, Glimelius B et al. (1987) Magnetic resonance imaging in diffuse malignant bone marrow diseases. Acta Radiol [Diagn] (Stockh) 28:199–205

Olson DO, Shields AF, Scheurich CJ, Porter BA, Moss AA (1986) Magnetic resonance imaging of the bone marrow in patients with leukaemia, aplastic anemia and lymphoma. Invest Radiol 21:540–546

Paling MR, Brookeman JR, Mugler JP (1987) Tumour detection with phase-contrast imaging: an evaluation of clinical potential. Radiology 162:199–203

Pennock JM, Bydder GM, Young IR (1986) Distinction between red and yellow bone marrow: normal appearances and applications in clinical practice. In: Proceedings of the Fifth Annual Meeting of the Society of Magnetic Resonance in Medicine, Montreal (Society of Magnetic Resonance in Medicine, Berkeley), pp 1161–1162

Petasnick JP, Turner DA, Charters JR, Gitelis S, Zacharias CE (1986) Soft-tissue masses of the locomotor system: comparison of MR imaging with CT. Radiology 160:125–133

Pettersson H, Gillespie T, Hamlin DJ et al. (1987) Primary musculoskeletal tumours: examination with MR imaging compared with conventional modalities. Radiology 164:237–241

Prendergast DJ, Hickey DS, Jenkins JPR, Isherwood I (1987) Increased potential for tissue discrimination in quantitative magnetic resonance imaging. Br J Radiol 60:1142–1143

Quencer RM, Sheldon JJ, Post MJD et al. (1986) MRI of the chronically injured cervical spinal cord. AJR 147:125–132

Radda GK, Bore PJ, Rajagopalan MA (1984) Clinical aspects of ^{31}P NMR spectroscopy. Br Med Bull 40:155–159

Reicher MA, Hartzman S, Bassett LW, Mandelbaum B, Duckwiler G, Gold RH (1987) MR imaging of the knee. Part I – traumatic disorders. Radiology 162:547–551

Reynolds H, Carter SW, Murtagh FR, Rechtine GR (1987) Cervical rheumatoid arthritis: value of flexion and extension views in imaging. Radiology 164:215–218

Ridgway JP, Turnbull LW, Smith MA (1987) Demonstration of pulsatile cerebrospinal fluid flow using magnetic resonance phase imaging. Br J Radiol 60:423–427

Ross BD, Cox IJ, Pennock J et al. (1987) Osteosarcoma and other neoplasms of bone: a possible contribution of phosphorus-31 magnetic resonance spectroscopy to therapeutic monitoring. Br J Radiol 60:810

Rubin JM, Aisen AM, DiPietro MA (1986) Ambiguities in MR imaging of tumoral cysts in the spinal cord. J Comput Assist Tomogr 10:395–398

Rubin JB, Enzmann DR, Wright A (1987) CSF-gated MR imaging of the spine: theory and clinical implementation. Radiology 163:784–792

Rubin JI, Gomori JM, Grossman RI, Gefter WB, Kressel HY (1987) High-field MR imaging of extracranial hematomas. AJR 148:813–817

Saunders RD, Smith H (1984) Safety aspects of NMR clinical imaging. Br Med Bull 40:148–154

Seegar LL, Ruszkowski JT, Bassett LW, Kay SP, Kahmann RD, Ellman H (1987) MR imaging of the normal shoulder: anatomic correlation. AJR 148:83–91

Sherman JL, Barkovich AJ, Citrin CM (1987) The MR appearance of syringomyelia: new observations. AJR 148:381–391

Stafford SA, Rosenthal DI, Gebhardt MC, Brady TJ, Scott JA (1986) MRI in stress fracture. AJR 147:553–556

Stoller DW, Martin C, Crues JV, Kaplan L, Mink JH (1987) Meniscal tears: pathologic correlation with MR imaging. Radiology 163:731–735

Sundaram M, McGuire MH, Schajowicz F (1987) Soft-tissue masses: histologic basis for decreased signal (short T_2) on T_2-weighted MR images. AJR 148:1247–1250

Sutton D (ed.) A textbook of radiology and imaging, 4th edn. Churchill Livingstone, Edinburgh

Tarr RW, Drolshagen LF, Kerner TC, Allen JH, Partain CL, James AE (1987) MR imaging of recent spinal trauma. J Comput Assist Tomogr 11:412–417

Taylor DJ, Styles P, Matthews PM et al. (1986) Energetics of human muscle: exercise-induced ATP depletion. Magn Reson Med 3:44–54

Thomsen C, Sørensen PG, Karle H, Christoffersen P, Henriksen O (1987) Prolonged bone marrow T_1-relaxation in acute leukemia. In vivo tissue characterization by magnetic resonance imaging. Magn Reson Imaging 5:251–257

Totty WG, Murphy WA, Lee JKT (1986) Soft-tissue tumours: MR imaging. Radiology 160:135–141

Turnbull LW, Ridgway JP, Smith MA, Best JJK (1987) Magnetic resonance flow imaging: a possible method for distinguishing communicating syringomyelia from cystic intraspinal lesions. Br J Radiol 60:517–518

Turner DA, Prodromos CC, Petasnick JP, Clark JW (1985) Acute injury of the ligaments of the knee: magnetic resonance evaluation. Radiology 154:717–722

Unger EC, Glazer HS, Lee JKT, Ling D (1986) MRI of extracranial hematomas: preliminary observations. AJR 146:403–407

Vanel D, Lacombe M-J, Couanet D, Kalifa C, Spielmann M, Genin J (1987) Musculoskeletal tumours: follow-up with MR imaging after treatment with surgery and radiation therapy. Radiology 164:243–245

Weekes RG, Berquist TH, McLeod RA, Zimmer WD (1985) Magnetic resonance imaging of soft-tissue tumours: comparison with computed tomography. Magn Reson Imaging 3:345–352

Wehrli FW, MacFall JR, Newton TH (1983) Parameters determining the appearance of NMR images. In: Newton TH, Potts DG (eds) Modern neuroradiology: advanced imaging techniques. Clavadel Press, San Anselmo, pp 81–117

Weiss KL, Beltran J, Shamam OM, Stilla RF, Levey M (1986a) High-field MR surface-coil imaging of the hand and wrist. Part I: normal anatomy. Radiology 160:143–146

Weiss KL, Beltran J, Lubbers LM (1986b) High-field MR surface-coil imaging of the hand and wrist. Part II: pathologic correlations and clinical relevance. Radiology 160:147–152

Westesson P-L, Katzberg RW, Tallents RH, Sanchez-Woodworth RE, Svensson SA, Espeland MA (1987) Temporomandibular joint: comparison of MR images with cryosectional anatomy. Radiology 164:59–64

Williams AL, Haughton VM, Pojunas KW, Daniels DL, Kilgore DP (1987) Differentiation of intramedullary neoplasms and cysts by MR. AJR 149:159–164

Worthington BS, Szypryt P, Hardy J, Mulholland RC (1987) The diagnosis of disc space infection induced in an animal model; a comparison between MR imaging and radio-isotope bone scanning. In: Proceedings of the Sixth Annual Meeting of the Society of Magnetic Resonance in Medicine, New York (Society of Magnetic Resonance in Medicine, Berkeley) p 261

Zimmer WD, Berquist TH, McLeod RA et al. (1985) Bone tumours: magnetic resonance imaging versus computed tomography. Radiology 155:709–718

13 Skeletal Scintigraphy

C.S.B. Galasko

Introduction 181
The Mechanism of Uptake 184
The Normal Scintigram 184
  Child and Adolescent 187
  Adult 187
  Bladder Uptake 187
  Renal Uptake 187
  Artefacts 188
The Abnormal Scintigram 189
Indications for Skeletal Scintigraphy 190
Tumours 190
  Skeletal Metastases 190
  Primary Tumours of Bone 190
The Arthritides 192
  Polyarthritis 194
  Osteoarthritis 195
  Ankylosing Spondylitis 195
  Miscellaneous Conditions 196
Infection 196
  Acute Osteomyelitis 196
  Chronic Osteomyelitis 198
  Tuberculosis Infection 200
  Pyogenic Spondylitis and Discitis 200
  Septic Arthritis 200
  Infected Implants 200
Metabolic Disease of Bone 201
  Paget's Disease 201
  Hyperparathyroidism 202
  Osteomalacia 202
  Renal Osteodystrophy 202
  Osteoporosis 203
  Transient Osteoporosis 204
Miscellaneous Conditions 204
  Fractures 204
  Spondylolysis 204
  Bone Graft 204
  Avascular Necrosis 204
  Reflex Sympathetic Dystrophy 205
The Future 205
References 205

Introduction

Skeletal scintigraphy is a most valuable technique of imaging the skeleton. It has one major advantage over all other imaging techniques, and that is the possibility of imaging the entire skeleton. Unlike other imaging techniques the amount of radiation is not related to the extent of the investigation. The radiation is due to the radiopharmaceutical which is injected intravenously. Therefore, the philosophy of requesting a skeletal scintigram is totally different

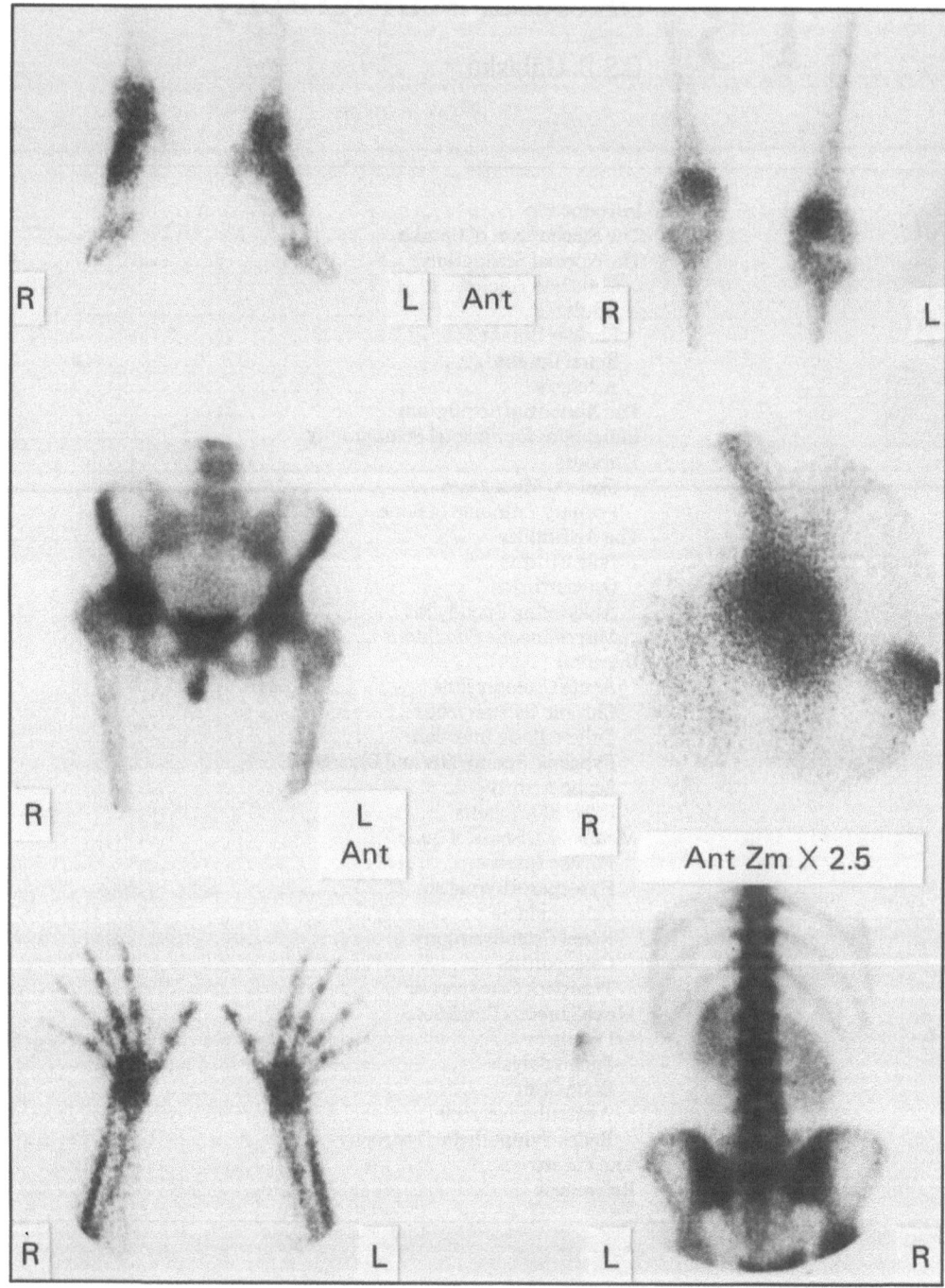

Fig. 13.1. Patient who presented with arthritis of her right hip. To evaluate a polyarthropathy, images must be taken of all the peripheral joints, as well as the axial skeleton. This illustration shows the images of her ankles and feet, knees, hips, hands and wrists, as well as her spine. In addition, she had scintigrams taken of her shoulders, elbows and the rest of her axial skeleton.

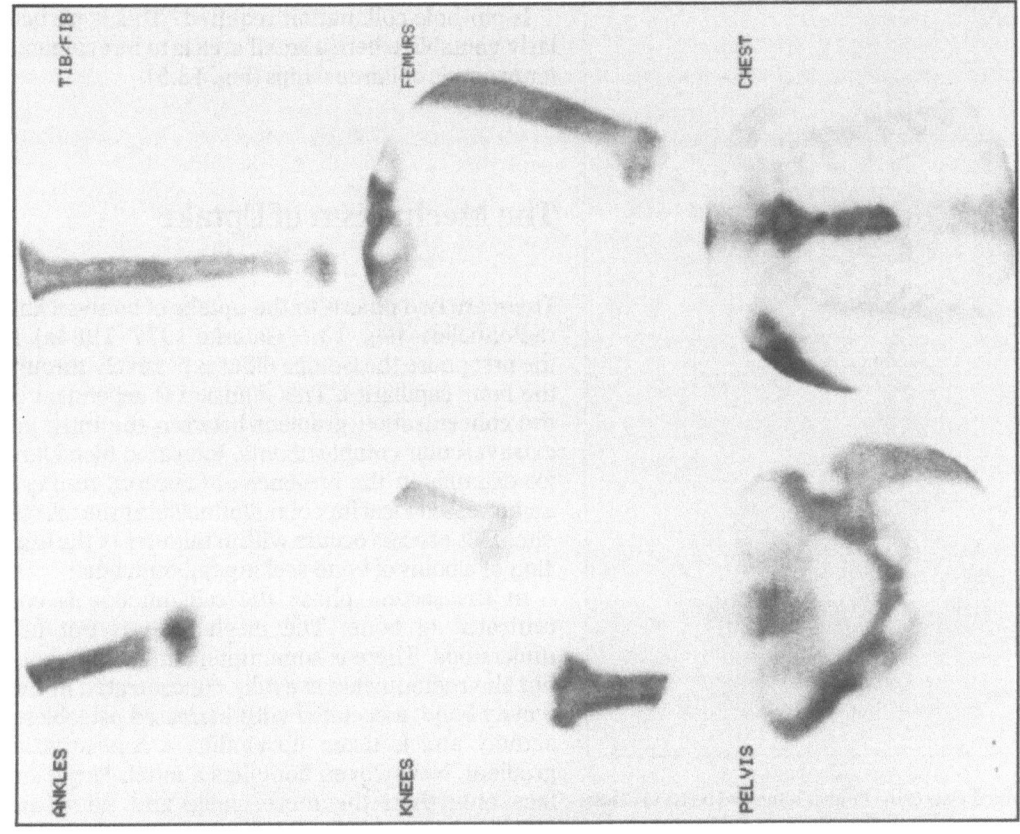

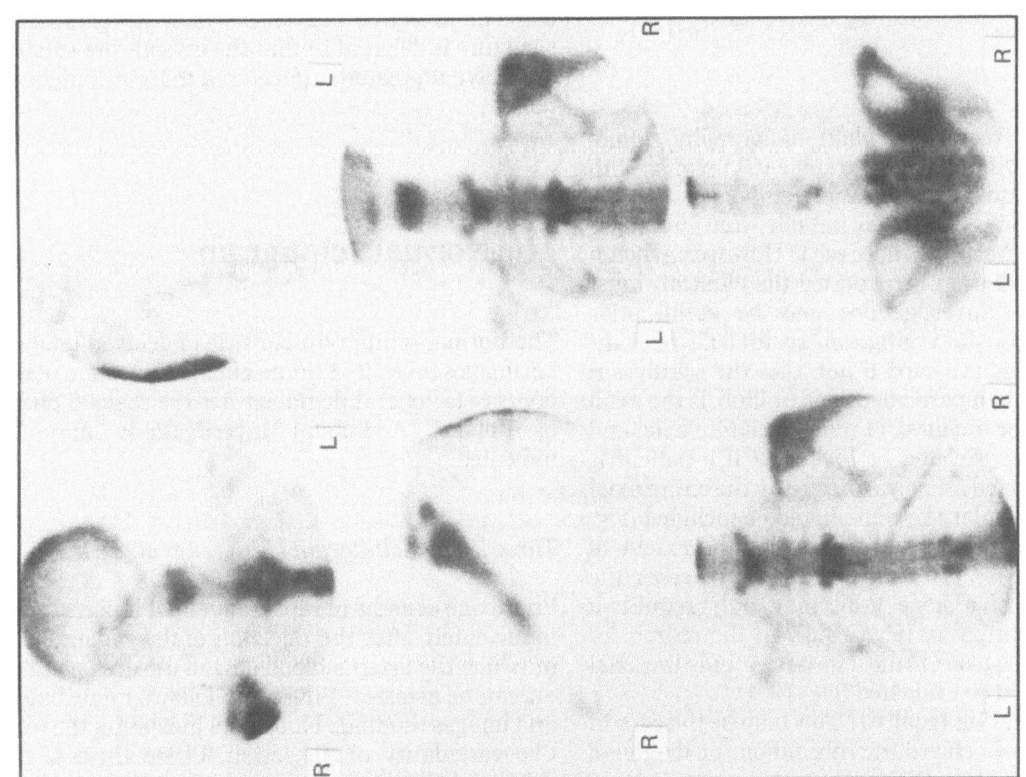

Fig. 13.2a,b. Paget's disease. Scintigram of the axial plus appendicular skeleton. Note the increased uptake in the right humerus, left femur, right tibia, right os calcis, sternum ("tie" sternum), as well as in the pelvis, spine and skull.

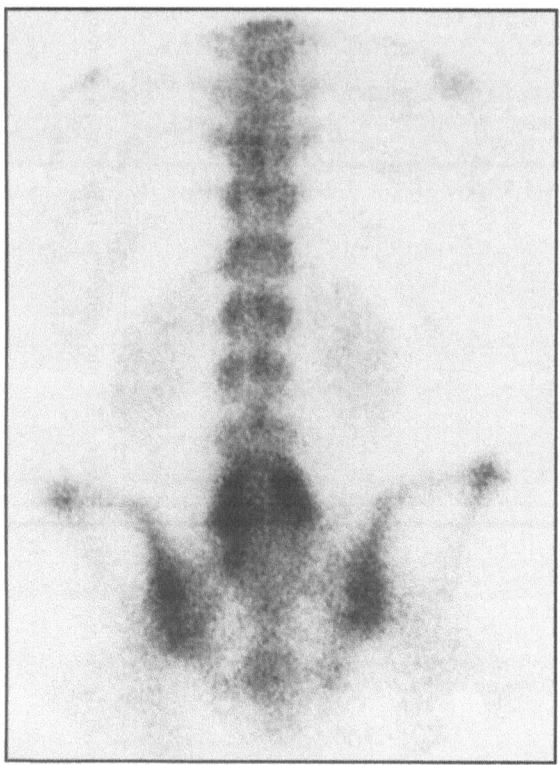

Fig. 13.3. Localized view of the lumbar spine and pelvis to assess L5 S1 fusion for spondylolisthesis.

to that for requesting plain radiography, tomograms, or computed tomographic (CT) scans. With these techniques the minimum number of investigations is usually requested initially, and investigations are increased as necessary. However, when a skeletal scintigram is requested the clinician must decide what investigations may be useful prior to requesting the scintigram, so that all relevant investigations are carried out. Can the scintigram be localized to a particular bone or limb, is the axial skeleton to be included, or must the entire axial and appendicular skeleton be included? If a patient is being evaluated for polyarthropathy the entire axial and appendicular skeleton should be included (Fig. 13.1), as is the case in evaluating the extent of Paget's disease of bone (Fig. 13.2), whereas the evaluation of a bone graft may only require a localized scintigram (Fig. 13.3). In the search for skeletal metastases, in most instances, only the axial skeleton need be evaluated (Fig. 13.4).

Is quantitation required? This may be the case in evaluation of delayed fracture union, or diagnosis of ankylosing spondylitis.

Is pin-hole collimation required? This is particularly valuable where a small area is to be evaluated, for example childrens' hips (Fig. 13.5).

The Mechanism of Uptake

There are two phases to the uptake of bone-seeking radionuclides (Fig. 13.6, Galasko 1977, 1984a). In the first phase the isotope diffuses passively through the bone capillaries. This diffusion is dependent on the concentration gradient between the intra and extravascular compartments. Increased blood flow, for example in the presence of infection, results in an increased local flux of radionuclide at the affected site. This process occurs within minutes of the injection of a bolus of bone-seeking radionuclide.

In the second phase the radionuclide is concentrated in bone. The mechanism is not fully understood. There is some uptake in normal bone, but the radionuclide is avidly concentrated in new woven bone, associated with increased osteoblastic activity and is taken up against a concentration gradient. New woven bone has a much larger surface area than the more stable and established lamellar bone, it is lined by plumper and metabolically more active osteoblasts and the crystalline structure is different in that the crystals are smaller and have a greater surface area than in immature bone.

The Normal Scintigram

The normal scintigram consists of delayed images, i.e. images taken 2–3 hours after the injection of the bolus of isotope; it demonstrates the skeletal phase of uptake. Additional investigations may be indicated.

Three Phase Scintigram (Maurer et al. 1981)

Phase one consists of rapid sequential images taken immediately after the injection of the radionuclide in which the arterial blood flow to the area of interest can be assessed. Phase two follows immediately and images the static blood pool indicating the relative vascularity of the lesion. Phase three is the delayed skeletal image.

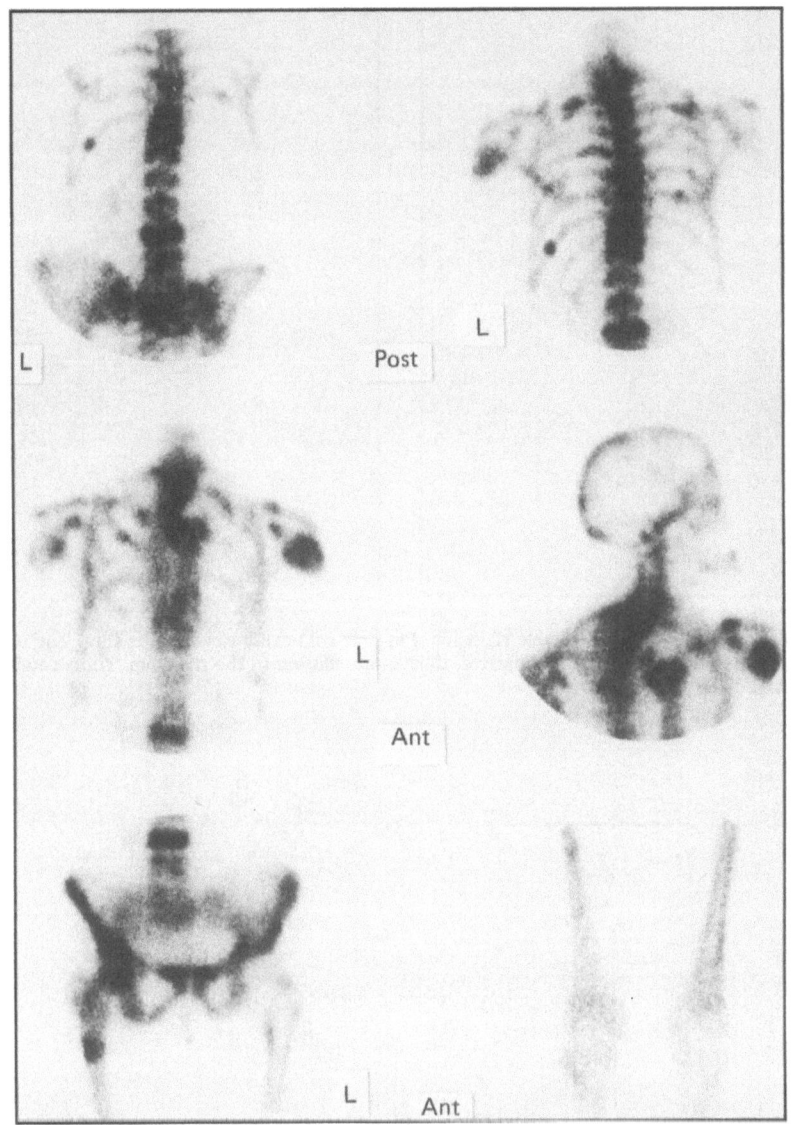

Fig. 13.4. Patient with advanced mammary carcinoma, who had undergone a left total hip replacement arthroplasty for a pathological fracture of the left femoral neck. The scintigram of the axial skeleton and femora shows multiple metastases affecting the spine, rib cage, proximal humeri, pelvis and right femur. Virtually the entire dorsal spine is affected, giving a "superscan" appearance of this area.

Blood pool images are particularly useful when infection is suspected.

Joint Imaging

If a patient is being evaluated for polyarthropathy, specific images of the hands and wrists, elbows, shoulders, knees, ankles and feet may be required.

Pin-hole Collimator Views

These provide greater definition of small areas. They are particularly useful for examination of the hips in a child, the hands or wrists, or a localized area, e.g. if an osteoid osteoma is suspected.

Quantitation

This may be provided either in the form of a ratio, or of an uptake profile.

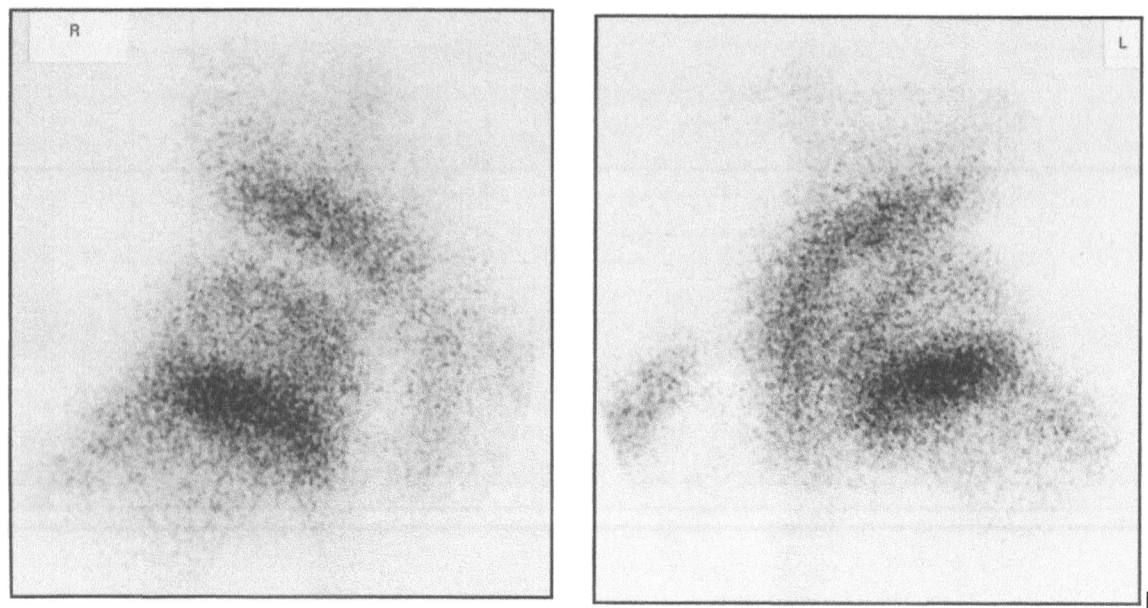

Fig. 13.5a,b. Child who presented with an irritable right hip. Pin-hole collimator views of the hips. The uptake is normal. The area of increased uptake is in the capital physis; however, there is an effusion in the right hip. These details could not be made out on the standard image of the pelvis.

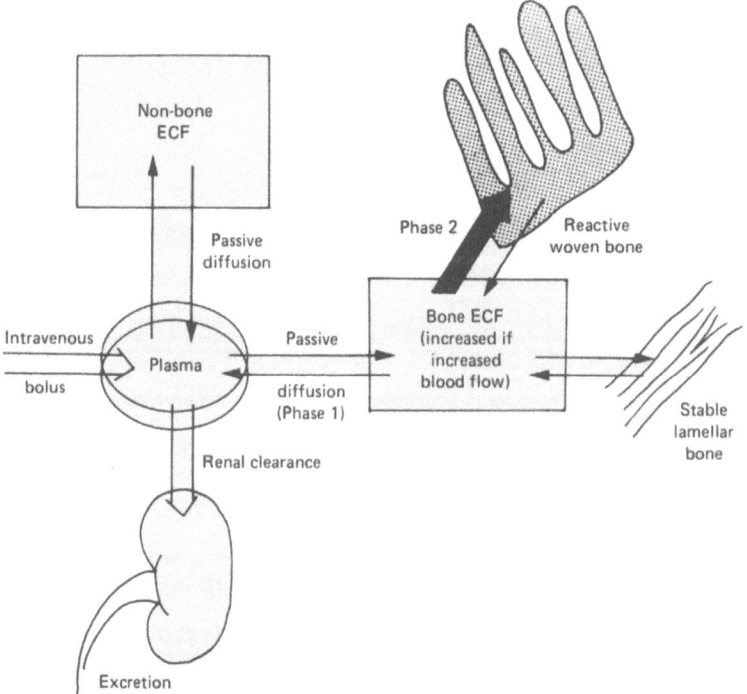

Fig. 13.6. The mechanism of uptake of bone-seeking radionuclides. Uptake occurs in two phases. In the first phase, isotope diffuses passively from the vascular compartment to the bone extracellular fluid (ECF) compartment. If there is an increase in vascularity, this will result in an increased amount of isotope in the bone ECF. This occurs within minutes of the intravenous injection of a bolus of radionuclide and is due to passive diffusion across the capillary pores. In phase 2, the radionuclide is selectively concentrated in reactive new immature bone. This occurs against a concentration gradient, is an active process and takes some hours, the time depending on the isotope.

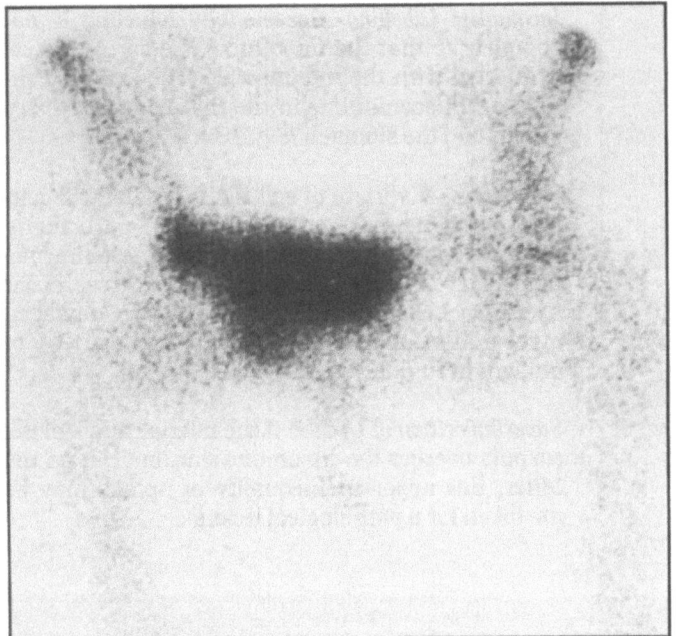
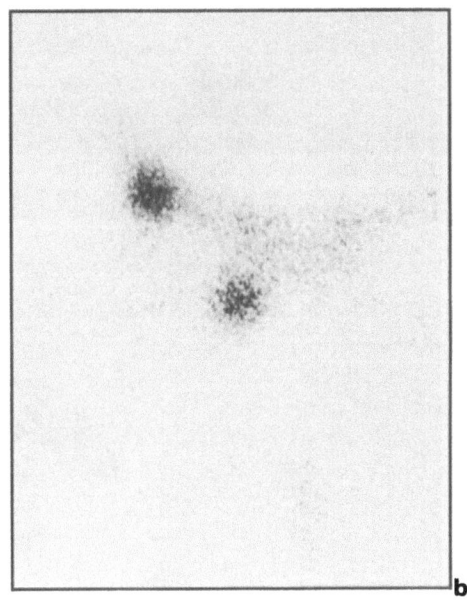

Fig. 13.7a,b. Patient with a right total hip arthroplasty, who developed pain in her right groin. Radiographs were normal. **a** ^{99m}Tc-MDP skeletal scintigram showing possible increased uptake in the right pelvis. However, the appearance is masked by isotope in the bladder. **b** Pin-hole collimator view of the right hip after catheterization. There are two areas of increased uptake in the superior and inferior pubic rami. The CT scans of the areas of increased uptake show that they were due to stress fractures in the pubic rami. The total hip replacement arthroplasty was satisfactory.

Child and Adolescent

The growth plates are seen as areas of increased uptake. In younger children they are more globular (Fig. 13.16) (unless imaged with a pin-hole collimator), whereas in older children they are flatter. It is particularly difficult to evaluate areas adjacent to the growth plates and pin-hole collimator views may be required.

Adult

In the adult the skeletal definition is usually better. Normally the uptake in the dorsal and lumbar spine is greater than in the sacrum or cervical spine. The sacroiliac joints, anterior superior iliac spines and anterior wing of the ilium show up as areas of increased uptake. Often the shoulder joints show up as areas of increased uptake as do the inferior angles of the scapulae. The sternoclavicular area may also demonstrate an apparently increased uptake. The shoulder on the dominant side frequently concentrates more isotope than the contralateral joint. Any joints subjected to increased stress may show an increased uptake of radionuclide, even in the absence of any radiographic abnormality. In the older patient there is often some loss of definition, possibly due to osteoporosis. Frequently, there is increased uptake in the cervical area due to calcification of the tracheal and laryngeal cartilages. There may be detectable uptake in the costal cartilages.

Bladder Uptake

The bone-seeking radionuclides are excreted in the urine. The more full the bladder the larger the bladder image and the poorer the visualization of the pelvis. If pathology in the pelvis is suspected the patient may have to be catheterized before the pelvis is imaged (Fig. 13.7).

Renal Uptake

The renal outline should be examined. Absent or very faint renal images may indicate a superscan, i.e. abnormally high, but symmetrical uptake in the skeleton which may occur in metabolic bone disease, as well as in patients with multiple diffuse

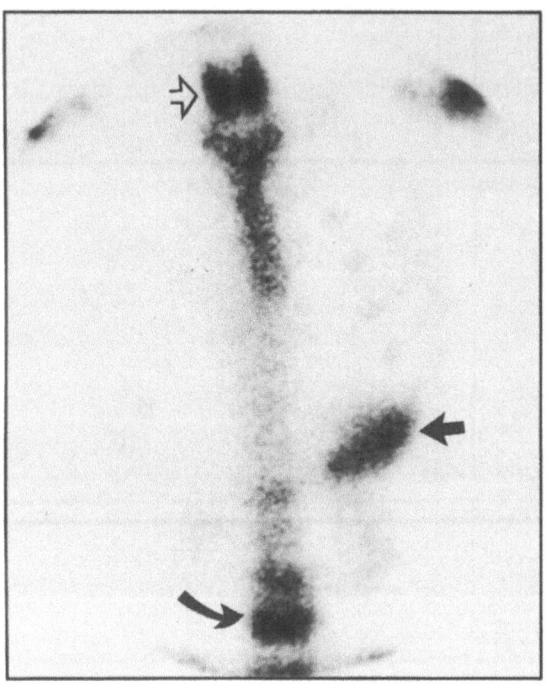

Incomplete Labelling. Occasionally labelling is not complete so that the unbound ^{99m}Tc-pertechnetate is injected with the radionuclide. The free pertechnetate will accumulate in the thyroid, the salivary glands and the stomach (Fig. 13.8).

Soft Tissue. A variety of soft tissue lesions will concentrate bone-seeking radionuclides, particularly the ^{99m}Tc-phosphate compounds. These include metastatic calcification in the lungs, areas of fat necrosis, hepatic metastases, acutely damaged myocardium and skeletal muscle, a variety of malignant tumours, and amyloid.

Superimposition of Uptake. If the inferior angle of the scapula overlies the rib on one side, but not on the other, this apparent inequality of uptake may be mistaken for a pathological lesion.

Fig. 13.8. Patient with staphylococcal osteomyelitis of the lumbar spine. Labelling was not complete and unbound ^{99m}Tc pertechnetate was injected with the ^{99m}Tc-MDP. Note the uptake in the thyroid (*open arrow*) and stomach (*closed arrow*) due to the unbound pertechnetate, as well as the area of increased uptake in the infected spine (*curved arrow*).

Table 13.1. Causes of increased uptake of bone-seeking radionuclides

A.	*Malignant disease*
	Skeletal metastases
	Primary malignant bone tumours
	Soft tissue metastases from osteosarcoma
B.	*Benign bone lesions*
	Benign tumours associated with new bone formation
	Infection – acute or chronic
	Arthritides – including rheumatoid arthritis, osteoarthritis, etc.
	Fractures and osteotomies
	Bone grafts
	Paget's disease
	Miscellaneous – including osteomalacia, hypertrophic pulmonary osteoarthropathy, etc.
C.	*Normal growth plates (in children)*
D.	*Soft tissue lesions*
	Metastatic calcification
	Shin splints
	Abscess and chronic inflammation[1]
	Infarction, expecially cerebral and cardiac[1]
	Neoplasia, e.g. neuroblastoma[1]
	Renal parenchyma[1]
E.	*Artefacts*
	Site of injection
	Urine
	Bladder diverticulum
	Unbound ^{99m}Tc-pertechnetate
	Superimposition of uptake

[1]Very occasional.

skeletal metastases. Pelvic or ureteric obstruction, unilateral functional impairment of the kidney etc. may be diagnosed unexpectedly on a skeletal scintigram.

Artefacts

Foci of Increased Uptake

Site of Injection. This probably is the commonest artefact producing a focus of increased uptake.

Urine. Urine at the external meatus, on the thigh, or any other site can present as an area of increased uptake. This is particularly important in an incontinent patient and contaminated clothes may provide a difficult diagnostic problem.

Bladder Diverticulum. This may simulate metastatic involvement of the anterior pelvis.

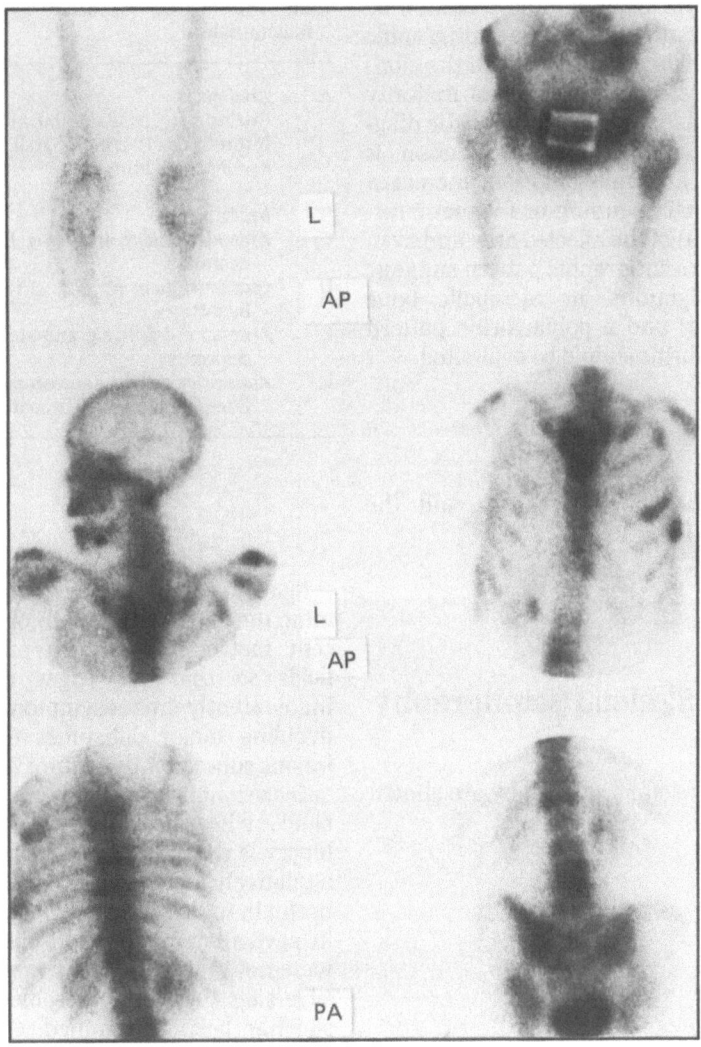

Fig. 13.9. Patient with disseminated mammary carcinoma. There are multiple areas of increased uptake in the rib cage, spine, pelvis and proximal left femur, due to metastatic involvement. The area of diminished uptake over the bladder, on the anterior pelvic view, was due to a buckle the patient was wearing.

Foci of Decreased Uptake

Metal Objects. These may be extrinsic or intrinsic and include pendants, buckles, coins, external splints, and implants used for internal fixation or replacement (Fig. 13.9).

Equipment Failure. Abnormalities in the crystal or photomultiplier tubes may be responsible for areas of apparently diminished uptake. This will be seen in every view and is particularly noticeable when several views are obtained with a gamma camera.

The Abnormal Scintigram

Increased Uptake

The usual abnormality is an area of increased uptake, and may have many causes (Table 13.1; Fig. 13.10). It is virtually impossible to make a diagnosis from the scintigraphic examination of a single area. Paget's disease, if extensive, has a unique pattern, and multiple skeletal metastases can usually be diagnosed if multiple views of the skeleton are obtained. However, the exact pathology cannot be diagnosed from the scintigram and the scintigraphic findings must be considered together with the clinical findings and radiographs. In the vast majority of instances this combination will provide the diagnosis, but occasionally further investigation is required (Fig. 22.11). Localized foci of increased uptake may require CT scanning or magnetic resonance imaging (MRI) of the affected area and even a biopsy; a metabolic scintigraphic pattern suggests that further investigations for metabolic bone disease are indicated; and a polyarthritic pattern suggests that polyarthritis should be evaluated.

Decreased Uptake

Decreased uptake occasionally occurs and the causes are shown in Table 13.2.

Indications for Skeletal Scintigraphy

The indications for skeletal scintigraphy are shown in Table 13.3.

Tumours

Skeletal Metastases

The detection of skeletal metastases is probably the commonest indication for skeletal scintigraphy. Furthermore, skeletal scintigraphy is the most accurate and sensitive method currently available for detecting skeletal metastases (Chap. 22). Usually it is indicated in the diagnosis of a symptomatic lesion and in assessing the extent of dissemination of the neoplasm. Its use in the assessment of a patient with apparently "early" cancer to stage the disease before starting treatment, is more controversial (Chap. 22). Skeletal scintigraphy has been used in mammary carcinoma, prostatic carcinoma, and bronchial carcinoma, but the detection rates have varied at different centres (Galasko 1984b). Occasional studies have been carried out in patients with thyroid carcinoma, neuroblastoma, carcinoma of the cervix, and malignant melanoma (Galasko 1984b).

Table 13.2. Causes of decreased uptake of bone-seeking radionuclides

A.   *Artefacts*
     Extrinsic, e.g. pendants, buckles, coins, splints
     Intrinsic, e.g. Harrington rods, plates, prostheses
     Equipment failure

B.   *Irradiation*

C.   *Avascular lesions*, including Perthes' disease, avascular necrosis

D.   *Occasional tumours* (Fig. 13.10), including occasional metastases

E.   *Anatomical defects*, e.g. amputation, congenital anomalies, deformity

F.   *Absence of activity* (autoamputation), e.g. scleroderma, Buerger's disease, neuropathy

Skeletal scintigraphy is frequently used to determine the extent of a lesion, or the presence of adjacent metastases prior to planning radiotherapy fields so that the edges of the field do not inadvertently cross asymptomatic metastases, thus avoiding major difficulties if these neighbouring lesions subsequently require treatment.

Occasionally a patient presents with metastatic cancer where no obvious primary can be found and biopsy is required. The presenting lesion may be in a relatively inaccessible site. Skeletal scintigraphy is useful in indicating the extent of dissemination and in particular may demonstrate metastases, which were not radiographically apparent, at more accessible sites that are preferable for biopsy. Once the site has been determined, CT or MRI can more accurately localize the metastasis.

Serial scintigrams are probably more accurate than any other method currently available for assessing the response of skeletal metastases to treatment (Fig. 13.11, Chap. 22), although serial CT or MRI of selected metastases may prove to be the treatment of choice in the future.

The results of skeletal scintigraphy in multiple myeloma are poor (Woolfenden et al. 1980), probably because many of the lesions do not provoke an osteoblast reaction, but the investigation appears to be more useful in the lymphomata.

Primary Tumours of Bone

Skeletal scintigraphy has not been used as extensively in primary bone tumours as in metastatic disease, but is an important investigation. Its uses in primary bone tumours are shown in Table 13.3.

Table 13.3. Indications for skeletal scintigraphy

A. *Tumours*
    1. Skeletal metastases
            Detection
                Diagnosis of a painful lesion
                Assessment of extent of metastatic involvement
            Staging of apparently "early" cancer
            Planning radiotherapy fields
            Locating suitable biopsy sites
            Assessment of response to therapy
            Differentiation of pathological from traumatic fracture
    2. Primary tumours of bone
            Location of benign tumours
            Assessment of malignant tumours
                Extent of primary lesion
                "Skip" lesions
                Distant dissemination
                Recurrence
            Detection of multicentric tumours
            Detection of malignant change, e.g. diaphyseal aclasis

B. *Arthritides*
    1. Polyarthritis
            Early diagnosis
            Distribution of joint involvement
            Assessment of response to treatment
    2. Ankylosing spondylitis
            Diagnosis
            Assessment of response to treatment
    3. Miscellaneous
            Psychogenic arthralgia
            Leprosy
            Haemophilic arthropathy

C. *Infection*
    1. Acute osteomyelitis
            Diagnosis
            Detection of multicentric lesions
            Assessment of response to treatment
    2. Chronic osteomyelitis
            Assessment of recurrent "flare-up"
            Brodie's abscess
    3. Tuberculosis
            Assessment of recurrence
    4. Discitis
    5. Septic arthritis
    6. Infected implants

D. *Metabolic disease of bone*
    1. Paget's disease
            Extent of skeletal involvement
            Assessment of response to treatment
    2. Hyperparathyroidism
            Extent of skeletal involvement
    3. Osteomalacia
    4. Renal osteodystrophy
    5. Transient osteoporosis

E. *Fractures*
    Assessment of fracture healing
    Diagnosis of stress fractures
    Diagnosis of scaphoid, proximal femoral fractures
    Development of avascular necrosis

F. *Miscellaneous*
    Spondylolysis
    Bone grafts
    Avascular necrosis
    Reflex sympathetic dystrophy

Scintigraphy cannot diagnose the tumour type, but it may be particularly useful in the detection and location of some primary tumours, as well as multicentric tumours.

Figure 13.12 shows the scintigram of an adolescent boy who had complained of back pain for three years. His radiographs were normal as were the serological investigations that had been carried out. Before labelling him as hysterical an orthopaedic opinion was sought. A scintigram was requested which showed an area of increased uptake in L5. CT confirmed the diagnosis of an osteoid osteoma. Surgical removal of the lesion was made easier by using a sterilizable probe (Szypryt et al. 1987), the patient having been given ^{99m}Tc-MDP 3 hours prior to surgery. The area of increased uptake, as detected by the probe at surgery, was removed from the pedicle of L5. Post-operatively his pain disappeared completely and the scintigraphic appearance of his spine reverted to normal. Szypryt and colleagues (1987) have shown that a cadmium telluride crystal mounted in a collimator 10 mm in diameter with a 3 mm window was more sensitive than the sodium iodide detector previously used.

Osteosarcoma may occasionally be multicentric. The primary tumour is usually diagnosed on radiograph, but scintigraphy may be extremely useful in the diagnosis of a multicentric tumour.

Scintigraphy may be very useful in demonstrating the extent of a primary malignant tumour, but is not as accurate as CT or MRI in indicating the soft tissue spread of an osteosarcoma. It may be useful in defining the extent of medullary extension, but MRI is probably more accurate as scintigraphy may suggest involvement beyond the histological limit, probably because of surrounding inflammatory changes. Soft tissue metastases may show up as areas of increased uptake on the scintigram, if they are associated with new bone formation (Fig. 13.13). Single photon emission computed tomography (SPECT) may improve the detection of pulmonary metastases from osteosarcoma (Kirk and Schulz 1987), but probably is less sensitive than CT.

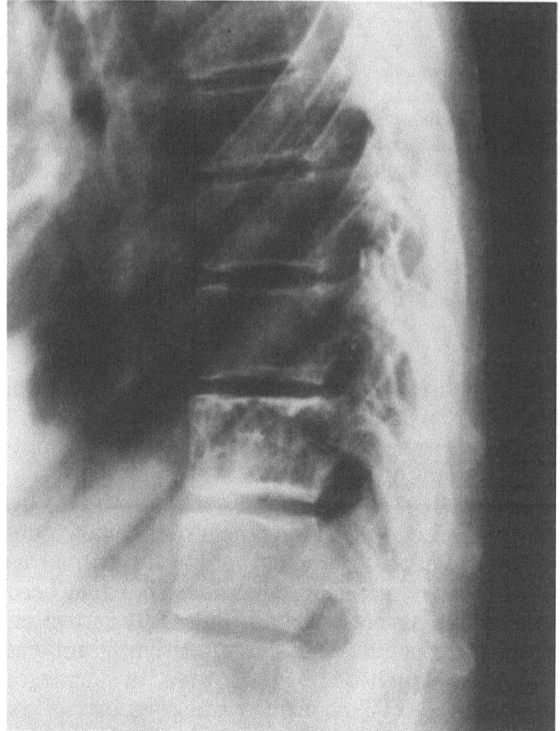
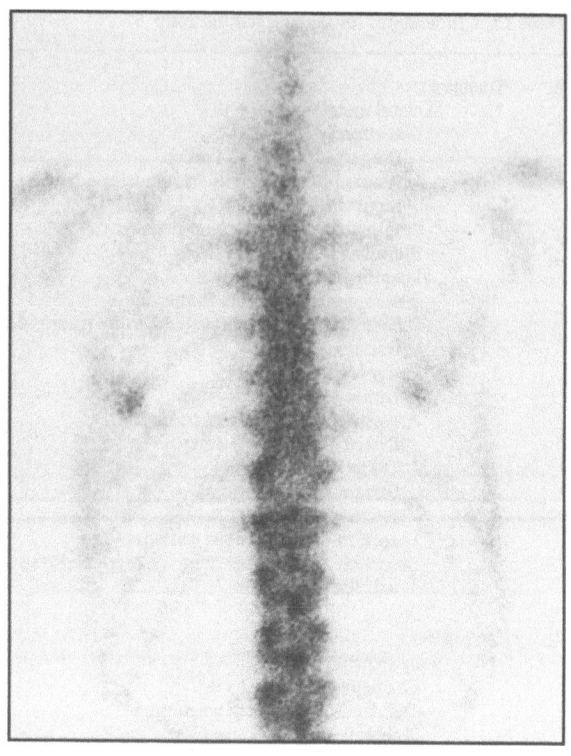

Fig. 13.10a,b. Fibrosarcoma of D10. The patient presented with back pain. a Lateral radiograph of the spine showing a lesion involving the body of D10. b ^{99m}Tc-MDP scintigram. There is diminished uptake in the body of D10. The CT scan showed some destruction within the vertebral body, but the diagnosis could not be made from the investigations, and a needle biopsy was required. This was carried out under radiographic control.

The humeral lesion shown in Fig. 13.13 is too extensive for local resection, whereas if the osteosarcoma is localized it may be ideally suited for local excision and prosthetic replacement (Chap. 21).

Skeletal scintigraphy may be useful in the detection of malignant change. For example it has been suggested that patients with diaphyseal aclasis should have an annual scintigram. Any lesion associated with increased activity should be removed because of the risk that that particular osteochondroma may be undergoing malignant change. Calcification of the cartilaginous cap can also be associated with increased uptake.

Scintigraphy may also be useful in the detection of local recurrence, either following amputation or prosthetic replacement. However, following prosthetic replacement, the uptake is often increased for up to 12 months.

Because of its non-specificity, scintigraphy cannot be used to detect malignant change in Paget's disease.

Although scintigraphy does not allow a positive diagnosis of tumour type, it is of value to determine the extent of a primary malignant tumour, the presence of some tumours such as osteoid osteoma, to identify skip lesions, and to detect spread.

The Arthritides

There are two groups of isotopes that can be used to examine joints.

1. Those isotopes that are localized in inflamed synovium

2. Bone seeking isotopes which will localize in periarticular bone

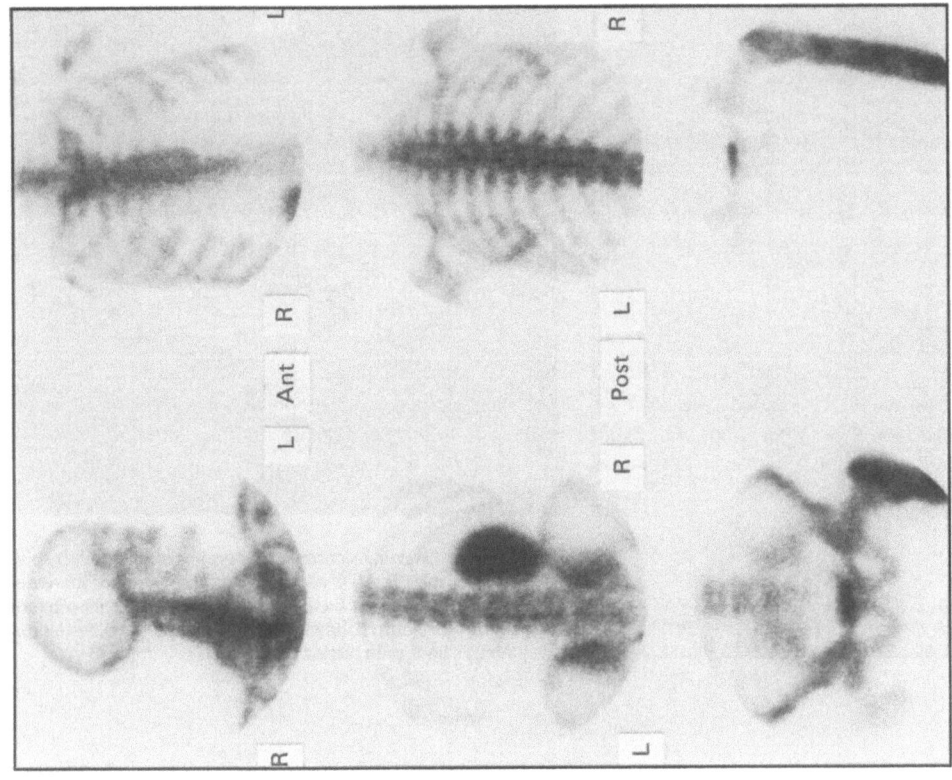

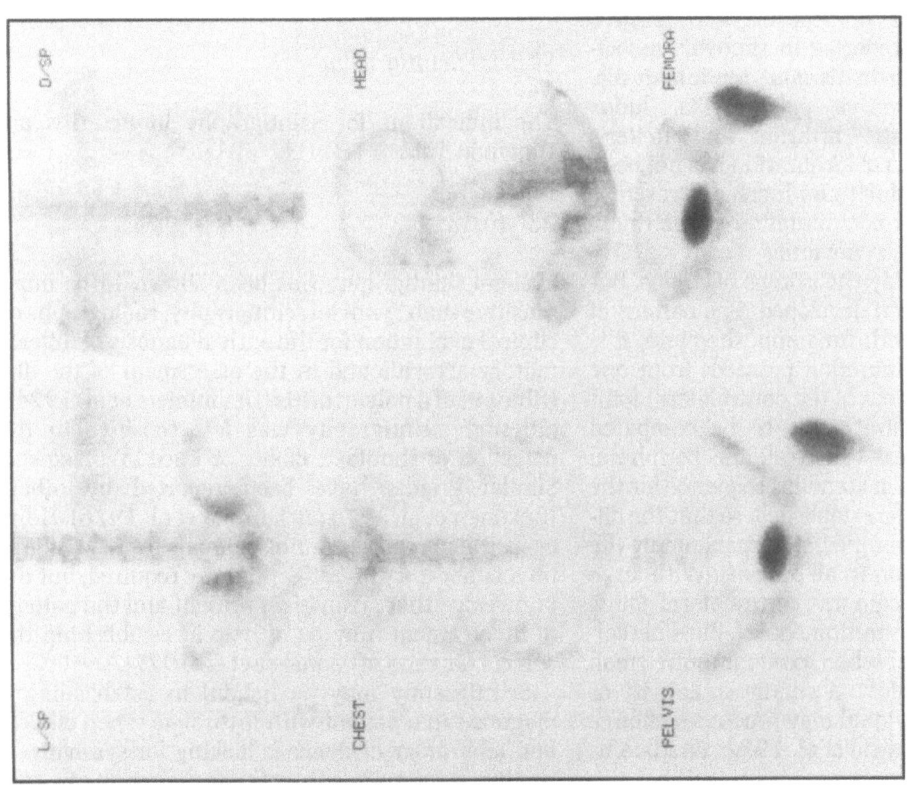

Fig. 13.11a,b. Patient with carcinoma of the rectum. ^{99m}Tc-MDP scintigram. a Patient complained of pain affecting his left lower limb. Scintigraphy showed a metastasis in the proximal left femur. b The patient did not respond to therapy. Repeat scintigram taken 7 months later showed complete involvement of the left femur. He also had developed a metastasis in the proximal left tibia.

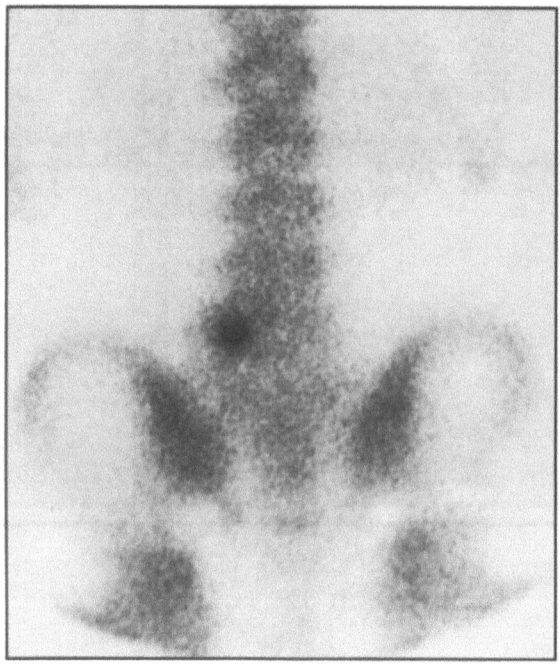

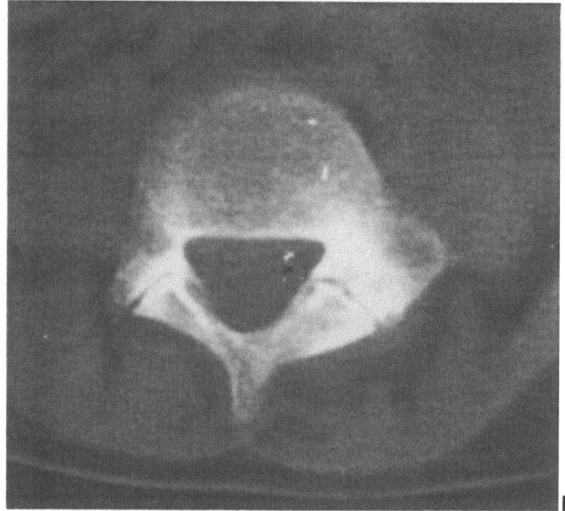

Fig. 13.12a,b. Osteoid osteoma. Radiographs of the lumbar spine were normal. **a** ^{99m}Tc-MDP skeletal scintigram showed increased uptake on the left of L5. **b** CT scan showed the osteoid osteoma close to the facet joint. Following removal of the osteoid osteoma, this patient's back pain settled completely.

Synovial Uptake

The localization of the radiopharmaceutical in the synovial membrane is non-specific and positive localization has been reported in synovitis associated with rheumatoid arthritis, gout, septic arthritis, osteoarthritis, seronegative polyarthritis, lupus erythematosus, psoriatic arthritis and Reiter's disease. The mechanism of localization has not been defined, but is largely due to an increased vascular pool and extravascular accumulation in the thickened and inflamed synovium. Today ^{99m}Tc-pertechnetate is probably the isotope of choice, but other isotopes have been developed, The pattern of localization changes with time and, therefore, it is essential that the examination proceeds from one joint to the identical view of the contralateral joint if the degree of localization is to be compared between the two sides. When all the peripheral joints are being studied a standard sequence for the different views should be established, so that the different joints will be examined at approximately the same time after injection in all patients. With large field of view gamma cameras contralateral joints often can be examined simultaneously. Pin-hole collimation may be useful when examining the small joints of the hands or feet. A change in activity or occupation of the individual may produce a change in the scintigram (Maxfield et al. 1972; Boerbooms and Buys 1978).

However, synovial scintigraphy is probably less sensitive than skeletal scintigraphy in the assessment of arthritis.

Skeletal Scintigraphy

The indications for scintigraphy in arthritis are shown in Table 13.3.

Polyarthritis

Skeletal scintigraphy has been shown to be more sensitive than synovial scintigraphy, radiographs or clinical evaluation for the early diagnosis of inflammatory arthritis and in the assessment of the distribution of a polyarthritis (Desaulniers et al. 1974), although scintigraphy was less sensitive in the detection of shoulder, elbow or knee involvement. Similar results have been reported by others (Rekonen et al. 1974; Bekerman et al. 1976). However, the diagnosis cannot be made from scintigraphy. Laboratory investigations are required, but the knowledge that synovitis is present and the pattern of involvement may be of help in establishing the correct diagnosis (Dequeker et al. 1977).

Scintigraphy may be helpful in establishing a diagnosis in a patient with arthralgia when clinical and laboratory evidence is lacking for synovitis. A positive scintigram supports the diagnosis of a true

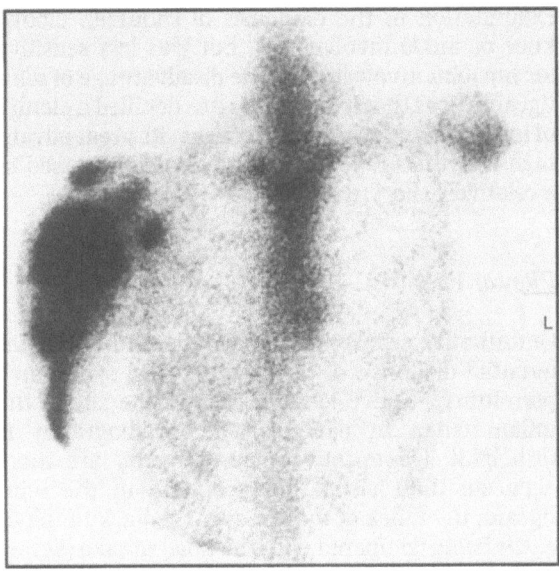

Fig. 13.13. 99mTc-MDP scintigram of the anterior chest wall and proximal right humerus in a patient with an osteosarcoma. The tumour can be seen on the scintigram; in addition, there was intramedullary extension along the humeral shaft, a deposit in the acromion and axillary node involvement. This tumour is too advanced for local resection and prosthetic replacement.

arthropathy, whereas a normal scintigram may support the diagnosis of a psychogenic arthralgia (McCarty et al. 1970).

Serial scintigraphy has been used to evaluate the response to treatment (Desaulniers et al. 1974; Sturrock et al. 1974). There probably is no indication for serial scintigraphy in the routine assessment of patients with polyarthritis, but it may be useful when evaluating new drugs, or when the clinical criteria are equivocal.

Joint scintigraphy is particularly useful in patients with arthralgia where a psychogenic element is suspected; in the diagnosis of monoarticular arthritis; in determining whether a patient with monoarticular arthritis has asymptomatic polyarthritis; and in assessing the extent of polyarthritis. It is more helpful than a radiographic survey in assessing the extent and activity of the disease, but is of no value in the differential diagnosis of arthritis except where the pattern of joint involvement may help make the diagnosis.

Osteoarthritis

Joint scintigraphy plays little role in the diagnosis of osteoarthritis, although osteoarthritis is associated with increased uptake of bone-seeking radio-

nuclide. Its main use is in the knee, in the preoperative assessment of a patient considered for an unicompartmental replacement. It may indicate that other compartments are affected, even though the radiographs suggest the disease is limited to one compartment. However, it is less accurate that arthroscopy and the decision as to whether a unicompartmental or total knee arthroplasty should be carried out is more likely to be based on the arthroscopic findings, or the findings at surgery, rather than a pre-operative scintigram.

Ankylosing Spondylitis

The diagnosis is often difficult to make in the early stages; it is helped by determining whether the individual possesses the HLA–B27 antigen. Once characteristic changes occur in the sacroiliac joints and the spine, the disease can be diagnosed readily on radiographs. Although symptoms can be improved by treatment, the radiographic changes do not improve and may progress.

There are two indications for scintigraphy in ankylosing spondylitis.

1. In the diagnosis of early symptomatic disease scintigraphic examination of the sacroiliac joints and particularly quantitative estimation of their uptake, may indicate a sacroiliitis many months or years before radiographic changes appear. It also may be useful in those patients who do not develop erosive or sclerotic changes and suffer for years with chronic backache and no definite diagnosis. The usual method is to determine the sacroiliac index by calculating the uptake over the sacroiliac joint and the sacrum. However, it must be appreciated that the technique is not specific and that an abnormally high ratio is not diagnostic of ankylosing spondylitis. Many patients with other diseases associated with backache such as Reiter's syndrome, psoriatic arthropathy, or inflammatory bowel disease may have a sacroiliitis and some patients with elevated indices have not yet shown any evidence of inflammatory sacroiliitis. The technique is of little value in children or adolescents because of the normal marked uptake by the sacroiliac region in this age group. The ratio may also be elevated in patients with low back pain, but no evidence of ankylosing spondylitis. This may reflect a forme fruste sacroiliitis.

2. Serial scintigraphy, and particularly serial quantitative estimations, give a useful indication of the response to treatment. When sclerotic changes are present radiographically, there are no clinical or laboratory methods to relate exacerbations of low

back pain to inflammatory activity in the sacroiliac joints, nor to disassociate them from the mechanical sequelae of the disease. Scintigraphy may be an objective method of assessing the short-term therapy of inflammatory sacroiliitis.

Miscellaneous Conditions

Leprosy

Scintigraphy may be more sensitive than radiography in indicating joint involvement (Goergen et al. 1976).

Synovial Rupture

Although joint scintigraphy is less invasive than arthrography, the latter investigation is the more reliable.

Gout

Scintigraphy is of no help in making the diagnosis, but may be useful in indicating which joints are involved. The scintigraphic pattern can easily be confused with rheumatoid arthritis, but the diagnoses can be separated by laboratory investigation. Serial scintigraphy may be useful in assessing the response to therapy and may show that, although the patient is asymptomatic, some residual synovitis persists.

Reiter's Disease

Scintigraphy may help in the early differentiation of Reiter's disease from rheumatoid arthritis, which may be difficult on clinical, radiographic and laboratory investigations. In Reiter's disease the predominant localization in the knee corresponds with site of tendon insertion and there is an increased uptake in the Achilles tendon, which also occurs with ankylosing spondylitis. Patients with rheumatoid arthritis may show localization in tendons, but the degree of localization is usually less and the typical pattern is of knee and tarsal joint involvement.

Haemophilic Arthropathy

Cambouroglou et al. (1976) found that scintigraphy was more sensitive than clinical or radiographic examination in the diagnosis of shoulder, elbow, knee or ankle involvement, but was less sensitive for hip joint involvement. The disadvantage of scintigraphy was that it did not give as detailed a picture of joint damage as the radiographs; its great advantage was that all joints could be safely assessed in a relatively short period.

Plantar Fasciitis

Quantitative scintigraphy may be useful in the differential diagnosis of the "painful heel syndrome" permitting positive identification of the site of the inflammation in patients where radiography is unhelpful. Quantitative measurements are more accurate than visual interpretation of the scintigram, the index of uptake over the back of the os calcis being compared with the tibial uptake (Sewell et al. 1980).

Pigmented Villonodular Synovitis

This is associated with periarticular osteoporosis and increased radionuclide uptake, usually affecting only one joint. In late cases lytic areas of bone destruction become obvious.

Neuropathic Arthropathy

The radiographic features are usually diagnostic. Scintigraphy shows increased uptake in the affected joints, but is of little additional value.

Infection

The indications for skeletal scintigraphy are shown in Table 13.3.

Acute Osteomyelitis

The classical manifestations of osteomyelitis have changed, possibly associated with an increased improvement in nutrition and social factors. In a recent survey we found that only four of 14 patients, in whom osteomyelitis was diagnosed, showed the classical symptoms of toxaemia, severe pain, exquisite tenderness and a very high pyrexia. Most patients presented with localized pain and tenderness and many were apyrexial. The white count

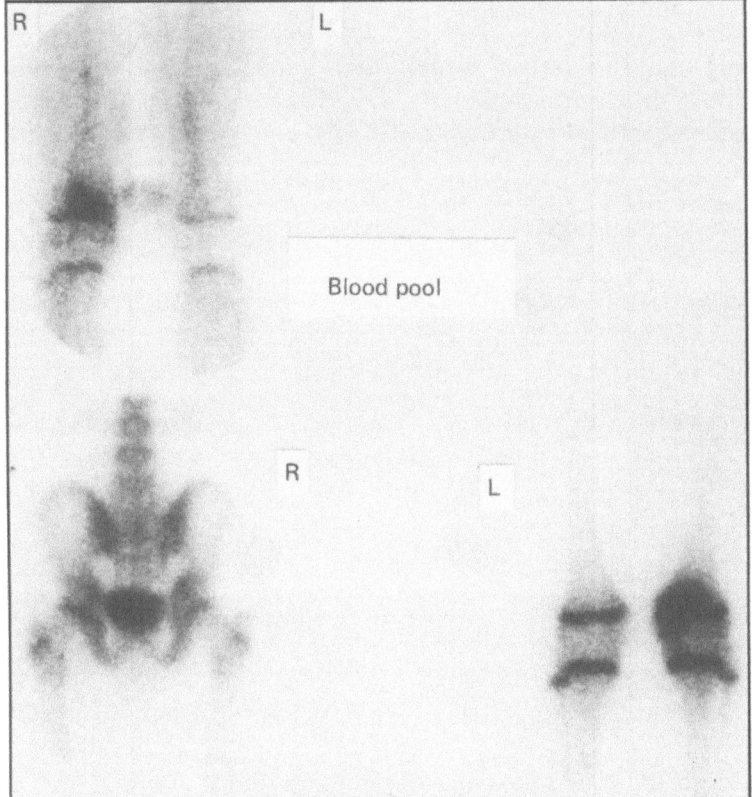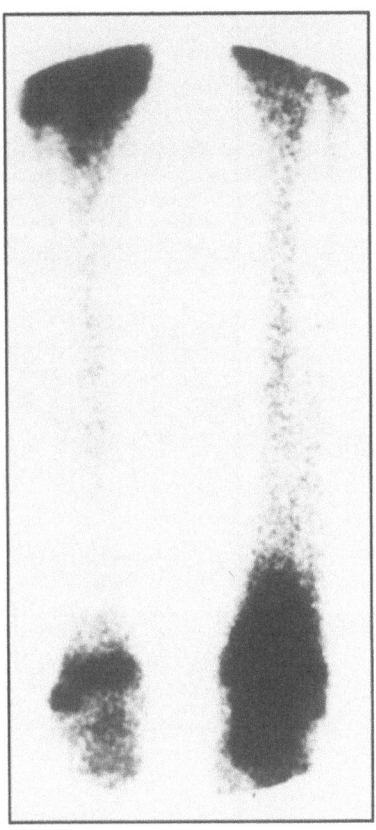

Fig. 13.14 (*left*). Early acute osteomyelitis of the distal right femur. The area of the increased uptake in the metaphysis can be seen both on the blood pool and the delayed images (^{99m}Tc-MDP).

Fig. 13.15 (*right*). Patient with multicentric acute osteomyelitis. There is a focus in the proximal right tibia, and the distal left tibia (^{99m}Tc-MDP scintigram). The radiographs were normal.

may not be elevated, but the erythrocyte sedimentation rate was raised in all, albeit only moderately in some. It often is extremely difficult to localize the site of infection on clinical examination. The initial radiographs are usually normal. Soft tissue swelling, followed by localized osteoporosis may be seen within days, but subperiosteal new bone and other skeletal changes are not seen for 10 to 14 days. Skeletal scintigraphy is particularly useful in this group of patients.

Early diagnosis of acute osteomyelitis is important, since the earlier treatment is instituted the less the risk of the potentially crippling complications from the infection. If osteomyelitis is present a more prolonged course of antibiotics is required than for a soft tissue infection.

Skeletal scintigraphy usually shows increased uptake within 24 hours (Duszynski et al. 1975, Figs 13.14, 13.15) but may be negative during the first few hours. There is an increase in both the vascular phase and skeletal phase. The latter may help differentiate an osteomyelitis from a cellulitis. In a soft tissue infection there is an increased uptake in the vascular phase, but the skeletal phase is normal (Fig. 13.16).

Combining skeletal scintigraphy with either ^{67}Gallium scintigraphy, or ^{111}In tagged white cell scintigraphy may be more accurate than skeletal scintigraphy alone. White cells are localized in infections and are not dependent on the reaction of bone to infection with increased osteoblast activity. Focal increased uptake of bone-seeking radionuclide adjacent to a growth plate in children is subtle and could escape detection. Here ^{67}Gallium or ^{111}In tagged white cells may be particularly useful (Lisbona and Rosenthall 1977).

Scintigraphy is not particularly useful in patients with fulminating osteomyelitis. These children require urgent surgical drainage and frequently it is not possible to obtain a skeletal scintigram prior

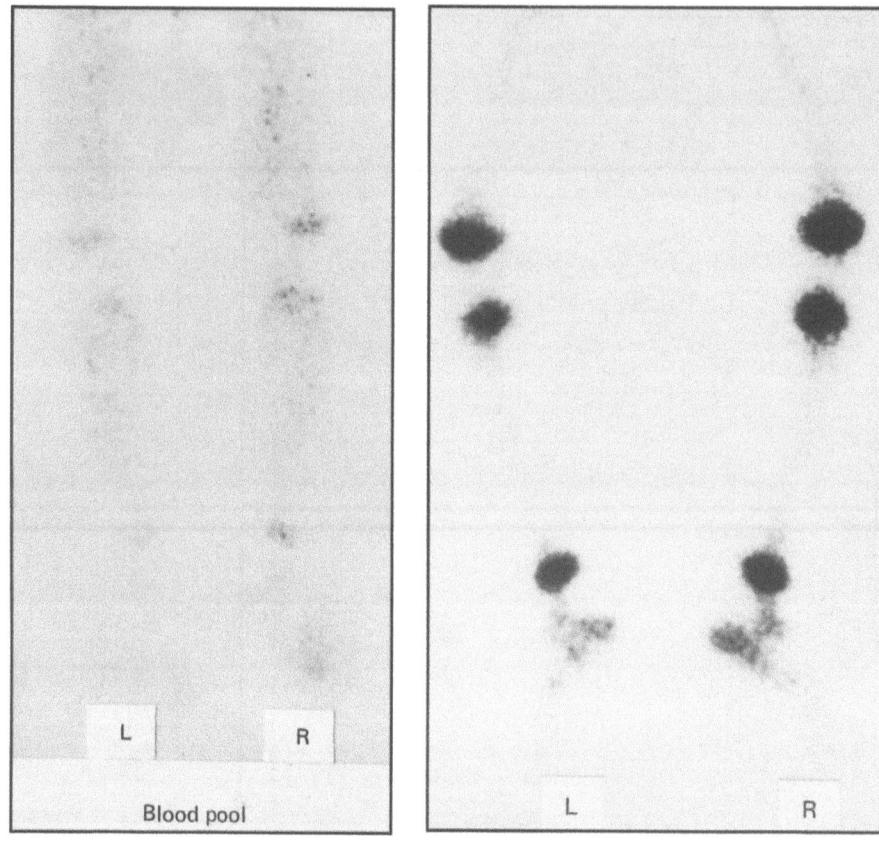

Fig. 13.16a,b. Infant with cellulitis affecting the right great toe. (^{99m}Tc-MDP scintigram). a Blood pool image. There was increased uptake over the right great toe. b Delayed skeletal image. The uptake was normal.

to surgery. However, skeletal scintigraphy is particularly useful in patients who present with the less acute form of osteomyelitis. They are treated with antibiotics, after a blood culture has been taken, and if they do not improve significantly within 12 to 24 hours, surgical intervention may be necessary. Skeletal scintigraphy is particularly useful in localizing the site of exploration (Figs 13.14, 13.15). The scintigram is usually abnormal within 24 hours. In contrast, scintigraphy is unreliable in neonates (Ash and Gilday 1980). In some instances the scintigram remains normal even though a lytic lesion and extensive periosteal new bone formation is evident on radiography. Occasionally serial skeletal scintigraphy may be useful in assessing the response to treatment. The latter is usually monitored by the clinical progress and improvement in the erythrocyte sedimentation rate. Scintigraphy is indicated if the latter fails to respond. With treatment the increased uptake gradually diminishes, although this may take several months. If the patient is not responding to treatment, the area of increased uptake may enlarge, or other foci may be seen.

Chronic Osteomyelitis

Often the radiographs do not relect whether a chronic osteomyelitis is quiescent or complicated by an acute recurrence, and frequently are unhelpful in patients with chronic osteomyelitis who present with pain over the affected bone, unless a new sequestrum is seen. If a sinus has developed, a sinogram will indicate the depth of the infection. Scintigraphy may help determine whether the pain is due to an infection (Fig. 13.17), and whether the infection is in the soft tissues or is due to an acute "flare-up" of the chronic osteomyelitis. Skeletal

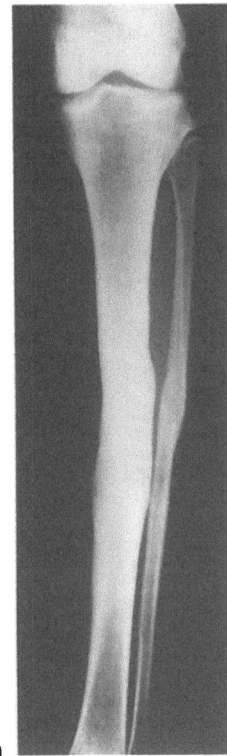
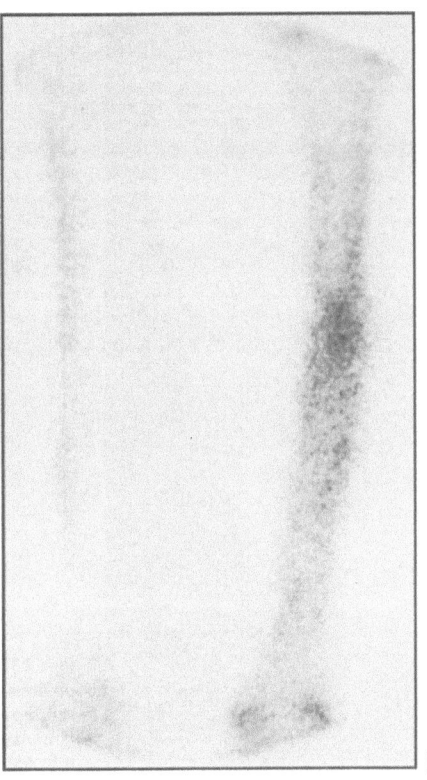

Fig. 13.17a,b. Patient with healed compound fracture of the left tibia, who presented with pain. **a** Radiographs showed no cause for the pain. **b** 99mTc-MDP scintigram. There is increased uptake at the site of the pain. Exploration at this site revealed an infected cavity.

scintigraphy will show an area of increased uptake at the site of recrudescence of the chronic osteomyelitis, but the delayed image will be normal if there is a soft tissue infection, or another cause for the pain. 67Gallium, or 111In tagged white cell scintigraphy usually localizes the site of infection, whether it arises from bone or not, and helps differentiate infection from other causes of pain.

Brodie's Abscess

These patients present with localized pain. The lesion is usually evident radiographically, but if it is normal a skeletal scintigram is indicated. It may

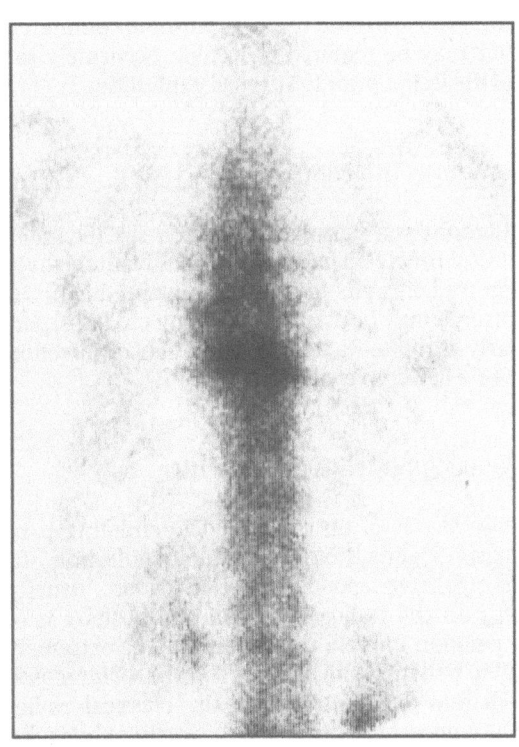

Fig. 13.18. Patient with reactivated tuberculosis. This patient had previously been treated for tuberculosis, and presented with a recurrence of back pain. Radiographs showed no obvious recurrence of infection. 99mTc-MDP scintigram showed increased uptake, suggesting reactivation of the disease. The diagnosis was confirmed by biopsy.

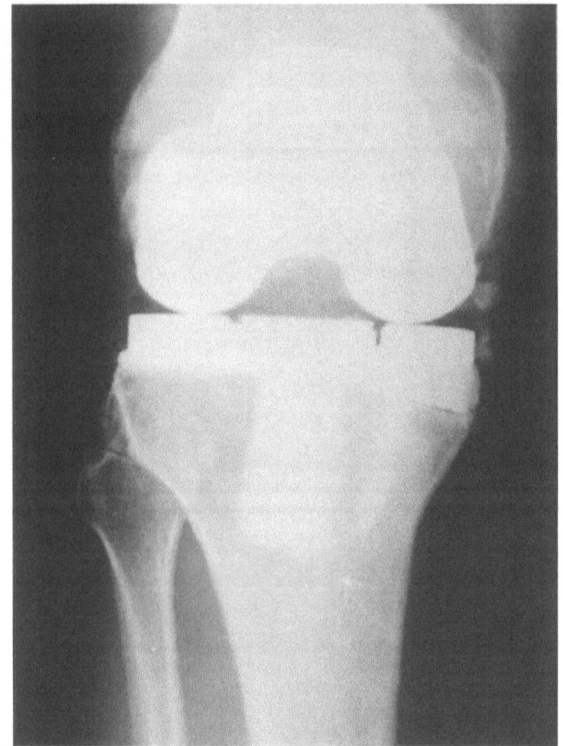

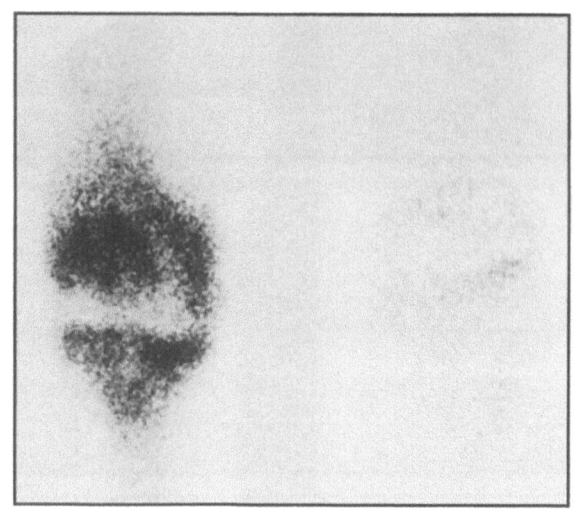

Fig. 13.19a,b. Loose total knee arthroplasty. a There was no obvious loosening or infection on the radiograph. b ^{99m}Tc-MDP scintigram showed increased uptake affecting all three components. At surgery, the implant was found to be loose, but not infected.

not be possible accurately to localize the site of the abscess on plain radiographs or on a skeletal scintigram, even with the use of a pin-hole collimator, and CT may be required to localize accurately the site of the lesion prior to surgical exploration.

Tuberculosis Infection

Scintigraphy is a sensitive, albeit non-specific index of skeletal involvement, but has no advantage over routine radiographs in establishing the diagnosis. However, it may be useful in assessing progress, particularly in patients with reactivation of infection (Fig. 13.18, Kemp et al. 1973).

Pyogenic Spondylitis and Discitis

Scintigraphy is of no value in differentiating pyogenic spondylitis from tuberculous infection. In acute pyogenic spondylitis changes are usually evident on the radiographs and scintigraphy is of little addition value. However, it may be extremely useful in patients with discitis. The area of increased uptake may be found before the classical radiographic appearance of disc narrowing in a child who

is generally fretful and with vague generalized spinal tenderness. Where there are obvious radiographic changes scintigraphy is of little diagnostic value.

Septic Arthritis

Radiographic changes occur late and skeletal scintigraphy is extremely useful in localizing the site of infection. The skeletal image may show the increased uptake as early as 24 hours after the onset of symptoms (Gilday et al. 1975). Pin-hole collimator views are particularly useful in children suspected of septic arthritis affecting a hip joint. The usual pattern is increased uptake on both sides of the joint. Although scintigraphy is helpful in making the diagnosis, it does not replace the need for joint aspiration, but may indicate the site of infection.

Infected Implants

Although infrequent, pain is an important complication of implants, particularly joint arthroplasty. It may indicate loosening or infection. The treatment varies, depending on the cause of the pain, and it is important to try and reach a diagnosis before

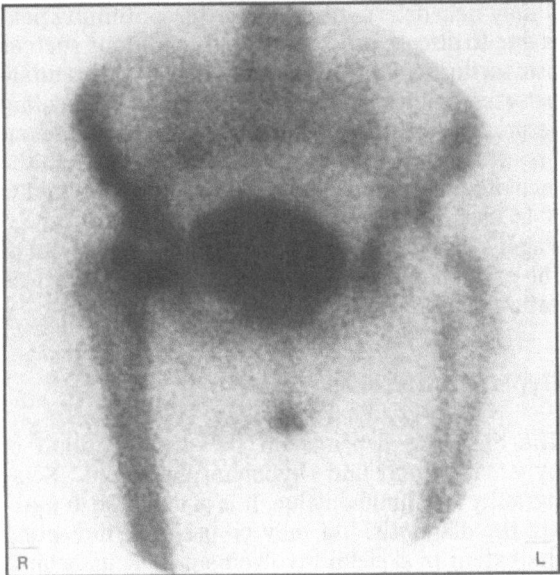 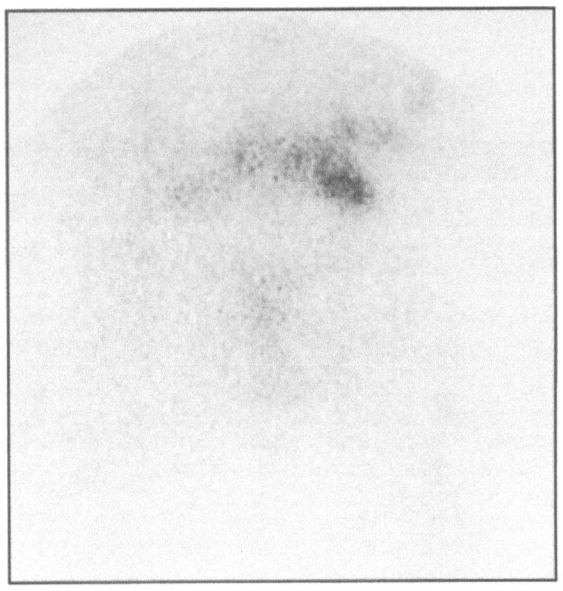

Fig. 13.20a,b. Infected Charnley total hip arthroplasty. Only the acetabular component was infected. The radiographs appeared normal, without any obvious sign of infection. **a** ^{99m}Tc-MDP scintigram. There may have been a focus of increased uptake at the inferior angle of the acetabulum. The increased uptake in this opposite (right) hip was due to osteoarthritis. **b** ^{111}In-tagged white cell scintigram. There was an obvious focus of increased uptake at the inferior angle of the acetabulum. Infection at this site was confirmed at surgery.

re-exploring the implants. Blood count, erythrocyte sedimentation rate, joint aspirate and radiographs may indicate the cause of the pain. Skeletal scintigraphy may also be useful in detecting loosening and/or infection.

The uptake of bone-seeking isotopes in the region of a prosthesis is usually increased for 9 to 12 months following its insertion. This is due to the normal healing response and, therefore, skeletal scintigraphy is usually of little help in the first year following surgery. Loosening and/or infection is associated with increased uptake of the radionuclide. Under both circumstances there is increased uptake on the skeletal image (Figs 13.19, 13.20), the area of increased uptake being limited to the site of infection or loosening. If the implant is infected there is also increased uptake on the vascular phase, which is not seen in the presence of aseptic loosening. It may be possible to differentiate these two complications by combining a two or three phase skeletal scintigram with either ^{67}Ga or ^{111}In tagged white blood cell scintigraphy (Mountford et al. 1986). In the presence of infection, increased uptake will be noted on both phases of the skeletal scintigram, as well as on the ^{67}Ga or ^{111}Indium tagged scintigram, whereas if the pros-

thesis is loose, but not infected, increased uptake will only be seen on the skeletal image. However, often it is not possible to differentiate between these complications prior to revision surgery.

Metabolic Disease of Bone

The indications for scintigraphy are shown in Table 13.3.

Paget's Disease

Scintigraphy may be useful in establishing the extent of skeletal involvement and in the assessment of response to treatment.

There is no correlation between the biochemical findings and the degree of skeletal involvement. Many of the lesions are asymptomatic and early lesions may not be obvious radiographically. Skeletal scintigraphy is more sensitive than a radiographic skeletal survey in determining the extent of

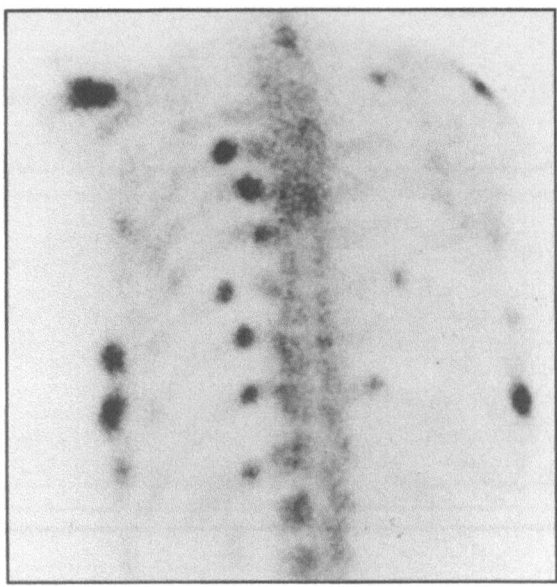

Fig. 13.21. Osteomalacia. The multiple areas of increased uptake in the rib cage were due to pseudo-fractures (Looser's zones). The differential diagnosis was of multiple fractures (Fig. 13.22) or skeletal metastases. Radiographs must be taken of the areas with foci of increased uptake to make the diagnosis.

the disease, but is not helpful in detecting sarcomatous change because of the high uptake of radionuclide in Pagetoid bone with or without this complication.

The scintigraphic appearance of Paget's disease is frequently typical, the "V" front being characteristic. Enlarged, bowed bones are also characteristic.

Serial skeletal scintigraphy is more sensitive than serial radiographic skeletal surveys in assessing the response to treatment (Goldman et al. 1975), although in most patients serial measurements of serum alkaline phosphatase and urinary hydroxyproline are sufficient. However, in controlled trials serial scintigraphy may be of value, particularly if quantitative measurements, comparing the uptake in involved and normal bone, are used.

The combination of scintigraphy and radiology probably demonstrates a wider spectrum of disease than either technique alone. This may represent differing phases of the underlying pathological process. In particular, scintigraphy is useful in detecting early lesions which may be symptomatic and, therefore, it may be possible to initiate treatment in appropriate patients at an earlier stage of the disease. Secondly, scintigraphy gives a more accurate assessment of the extent of the disease. Thirdly,

it may help determine whether the continuing pain is due to disease or to associated conditions such as osteoarthritis. Fourthly, it may help to differentiate between continued disease activity and the healing response in those patients who demonstrate an apparent biochemical resistance to treatment in the face of a maintained clinical improvement. Finally, it is useful in assessing the response of localized Paget's disease to treatment, and may be helpful in the early diagnosis of recurrence following the cessation of therapy.

Hyperparathyroidism

The diagnosis depends on the demonstration of hypercalcaemia and hypophosphataemia. Scintigraphy is of limited value. It is of no value in making the diagnosis, but may be useful in indicating the extent of skeletal involvement. It is associated with a significantly increased 24-hour retention of ^{99m}Tc-diphosphonate (Fogelman et al. 1978a).

Osteomalacia

Scintigraphy may be useful in assessing patients with osteopenia and may help in differentiating osteomalacia from other causes of decreased bone density. The classical scintigraphic appearance is virtually diagnostic (Fig. 13.21), but frequently these changes are not present. There is an increase in the bone to soft tissue ratio which is not always apparent from the scintigram, but can be assessed from quantitative measurement. The commonest abnormalities are increased uptake by the long bones and wrists, prominence of the calvarium and mandible, beading of the costochondral junction, and increased uptake by the sternum particularly at its margins ("tie") sternum (Fogelman et al. 1978b) but these abnormalities are not specific and may occur in renal osteodystrophy. There is increased 24-hour whole body retention of ^{99m}TC-diphosphonate (Fogelman et al. 1978a). The most significant finding is localized areas of increased uptake due to pseudo-fractures. These may be mistaken for metastatic disease, particularly as the pseudo-fractures may not be apparent on radiographic examination unless coned views are obtained. Renal images may be faint possibly due to increased skeletal uptake.

Renal Osteodystrophy

The changes are mainly a combination of hyperparathyroidism and osteomalacia and this is

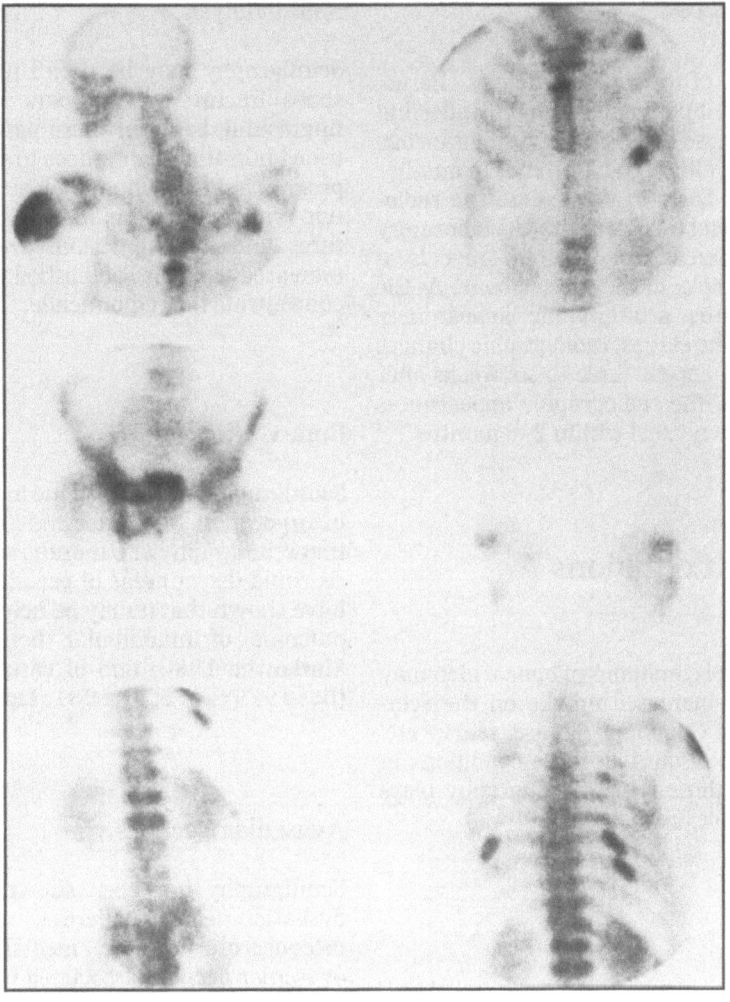

Fig. 13.22. Patient with multiple fractures, including ribs, proximal right humerus, right superior and inferior pubic rami, first and second lumbar vertebrae and sternum. The differential diagnosis was metastatic disease.

reflected in the scintigraphic appearance. Scintigraphy is useful in that it indicates the extent and severity of the osteodystrophy, but is not of diagnostic help. The scintigraphic appearances tend to revert to normal following treatment.

Osteoporosis

Scintigraphy is of no value in the assessment of patients with generalised osteoporosis, but may occasionally be helpful in differentiating osteoporosis from osteomalacia, and in differentiating multiple vertebral crush fractures due to osteoporosis from metastatic carcinoma.

The diagnosis of osteoporosis can best be made on bone morphometry on an iliac crest biopsy, but radiographic morphometry (Chap. 17), photon absorptiometry (Chap. 18), or dual energy CT (Chap. 19) may obviate the need for biopsy. The scintigraphic appearance is usually one of decreased uptake with loss of anatomical detail.

There is a significant increase in uptake in crush fractures less than six months old, the uptake gradually returning to normal. In metastatic disease there usually are multiple foci of increased uptake, whereas in osteoporosis there may be differing degrees of uptake, suggesting that some of the crushed vertebrae are old.

Transient Osteoporosis

This is a condition of unknown aetiology characterized by severe joint pain and commonly affecting a hip joint. The disease is self-limiting, spontaneous recovery occurring, although recurrence in another joint may develop. Early in the disease the radiographs appear normal together with the laboratory investigations, whereas scintigraphy reveals a marked increase uptake in the affected bone. As the disease regresses the scintigraphic appearances return to normal. The earliest radiographic changes of demineralization appear three to six weeks after the first symptoms, the radiographic appearances usually returning to normal within 2–6 months.

Miscellaneous Conditions

There are a variety of conditions of bone which may be associated with increased uptake on the scintigram, for example Gaucher's disease, scurvy etc. It is not possible to discuss all these conditions in this chapter; only those where scintigraphy plays a more important role are included.

Fractures

The indications for skeletal scintigraphy are shown in Table 13.3. Serial skeletal scintigraphy with quantitation may be a useful technique to judge fracture union and differentiate fractures that are likely to go on to delayed or non-union (Alberts et al. 1987; Smith et al. 1987, Fig. 13.22).

Scintigraphy may also be of value in the early diagnosis of stress fractures. The fracture may not be seen on early radiographs and the callus may only be seen after an interval of 2–3 weeks.

Occasionally, scintigraphy may be of value in the diagnosis of a fracture of the scaphoid (King and Turnbull 1981) or the femoral neck in elderly patients (Colhoun et al. 1987; Fairclough et al. 1987) when the radiographic examinations appear normal.

Scintigraphy may also be of value in evaluating the extent of skeletal trauma in the child abuse syndrome (Jaudes 1984), although skull fractures may not be associated with increased uptake (Haase et al. 1980, Chap. 27).

Spondylolysis

Scintigraphy may be useful in detecting a recent stress fracture in the pars interarticularis, distinguishing between those patients with an established non-union and those in whom healing is still progressing and who may benefit from immobilization (van den Oever et al. 1987). Recent stress fractures and healing lesions were associated with increased uptake. Established non-unions did not concentrate the radionuclide.

Bone Graft

Scintigraphy may be of value in assessing bone graft incorporation. McMaster and Merrick (1980) found that scintigraphy at 6 months after fusion for scoliosis could detect areas of pseudarthrosis and others have shown that it may be helpful in predicting the outcome of mandibular bone grafts (Lee and Markowitz 1980) and of vascularized bone grafts (Bos 1979; Dee et al. 1981; Lipson et al. 1981).

Avascular Necrosis

Scintigraphy has been shown to be of value in dysbaric necrosis, Perthes' disease, idiopathic osteonecrosis of the medial femoral condyle, avascular necrosis associated with renal transplantation or steroids, and avascular necrosis following a fracture. The early appearance is one of diminished uptake (Fig. 13.23), but this is probably only seen in very early Perthes' disease, or following a femoral neck fracture. The usual pattern is one of increased uptake, which may be patchy and associated with "creeping substitution" and repair of the avascular segment. The scintigraphic changes (both diminished and increased uptake) usually precede the radiographic changes by weeks or even months. In patients with fractures of the femoral neck, scintigraphy is not sufficiently reliable to determine whether the head is avascular immediately after the fracture, although a scintigram carried out 4 weeks after internal fixation of the fracture is of prognostic significance. Bauer et al. (1980) found that normal or enhanced uptake of ^{99m}Tc-MDP within the first 4 weeks following fracture was associated with uncomplicated healing, whereas non-union and late segmental collapse was associated with reduced uptake, although some patients with diminished uptake went on to uncomplicated union.

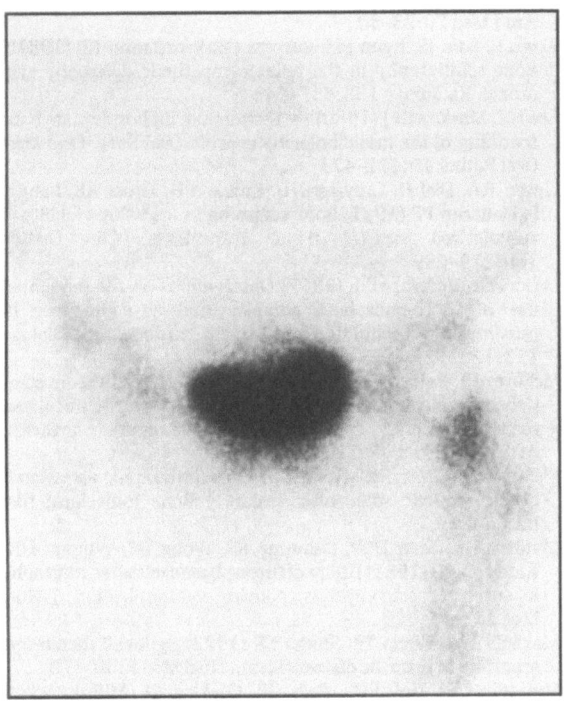

Fig. 13.23. Transcervical fracture of the left femur. The femoral head was avascular. There was increased uptake at the site of the fracture.

Reflex Sympathetic Dystrophy

The radiographic appearances are primarily those of demineralization, although osteoid is laid down. Skeletal scintigrams frequently show changes before the radiographs, the characteristic finding being an increased periarticular uptake in the involved region. The uptake is increased on the vascular phase, as well as the skeletal phase. Although the condition usually involves the distal end of an extremity, it may be localized to a single bone e.g. the patella. Serial scintigraphy may provide a method of predicting therapeutic response (Kozin et al. 1981a,b).

The Future

The past 20 years has seen considerable advances in skeletal scintigraphy, with the development of new radiopharmaceuticals and greatly improved imaging devices. The development of the ^{99m}Tc-compounds made skeletal scintigraphy easily available and the use of the ^{99m}Tc-diphosphonates has lead to improved images.

The development of the gamma camera revolutionized scintigraphy. Large field of view cameras were especially useful in skeletal scintigraphy.

Despite the development of CT and MRI, scintigraphy still has an important role in the investigation of skeletal abnormalities, particularly in its ability to evaluate the entire skeleton or all the joints in a short period, and detect infection within 24 hours.

The relatively recent development of emission computer tomography has increased markedly the anatomic precision of scintigraphy and decreased the size of lesion that can be detected, but CT gives greater anatomical accuracy.

Acknowledgements. Figures 13.6, 13.13 and 13.21 are reproduced with permission from Galasko CSB, Weber DA (eds) (1984) Radionuclide scintigraphy in orthopaedics. Churchill Livingstone, Edinburgh.

References

Alberts KA, Dahlborn M, Ringertz H (1987) Sequential scintimetry after femoral neck fracture. Methodologic aspects and prediction of healing complications. Acta Orthop Scand 58:217–222

Ash JM, Gilday DL. (1980) The futility of bone scanning in neonatal osteomyelitis: concise communication. J Nucl Med 21:417–420

Bauer G, Weber DA, Ceder L et al. (1980) Dynamics of technetium-99m methylenediphosphonate imaging of the femoral head after hip fracture. Clin Orthop 152:85–92

Bekerman C, Genant HK, Hoffer PB, Kozin F, Ginsberg M (1976) Radionuclide imaging of the bones and joints of the hand. A definition of normal and a comparison of sensitivity using ^{99m}Tc pertechnetate and ^{99m}Tc-diphosphonate. Radiology 118:653–659

Boerbooms Agnes MTh, Buys WCAM (1978) Rapid assessment of ^{99m}Tc-pertechnetate uptake in the knee joint as a parameter of inflammatory activity. Arthritis Rheum 21:348–352

Bos KE (1979) Bone scintigraphy of experimental composite bone grafts revascularized by microvascular anastomoses. Plast Reconstr Surg 64:353–360

Cambouroglou G, Papathanassiou B, Koutoulidis C, Bossinakou I, Mandalaki T (1976) Haemophilic arthropathy surveyed with whole-body gamma camera scintigraphy. Acta Orthop Scand 47:607–612

Colhoun EN, Johnson SR, Fairclough JA (1987) Bone scanning for hip fracture in patients with osteoarthritis: brief report. J Bone Joint Surg [Br] 69:848

Dee P, Lambruschi PG, Hiebert JM (1981) The use of Tc-99m MDP bone scanning in the study of vascularized bone implants: concise communication. J Nucl Med 22:522–525

Dequeker J, Goddeeris T, De Roo M, Boeckx L (1977) Comparison of technetium uptake in small joints with other indices of inflammation in rheumatoid arthritis. Eur J Nucl Med 2:269–271

Desaulniers M, Fuks A, Hawkins D, Lacourciere Y, Rosenthall L (1974) Radiotechnetium polyphosphate joint imaging. J Nucl Med 15:417–423

Duszynski DO, Kuhn JP, Afshani E, Riddlesberger MM Jr (1975) Early radionuclide diagnosis of acute osteomyelitis. Radiology 117:337–340

Fairclough J, Colhoun E, Johnston D, Williams LA (1987) Bone scanning for suspected hip fractures. A prospective study in elderly patients. J Bone Joint Surg [Br] 69:251–253

Fogelman I, Bessent RG, Turner JG, Citrin DL, Boyle IT, Greig WR (1978a) The use of whole body retention of Tc-99m diphosphonate in the diagnosis of metabolic bone disease. J Nucl Med 19:270–275

Fogelman I, McKillop JH, Bessent RG, Boyle IT, Turner JG, Greig WR (1978b) The role of bone scanning in osteomalacia. J Nucl Med 19:245–248

Galasko CSB (1977) The mechanism of uptake of bone-seeking isotopes by skeletal metastases. In: Medical radionuclide imaging, Vol. II. I A E A, Vienna, pp 125–134

Galasko CSB (1984a) The pathophysiological basis for skeletal scintigraphy. In: Galasko CSB, Weber DA (eds) Radionuclide scintigraphy in orthopaedics, Churchill Livingstone, Edinburgh, pp 34–53

Galasko CSB (1984b) Tumours. In: Galasko CSB, Weber DA (eds) Radionuclide scintigraphy in orthopaedics, Churchill Livingstone, Edinburgh, pp 65–109

Gilday DL, Paul DJ, Paterson J (1975) Diagnosis of osteomyelitis in children by combined blood pool and bone imaging. Radiology 117:331–335

Goergen TG, Resnick D, Lomonaco A, O'Dell CW Jr (1976) Radionuclide bone-scan abnormalities in leprosy: Case reports. J Nucl Med 17:788–790

Goldman AB, Braunstein P, Wilkinson D, Kammerman S (1975) Radionuclide uptake studies of bone: a quantitative method of evaluating the response of patients with Paget's disease to diphosphonate therapy. Radiology 117:365–369

Haase GM, Ortiz VN, Sfakianakis GN, Morse TS (1980) The value of radionuclide bone scanning in the early recognition of deliberate child abuse. J Trauma 20:873–875

Jaudes PK (1984) Comparison of radiography and radionuclide bone scanning in the detection of child abuse. Pediatrics 73:166–168

Kemp HBS, Johns DL, McAlister J, Godlee JN (1973) The role of fluorine-18 and strontium-87m scintigraphy in the management of infective spondylitis. J Bone Joint Surg [Br] 55:301–311

King JB, Turnbull TJ (1981) An early method of confirming scaphoid fracture. J Bone Joint Surg [Br] 63:287

Kirk GA, Schulz EE (1987) Usefulness of SPECT in evaluating osteosarcoma metastases to the lung. Clin Nucl Med 12:356–358

Kozin F, Ryan LM, Carrera GF, Soin JS, Wortmann RL (1981a) The reflex sympathetic dystrophy syndrome (RSDS). III. Scintigraphic studies, further evidence for the therapeutic efficacy of systemic corticosteroids and proposed diagnostic criteria.

Am J Med 70:23–30

Kozin F, Soin JS, Ryan LM, Carrera GF, Wortmann RL (1981b) Bone scintigraphy in the reflex sympathetic dystrophy syndrome. Radiology 138:437–443

Lee HK, Markowitz J (1980) 99mTechnetium diphosphonate bone scanning of the mandibular bone graft. Oral Surg, Oral Med, Oral Pathol 49:471–473

Lipson RA, Dief H, Greyson ND, Kawano H, Gross AE, Langer F, Halloran PF (1981) Bone scanning in assessing viability of vascularized skeletal tissue transplants. Clin Orthop 160:279–289

Lisbona R, Rosenthall L (1977) Observations on the sequential use of 99mTc-phosphate complex and 67Ga imaging in osteomyelitis, cellulitis and septic arthritis. Radiology 123:123–129

McCarty DJ, Polcyn RE, Collins PA (1970) 99mTechnetium scintiphotography in arthritis II. Its nonspecificity and clinical and roentgenographic correlations in rheumatoid arthritis. Arthritis Rheum 13:21–32

McMaster MJ, Merrick MV (1980) The scintigraphic assessment of the scoliotic spine after fusion. J Bone Joint Surg [Br] 62:65–72

Maurer AH, Chen DCP, Camargo EE, Wong DF, Wagner HN, Alderson PO (1981) Utility of three-phase skeletal scintigraphy in suspected osteomyelitis: concise communication. J Nucl Med 22:941–949

Maxfield WS, Weiss TE, Shuler SE (1972) Synovial membrane scanning in arthritic disease. Semin Nucl Med 2:50–70

Mountford PJ, Hall FM, Wells CP, Coakley AJ (1986) 99mTcm-MDP, 67Ga-citrate and 111In-leukocytes for detecting prosthetic hip infection. Nucl Med Comm 7:113–120

Rekonen A, Kuikka J, Oka M (1974) Measurement of joint inflammation. Local 99mTc indices of knees, hands, elbows and feet. Scand J Rheumat 3:75–78

Sewell JR, Black CM, Chapman AH, Statham J, Hughes GRV, Lavender JP (1980) Quantitative scintigraphy in diagnosis and management of plantar fasciitis (calcaneal periostitis): concise communication. J Nucl Med 21:633–636

Smith MA, Jones EA, Strachan RK, Nicoll JJ, Best JJK, Tothill P, Hughes SPF (1987) Prediction of fracture healing in the tibia by quantitative radionuclide imaging. J Bone Joint Surg [Br] 69:441–447

Sturrock RD, Nicholson R, Wojtulewski JA (1974) Technetium counting in rheumatoid arthritis: evaluation in the small joints of the hand. Arthritis Rheum 17:417–420

Szypryt EP, Colton CL, Hardy JG (1987) Intra-operative bone scanning in orthopaedics. In: Noble J, Galasko CSB (eds) Recent developments in orthopaedic surgery, Manchester University Press, Manchester, pp 62–65

van den Oever M, Merrick MV, Scott JHS (1987) Bone scintigraphy in symptomatic spondylolysis. J Bone Joint Surg [Br] 69:453–456

Woolfenden JM, Pitt MJ, Durie BGM, Moon TE (1980) Comparison of bone scintigraphy and radiography in multiple myeloma. Radiology 134:723–728

14 Isotope Techniques in the Investigation of Diseases of Joints

M.V. Merrick

Introduction 207
Administered Tracers 207
   General Properties 207
   Water and Blood-Pool Markers 208
   Bone-Seeking Tracers 209
   Markers of Inflammatory Processes 209
   Arthrography 209
   Gamma Ray Sources 210
   Neutron Sources 211
Rheumatoid Arthritis 211
   Extra-articular Manifestations of Rheumatoid Arthritis 215
   Occult Fractures and Osteoporosis 215
Ankylosing Spondylitis 215
Miscellaneous Arthropathies 217
   Other Connective Tissue Diseases 217
   Low Back Pain 217
   Reflex Sympathetic Dystrophy Syndrome 217
   Degenerative Joint Disease 218
   Avascular Necrosis 218
References 218

Introduction

The diagnosis of diseases of joints is usually made from the clinical findings, serological investigations, and the radiographic appearance. Plain radiographs usually suffice. For example, rheumatoid arthritis is suspected from the clinical findings, particularly the type of joint involvement. The diagnosis is confirmed by the serological tests. Radiographs may show the classical erosions, but these are relatively late findings. The severity of joint involvement is often graded by the radiographic appearance. However, it is unusual for patients to have radiographic surveys to determine the extent of their joint involvement, nor is it desirable to carry out such surveys, on a regular basis, to assess patients' progress. Therefore, much work has been carried out in an attempt to find other methods of assessing joint function in the arthropathies, as an aid in the differential diagnosis and particularly to assess the extent of the joint involvement. Most of this work has involved the development of isotope techniques, employing a variety of both physical and physiological processes. If these methods are to be applied and interpreted correctly it is important to have a clear understanding of their scientific basis. They may be considered under three general headings.

1. Those involving the administration of a radioactive tracer to the patient
2. Those employing radioisotopes as an external source of gamma rays, because a beam of constant and defined properties is required
3. Neutron irradiation of the patient, in order to make radioactive stable elements which are present either naturally or as the result of pathological processes

Administered Tracers

General Properties

A number of tracers have been used to assess regional blood volume and permeability, the objective being to obtain a numerical measure of the physical signs of inflammation. With all isotopic investigations, constraints are imposed by the properties of available nuclides. The usual intention, when administering a radioactive tracer to a patient, is to detect its local concentration by non-invasive means, for example by using an externally placed radiation detector. For this to be possible it is necessary for gamma-rays to be emitted, which can be detected outside the patient. Beta particles have a mean path of only a few millimetres in tissue and, therefore, can be detected only if they originate from the skin. Radiation damage results from radiation energy being absorbed within the patient rather than escaping. As beta particles are stopped very close to their origin, all of their energy is dissipated locally in the tissue. They are thus undesirable, as well as being unsuitable for *in vivo* diagnostic purposes. Beta-emitting isotopes, therefore, are not employed for *in vivo* imaging investigations, although they do have some therapeutic uses, when the objective is to deliver a large dose of radiation to a small defined volume.

Alpha particles are similar to helium nuclei and carry two positive charges, in contrast to the one negative charge of the beta particle. As a consequence of their greater charge and greater mass they deposit more energy locally, doing more damage and penetrating an even shorter distance in tissue. Alpha-emitting isotopes are very undesirable and have no diagnostic or therapeutic applications.

Isotopes which emit gamma-rays are therefore used. Even here there are considerable restrictions as, if the gamma-rays are of too low an energy, they will be absorbed whereas if they are of too high energy, although they will escape from the body, they will not be efficiently detected by conventional imaging equipment. In practical terms the useful limits are not less than 50 keV and not more than 500 keV. Relatively few elements have radioactive isotopes which are able to meet these constraints, namely a pure gamma emitter of suitable energy, with no alpha or beta particles. It is sometimes necessary to resort to isotopes with both gamma and beta emissions, and frequently unphysiological tracers, which have been incorporated into chemical compounds that act as analogues of normal substrates are used.

Water and Blood-Pool Markers

The tracers which have been used in the study of joint disease can be considered under two headings:

1. Those which demonstrate regional blood volume. The best for this purpose are red cells, to which a number of isotopes can be attached by a variety of techniques. The only system commonly employed clinically in arthropological studies is autologous red cells labelled with ^{99m}Tc. Technetium is chosen because it has convenient physical properties, combining a short half-life, a gamma-ray of appropriate energy and no beta particles. It can be made to label erythrocytes by "pre-tanning" the cells with a tin salt such as stannous pyrophosphate, which binds to the cell surface. Pertechnetate, when added to cells which have been thus prepared, is reduced – stannous tin is a reducing agent – and becomes attached to the cell membrane. This technique has many other clinical applications and is generally available. Although not giving primary diagnostic information in joint disease, it is sometimes employed in order to correct for variations in blood volume found in the course of other investigations.

2. Tracers whose distribution is related to capillary permeability. By employing compounds with different molecular sizes it may be possible to obtain some information about differential permeability. Sodium pertechnetate has been widely employed, although not ideal because its behaviour is complex.

Technetium is taken up by those tissues which trap iodide namely the thyroid, salivary glands, gastric mucosa and choroid plexus. Circulating pertechnetate is mostly bound to albumin, although some is present as the free ion. It is excreted via the kidneys and secreted by the gastric mucosa, the latter being the principal pathway of excretion. If trapping is blocked by a drug such as perchlorate, the distribution of pertechnetate approximates to the chloride space, i.e. the distribution of extracellular water, but it is not an exact representation as it is partially protein-bound. It is well established that areas of inflammation, where the extracellular water content is increased, show a higher concentration of pertechnetate. This has been used as a means of demonstrating the extent and the activity of rheumatoid arthritis.

The only other radionuclide to have been widely used for this purpose in joint disease is ^{113m}In. It forms very stable chelates with transferrin and other metal-binding proteins and indium transferrin is rapidly formed following intravenous injection of sub-microgram quantities of any simple indium salt. Transferrin is of fairly high molecular weight and its initial distribution approximates to the intravascular space. However, at equilibrium the transferrin space is appreciably larger than the intravascular space. It has been used as an alternative to red cells to distinguish between blood volume and extravascular water, but unfortunately indium binds strongly to other metal-binding proteins, the most significant of which is lactoferrin, present in high concentration in many inflammatory tissues. Consequently at equilibrium the concentration of indium at an inflammatory site may be higher than can be accounted for purely on the basis of blood or extracellular volume (Merrick et al. 1973; Sayle et al. 1983).

Other tracers which have been employed, but are not in general use, include sodium iodide, iodinated human serum albumin and xenon.

Bone-seeking Tracers (Chap. 13)

A large number of radioactive tracers accumulate in the skeleton. There are no suitable radioactive isotopes of calcium or phosphorus. Strontium was used formerly but no strontium isotope has ideal properties, although ^{85}Sr is the best available tracer for longterm turnover studies of bone mineral. It has a number of serious shortcomings, in particular a faster rate of excretion than calcium and slower absorption from the gut. The only compounds now widely used for imaging are ^{99m}Tc complexes with a variety of phosphate compounds, particularly the diphosphonates. Recently a number of newer diphosphonates have been introduced including methylene diphosphonate (MDP) and methane hydroxydiphosphonate (HMDP).

The usual criterion for selection of a compound has been rapid and high uptake into the normal skeleton and prompt excretion from all other tissues. However one compound (dimethylaminomethylene diphosphonate – DMAD), which has a relatively lower uptake into the normal skeleton, gives a higher contrast between normal and abnormal areas of the skeleton and detects more abnormalities (Rosenthall et al. 1982) than MDP. The whole question has thus been thrown open and it is unclear at the present time which is the best agent for skeletal imaging, or indeed if there is a single best agent for all purposes.

Imaging immediately after injection, before much of the activty has been incorporated into the skeleton, gives a picture very comparable to that obtained with pertechnetate (Domljan and Dodig 1984). It is thus possible to obtain a picture both of the blood pool and of the bone uptake from a single administration of tracer by imaging at different times (Chap. 13).

Markers of Inflammatory Processes

Apart from those which demonstrate blood volume and extracellular fluid, some compounds are taken up in high concentration in areas of chronic inflammation and rheumatoid activity. These include simple salts of gallium (McCall et al. 1983), indium (Sayle et al. 1983) and ^{99m}Tc liposomes (Williams et al. 1986). Although the mechanism is not entirely clear, there is evidence that a number of factors are working synergistically. Gallium is closely related to indium and both are bound by transferrin (Gunasekera et al. 1972; Merrick et al. 1973). In the presence of inflammation there is increased capillary permeability, allowing the metal–protein complex to diffuse out of the circulation. Lactoferrin, present in high concentration in chronic inflammation, will strip gallium from transferrin, resulting in local accumulation (Weiner et al. 1981). Intracellular incorporation also occurs, especially in moribund cells with abnormally permeable cell walls and, in the presence of infection, there may be some uptake into bacteria. The accumulation is therefore a combination of abnormal permeability, increased local binding and, to a lesser extent, increased cellular uptake. The process is non-specific and does not distinguish between infective and non-infective inflammatory processes. Uptake occurs most constantly in chronic inflammation.

Gallium may be less useful for the detection of acute infection where labelled white cells can be employed (Coakley and Mountford 1986). The label most commonly used is ^{111}In, bound either to oxine or tropolone. More recently ^{99m}Tc HMPAO ((d,l) hexamethyl propylene amine oxime) has been suggested as an alternative. As neither of these is a specific ligand for white cells, a pure preparation of the cells must first be obtained. This is a highly skilled, time-consuming and technically demanding operation which is not universally available because of the difficulty of separating cells without devitalizing them. Although a good technique for the detection of occult sites of acute pyogenic infection, its role in the management of rheumatic diseases is less well-established. It has been proposed as an index of disease activity (Uno et al. 1986), although there is no evidence that it has any advantage over the numerous more readily available indices. It does not appear to distinguish reliably between rheumatoid activity and acute infection.

Arthrography (see also Chap. 3)

The joint space may be imaged directly by a number of techniques. There are no tracers which are incorporated to any useful extent into cartilage. Gross increase in volume of the synovial fluid, for example as the result of a Baker's cyst, can be imaged by intravenous injection of pertechnetate (Greyson 1979). This technique had a brief vogue, but has little practical application, the injection of a radio-opaque dye (Chap. 3) being the optimum investigation. Other workers have suggested the direct intra-articular injection of a non-absorbable substance such as technetium sulphur colloid, in order to demonstrate its distribution prior to the administration of therapeutic agents such as ^{32}P chromic phosphate (Abdel-Dayem et al. 1981).

Intra-articular injection of ^{133}Xe (xenon) solution has been used to measure blood flow to large joints (Dick et al. 1970). This is only one use of a method which is of fairly general application. However, it suffers from a number of serious theoretical disadvantages, in particular that it tends to overestimate flow in areas of low flow rate, as the rate of diffusion may exceed the rate of wash-out. For this reason the technique has not achieved widespread popularity. It nevertheless remains the best available method of measuring blood flow to a joint.

An alternative approach suggested by Wallis et al. (1983) involved the simultaneous injection of ^{131}I-labelled radioiodinated human serum albumin and ^{123}I-sodium iodide into the knees of patients with effusions. The apparent volume of distribution of the two tracers was measured by taking fluid samples 1 hour and 24 hours later. From this the clearance rate of the protein, which was interpreted as effective synovial lymph flow, and small solutes, interpreted as synovial blood flow, were calculated. Differences were observed between patients with osteoarthritis and those with rheumatoid arthritis, the latter having the greater effective lymph flow but a smaller effective blood flow than the former.

Gamma-Ray Sources

Single Photon Absorptiometry

The quantity of mineral present in bone can be estimated by measuring the extent to which a beam of X-rays passing through the bone is attenuated. Because absorption is critically dependent on the X-ray energy, the stability required of the output from the X-ray generator when obtaining measurements is much greater than is required for other radiological applications. In practice it is often simpler and more convenient to employ the unvarying monochromatic beam of X-rays originating from a radioactive source than the continuous and inconstant

spectrum from an X-ray tube. A large number of techniques have been described (Wahner et al. 1984a,b). One of the best for measurement of the peripheral skeleton employs ^{125}I, which emits a single gamma ray of 25 keV, as the source. At this energy small differences in the mineral content of bone make an appreciable difference in absorption of the gamma-rays. It is well-established as an accurate method of measuring mineral content in bones such as those of the forearm, which have a limited amount of soft tissue surrounding them.

Dual Photon Absorptiometry

A gamma-ray of this energy is absorbed to such a high extent that it cannot be used for measuring mineral content in the spine, which clinically is usually of much more interest. The difficulty is compounded because the soft tissues overlying the spine are not homogeneous, as a result of the presence of moving, gas-containing viscera such as the stomach and colon. To overcome this, techniques have been developed which simultaneously use gamma-rays of two energies, a lower one giving a high contrast between bone and soft tissue and a higher energy which distinguishes poorly between bone and soft tissue but does differentiate soft tissue and air. The best isotope for this purpose is Gadolinium-153 which emits two gamma-rays, one of 40 keV and the second of 110 keV. These are both close to the theoretical optimum for this purpose whilst, because one isotope is emitting both gamma-rays, the proportion of the two remains constant. The 40 keV gamma-ray of gadolinium is inconvenient for use with some equipment. It, therefore, is sometimes preferable to use a slightly higher energy, such as the 60 keV gamma-ray of americium-241, combined with the 140 keV gamma-ray of ^{99m}Tc. When two isotopes are used it is necessary to correct for the differential rates of decay (LeBlanc et al. 1986).

X-ray Fluorescence Analysis

X-ray fluorescence analysis has been used to a limited extent in vivo. When any atom interacts with an incident X-ray photon, some of the energy absorbed is dissipated by the emission of a new gamma-ray, the energy (wavelength) of which depends on the atomic number of the element interacting with the incident photon, being higher for heavier elements. For lighter elements the energy emitted is so low that these characteristic X-rays, as they are called, are absorbed within a few millimetres of their source. Some heavier elements can be assayed in vivo, provided that they are not too deeply situated. It is possible to assay calcium in the cortex of a superficial bone such as the tibia. The principal application of this technique is in the detection and measurement of heavy metals, particularly lead in bone (Somervaille et al. 1985).

Neutron Sources

The quantity of calcium and of some other elements present in bone can be measured directly by neutron activation. When any stable element is irradiated by low energy (thermal) neutrons, some of the neutrons are incorporated into nuclei, making radioactive some of the naturally occurring stable atoms. The amount and type of radioactivity induced depends on the elements present and the energy and strength of the neutron beam. Because the composition of tissue is known in general terms, it is possible to calculate the amount of calcium present from the amount of induced radioactivity, provided that the characteristics of the incident neutron beam are known. Correction must be made for radioactive sodium, potassium, phosphorus etc. inevitably formed at the same time (Smith 1982).

This is a well-established technique, and is undoubtedly the best method available for measuring the total body content of calcium. It is less useful for obtaining information about the amount of calcium present in a part or region, as the volume irradiated cannot be precisely defined. Nevertheless, it has been used successfully for longitudinal studies. Bone mineral measurements by absorptiometry give a lower radiation dose than neutron activation and permit regional measurements of bone mineral. In principle, bone mineral and bone calcium are not interchangeable. However the two are closely related, and for many clinical purposes the measurement of bone mineral is more useful than that of bone calcium. Sources of neutrons which have been employed include californium-252, plutonium/beryllium, cyclotrons or atomic reactors.

Rheumatoid Arthritis

The diagnosis is based on the clinical, serological and radiographic examination. Scintigraphic methods are not used in the primary diagnosis of this condition, but a number of methods have been advocated to determine the extent and activity of the disease. Whereas the majority of early papers employed pertechnetate, most of the more recent ones have used bone imaging agents such as MDP. The technique with pertechnetate is to administer up to 15 millicuries (600 MBq) of ^{99m}Tc sodium pertechnetate intravenously, following the administration of 200 mg sodium perchlorate to block thyroid and gastric mucosal uptake. Images of each joint are obtained starting 5 minutes after administration. In practice, providing sufficient time has been allowed for mixing and diffusion to occur, the appearances are little affected by time. Paired organs such as hands or feet wherever possible should be imaged together to ensure that a direct comparison can be made between the two sides. Where this is not possible, images should be obtained for equal times (not equal numbers of counts) and care should be taken when obtaining the photographic record that the factors have not been changed, so that the films are directly comparable.

In the normal subject, the distribution of activity is principally a function of the blood pool, which reflects the vascularity and bulk of soft tissue, especially muscle. Normal joints tend to be less active than adjacent muscular areas (Fig. 14.1). Abnormal joints show increased uptake due to hyperaemia which affects soft tissues, especially the synovium, as much as or more prominently than bone (Fig. 14.2). The uptake is sometimes visible as a rim around a less active area, the rim representing the synovium seen in profile and the less active area the joint where the synovium is seen *en face*. These appearances are easier to see in large joints such as the knee and shoulder than in small joints of the hand and foot.

When routine surveys are conducted using this technique, more joints may be found to be affected than are apparent clinically (McCarthy et al. 1970; Hays and Green 1972; John et al. 1982). Attempts have been made to improve the investigation by adding measurement to simple visual interpretation. Various methods have been used (Whaley et al. 1968; Katona et al. 1983), all essentially amounting to attempts to express the activity present in a joint as a fraction of the administered radioactivity. Although measurements of this sort are possible, in practice they have proved to have no advantage over simple parameters such as grip strength, the number of affected joints or ESR (Dequeker et al. 1977).

A more sophisticated approach, suggested by Bergmann and Kolarz (1976), involved the simultaneous administration of both pertechnetate and [113m]In transferrin. They employed a whole body counter and required the patient to be sufficiently

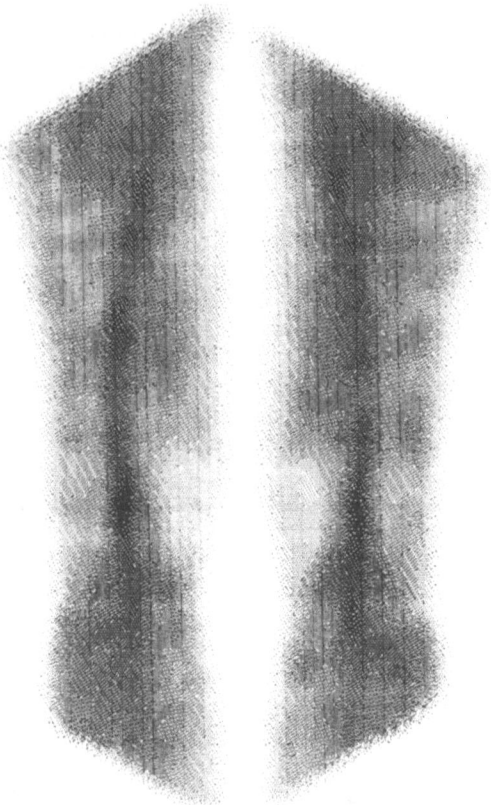

Fig. 14.1. Normal blood-pool of knees.

agile to be able to lie prone with arms extended above the head. They were thus able to obtain a one-dimensional profile of the distribution of radioactivity, and from the profile identify the regions corresponding to the feet, the knees, the elbows and the hands. Other joints could not be assessed by this method. It was assumed that the distribution of indium transferrin represented blood volume, while that of pertechnetate represented extracellular fluid. It would be possible to apply this method to peripheral joints by employing a suitably designed and relatively inexpensive part body counter, if it could be shown to be clinically useful.

They found the most useful index to be the ratio of ^{99m}Tc counts to ^{113m}In counts, which they considered to represent the ratio of extracellular fluid volume to blood volume, but they did not compare their results with the simple criteria used by Dequeker et al. (1977). Moreover, the assumption that indium transferrin remains intravascular is open to question. In the presence of acute inflammation, transfer of indium to lactoferrin in the inflammatory tissues is likely to occur. However, this may

take some hours and if the ratio is measured shortly after injection the error is probably not large. The clinical role of this technique is not established.

Desaulniers et al. (1974) compared pertechnetate with skeletal scintigraphy using one of the earlier technetium complexes, technetium polyphosphate. Imaging was started 2 hours after the polyphosphate or 30 minutes after the pertechnetate. More joints showed increased uptake of polyphosphate than of pertechnetate or were clinically involved by disease. Part of this difference was due to uptake of the polyphosphate in osteoarthritic joints, sites of trauma and erosions due to metabolic bone disease. It is of course well-established that bone imaging with the technetium complexes (Chap. 13; Fig. 14.3) is an extremely sensitive method for detecting sites of increased bone turnover, although it has a low specificity. For this reason skeletal scintigrams should always be interpreted in association with radiographs of affected areas. This high "false positive" rate is therefore not surprising.

Other workers have employed quantitative indices to reduce the subjectivity of interpretation. Park et al. (1977) developed an index which was the ratio of the activity in the region of an affected joint to that in an adjacent mid-shaft part of an unaffected long bone. This ratio varied with time but reached a plateau approximately 5 hours after administration of the tracer. Although higher ratios were found in patients with active rheumatoid arthritis than in controls, there was no sharp cut-off and many patients fell in the intermediate range. It, therefore, was not possible to distinguish rheumatoid from other forms of arthritis or other joint diseases.

Oka et al. (1983), using slightly more sophisticated equipment, elaborated this technique by comparing the highest activity at any point in an affected joint with the peak activity at any point in the contralateral unaffected side. They calculated these ratios both for MDP and for pertechnetate and found higher ratios with MDP than with pertechnetate in all joints with rheumatoid involvement. Patients with what they describe as "reactive arthritis" had ratios which were similar with the two compounds. The highest ratio was observed in a patient with septic arthritis. In addition to being limited to patients with an unaffected contralateral

Fig. 14.2a,b. Scintigram of knee of a patient with rheumatoid arthritis, which was not clinically active in this joint at the time of scintigraphy. c,d Scintigram of contralateral knee of the same patient, showing a ruptured Baker's cyst. e,f Arthrogram. This shows the extent of the cyst more accurately than the scintigram.

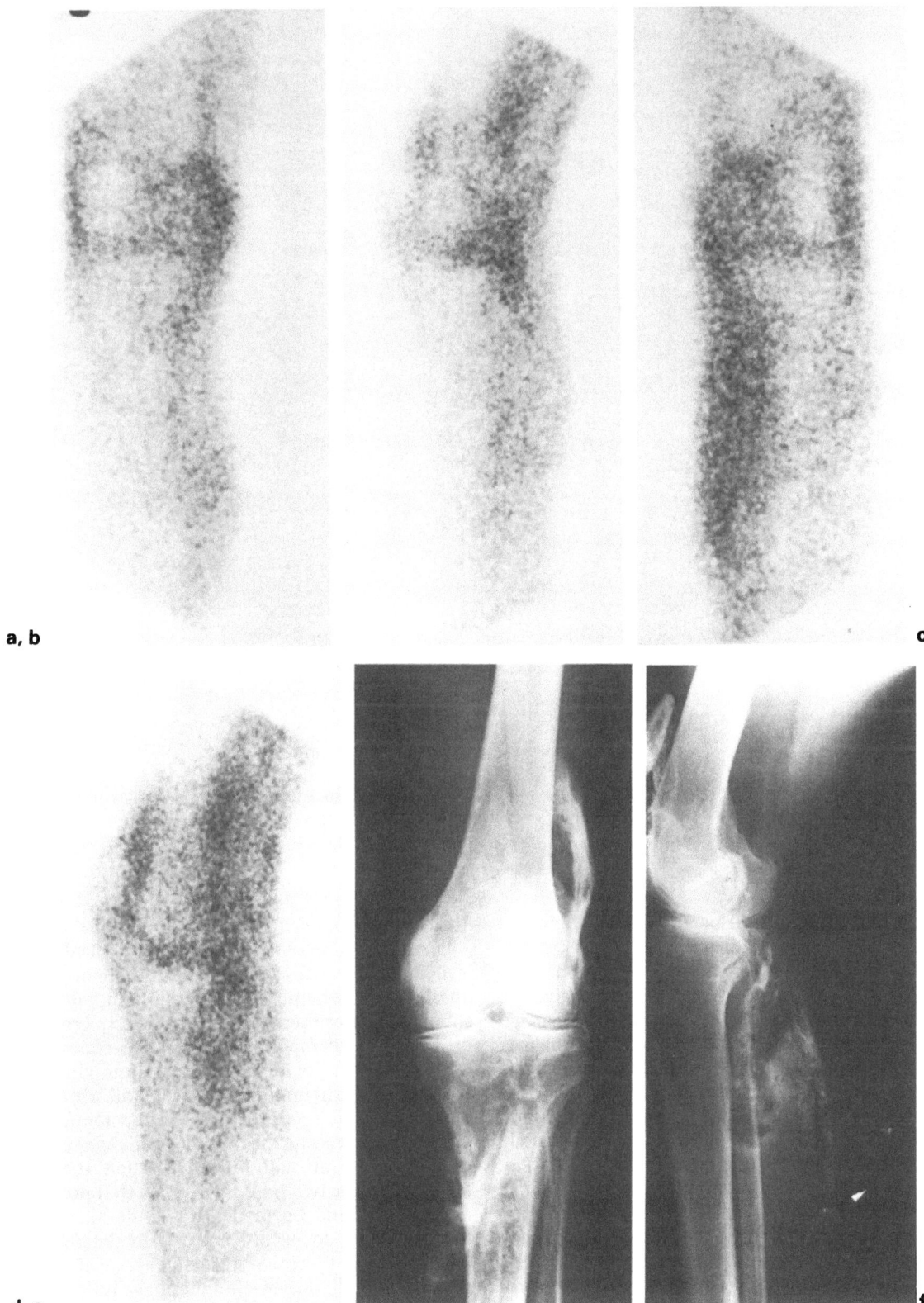

a, b

c

d, e

f

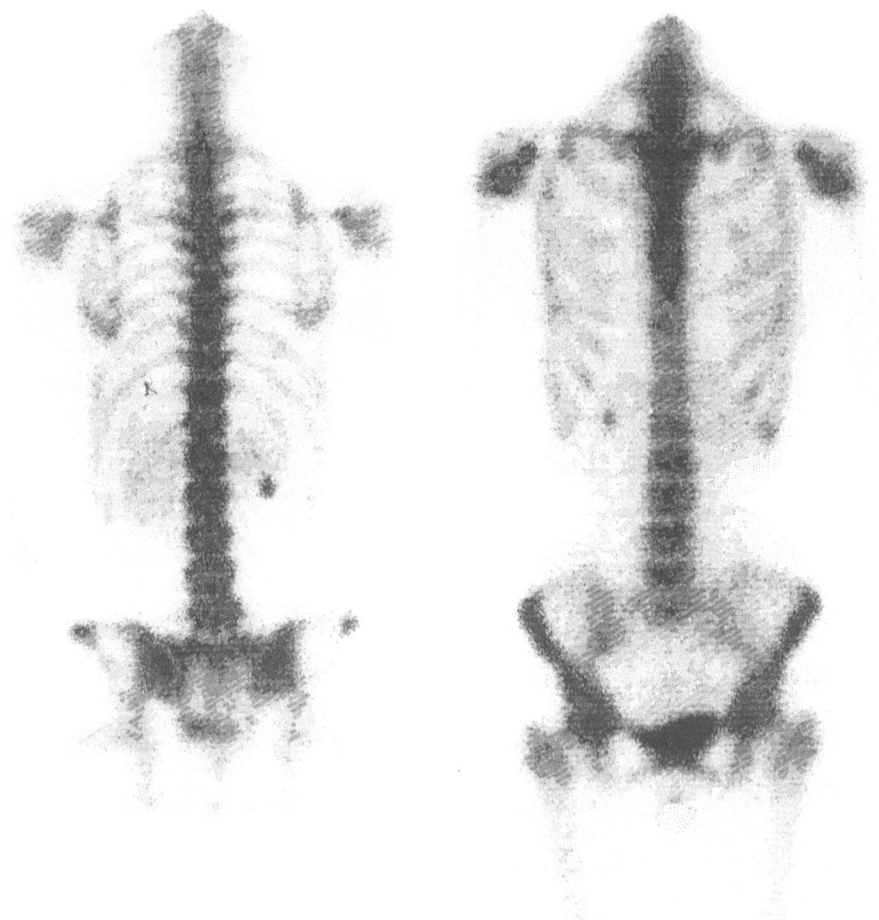

Fig. 14.3a,b. Normal image of the trunk. a Posterior image. The appearance is similar with any of the bone-seeking radiopharmaceuticals. b Normal anterior image.

joint, which could be used for comparison, this study suffered from the usual problem with preliminary reports, namely that two selected populations with well-established diagnoses were compared, giving a spuriously high specificity for the test. When carried out in mixed populations without an established diagnosis, the distinction became blurred and this ratio appears to be of little practical value.

A third approach has been that of Domljan and Dodig (1984) who performed imaging immediately after injection of MDP and again 3 hours later (Fig. 14.4). The early pictures resemble those obtained with pertechnetate, essentially showing blood pool, while the later showed regional bone turnover rate. This technique did not improve the sensitivity or the specificity of the investigation when compared with the double injection technique but had the virtue of requiring only a single injection of radioisotope

and could be completed on a single attendance.

Scintigraphic activity persists after clinical signs of activity have disappeared, and, therefore, it is questionable whether the scintigraphic findings should influence therapy (Oh et al. 1983). Coleman et al. (1982) compared joint-to-bone ratios with MDP with those obtained using gallium citrate in patients with rheumatoid arthritis and a number with suspected septic arthritis. They found that although on average the ratios for both agents were higher for patients with proven infection, the overlap between the two groups was such that no useful differential could be made. McCall et al. (1983) found gallium to be of some use in determining whether or not there was still active synovial inflammation. Overall, these techniques have little to offer in the management of the majority of patients with rheumatoid arthritis.

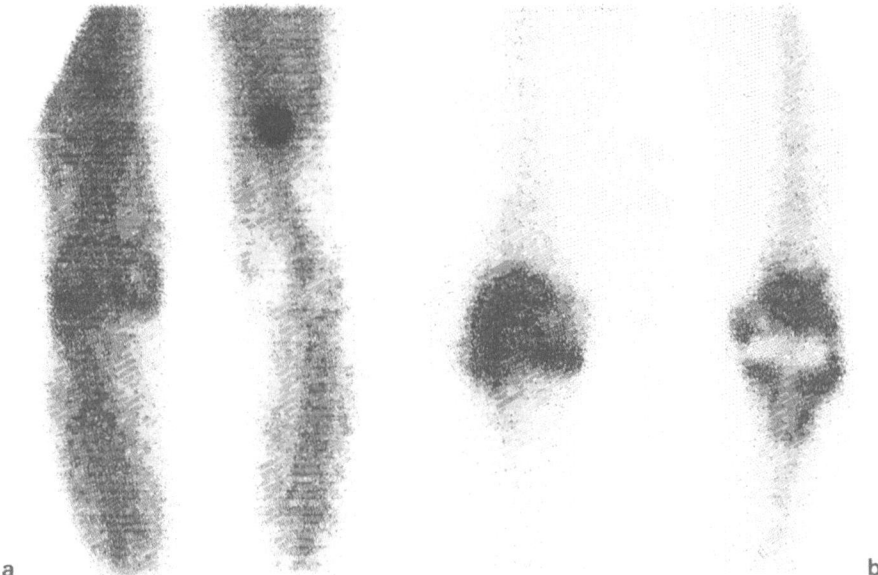

Fig. 14.4a,b. Patient with active rheumatoid arthritis. a Blood-pool picture of the knees. Active rheumatoid on the right, knee replacement on the left. Note inflamed synovium on the right, shown as two crescentic areas. b At 3 hours, the distribution of activity represents the rate of bone turnover. There is substantial uptake in both knees, that on the left suggesting that the prosthesis may be loose or infected.

Extra-articular Manifestations of Rheumatoid Arthritis

Pertechnetate is taken up in salivary glands and can be used both for imaging and assessment of function. Sodium pertechnetate 50–100 MBq (2.5–5 mc) is given intravenously. Sequential frames may be taken at the rate of one per minute for 20 minutes, or alternatively images may be taken at intervals over the next 30 minutes. Anterior and both oblique projections should be obtained in order to visualize the parotids and submandibular glands. In the normal subject there is higher uptake in the parotids than in the submandibular glands. Sublingual glands are normally not visualized, although there may be an appearance of visualization because of secreted activity pooling in the mouth. Stimulation by ingestion of sour or acidic compounds causes uptake to be discharged rapidly. Virtually all pathological processes result in a reduced accumulation of pertechnetate. This technique has been used in assessing salivary function in patients with rheumatoid arthritis (Janin-Mercier et al. 1982). Reduced salivary function is found in substantially more patients than present with clinical evidence of sicca complex. In some of these patients overt evidence of Sjogren's syndrome develops sub-

sequently. The technique may have some value in identifying patients at risk of subsequently developing overt Sjogren's syndrome.

Occult Fractures and Osteoporosis

Patients with rheumatoid arthritis, especially those on treatment with steroids, are at increased risk of osteoporosis with the development of stress fractures and avascular necrosis. These can be visualized by scintigraphy with MDP or other bone-seeking agents prior to there being overt radiological evidence of fracture (Schneider and Kaye 1975; Nixon 1984). The rate of mineral loss can be assessed by dual photon absorptiometry.

Ankylosing Spondylitis

In the late case, the diagnosis is made by the classical "bamboo spine" appearances on conventional radiographs. However, in the early case it is much more difficult to establish a diagnosis. The condition

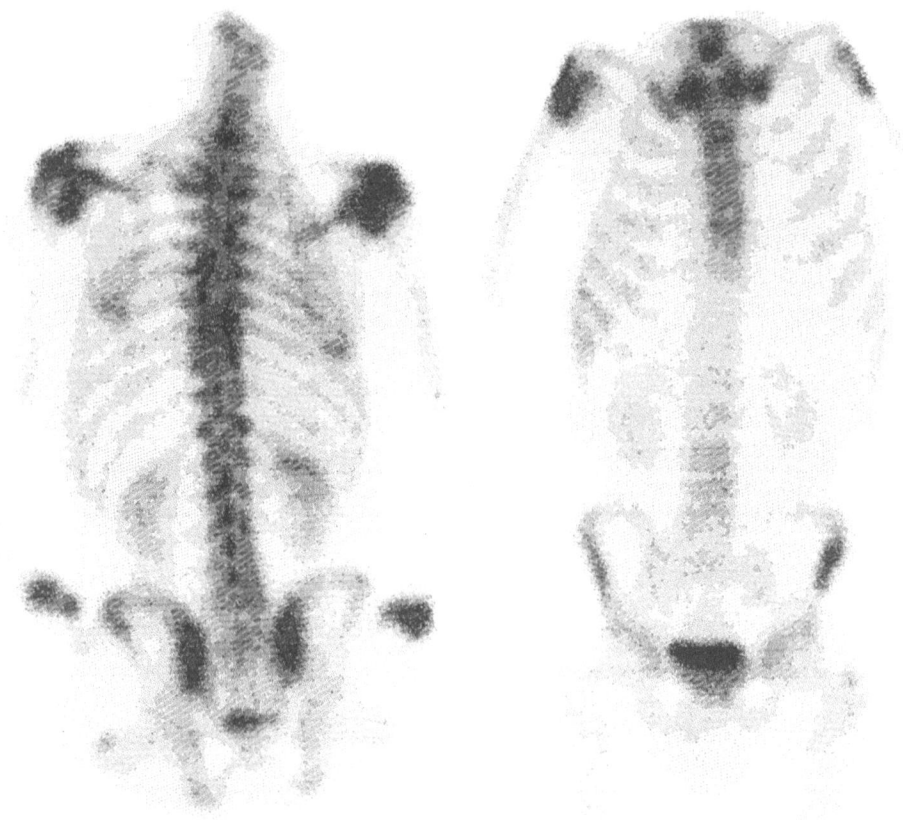

a   b

Fig. 14.5a,b. Patient with active rheumatoid arthritis. a Posterior image showing increased uptake at multiple apophyseal joints, especially in the thoracic spine, the shoulders and both wrists. A similar pattern is seen in the spine, in ankylosing spondylitis, but in the latter condition the sacroiliac joints are usually more active. b Anterior scintigram showing disease activity in the sterno-clavicular joints

is suspected from the classical history and examination of back pain and stiffness, particularly in a young adult male who is HLA-B27 positive. Radiographs of the spine may be normal, the earliest change being squaring of the vertebral bodies anteriorly.

Although a specific diagnosis cannot be made by scintigraphy, there are certain differences in the patterns of distribution of disease seen in ankylosing spondylitis and rheumatoid arthritis. In particular, involvement of peripheral and small joints is much less common in ankylosing spondylitis, while the more proximal and larger joints are more frequently involved. Other sites to be affected more often in ankylosing spondylitis are the sternoclavicular and manubriosternal joints (Lentle et al. 1977a). Because it is simple to image the entire skeleton, these patterns are more readily displayed scintigraphically than by radiography. The principal role of scintigraphy is in the differential diagnosis of the patient presenting with undiagnosed back or other pain, and in the evaluation of some complications.

In the spine, abnormal activity is commonly seen asymmetrically at multiple apophyseal joints. This is readily confused with the appearance of widespread metastatic disease, especially in patients presenting with back pain and no known antecedent disease (Fig. 14.5). It may be necessary to obtain transmission tomograms or CT scans to make a definitive diagnosis. It has been suggested that single photon emission tomography (Jacobsson et al. 1984) or ultra high resolution imaging (Bahk et al. 1987) may be a useful aid to differential diagnosis by localizing the site of increased uptake more precisely. A discitis, with increased uptake across the full width of the spine at the level of one or more intravertebral discs, is seen occasionally (Lentle et al. 1977a), especially in patients with early disease. It is often necessary to perform tomography to differentiate it from collapse of the upper portion of a vertebral body. Scintigraphy is particularly valuable in establishing the cause of pain recurring in apparently inactive sites, where fractures may be followed by pseudarthrosis (Park et al. 1980).

Perhaps the most important and characteristic feature of ankylosing spondylitis is involvement of the sacroiliac joints. A number of methods have been described for obtaining a numerical assessment of disease activity at this site (Lentle et al. 1977b; Namey et al. 1977a; Dequeker et al. 1978; Berghs et al. 1978; Ho et al. 1979; Pfannenstiel et al. 1980; Ayres et al. 1981; Snaith et al. 1982). All the methods involve calculating a ratio between activity in the sacroiliac region and that in an "inactive" region of bone such as the sacrum or, in one case, the iliac crest. The various methods were compared by Davies et al. (1984). That proposed by Ayres et al., which used an isocount contour to define the sacroiliac region, had a smaller variance and a larger mean difference between groups than the others. Nevertheless with all methods there was a substantial overlap between patients and control groups.

Bennett et al. (1984) found that the ratio fell with increasing age and that whilst it was more sensitive than thermography, scintigraphy was of little or no value as a primary diagnostic criterion. Nevertheless Dunn et al. (1984) found that the method was sufficiently reproducible to be used for assessing response to treatment by serial studies in the same individual. They compared a number of indices and found that the sacroiliac ratio, measured by a method similar to that of Ayres et al. (1981) gave the best independent correlation with the patient's subjective report of the severity of symptoms. Even so it is doubtful whether it gave any additional useful information beyond that obtained from a careful clinical history.

Ankylosing spondylitis is commonly associated with a form of inflammatory bowel disease resembling ulcerative colitis, which may also affect the terminal ileum. The most sensitive and also the simplest test to identify ileal dysfunction resulting from involvement is to measure how much of a tracer dose of [75]SeHCAT is retained one week after oral administration of a capsule containing 0.4 MBq (10 μCi) (Merrick 1988). [75]SeHCAT is the taurine conjugate of a synthetic trihydroxy bile acid containing the gamma-emitting radionuclide [75]Se. It resembles taurocholate in most respects, the principal exception being that it is much more resistant to bacterial deconjugation, and is a specific marker for the functional integrity of the mucosa in the terminal ileum. In the normal subject more than 15% of the administered activity is still present after one week. A retention of less than 8% indicates involvement of the terminal ileum.

Miscellaneous Arthropathies

Other Connective Tissue Diseases

Scintigraphic techniques have no established role in the differential diagnosis or management of articular manifestations of other connective tissue diseases. Namey and Rosenthall (1977b) described one case of systemic sclerosis in whom there was substantially increased uptake of ^{99m}Tc pyrophosphate around all joints examined, even though there was no radiographic or clinical abnormality at any of them. They hypothesized that this might be due to absorption onto immature collagen. Unfortunately no other cases or follow up have been reported.

Low Back Pain

Low back pain may be due to many causes other than ankylosing spondylitis (Chap. 25). Agnew et al. (1982) found the sacroiliac ratios to be elevated in patients with back pain and inflammatory bowel disease, whilst Chisin et al. (1984) observed asymmetrically raised values in young military recruits subjected to unaccustomed physical stress. The ratio was also elevated on one or both sides in some patients with back pain for which no specific cause could be identified. Ayres et al. (1981) pointed out that there was no good criterion for defining which patients with symptoms and a raised sacroiliac ratio were "false positives". The index is not specific for ankylosing spondylitis, and these patients may have had joint or ligamentous stresses which were responsible both for the pain and the elevated ratio. This is in keeping with the correlation between the ratio and symptoms found by Dunn et al. (1984). It is possible to speculate that a normal sacroiliac ratio in patients with back pain indicates a non-bony origin of their symptoms. Van den Oever et al. (1987) demonstrated that scintigraphy was the best method of deciding whether a spondylolysis was recent, and might therefore respond to conservative management, or whether there was established non-union. They found one case in which the scintigraphic changes preceded radiological spondylolysis. Scintigraphic findings should not be dismissed as "false positive" merely on the basis of the non-visualization of the abnormality on radiographs.

Reflex Sympathetic Dystrophy Syndrome

The reflex sympathetic dystrophy syndrome (RSDS) is essentially a clinical diagnosis based on the characteristic combination of pain and tenderness, vasomotor instability, swelling of the affected parts and dystrophic skin changes. The aetiology is poorly understood but one common feature is bone reabsorption which radiographically is indistinguishable from that found in disuse osteoporosis. The scintigraphic features have been described by Kozin et al. (1981). There is increased blood flow compared with the contralateral side. Blood-pool images obtained with a blood-pool marker or immediately after injection of a bone-seeking tracer show increased blood volume in the affected part, whilst late images with any bone agent show increased uptake around joints. Symmetry of uptake in affected limbs may be affected by concurrent disease such as healing fractures or osteoarthritis. The condition may be distinguished from rheumatoid arthritis, in which symmetrical involvement of all joints in an affected limb is uncommon (Helliwell et al. 1984).

The sensitivity of scintigraphy is similar to that of radiography, but scintigraphy is said to be more specific. However the population upon which this conclusion was based had an atypically high *a priori* probability of having RSDS and therefore this may not be the case in less highly selected populations. Similar appearances have been reported following sympathetic denervation (Lentle et al. 1977c), in migratory osteolysis (Strashun and Chayes 1979) and in diabetic osteoarthropathy, although the latter tends to be more asymmetrical (Eymontt et al. 1981).

Degenerative Joint Disease

The diagnosis is made on plain films and first pass and blood-pool images are normal. The appearance on the late skeletal image does not correlate with the radiographic findings, especially with respect to osteophyte formation. Scintigraphic abnormalities tend to be most marked in the earlier stages, when radiographic changes are absent or limited to reduction of the width of the joint space, and may be essentially normal in the presence of gross osteophytes. Osteophytes are an adaptive response to a changed pattern of stresses to which the joint is subjected and their effect is to increase the load-bearing area and thus to reduce the peak load per unit volume of bone. Bone turnover is greatest whilst these adaptations are in progress. If they are successful in reducing the load, the rate of turnover returns to normal. Continued increased uptake indicates that adaptation is incomplete.

It is logical to assume that there should be a better correlation between the scintigraphic appearance and clinical symptoms than with the radiographic appearance. Although there is a clinical impression that this is the case, such an association has never been formally proven. Thomas et al. (1975) found that scintigraphy was more accurate than radiography, arthrography or clinical examination in assessing the distribution and severity of osteoarthritis of the knee, and suggested that it provided a useful means of deciding the most appropriate surgical approach. In other large joints, such as the hip, scintigraphy may have a useful role in displaying the distribution of active involvement. It is less useful in smaller joints where there are fewer therapeutic options and such detailed information about the distribution of the disease process is less relevant. In practice, resolution limits of imaging equipment is no longer a limiting factor. Patterns of uptake in complex joints such as the ankle and mid-tarsal joints may require multiple projections or tomography, which can be time-consuming.

Avascular Necrosis (See Chap. 28)

References

Abdel-Dayem HM, Barodawala Y, Papademetriou T (1981) Scintigraphic arthrography: a new imaging procedure. Clin Nucl Med 6:246–248

Agnew JE, Pocock DG, Jewell DP (1982) Sacroiliac joint uptake ratios in inflammatory bowel disease: relationship to back pain and to activity of bowel disease. Br J Radiol 55:821–826

Ayres J, Hilson AJW, Maisey MN, Laurent R, Panayi GS, Saunders AJ (1981) An improved method for sacro-iliac joint imaging: a study of normal subjects, patients with sacro-iliitis and patients with low back pain. Clin Radiol 32:441–445

Bahk YW, Kim OH, Chung SK (1987) Pinhole collimator scintigraphy in differential diagnosis of metastasis, fracture and infections of the spine. J Nucl Med 28:447–451

Bennett RJM, Grennan DM, Johns CW, Taylor L, Brown JDK (1984) A comparative evaluation of thermography and scintigraphy in the assessment of sacroiliitis. Int J Nucl Med Biol 11:42–45

Berghs H, Remans J, Drieskens L, Kiebooms L, Polderman J (1978) Diagnostic value of sacroiliac joint scintigraphy with 99m technetium pyrophosphate in sacroiliitis. Ann Rheum Dis 37:190–194

Bergmann H, Kolarz G (1976) Pertechnetate uptake of joints in rheumatoid arthritis. Eur J Nucl Med 1:205–210

Chisin R, Milgrom C, Margulies J, Giladi M, Stein M, Kashtan H, Atlan H (1984) Unilateral sacroiliac overuse syndrome in military recruits. Br Med J 289:590–591

Coleman RE, Samuelson CO, Baim S, Christian PE, Ward JR (1982) Imaging with Tc99m MDP and Ga-67 citrate in patients with rheumatoid arthritis and suspected septic arthritis: concise communication. J Nucl Med 23:479–482

Coakley AJ, Mountford PJ (1986) Indium-111 leucocyte scanning – underused? Br Med J 293:973–974

Conklin JJ, Alderson PO, Zizic TM, Hungerford DS, Densereaux JY, Gober A, Wagner HN (1983) Comparison of bone scan and radiograph sensitivity in the detection of steroid induced ischaemic necrosis of bone. Radiology 147:221–226

Davis MC, Turner DA, Charters JR, Golden HE, Ali A, Fordham EW (1984) Quantitative sacroiliac scintigraphy: the effect of method of selection of region of interest. Clin Nucl Med 9:334–340

Dequeker J, Goddeeris T, De Roo M, Boeckx L (1977) Comparison of technetium uptake in small joints with other indices of inflammation in rheumatoid arthritis. Eur J Nucl Med 2:269–271

Dequeker J, Goddeeris T, Walravens M, De Roo M (1978) Evaluation of sacro-iliitis: comparison of radiological and radionuclide techniques. Radiology 128:687–689

Desaulniers M, Fuks A, Hawkins D, Lacourciere Y, Rosenthall L (1974) Radiotechnetium polyphosphate joint imaging. J Nucl Med 15:417–423

Dick WC, Shenkin A, Freeman P, Nuki G, Whaley K, Buchanan WW (1970) Effect of synovectomy on the clearance of radioactive xenon (^{133}Xe) from the knee joint of patients with rheumatoid arthritis. J Bone Joint Surg [Br] 52:70–76

Domljan Z, Dodig D (1984) The value of early and late ^{99m}Tc-methylene diphosphonate scintigrams of hands in patients with rheumatoid arthritis and other inflammatory rheumatic diseases. Z Rheumatol 43:167–170

Dunn NA, Mahida BH, Merrick MV, Nuki G (1984) Quantitative sacroiliac scintiscanning: a sensitive and objective method for assessing efficacy of nonsteroidal anti-inflammatory drugs in patients with sacroiliitis. Ann Rheum Dis 43:157–159

Eymontt MJ, Alavi M, Dalinka MK, Kyle GC (1981) Bone scintigraphy in diabetic osteoarthropathy. Radiology 140:475–477

Greyson ND (1979) Radionuclide bone and joint imaging in rheumatology. Bull Rheum Dis 30:1034–1038

Gunasekera SW, King LJ, Lavender PJ (1972) The behaviour of tracer gallium-67 towards serum proteins. Clin Chim Acta 39:401–406

Hays MT, Green FA (1972) The pertechnetate joint scan. I. Timing. Ann Rheum Dis 31:272–277

Helliwell M, Shaban R, Ellis RM (1984) Bone scintigraphy in benign bone disease. Br Med J 288:797

Ho G, Sadovnikoff N, Malhotra CM, Claunch BC (1979) Quantitative sacroiliac joint scintigraphy. A critical assessment. Arthritis Rheum 22:837–844

Jacobsson H, Larsson SA, Vesterskold N, Lindvall N (1984) The application of single photon emission computed tomography to the diagnosis of ankylosing spondylitis of the spine. Br J Radiol 57:133–140

Janin-Mercier A, Sauvezie B, Ristori JM, Betail G, Veyre A, Rampon S (1982) Histological and immunological study in patients with rheumatoid arthritis showing isolated abnormalities of salivary scintigraphy. J Clin Immunol 2:282–288

John M, John V, Oppermann J, Gabriel R, Petters W (1982) Die diagnostische Bedeutung der ^{99m}Tc Pertechnetat-Profilographie bei der juvenilen chronischen Arthritis. Radiol Diagn 23:679–684

Katona G, Burgos R, Zimbron A (1983) Sequential quantitative joint scintigraphy in the investigation of anti-inflammatory effects of piroxicam. Eur J Rheum Inflam 6:63–72

Kozin F, Soin JS, Ryan LM, Carrera GF, Wortmann RL (1981) Bone scintigraphy in the reflex sympathetic dystrophy syndrome. Radiology 138:437–443

LeBlanc AD, Evans HJ, Marsh C, Schneider V, Johnson PC, Jhingran SG (1986) Precision of dual photon absorptiometry measurements. J Nucl Med 27:1362–1365

Lentle BC, Russell AS, Percy JS, Jackson FI (1977a) Scintigraphic findings in ankylosing spondylitis. J Nucl Med 18:524–528

Lentle BC, Russell AS, Percy JS, Jackson FI (1977b) The scintigraphic investigation of sacroiliac disease. J Nucl Med 18:529–533

Lentle BC, Glazebrook GA, Percy JS, Jackson FI (1977c) Sympathetic denervation and the bone scan. Clin Nucl Med 2:276–278

McCall IW, Sheppard H, Haddaway M, Park WM, Ward DJ (1983) Gallium-67 scanning in rheumatoid arthritis. Br J Radiol 56:241–243

McCarthy DH, Polcyn RE, Collins PA (1970) ^{99m}Tc technetium scintiphotography in arthritis. Arthritis Rheum 13:11–32

Merrick MV, Gunasekera SW, Lavender JP, Nunn AD, Thakur ML, Williams ED (1973) The use of indium-111 for tumour localisation. Medical Radioisotope Scintigraphy vol. 2. IAEA, Vienna, pp 721–729

Merrick MV (1988) Bile acid malabsorption. Ann Dig Dis 6:159–169

Namey TC, McIntyre J, Buse M, LeRoy EC (1977a) Nucleographic studies of axial spondarthritides. I. Quantitative sacroiliac scintigraphy in early HLA-B27-associated sacroiliitis. Arthritis Rheum 20:1058–1064

Namey TC, Rosenthall L (1977b) Generalized periarticular uptake of ^{99m}Tc-pyrophosphate in progressive systemic sclerosis. Clin Nucl Med 2:26–28

Nixon JE (1984) Early diagnosis and treatment of steroid induced avascular necrosis of bone. Br Med J 288:741–744

Oh BK, MacFarlane JD, Goei The HS, Pauwels EKJ (1983) Sequential joint scintigraphy in rheumatoid arthritis. Clin Rheumatol 2:45–51

Oka M, Mottonen T, Rekonen A (1983) A comparison of ^{99m}Tc-MDP and ^{99m}Tc-pertechnetate by computerized quantitative joint scintigraphy. Scand J Rheumatol 12:46–48

Park HM, Terman SA, Ridolfo AS, Wellman HN (1977) A quantitative evaluation of rheumatoid arthritic activity with Tc-99m HEDP. J Nucl Med 18:973–976

Park WM, McCall IW, Spencer D (1980) Bone scanning in the detection of spinal pseudarthrosis in ankylosing spondylitis. Nucl Med Communications 1:167

Pfannenstiel P, Semmler U, Adam W, Halbsguth A, Bandilla K, Berg D (1980) Comparative study of quantitating ^{99m}Tc-EHDP uptake in sacroiliac scintigraphy. Eur J Nucl Med 5:49–55

Rosenthall L, Stern J, Arzoumanian A (1982) A clinical comparison of MDP and DMAD. Clin Nucl Med 7:403–406

Sayle BA, Balachandran S, Rogers CA (1983) Indium-111 chloride imaging in patients with suspected abscesses. J Nucl Med 24:1114–1118

Schneider R, Kaye JJ (1975) Insufficiency and stress fractures of the long bones occurring in patients with rheumatoid arthritis. Radiology 116:595–599

Smith MA (1982) Neutron activation analysis: choice of site, precision and accuracy. In: Jequeker J, Johnston CC Jr (eds) Non-invasive bone measurements: methodological problems. IRL Press, Oxford, Washington, pp 77–83

Somervaille LJ, Chettle DR, Scott MC (1985) In vivo measurement of lead in bone using x-ray fluorescence. Phys Med Biol 30:929–943

Snaith ML, Galvin SE, Short MD (1982) The value of quantitative radioisotope scanning in the differential diagnosis of low back pain and sacroiliac disease. J Rheumatol 9:435–440

Strashun A, Chayes Z (1979) Migratory osteolysis. J Nucl Med 20:129–132

Thomas RH, Resnick D, Alazraki NP, Daniel D, Greenfield R (1975) Compartmental evaluation of osteoarthritis of the knee. A comparative study of available diagnostic modalities. Radiology 116:585–594

Uno K, Matsui N, Nohira K et al. (1986) Indium-111 leucocyte imaging in patients with rheumatoid arthritis. J Nucl Med 27:339–344

van den Oever M, Merrick MV, Scott JHS (1987) Bone scintigraphy in symptomatic spondylolysis. J Bone Joint Surg [Br] 69:453–456

Wahner HW, Dunn WL, Riggs BL (1984a) Assessment of bone mineral. Part 1. J Nucl Med 25:1134–1141

Wahner HW, Dunn WL, Riggs BL (1984b) Assessment of bone mineral. Part 2. J Nucl Med 25:1241–1253

Wallis WJ, Simkin PA, Foster DM, Nelp WB (1983) Pathophysiology of synovial effusions: intraarticular volume, metabolism and clearance kinetics. J Nucl Med 24:p 85 (abs)

Weiner R, Hoffer PB, Thakur ML (1981) Lactoferrin: its role as a ^{67}Ga-binding protein in polymorphonuclear leukocytes. J Nucl Med 22:32—37

Whaley K, Pack AI, Boyle JA, Dick WC, Downie WW, Buchanan WW, Gillespie FC (1968) The articular scan in patients with rheumatoid arthritis: A possible method of quantitating joint inflammation using radio-technetium. Clin Sci 35:547–552

Williams BD, O'Sullivan MM, Saggu GS, Williams KE, Williams LA, Morgan JR (1986) Imaging in rheumatoid arthritis using liposomes labelled with technetium. Br Med J 293:1143–1144

15 Ultrasound of the Axial Skeleton

R.W. Porter

Introduction 221
   Accuracy and Precision 221
   Reproducibility 221
Anatomical Relevance 221
Clinical Relevance 223
   Patient Management 223
   Neurogenic Claudication 224
   Isthmic spondylolisthesis 224
   Intra-operative Ultrasonography 224
   Spinal Muscle Measurement 225
Epidemiology 225
References 228

Introduction

A method of measuring the oblique sagittal diameter of the spinal canal was introduced in 1978 (Porter et al. 1978) and many thousands of patients and volunteer subjects have now been examined. The technique employs a two-dimensional display of echoes, the B-scan (Fig. 15.1) demonstrating vertebral body and laminar echoes. The distance between the reflecting surfaces of these echoes can be measured from the B-scan with electronic calipers (Asztély 1983) or more precisely from an A-scan display at any one particular level (Fig. 15.2) but there has been much debate about the accuracy and precision, reproducibility, and relevance of the measurements.

Accuracy and Precision

It has been suggested that it is not technically possible for ultrasound to measure to a precision of less than half a wavelength. Using a 1.5 Mhz transducer, half a wavelength is 0.5 mm. This is the range resolution, i.e. it is not possible to differentiate two surfaces closer together than this. The limitations of range resolution, however, do not mean that the accuracy of linear measurement between two widely separated surfaces is also so limited. In practice, a 1.5 Mhz transducer allows for detection of 0.05 mm movement of a reflecting surface fixed to a micrometer screw gauge (Hammond 1984). Such accuracy is highly acceptable for spinal measurement.

Reproducibility

Some have criticized the method on the grounds of poor reproducibility (Stockdale and Finlay 1980; Finlay et al. 1981), although with care and time we have been able to obtain a mean reproducibility of less than 0.5 mm (Hibbert et al. 1981). Others have found less acceptable mean reproducibility (up to 1.29 mm, Legg and Gibbs 1984; Hammond 1984). Battie et al. (1986) recorded an intra-observer error of 0.65 mm, and found the technique helpful in identifying subjects with wide or narrow canals. A discrepancy of 0.5 mm is not inconsiderable in the vertebral canal where linear measurements can range from 11 to 18 mm, but is probably adequate for epidemiological studies.

Anatomical Relevance

The exact origin of the echoes is uncertain. The current impression is that they originate from the cranial aspect of the posterior surface of the vertebral bodies and from the posterior margin of

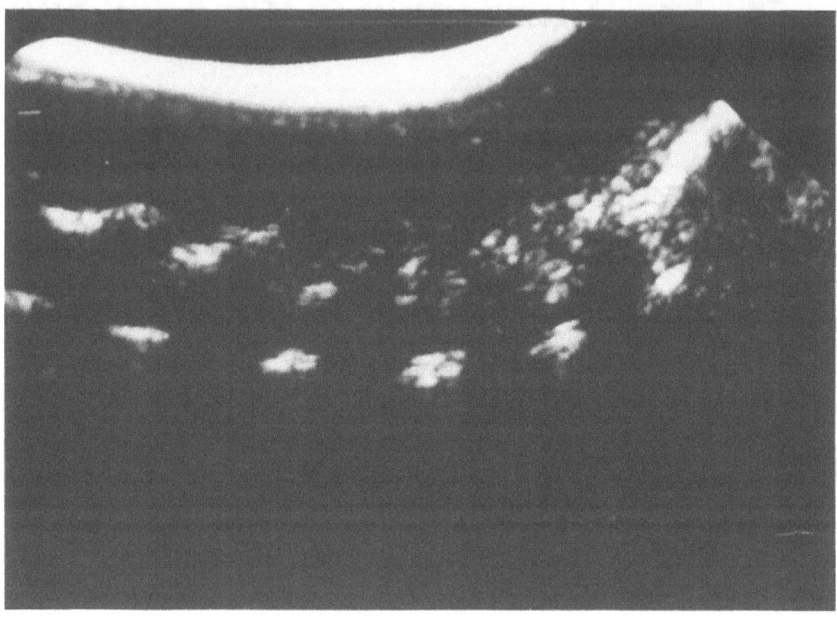

Fig. 15.1. B-scan display showing echoes from the bodies of five lumbar vertebrae and the sacrum, and laminar echoes with the continuous echo from the sacral lamina. The patient is prone, with the cranial vertebrae on the left.

the spinal canal at the cranial lip of the lamina (Fig. 15.3). Much of the sound must enter the canal through the ligamentum flavum. Asztély (1983) and Kadziolka and coworkers (1981) concluded from cadaveric work that echoes originated from the boundaries between the dural sac and surrounding tissues at the level of the intervertebral disc. This could be the echo from the posterior boundary, where the dura and the cranial lip of the lamina are closely opposed, but if the dura were the echo from

the anterior boundary, we would have expected to obtain a gross reduction of measurements in the presence of a large disc herniation. Engel et al.

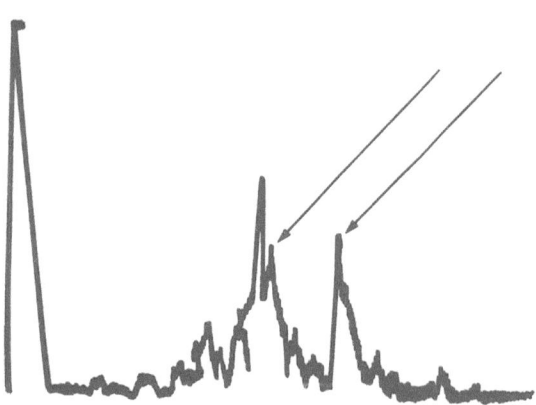

Fig. 15.2. A-scan display at one vertebral level. The *first arrow* (at the left) points to the echo reflected from the posterior canal and the *second arrow* (to the right) from the posterior aspect of the vertebral body.

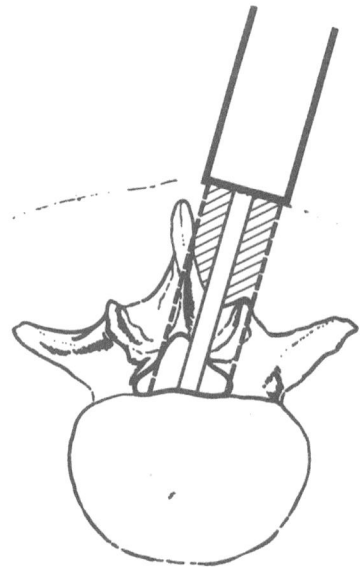

Fig. 15.3. Diagram to show the fifteen degree sagittal scanning plane, and the sound entering the canal through the interlaminar space.

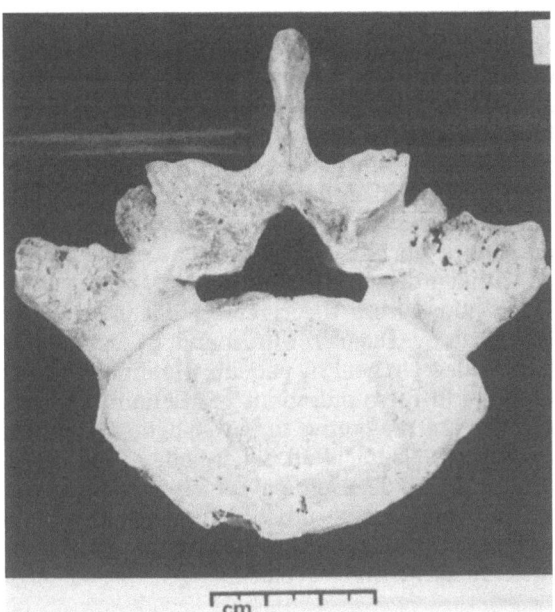

Fig. 15.4. A photograph showing a fifth lumbar vertebra with a shallow trefoil vertebral canal. Approximately fifteen per cent of canals at L5 are trefoil (Eisenstein 1980).

(1986) recognized a third soft tissue interface between the two bony interfaces – the "triple density" sign – and found this to be 89% sensitive and 100% specific for disc herniation in patients who subsequently underwent surgery. Hammond (1984) concluded that the main echoes arose from both bony and soft tissues of the spine, and that the operator could accentuate or diminish the echoes by altering the scanning plane or the method of signal processing. It must be recognized that the ultrasound beam is an area of sound varying with the focus of the transducer and that it must inevitably average to a point measurement, thus adding further doubt about which point is actually being measured.

Clinical Relevance

There is no debate about the clinical relevance of the shallow vertebral canal (Fig 15.4). Following the early papers of Sarpyener (1945), Verbiest (1954) and Van Gelderen (1958), others have confirmed that a variety of back pain syndromes are related to spinal pathology in the presence of an already small canal (Epstein et al. 1962; Salibi 1976; Porter et al. 1980). Edwards and La Rocca (1985) showed that 71% of patients with back pain and degenerative change had mean sagittal canal diameters below the mean.

What is at issue is whether ultrasound linear measurements are sufficiently accurate and reproducible to be clinically useful. Howie and colleagues (1983) discarded the technique because the preoperative measurements bore no relationship to the observed level of pathological problem found at surgery. If indeed bony parameters are being measured, it is unlikely that ultrasound will show the clinical level of significant pathology, which is more often a combination of bone and soft tissue encroachment. They noted, but failed to comment upon, the fact that half their operated patients had vertebral canals in the bottom 10% of their "normal values" obtained from healthy volunteers.

Forsberg and Wallöe (1982) reported that B-scan measurements for their patients, who had made a poor recovery from disc surgery, were narrower than those who had recovered uneventfully.

We have found ultrasound measurements to be meaningful in certain clinical situations, and the results of population studies to be valuable epidemiologically. The uncertainties of the technique, however, have meant that the criticisms have been largely accepted and it is not a diagnostic aid that has yet received general acceptance.

Patient Management

The attraction of ultrasound as a diagnostic tool lies in its simplicity and safety for the patient (Fig. 15.5).

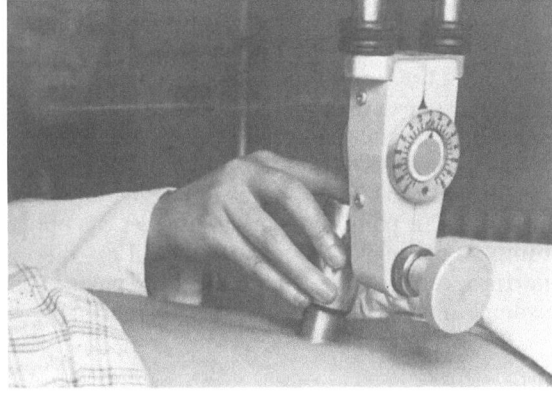

Fig. 15.5. The patient lies prone, and a 1.5 Mhz transducer moves along the lumbar spine just lateral to the spinous processes until an acceptable B-scan display is developed. The canal size is maximized before the scanning plane is accepted.

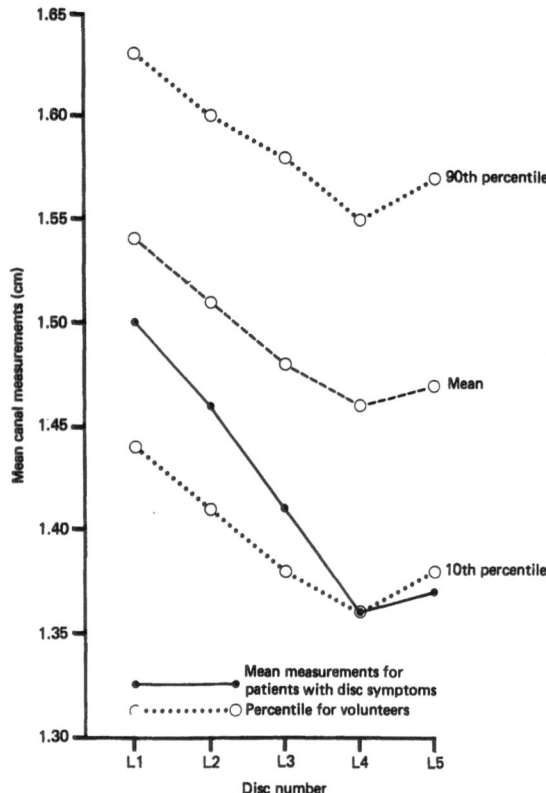

Fig. 15.6. A graph showing the mean canal measurements by ultrasound for 151 patients with disc symptoms fulfilling McCulloch's criteria (1977), compared with means and percentiles for age and sex-matched volunteers.

We routinely scan every patient with back pain and whilst recognizing the margin of error in the results, are usually able to comment on the significance of space in the spinal canal. A patient with recurrent episodes of back pain, listing to one side, but without sciatic pain, may have a disc protrusion but be fortunate enough to have an adequate spinal canal protecting the nerve root, whilst a patient with leg pain and poor straight leg raising, and a narrow canal is vulnerable (Fig. 15.6).

Many patients with rising expectations about health, want to know as much as possible about the source of this pain. Ultrasound provides the opportunity to discuss questions in a logical manner. A narrow canal with an unstable segment, for example, makes talk about dural pain sensible.

Neurogenic Claudication

There are many factors responsible for the symptoms of neurogenic claudication in addition to

a shallow spinal canal. These include soft tissue encroachment, segmental movement and vascular insufficiency. The narrow canal, however, is an essential factor. If the possibility of surgery is contemplated, myelography or a CT scan is essential, but there are some patients not sufficiently disabled for surgery, or with inappropriate signs, where ultrasound may be helpful. An ultrasound scan with measurements in the upper percentiles would suggest a diagnosis other than neurogenic claudication.

Pulsations from the cerebrospinal fluid can be identified by Doppler ultrasound at each interlaminar level in healthy patients (Hammond 1984). Changes in these pulsations in relation to posture and exercise may prove to have diagnostic value in neurogenic claudication, where one of the vexing problems is to determine at which of several levels is the pathological process responsible for the symptoms. Unnecessarily extensive surgical decompression may then be avoided.

Isthmic Spondylolisthesis

Forward displacement of the proximal vertebral body is usually obvious from the B-scan echoes (Fig. 15.7). The displacement may be more apparent on ultrasound than radiographically, perhaps because it is accentuated by the forward rotation of the body. The canal measurements are generally wider than in patients without a lysis, partly because the displaced lamina increases the sagittal diameter, and also because the canal in spondylolisthesis is usually dome-shaped and rarely trefoil.

Hammond (1984) attempted to identify the unstable spondylolysis by measuring the sagittal diameter of the canal by ultrasound before and after torsion or flexion of the lumbar spine, but his results were equivocal. Ultrasound has its limitations, even if one accepts a fair degree of accuracy, reproducibility and anatomical relevance. It has not been shown to help in the prediction of outcome of an episode of back pain, or the likelihood of a recurrence within 12 months (Drinkall et al. 1984), nor will it make the diagnosis of the level of significant pathology. It does draw attention to space in the spinal canal, however, and even with its limitations can be a useful clinical tool.

Intra-operative Ultrasonography

Ultrasound is being used intra-operatively to investigate extra-dural cord or root impingment and intradural and intra-medullary spinal cord pathology

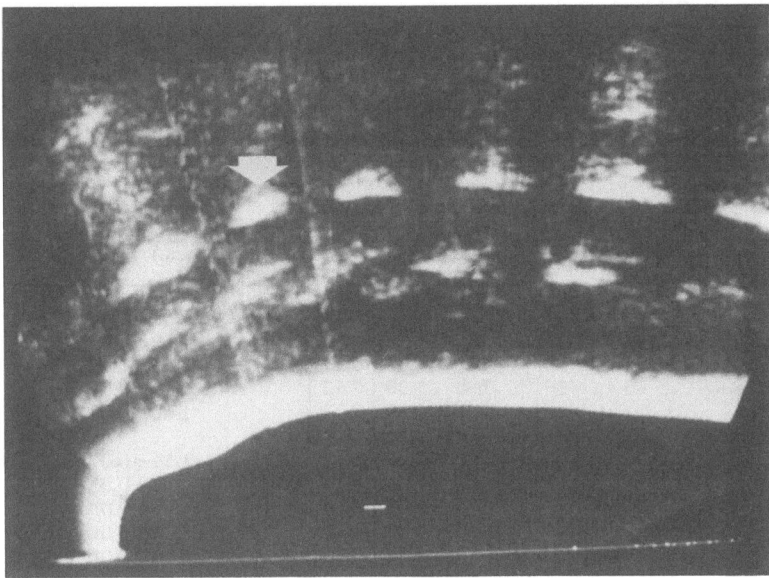

Fig. 15.7. B-scan display of a patient with an isthmic spondylolisthesis, the body of L5 (arrowed) is displaced forwards. The patient is prone, with the cranial vertebrae on the left.

(Dohrmann and Rubin 1982; Knake et al. 1983; Eismont et al. 1984; Montalvo et al. 1984; Quencer et al. 1984). After laminar excision the wound is filled with Ringer's lactate solution and the spine examined with a real-time machine, the sterile probe being covered with sterile lubricant within a plastic cover.

Following spinal trauma the degree of anterior bony encroachment and stenosis can be identified. Fragments of a sequestered disc, otherwise hidden, can be located and the extra-medullary masses and intra-medullary cavities demonstrated. Matsuzaki et al. (1987) found real-time intra-operative ultrasonography helpful in localizing intramedullary cord tumours. In the surgical treatment of spinal stenosis, they did not find that a return of pulsations meant that the spine was fully decompressed.

Endoscopic ultrasonography is a further extension of this principle (Cotton et al. 1985) and with an ultrasound transducer incorporated into the tip of a myeloscope it may soon be possible to examine the contents of the spinal canal from within.

Spinal Muscle Measurement

There is increasing interest in the morphology of the spinal muscles (Bogduk and MacIntosh 1984), their role in the many back pain syndromes, and in muscle atrophy and recovery after surgery. The cross-sectional area of muscle can be measured by real-time ultrasound with a high degree of repeatability (Stokes and Young 1986) and where the research studies need an inexpensive non-invasive method of measurement, ultrasound is the first choice.

Epidemiology

Ultrasound results have suggested that the antero-posterior diameter of the spinal canal is an important factor in most patients with back pain. In a general practice study (Drinkall et al. 1984) it was found that patients attending with back pain had significantly smaller sagittal oblique spinal canal measurements than a randomized group of matched controls who had never attended with back pain. Patients attending hospital with back pain, when compared with volunteers of similar age, also tended to have narrower canals, 39% of clinic patients, 43% of those admitted, and 46% of those having spinal surgery being below the tenth percentile of the volunteers (Fig. 15.8).

An industrial study (Macdonald et al. 1984; Fig. 15.9) showed that 37% of the days lost from work by a group of coal miners aged over 50 years was by the 10% of men whose canals were the nar-

Table 15.1. Comparison of ultrasound canal measurements in patients with symptomatic disc lesion, root entrapment syndrome and neurogenic claudication

						Controls (volunteer subjects)		Patients below percentile (%)		
Clinical Diagnosis	Number	% Male	Age (years)	Mean canal measurements (cm)		Age range	Mean canal measurements (cm)	5th	10th	50th
Disc lesion	173	71.8	33.6±6.6	L.1	1.53±0.13	20–50 (n=547)	1.54±0.08	36.4	41.0	82.7
				L.2	1.49±0.13		1.52±0.08			
				L.3	1.43±0.12		1.49±0.07			
				L.4	1.38±0.11		1.46±0.08			
				L.5	1.38±0.12		1.48±0.08			
Neurogenic claudication	134	70.1	50.8±10.7	L.1	1.48±0.11	40–60 (n=197)	1.54±0.07	42.5	56.7	85.1
					1.44±0.11		1.51±0.08			
					1.38±0.10		1.47±0.08			
					1.33±0.10		1.45±0.08			
					1.33±0.12		1.46±0.08			
Root entrapment syndrome	250	52.7	51.3±7.8		1.51±0.10	40–60 (n=197)	1.54±0.07	21.2	30.0	67.2
					1.48±0.10		1.51±0.08			
					1.43±0.09		1.47±0.08			
					1.49±0.10		1.45±0.08			
					1.41±0.10		1.46±0.08			

Table 15.2 Comparison of ultrasound canal measurements in patients with vertebral displacement

					Controls (volunteer subjects)		Patients below percentile (%)		
Diagnosis	Number	% Male	Age (years)	Mean canal measurements (cm)	Age range	Mean canal measurements (cm)	5th	10th	50th
Retro-spondylolisthesis	56	62.1	45.5±12.4	1.48±0.09	30–60 (n=557)	1.54±0.07	21.4	42.9	89.3
				1.45±0.09		1.51±0.07			
				1.41±0.08		1.48±0.08			
				1.38±0.08		1.45±0.08			
				1.39±0.06		1.47±0.08			
Degenerative spondylolisthesis	65	28.4	61.3±10.3	1.48±0.09	50–65 (n=124)	1.54±0.08	23.1	32.3	78.5
				1.45±0.09		1.51±0.08			
				1.42±0.08		1.47±0.09			
				1.39±0.09		1.45±0.08			
				1.39±0.10		1.47±0.08			
Isthmic spondylolisthesis	89	64.4	39.3±13.5	1.52±0.09	30–50 (n=315)	1.54±0.07	16.9	24.7	67.4
				1.49±0.09		1.52±0.07			
				1.46±0.07		1.49±0.07			
				1.44±0.09		1.46±0.08			
				1.43±0.11		1.47±0.07			

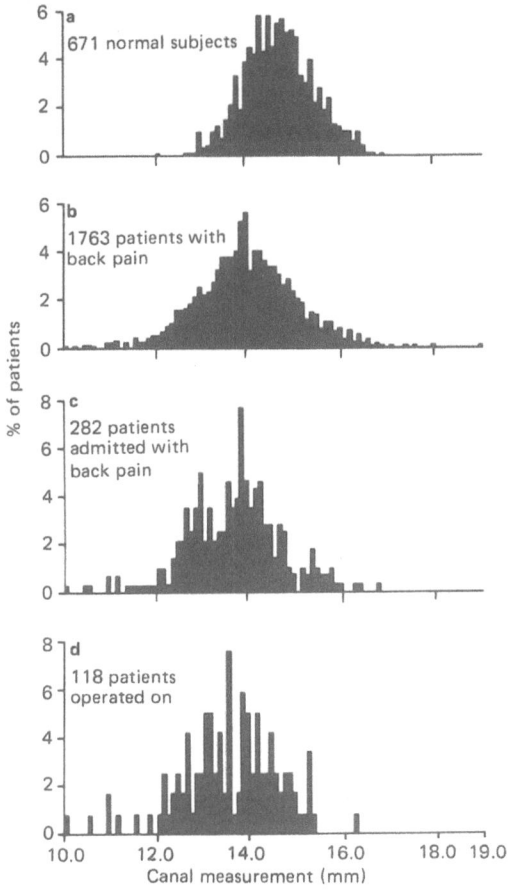

Fig. 15.8. Histograms comparing canal measurements at L5 in volunteer asymptomatic subjects (a), patients attending hospital with back pain (b), those admitted (c), and those requiring spinal surgery (d).

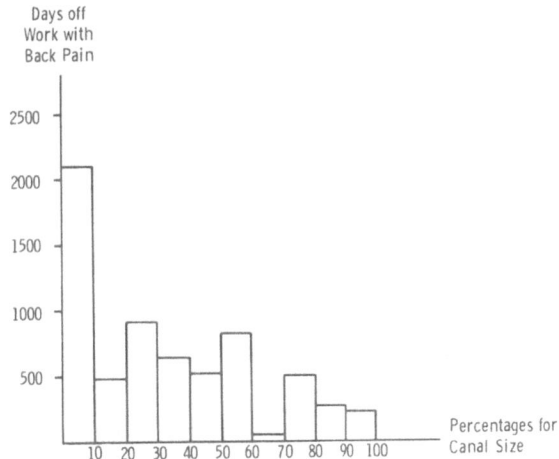

Fig. 15.9. Histogram showing days lost from work compared with canal size at L5 in 191 50-year-old miners.

rowest. In the 3 years after measurement, the men who took early retirement had significantly narrower canals than those who stayed at work. It seems that the canal size as measured by ultrasound has some value in predicting those most vulnerable to back pain. The implications for occupational health are important.

Population studies using ultrasound in back pain syndromes have been helpful in evaluating their pathogenesis. Of patients with symptomatic disc lesions, 41% had canal measurements below the tenth percentile for asymptomatic volunteers (Table 15.1) suggesting that for many, canal size is an important factor in the pain mechanism. This is more significant in older patients whose back pain restricted walking distance; 57% were below the tenth percentile. In root entrapment syndrome, where the lesion is more lateral in the root canal

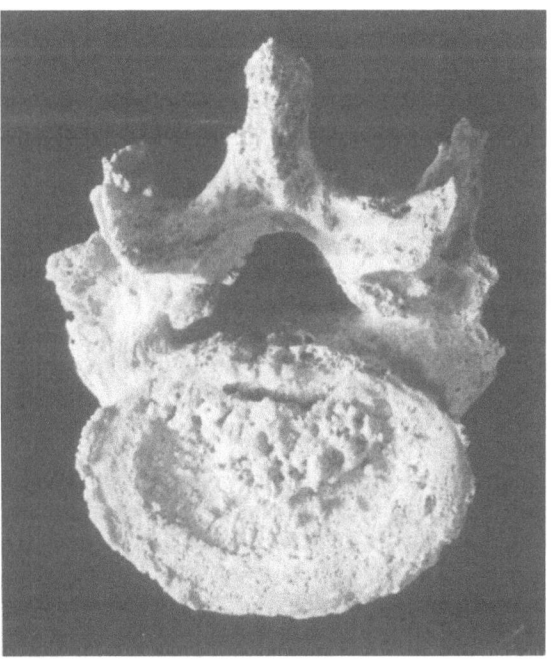

Fig. 15.10. Photograph of fifth lumbar vertebra showing degenerative change in the left root canal. Added soft tissue encroachment would readily precipitate symptoms. The size of the central canal does not assume great significance.

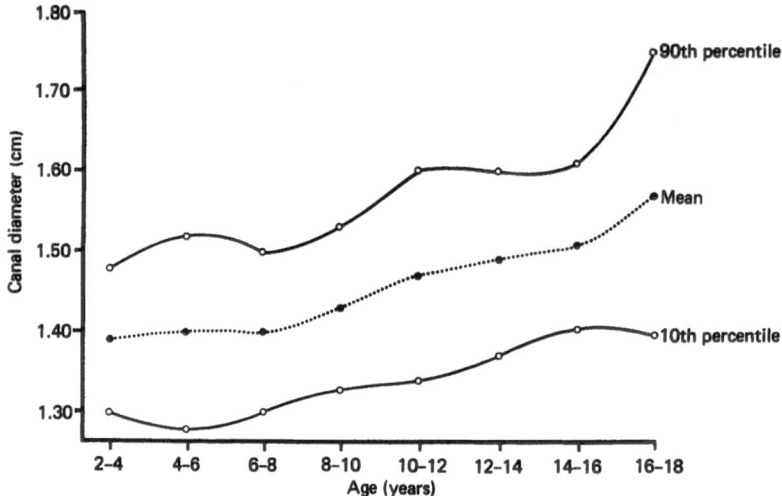

Fig. 15.11. Graph of the mean and percentile 15 degree oblique sagittal diameter of the canal at L5 plotted against age for 150 children.

(Fig. 15.10), only 30% had central canal measurements below the tenth percentile.

In back pain syndromes associated with vertebral displacement, the canal size as measured by ultrasound seems to have variable significance. It assumes greater importance when pain is associated with retrolisthesis or rotationary displacement (43% below the tenth percentile), some importance in degenerative spondylolisthesis, and less in isthmic spondylolisthesis (Table 15.2).

Ultrasound measurements of the cervical spinal canal can be useful in population studies, where an entirely non-invasive method may be preferable to radiography. We have measured 254 young volunteers and shown a good correlation between cervical and lumbar canals especially at the lower cervical and lumbar levels (Table 15.3). This may be one factor in the common association between symptomatic cervical and lumbar spondylosis (Edwards and La Rocca 1985).

Ultrasound provides the opportunity to investigate the growing spinal canal. Children are easier to measure than adults and Fig. 15.11 shows the mean and percentiles for 150 children. The relatively large sagittal diameter of the infant's canal indicates that its growth is accomplished early in development. It may be a marker in later life of infantile malnutrition. The canal could prove to be an indicator of health status, and its measurement by non-invasive technique valuable (Clark et al. 1985; Porter and Pavitt 1987; Porter et al. 1987).

Table 15.3. Correlation between measurements of cervical and lumbar vertebral canal in 254 young volunteer subjects

	C2	C3	C4	C5	C6	C7
L1	0.18	0.16	0.18	0.22	0.22	0.21
L2	0.19	0.21	0.24	0.28	0.28	0.29
L3	0.18	0.21	0.23	0.26	0.27	0.28
L4	0.20	0.23	0.25	0.28	0.28	0.29
L5	0.23	0.23	0.24	0.28	0.29	0.32

There is no doubt that the space within the spinal canal is of great clinical significance. An individual with a shallow canal, and especially a trefoil-shaped canal at L5, has a highly vulnerable back, and is at risk. The question still to be answered is whether such an individual can reliably be identified using ultrasound.

References

Asztély M (1983) Lumbar sonography: a comparative radiological study. Thesis: Departments of diagnostic radiology and orthopaedic surgery, University of Goteborg, Sweden

Battie MC, Hanson TH, Engel JM, Zeh J, Bigos SJ, Spengler DM (1986) The reliability of measurements of the lumbar spine using ultrasound B-scan. Spine 11:144–148

Bogduk N, MacIntosh JE (1984) The applied anatomy of the thoraco lumbar fascia. Spine 9:164–170

Clark GA, Panjabi MM, Wetzel FT (1985) Can infant malnutrition cause adult vertebral stenosis? Spine 10:165—170

Cotton PB, Shorvon PJ, Lees WR (1985) Endoscopic ultrasonography: a new look from within. Br Med J 290:1373

Drinkall JN, Porter RW, Hibbert CS, Evans C (1984) The value of ultrasonic measurement of spinal canal diameter in general practice. Br Med J 288:121–122

Dohrmann GJ, Rubin JM (1982) Intra-operative ultrasound imaging of the spinal cord: syringomyelia, cysts, and tumours – a preliminary report. Surg Neurol 18:395–399

Edwards WC, La Rocca SH (1985) The developmental segmental sagittal diameter in combined cervical and lumbar spondylosis. Spine 10:42—49

Eisenstein S (1980) The trefoil configuration of the lumbar vertebral canal. A study of South African skeletal material. J Bone Joint Surg [Br] 62:73–77

Eismont FJ, Green BA, Berkowitz BM, Montalvo BM, Quencer M, Brown MJ (1984) The role of intra-operative ultrasonography in the treatment of thoracic and lumbar spine fractures. Spine 9:782–787

Engel JM, Engel GM, Gunn DR (1986) Ultrasound of the spine in focal stenosis and disc disease. Spine 10:928–931

Epstein JA, Epstein BS, Lavine L (1962) Nerve root compression associated with narrowing of the lumbar spinal canal. J Neurol Neurosurg Psychiatry 25:165—176

Finlay D, Stockdale HR, Lewin E (1981) An appraisal of the use of diagnostic ultrasound to quantify the lumbar spinal canal. Br J Radiol 54:870–874

Forsberg L, Wallöe A (1982) Ultrasound in sciatica. Acta Orthop Scand 53:393–395

Hammond BR (1984) The detection of spondylolysis using lumbar sonography. PhD Thesis. University of Surrey

Hibbert CS, Delaygue C, McGlen B, Porter RW (1981) Measurement of the lumbar spinal canal by diagnostic ultrasound. J Radiol 54:905–907

Howie DW, Chatterton BE, Hone MR (1983) Failure of ultrasound in the investigation of sciatica. J Bone Joint Surg [Br] 65:144–147

Kadziolka R, Asztély M, Hanai K, Hansson T, Nachemson A (1981) Ultrasonic measurement of the lumbar spinal canal. The origin and precision of the recorded echoes. J Bone Joint Surg [Br] 63:504–507

Knake JE, Chandler WF, McGillicuddy JE et al. (1983) Intra-operative ultrasonography of intra-spinal tumours: initial experience. Am J Neuroradiol 4:1199–1201

Legg SJ, Gibbs V (1984) Measurement of the lumbar spinal canal by echo ultrasound. Spine 9:79–82

McCulloch JA (1977) Chemonucleolysis. J Bone Joint Surg [Br] 59:45–52

Macdonald EB, Porter R, Hibbert C, Hart J (1984) The relationship between spinal canal diameter and back pain in coal miners: ultrasonic measurement as a screening test? J Occup Med 26:23–28

Matsuzaki H, Hoshino M, Koyama I, Toriyama S (1987) Value of intraoperative ultrasonography in Spine surgery. Presented to Societe Internationale de Chirurgie Orthopedique et de Traumatologie, 17th World Congress, Munich

Montalvo BM, Quencer RM, Green BA, Eismont FJ, Brown MJ, Brost P (1984) Intra-operative sonography in spinal trauma. Radiology 153:125–134

Porter RW, Pavitt D (1987) The vertebral canal. Part 1: nutrition and development: an archaeological study. Spine 12:901–906

Porter RW, Wicks M, Ottewell D (1978) Measurement of the spinal canal by diagnostic ultrasound. J Bone Joint Surg [Br] 60:481–484

Porter RW, Hibbert C, Wellman P (1980) Backache and the lumbar spinal canal. Spine 5:99–105

Porter RW, Drinkall JN, Porter DE, Thorp L (1987) The vertebral canal. Part 2: Health and academic status. Spine 12:907–911

Quencer RM, Morse BMM, Green BA, Eismont FJ (1984) Intra-operative spinal sonography of soft tissue masses of the spinal cord and spinal canal. Am J Neuroradiol 5:507–515

Salibi BS (1976) Neurogenic claudication and stenosis of the lumbar spinal canal. Surg Neurol 5:269–272

Sarpyener MA (1945) Congenital stricture of the spinal canal. J Bone Joint Surg 27:70–79

Stockdale HR, Finlay D (1980) Use of diagnostic ultrasound to measure the lumbar spinal canal. J Radiol 53:1101–1102

Stokes M, Young A (1986) Measurement of quadriceps cross-sectional area by ultrasonography: a description of the technique and its applications in physiotherapy. Physiotherapy Practice 2:31–36

Van Gelderen V (1958) Ein Orthotisches (lordotisches) kauda syndrom. Acta Psychiatr Neurol Scand 23:57

Verbiest H (1954) A radicular syndrome from developmental narrowing of the lumbar vertebral canal. J Bone Joint Surg [Br] 36:230–237

16 Appendicular Ultrasound

D. Rickards

Introduction 231
Technique of Examination 231
Ultrasound Appearances 232
    Normal Condition 232
    Tumour 232
    Soft Tissue Trauma 233
    Neuromuscular Disease 235
    Tendons and Bones 238
    Hip Disorders in Children 238
    Muscular Infection and Inflammation 238
References 239

Introduction

Over the past decade, ultrasound has made an enormous impact on the radiologist's ability to image anatomy that is beyond the reach of plain film radiography. In the fields of obstetric care, upper abdominal and pelvic disease, ultrasound is not only an important, but frequently the only, diagnostic modality needed to achieve a diagnosis. There are, however, areas where ultrasound is known to be of limited or no value due mainly to the physical principles that govern the transmission of ultrasound. Imaging the adult brain, through an intact skull, pulmonary pathology through air-containing lung, and the large and small bowel may be cited as examples, but in air-free contiguous soft tissues ultrasound is excellent.

Appendicular muscle fulfils the necessary criteria for good ultrasound imaging. Furthermore, muscle is predominately superficial with easy access to ultrasound probes. Yet in no department in the author's experience is muscle ultrasound a significant part of radiological practice. Very few muscle complaints of course require any imaging at all. The majority of sports-mediated muscle sprains and bruises require little or no radiological input. In this chapter, the uses of ultrasound in the appendicular skeleton are discussed.

Technique of Examination

The choice of equipment and scanning technique depend upon which muscle or muscle group is under investigation. Limb muscles are superficially situated and longitudinally orientated. Although many ultrasound departments no longer have B-mode facilities available, such machines having been replaced with modern real-time linear array and sector scanners, the muscles of the limbs are ideally situated to B-mode scanning (Fig. 16.1). The whole length of muscle groups can be displayed on one scan. Probes of 3.5 or 5 MHz are used depending upon the depth of muscle under investigation, with coupling gel on the skin. For detail of most superficial muscle, a "stand-off" is used. This consists of either a water bath or commercially available solid gel block which acts as a "water-delay system" (Fornage et al. 1984). Transverse scanning is more difficult as the curvature of the limb has to be taken into account. Linear array real-time scanning is more suited to this orientation, again using 3.5 or 5 MHz probes either with coupling gel alone or in connection with a "stand-off".

Muscles are paired structures permitting comparison of one side with another, an advantageous feature if disease is suspected to be unilateral. Scans can be performed with the patient supine or erect

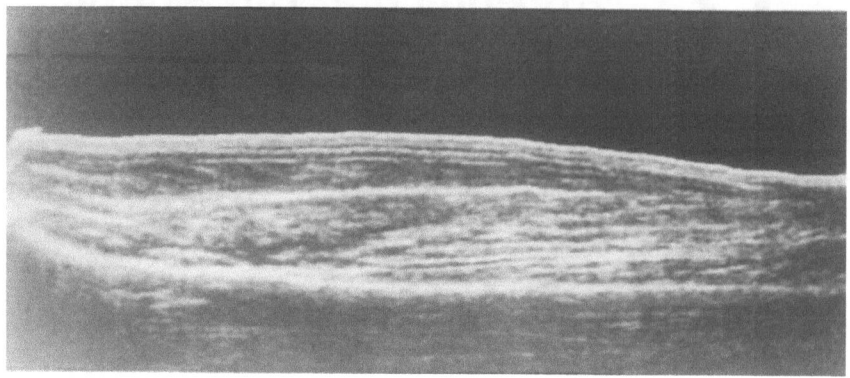

Fig. 16.1. B mode longitudinal scan. Muscles of the calf from knee to ankle.

and before and after exercise, if clinically appropriate. Using real-time equipment, localized areas of abnormality within muscle can be imaged in varying planes and at multiple angles permitting clear delineation within a few minutes.

Modern probe technology has extended the possible uses of appendicular ultrasound. Reports are now emerging on the applications of ultrasound in "small part" appendicular imaging. Higher frequency probes of 7.5 and 10 MHz have excellent spatial resolution and are ideal for imaging in great detail those structures just beneath the probe.

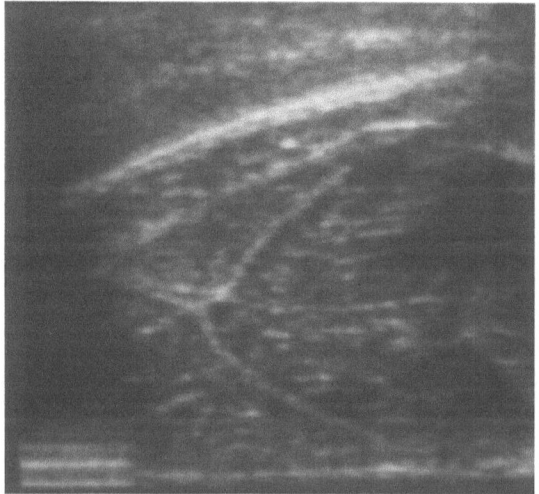

Fig. 16.2. Transverse section through adductor muscles of the thigh. Fat planes separate muscle groups from each other.

Ultrasound Appearances

Normal Condition

Individual muscle groups are separated by strongly reflective muscle fascia. Bone itself forms a bright echo and therefore echoes observed beyond bone are artefacts due to reverberation. Muscle itself has a rather pleniform appearance. Fat between muscle bundles and fascicles gives a streaky appearance (Fig. 16.2). Muscle itself is relatively echo-poor and the echogenicity of muscle groups at the same anatomical level in one limb can vary considerably, unlike that seen on cross-sectional computed tomography. Comparison with the muscles on the contralateral limb becomes important in determining the significance of this. Major arterial vessels can be clearly identified and the proximity of pathological processes to them identified.

Tumour

The role of radiology in the diagnosis and staging of soft tissue sarcoma in the appendicular skeleton is to locate disease and to assess its extent and nature. Irrespective of the imaging modality used, early diagnosis is essential as soft tissue sarcomas tend to be aggressive and to metastasize early. Prior to cross-sectional imaging with computed tomography and ultrasound, plain film radiology, tomography and xerography were the modalities of choice. Plain films of soft tissue are of limited value because

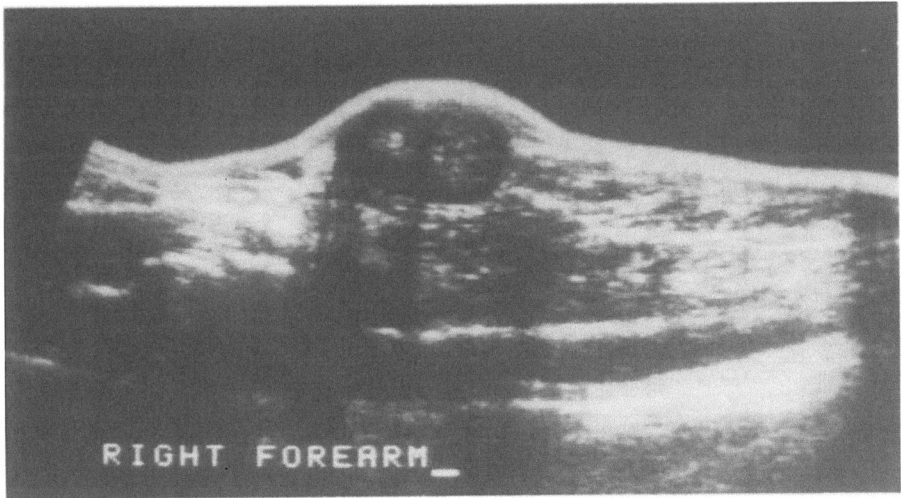

Fig. 16.3. Haemangiopericytoma. Well-defined lesion anterior to the elbow.

the inherent density of tumour and normal surrounding tissue is similar, though plain radiographs are of far greater value in the assessment of bone itself. Ultrasound has no role to play in the assessment of primary or secondary bone tumour except to image the extra-osseous soft tissue component, but this is usually of secondary importance to the extent of tumour in bone and in the medullary cavity. Ultrasound is capable of detecting the size, orientation and extent of soft tissue appendicular tumours much earlier than conventional radiological techniques and with greater accuracy than computed tomography. As with all ultrasound, the quality of the examination depends largely upon the operator and not on the equipment itself.

Musculoskeletal soft tissue tumours have a different echo pattern to surrounding normal tissue and the differentiation between solid, cystic and complex masses can usually be made. The ultrasound characteristics of soft tissue sarcoma are, however, not uniform. Such tumours may be relatively echo-poor or complex in consistency. Differentiation on echo pattern alone between benign and malignant tumours is of little value (Goldberg 1975). The ability of ultrasound to image in multiple planes provides good definition of the interface between normal and abnormal tissue which if absent suggests invasion by tumour into surrounding tissue. Ultrasound is limited in detecting tumours that arise adjacent to bone especially those that arise within the pelvis (Levine et al. 1979).

Any soft tissue appendicular mass should be subjected to ultrasound examination following plain film assessment. Much can be learned from a quick

and non-invasive technique which causes the patient minimal or no discomfort. If the interface between normal and abnormal tissue can be identified throughout the circumference of the abnormality, it does suggest that local surgery may be effective (Fig. 16.3). If, however, such interfaces are not seen, a more invasive tumour is likely to be beyond the scope of local excision treatment (Fig. 16.4). The diffuse interruption of normal anatomy (Fig. 16.5) without identifiable interfaces also suggests an invasive tumour even though it may be difficult to define the tumour itself. Ultrasound is valuable in the follow-up of tumour treated by chemotherapy or radiotherapy and in diagnosing recurrent tumour following local excision (Fig. 16.6). Radiotherapy planning is also enhanced by ultrasound. Benign soft tissue tumours are usually well described (Fig. 16.7) and lipomas are usually quite characteristic, having a highly reflective echo pattern. The relationships of tumours to the vascular bundle can be identified on real-time scanning. The ability to biopsy a lesion under ultrasound control is well established and is of equal importance in the appendicular skeleton as elsewhere.

Soft Tissue Trauma

There is increasing interest in the use of ultrasound in patients with muscle pain following sporting injuries. Sprains do not produce any detectable anatomical abnormality, but muscle tears and haematomas do and ultrasound is able to image such lesions.

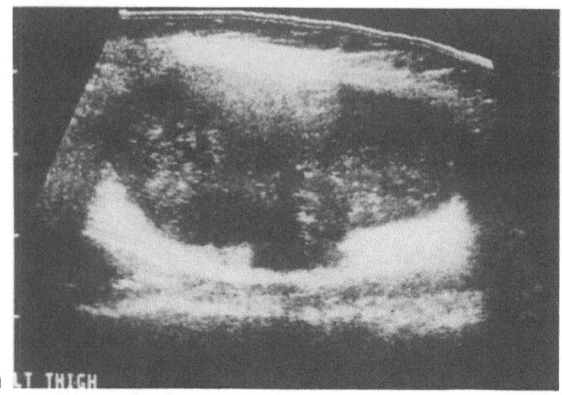

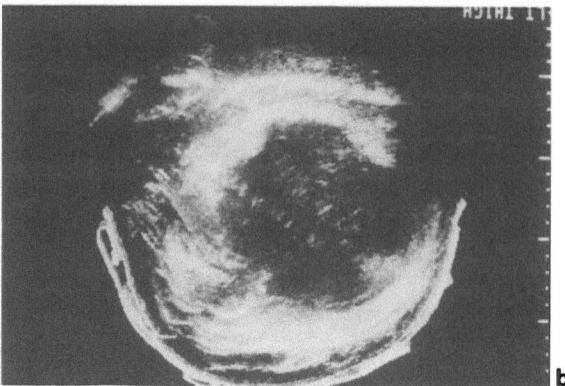

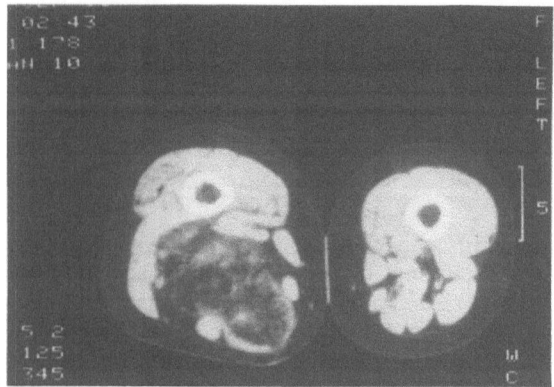

Fig. 16.4. a Transverse scan of upper thigh. **b** Longitudinal scan. Large infiltrative mass adjacent to femur beyond the scope of local excision. Malignant fibrous histiocytoma. **c** The CT appearance of the lesion.

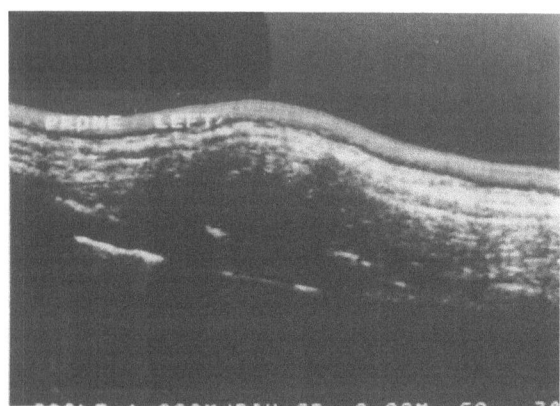

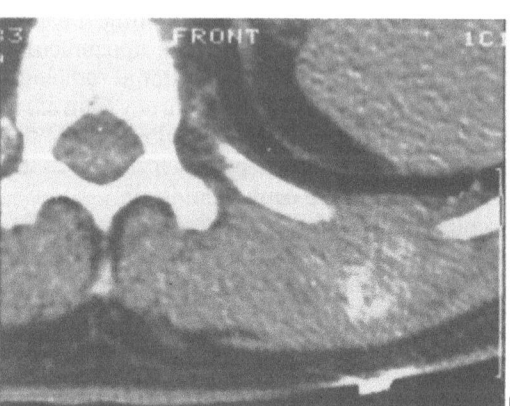

Fig. 16.5. a Longitudinal B mode scan of the erector spinae muscle. **b** CT scan. Ill-defined mass seen on ultrasound, interrupting the normal anatomy. Chondrosarcoma.

Collections of fluids or solid masses in the appendicular soft tissues have ultrasound characteristics similar to lesions elsewhere in the body. Their configuration tends to be more fusiform with a long axis in the direction of the muscle fibres. In common with haematomas in other sites, the ultrasound appearances alter with the age of the bleed (Wicks et al. 1978). In the initial stages, they may have a variable number of internal echoes, but are predominantly echo-poor (Fig. 16.8). After 4 weeks,

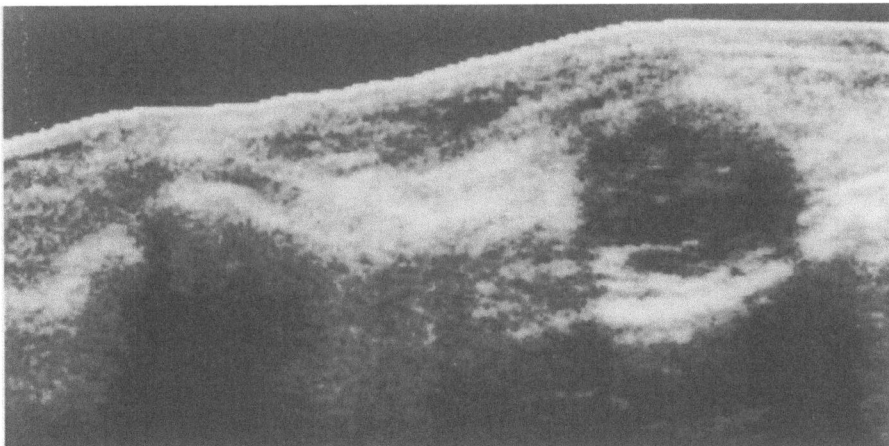

Fig. 16.6. Longitudinal B mode scan of left forearm. Well-defined low-echogenic soft tissue mass due to recurrent soft tissue sarcoma following local excision.

they tend to become more echo-free as the haematoma becomes more serous. They may become entirely echo-free mimicking simple cysts, resolve completely with no discernible sequelae, or heal with fibrosis and scarring. In the latter case, the scar appears as a dense echogenic area with poor through-transmission (Fig. 16.9).

The spectrum of ultrasound findings in haematoma is wide and such lesions can, therefore, have similar appearances to other pathological processes. The site of a haematoma, for example, may mislead and in the calf, a haematoma may mimick a popliteal artery aneurysm (Fig. 16.10), though such a lesion should demonstrate characteristic intrinsic rather than transmitted pulsations, unless the aneurysm is totally thrombosed (Silver et al. 1977). Baker's cysts appear as echo-free masses and may extend down the calf as far as the Achilles tendon. Such cysts can dissect into the gastrocnemius muscle and are difficult to distinguish clinically from deep vein thromboses. As the treatment of the two conditions is clearly different, the distinction between them is important and can be made by ultrasound (Slasky et al. 1982). Similarly, haematomas into the gastrocnemius muscle present with symptoms difficult to differentiate from thrombophlebitis. Ultrasonic demonstration of a predominately echo-poor lesion within muscle suggests the diagnosis of haematoma which can be confirmed by fine needle aspiration biopsy under ultrasound guidance (Shirkhoda et al. 1983). The resolution of haematoma can be monitored by serial ultrasound examination.

Rectus sheath haematomas are uncommon, but can be precipitated by sudden muscular exertion and can complicate sneezing, coughing and anticoagulant treatment (Hopper et al. 1983). Such lesions can mimick an acute abdomen and are difficult to diagnose by palpation (Spitz and Wyatt 1977). An echo-poor or echo-free ovoid mass confined to the rectus sheath readily establishes the diagnosis avoiding further unnecessary radiological investigation.

Muscle tears and ruptures can be demonstrated by ultrasound. Tears are usually associated with some degree of haemorrhage while ruptures cause retraction of muscle away from the site of injury, due either to avulsion from the origin or insertion or in the muscle bulk itself. It is not always easy to differentiate between the two, but ultrasound can help, certainly in distinguishing between partial and complete tear.

Neuromuscular Disease

Ultrasound has been used in the study of various neuromuscular disorders in an attempt to assess the extent of disease and its severity. The pathological changes in the muscle dystrophies are similar irrespective of the type of dystrophy. Damaged and atrophic muscle fibres ultimately disappear and are progressively replaced by fibrous tissue and fat cells. The fatty infiltration of muscle gives rise to characteristic ultrasound findings. The demonstration of echogenic muscles and the inability clearly to separate one muscle group from another because of obliteration of strongly reflective muscle fascia is

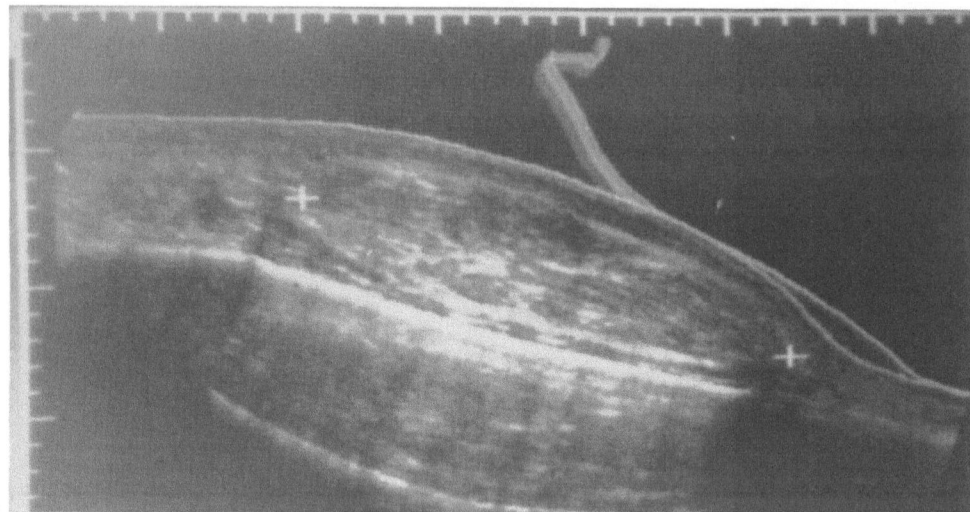

a

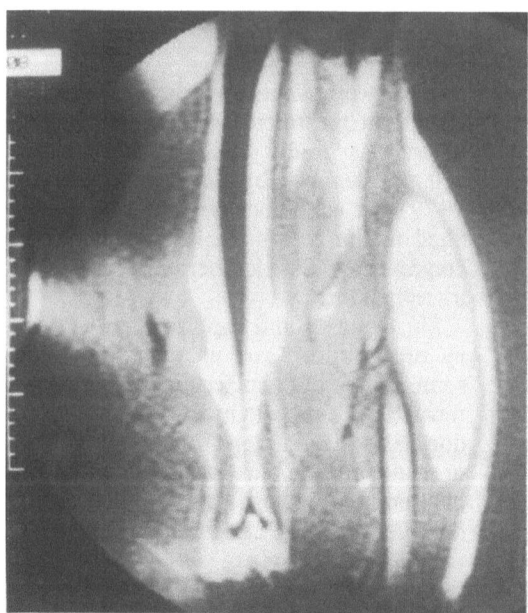

b

Fig. 16.7. a Well-defined soft tissue mass lying within the vastus lateralis muscle (*between caliper marks*). Reflective but disorganized echo pattern consistent with lipoma. b The coronal magnetic resonance section confirms the high intensity lipoma within the vastus lateralis muscle.

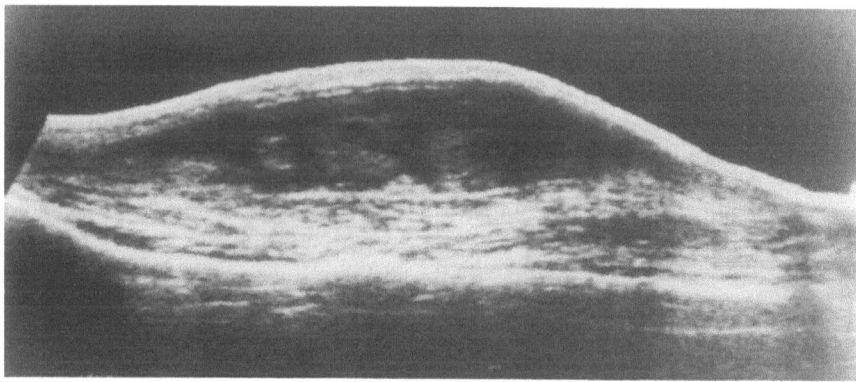

Fig. 16.8. Longitudinal B mode section through calf muscles. Large complex echo-soft tissue mass lying predominantly subcutaneously due to a large haematoma.

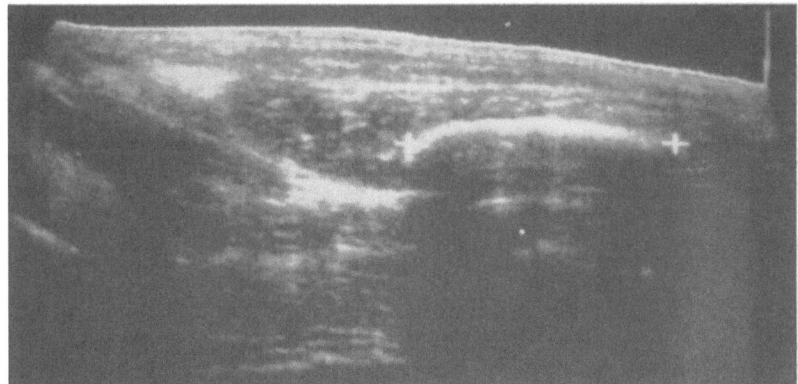

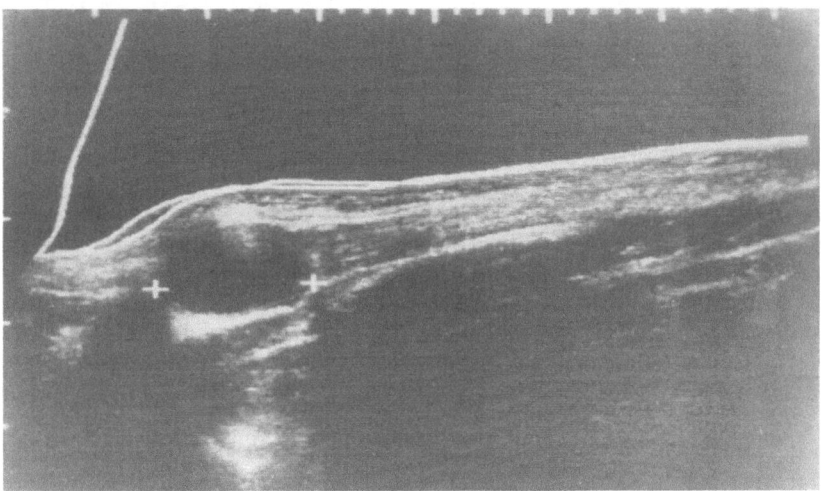

Fig. 16.9 (*top*). Longitudinal B mode section of the anterior thigh. The end result of a resolved haematoma. Highly reflective interface (*between calipers*) within the vastus medialis muscle due to healing with fibrosis and scarring.

Fig. 16.10 (*bottom*). Longitudinal B mode section posterior to the knee. Well defined echo-free lesion due to popliteal artery aneurysm.

common to all muscular dystrophies, especially in their late stages. Clinically, however, this observation is of limited use.

In children, however, the demonstration of abnormal musculature by ultrasound is of more clinical relevance. In those cases where symptoms of neuromuscular disease are mild and muscle function itself may be normal, ultrasound offers a non-invasive method for detecting abnormal muscle. In a study of 20 children with progressive muscular dystrophy, Kamala et al. (1985) demonstrated abnormal muscle echo patterns in all patients and attempted to grade the severity of muscle involvement with reference to the echogenicity of underlying bone. A good correlation was established between the ultrasound images and the pathological changes in the muscles of these children.

Ultrasound has been found to be of use in the assessment of the "floppy baby" (Heckmatt et al. 1982). Abnormalities were detected in the muscles of infants with spinal muscular atrophy and congenital dystrophy, but not in those with hypotonia of muscular origin. Such a distinction made quickly and non-invasively may defer further investigation and muscle biopsy. The detection of carriers of Duchenne muscular dystrophy is also possible by ultrasound examination of the thigh (Rott and Mulz 1983). The carrier condition is inferred by the demonstration of increased echoes within muscle.

Unlike computed tomography, ultrasound is able rapidly, and without ionizing radiation, to image all limb muscle groups in patients with neuromuscular disease. The ability of magnetic resonance, however, to image limb musculature in any plane and to identify very early fatty infiltration is of more clinical use. Nevertheless in the absence of magnetic resonance imaging equipment, ultrasound remains a useful and inexpensive modality.

Tendons and Bones

The development of 10 MHz "small parts" probes has allowed the ultrasound imaging of very small structures with excellent spatial resolution. Reports are now available of the use of such probes in the diagnosis of tendon pathology, a diagnosis that was hitherto the domain of arthrography. The evaluation of shoulder pain is currently under review. Lesions of the rotator cuff are common causes of shoulder pain and may be due to tendonitis, cuff strains or tears and calcified tendonitis. The biceps and supraspinatus tendon can be seen on ultrasound. Small effusions within the biceps tendon sheath are associated with tears of the biceps tendon and of the rotator cuff and are readily detected (Middleton et al. 1985). Partial and complete tears of the biceps tendon can be directly imaged as discontinuities of the echogenic pattern within the bicipital groove in the humeral head. Mack et al. (1985) report that in a comparative study between shoulder arthrography and ultrasound, 68 of 72 patients with shoulder pain were adequately imaged by ultrasound alone, eliminating the need for arthrography as a first-line investigation.

The Achilles tendon is prone to injury and the differentiation between tendonitis and partial tear is important. Tendonitis produces a thickened homogeneous tendon in which flecks of dystrophic calcification may be seen. Partial discontinuities within the tendon suggest incomplete tears which should prompt surgical repair to forestall total rupture (Fornage 1986). The role of ultrasound in complete tears is limited since the clinical assessment is usually sufficient.

Ultrasound has been used to assess the degree of femoral anteversion and of tibial torsion by imaging the bone interface of the femoral neck and the anterior aspect of the femoral condyles on a single B-mode scan and measuring the angle made between them (Moulton and Upadhyay 1982). Such techniques are difficult to reproduce and have little advantage over plain film radiography or computed tomography.

Hip Disorders in Children

Ultrasound may be an extremely useful modality for examining the hip in children and infants (Chap.

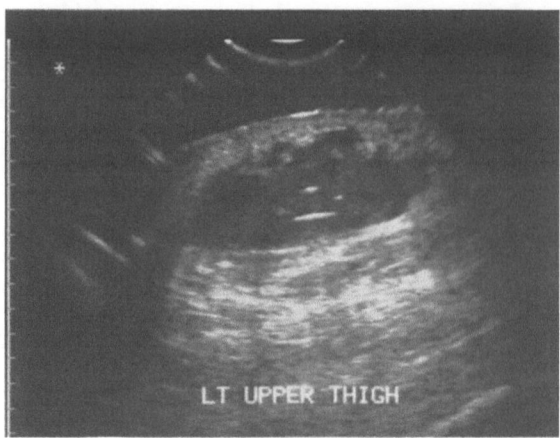

Fig. 16.11. Sector scan through upper thigh. Well-defined but irregular complex lesion lying within muscle. Large muscle abscess which was drained percutaneously.

27). The hip is not well seen on X-ray examination, because most of the femoral head, as well as acetabulum, is cartilaginous. Ultrasound may, therefore, be useful in the early detection of congenital dislocation of the hip (Berman and Klenerman 1986; Suzuki et al. 1987b), in assessing the shape of the acetabulum, in determining whether there is any fluid in the joint and in Perthes' disease (Suzuki et al. 1987a). Using ultrasound, Graf and Schuler (1986) have classified the hip into four types. Type 1a and 1b hips show an equally well-formed bony roof, but have varying morphologies of the cartilaginous roof. Both hips are regarded as physiological variants of a normally mature hip. The Type 2a hip is a physiolocally immature one in a patient under 3 months of age, whereas the Type 2b and 2c suggest some acetabular dysplasia. Type 3 and 4 hips are eccentric in which the femoral head is uncentred and the contour of the bony roof is poor.

In the assessment of the irritable hip in a child, ultrasound can image small joint effusions which can be of clinical importance.

Muscular Infection and Inflammation

Cellulitis can be difficult to separate from muscle abscess on clinical examination alone. An abscess in muscle on ultrasound resembles an abscess seen elsewhere in the body and appears as a complex lesion usually well defined and confined to muscle (Fig. 16.11). Such lesions can be biopsied under ultrasound control and drained if that procedure is deemed clinically appropriate. Cellulitis does not involve the muscle layers, but causes thickening of subcutaneous tissues. Polymyositis can be differentiated from superficial cellulitis on ultrasound, giving rise to blurring of fascial planes between muscle groups and rendering the muscles themselves more echo-poor.

References

Berman L, Klenerman L (1986) Ultrasound screening for hip abnormalities: preliminary findings in 1001 neonates. Br Med J 293:719–722

Fornage BD (1986) Achilles tendon: US examination. Radiology 159:759–764

Fornage BD, Rifkin MD, Touche DH, Segal PM (1984) Sonography of the patellar tendon: a preliminary experience. ARJ 143:179–182

Giyanani VL, Grozinger KT, Gerlock AJ, Mirfakhraee M, Husbands HS (1985) Calf haematoma mimicking thrombophlebitis: sonographic and computed tomographic appearance. Radiology 154:779–781

Goldberg BB (1975) Ultrasonic evaluation of superficial masses. J Clin Ultrasound 3:91–94

Graf R, Schuler P (1986) Sonography of the infant hip: an atlas (translated by Telger T). VCH Verlagsgesellschaft, Weinheim, pp. 1–276

Heckmatt JZ, Leeman S, Dubowitz V (1982) Ultrasound imaging in the diagnosis of muscle disease. J Paediatr 101:656–660

Hopper KD, Smazal SF, Ghaed N (1983) CT and Ultrasonic evaluation of rectus sheath haematoma: A complication of anticoagulant therapy. Milit Med 148:447–449

Kamala D, Suresh S, Githa K (1985) Real-time ultrasonography in neuromuscular problems of children. J Clin Ultrasound 13:465–468

Levine E, Lee KR, Neff JR, Maklad NF, Robinson RG, Preston DF (1979) Comparison of computed tomography and other imaging modalities in the evaluation of musculo-skeletal tumours. Radiology 131:431–437

Mack LA, Matsen FA, Kilcoyne RF, Davies PK, Sickler ME (1985) US evaluation of the rotator cuff. Radiology 157:205–209

Middleton WD, Reinus WR, Totty WG, Melson GL, Murphy WA (1985) US of the biceps tendon apparatus. Radiology 157:211–215

Moulton A, Upadhyay SS (1982) A direct method of measuring femoral anteversion using ultrasound. J Bone Joint Surg [Br] 64:469–472

Rott HD, Mulz D (1983) Duchenne's muscular dystrophy: carrier detection by muscle ultrasound. J Genet Hum 31:63–65

Shirkhoda A, Mauro MA, Staab EV, Blatt PM (1983) Soft tissue haemorrhage in haemophiliac patients. Radiology 147:811–814

Silver TM, Washburn RL, Stanley JC, Gross WS (1977) Gray scale ultrasound evaluation of popliteal artery aneurysms. AJR 129:1003–1006

Slasky BS, Lenkey JL, Skolnick ML, Campbell WL, Cover KL (1982) Sonography of soft tissues of extremities and trunk. Semin Ultrasound 3:288–303

Spitz HB, Wyatt GM (1977) Rectus sheath haematoma. J Clin Ultrasound 5:413–416

Suzuki S, Awaya G, Okada Y, Ikeda T, Tada H (1987a) Examination by ultrasound of Legg-Calve-Perthes Disease. Clin Orthop 220:130–136

Suzuki S, Awaya G, Wakita S, Maekawa M, Ikeda T (1987b) Diagnosis by ultrasound of congenital dislocation of the hip joint. Clin Orthop 217:171–178

Wicks JD, Silver TM, Bree RL (1978) Gray scale features of haematomas: an ultrasonic spectrum. AJR 131:977–980

Part 2:

Bone Mineral Studies

17 Bone Measurement by Conventional Radiographic Techniques

A. Horsman

Introduction 243
Radiographic Morphometry of Tubular Bones 243
   Sequential Radiographic Morphometry of Metacarpals 244
Measurement of Vertebral Body Wedging and Collapse 245
Grading Trabecular Architecture in the Proximal Femur 246
Age-Related Bone Loss and Fracture Risk 247
References 248

Introduction

Within a radiographic image of a bone there is an obvious qualitative relationship between optical density and bone tissue thickness. Experiments with stepwedge standards have been carried out since the turn of the century (Price 1901) and many variants of bone X-ray densitometry have been described in which attempts have been made to quantify that relationship (e.g. Colbert and Garrett 1969). The problems, however, are almost insuperable: X-ray beams are polychromatic and vary in intensity over the film both within and between exposures; the spectrum changes as the beam penetrates the body; much of the radiation reaching the film is scatter; radiographic film varies in its characteristics between batches; and film development tends to be variable.

In 1963 the advent of photon absorptiometry for bone mineral measurement (Cameron and Sorenson 1963) effectively removed the stimulus for further work on X-ray densitometry, but there was and still is a need to detect changes in bone shape and trabecular structures within bones. Although rectilinear scanning photon absorptiometers can produce transmission images of bones (Christiansen and Rødbro 1977), the spatial resolution is low;

better resolution can be achieved using bi-dimensional detectors (Horsman et al. 1977b), but the resulting images still lack detail.

In this chapter three methods of quantifying bone mass are described which capitalize on the high spatial resolution of radiographic images. None requires special X-ray facilities. Radiographic morphometry of tubular bones quantifies endosteal resorption and subperiosteal apposition and, with some refinements, can be used to follow changes in individual subjects; morphometry of vertebral bodies provides an objective measure of wedging and collapse and an overall score which represents the severity of spinal osteoporosis; and assessment of the presence or absence of trabecular arches in the proximal femur provides a semi-quantitative measure of bone loss in the potential fracture zone. Each method reveals some aspect or consequence of skeletal involution, and the relationship between age-related bone loss and increasing fracture risk is discussed in the last section.

Radiographic Morphometry of Tubular Bones

Radiographic morphometry is a simple technique well suited to the measurement of the cortical

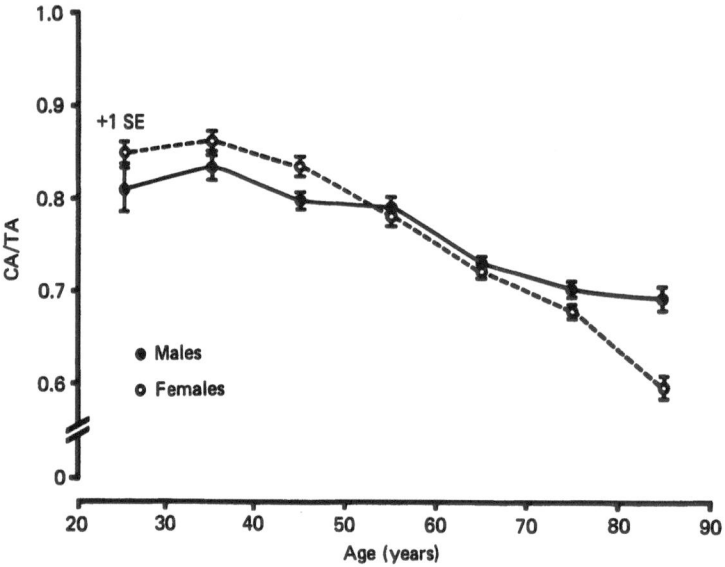

Fig. 17.1. Age-related changes in the cortical/total area ratio (CA/TA) of the second metacarpal. In young men, both CA and TA are greater than in young women, reflecting skeletal size differences; CA/TA is virtually independent of skeletal size.

diameters of the diaphyses of tubular bones (Horsman 1976a). Unlike photon absorptiometry, morphometry can quantify surface-specific processes but cannot reveal changes in bone tissue composition or losses due to intracortical resorption (Meema and Schatz 1970). Measurements are usually made at the mid-shaft of the bone, but other sites such as the proximal radius (Meema and Meema 1969) and calcar femorale (Horsman et al. 1982) have been investigated. Data on age-related changes in total bone width (TW), medullary width (MW), cortical width (CW = TW − MW) and other variables derived from the basic measurements are available for almost every tubular bone (Virtama and Helela 1969). However, because radiographs of the hand are easily taken and variations in positioning are minimal, attention has been concentrated on the second metacarpal (Barnett and Nordin 1960; Garn 1970).

When radiographs of the hand are to be used for metacarpal morphometry, film–focus distance should be standardized, but the results are not critically dependent on radiographic technique (Horsman 1976b). However, the position of the hand must be standardized, with the thumb abducted to reduce the thickness of the thenar eminence. The films should be measured using needle-tipped Vernier calipers with dial-gauge readout or alternatively a magnifying viewer and graticule. The subjectivity of the measurement procedure, which involves judging the positions of the periosteal and endosteal surfaces in the image, is a disadvantage,

but some control can be exercised over the technique by selecting from the outset a series of films to be used as a local standard (Adams et al. 1969; Dequeker 1972).

Cross-sectional morphometric data clearly demonstrate continuous net endosteal resorption from middle age onwards (MW increasing) and subperiosteal apposition (TW increasing) throughout life (Garn 1970). Longitudinal data (see below) are consistent with these observations (Nordin et al. 1979), although cross-sectional data might nonetheless contain a secular component. The combined result of the two surface processes is a decrease with age in both sexes in the fraction of the shaft volume occupied by compact bone. An estimate of this fractional volume (CA/TA) has been used as an index of osteoporosis (Nordin 1973) and is easily calculated from TW and MW if the metacarpal is assumed to have an annular cross-section (Horsman and Kirby 1972). Figure 17.1 shows the age-related changes in the CA/TA ratio of the second metacarpal. Young men tend to have slightly lower values of this ratio than young women, but the age-related decrease starts somewhat later and values in old age tend to be higher in males than in females.

Sequential Radiographic Morphometry of Metacarpals

Early longitudinal morphometric studies of bone loss in individuals (Garn et al. 1967; Adams et al. 1970) were severely limited by measurement error.

A more precise technique was described by Horsman and Simpson in 1975; the improvement is obtained by making duplicate observations of six bones rather than one observation of one bone.

The hands are radiographed on separate films, particular care being taken with positioning to avoid rotational errors (Armes et al. 1979). A series of films on one subject obtained over a period of time must subsequently be measured on one day by one observer. TW and MW at the mid-shafts of the second, third and fourth metacarpals of both hands are each measured twice. Measurement sites are marked on the first pair of films with reference to the metaphyses; on all other films they are located by superimposition on one of the first pair. Needle-tipped calipers can be used for the measurements, but the method is laborious and a semi-automated measurement system is preferable (Horsman et al. 1977c).

Evaluation of the results is straightforward. For each date, the mean cortical width and cortical area are calculated. Differences in mean cortical width and/or area between the two dates are then evaluated and can be expressed as rates, given that the time interval between the films is known. The errors of the method are such that in a post-menopausal female losing bone at the normal rate, a significant loss of bone can be detected in under 2 years (Horsman and Simpson 1975). However, individual results should not be overinterpreted because the error on the individual *rate* can be very large; it increases in proportion to the reciprocal of the observation period, because the measurement errors are absolute.

Sequential radiographic morphometry is a technically simple method better suited to long-term trials of the effect of treatment on age-related bone loss. Figure 17.2 shows, as an example, the results of a retrospective analysis of data on 120 normal post-menopausal females treated with ethinyl oestradiol in doses ranging from 5 to 50 μg/day; the mean observation period was 1.85 years, the whole analysis including 222 patient-years of observation (Horsman et al. 1983). The results demonstrated that the protective effect of this therapy was dose-dependent and also served to emphasize the large scale on which sequential studies must be carried out.

When groups of individuals are investigated, the group mean rate of change and its standard error can be calculated as usual from the individual rates; however, if the durations of observation differ widely between members of the group, this is not the optimum method of analysis. A cusum technique developed specifically for the analysis of sequential measurements on bones (Horsman et al. 1986), which takes into account variations in observation period, was used to calculate the standard errors shown in Fig. 17.2.

Measurement of Vertebral Body Wedging and Collapse

Although it is still common radiological practice to diagnose biconcavity, wedging and collapse of the vertebral bodies by visual assessment of lateral films, radiographic morphometry of the spine is a more objective approach which is not difficult to implement (Barnett and Nordin 1960; Kleerekoper et al. 1984). However, because artefacts due to obliquity are easily misinterpreted as biconcavity (it is impossible to obtain a normal projection of all vertebrae), quantification of biconcavity remains a problem (Dequeker 1972).

In practice, lateral lumbar and thoracic spine radiographs are taken from both sides using standardized radiographic factors (Horsman 1976b) and the films showing the clearest outlines of the vertebral bodies are selected for measurement. The four apices of each vertebral body are marked and the distances A, B, and E measured (see Fig. 17.3). The wedge angle, θ, is calculated as $2\sin^{-1}[(B-A)/2E]$. This is a slight approximation which can be avoided if a digitizer is used to provide exact coordinates of all four apices.

A vertebra can be classified as wedged if the value of θ lies beyond two standard deviations from its normal mean, established by measuring films of young normal people (Horsman 1976a). The same measurements can also be used to identify collapsed vertebrae (with deformations of both the anterior and posterior aspects of the cortex), which often have normal wedge angles. If its neighbours are neither wedged nor collapsed, a given vertebra might, for example, be classified as collapsed if its value of the ratio R is less than or equal to 0.9 times the mean value of R for its neighbours, where the ratio R is defined as $[(A+B)/2E]$. Such an algorithm can easily be extended to avoid using for reference any vertebra already known to be deformed.

Once wedged and collapsed vertebrae have been identified, a spine score, S, can be calculated which reflects the overall severity of spinal osteoporosis (Nordin et al. 1980). If W is the number of wedged and C the number of collapsed vertebrae (including any which are both wedged and collapsed), then $S = W + 2C$, where the multiplier 2 is an arbitrary

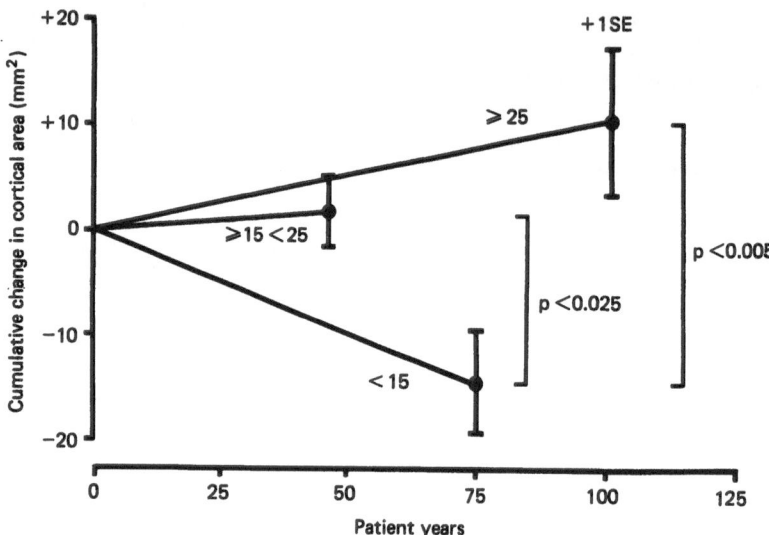

Fig. 17.2. Results of a sequential study of the effects of ethinyl oestradiol therapy on the mean cortical area of six metacarpals in normal post-menopausal females grouped according to dose (μg/day).

weighting factor. The spine score correlates inversely with trabecular bone density in iliac crest biopsies (Horsman et al. 1981) and with bone mineral content in the lumbar spine assessed by dual photon absorptiometry (A. Horsman and F. M. Armes unpublished data 1985).

Grading Trabecular Architecture in the Proximal Femur

In the femoral neck there are two main arches of trabeculae: the principal compressive group, which originates in the medial cortex, and the principal tensile group, which originates in the lateral cortex. The trabeculae are thickest and most closely packed in these arches where the stresses are maximal (Koch 1917); the secondary groups of trabeculae are structurally less important. With ageing, groups of trabeculae are resorbed in an order which is thought to be determined by their functional significance (Hall 1961).

In 1970 Singh and colleagues introduced a six-point scale for grading the trabecular patterns in the neck of the femur. Radiographs of the hip in 15° internal rotation are used. Trabecular bone loss

assessed by this method is greater in females than in males over 50 years. Unlike most other morphometric or densitometric variables the reduction in grade is not common to everyone, a large proportion of people having essentially normal grades even at age 80 (Singh et al. 1972). The age-dependence of the grade in normal females is shown in Fig. 17.4, together with observations on female femur fracture cases (Horsman et al. 1982). There is a marked reduction in grade in younger patients with proximal femoral fractures, but the difference between patients with and without fractures tends to diminish with age, in accordance with the model of bone loss and fracture risk described below (Horsman et al. 1985).

The subjectivity of the Singh grading scale is undoubtedly a disadvantage, but the method possesses the advantage of ease of implementation given routine diagnostic X-ray facilities and, with practice, grading can be reproducible and consistent between observers (Cooper 1985). Singh grading is a practicable method for epidemiological studies and could be used as a screening procedure to identify patients at high risk of femoral neck fracture. It has yet to be demonstrated that more sophisticated methods which measure bone mineral content in the femoral neck by dual photon absorptiometry (Mazess 1984) provide more accurate risk estimates.

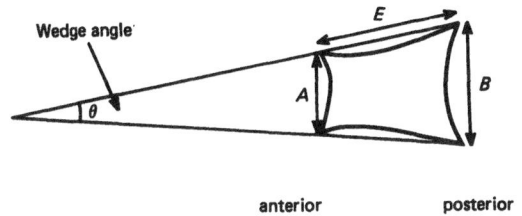

Fig. 17.3. Definition of the vertebral body wedge angle, θ. When A is greater than B (as in many normal lumbar vertebrae), the value of θ is negative.

Age-Related Bone Loss and Fracture Risk

The age-specific incidence of fractures of the proximal femur increases rapidly with advancing age in both sexes, but the fractures are more common in females than in males (Knowelden et al. 1964). Bone mass decreases with age in both sexes (Horsman 1976a), more rapidly in females than in males (Morgan 1973), and bone strength depends on bone mass (Currey and Horsman 1981). It is therefore generally accepted that a causative association between age-related bone loss and increasing fracture risk exists, although other age-related variables

such as increasing incidence of falls might be additional risk factors.

A model capable of explaining in semi-quantitative terms the relationship between amount of bone and fracture risk was first described by Newton-John and Morgan in 1968. A more recent approach enables evaluation of the characteristics of populations in which amount of bone in the young adult, age of onset of bone loss and subsequent bone loss all vary between individuals (Horsman et al. 1985). A linear model of bone loss is used to predict femoral fracture incidence and an exponential model to predict the age-specific incidence of fractures of the distal radius. The model is stochastic, and the age-specific incidence of fractures is calculated by simulating the effects of ageing a large cohort of individuals from 20 to 100 years. Every individual is randomly allocated a particular amount of bone at age 20, an age of onset of bone loss, and values of parameters which determine the subsequent bone loss. Fracture risk is assumed to be zero when the amount of bone is above a global threshold level, increasing progressively as the amount of bone falls below the threshold. From the individual fracture risks, fracture cases are identified as the cohort ages and fracture incidence is evaluated numerically.

By adjusting the mean values of the linear model parameters, predicted and observed age-specific

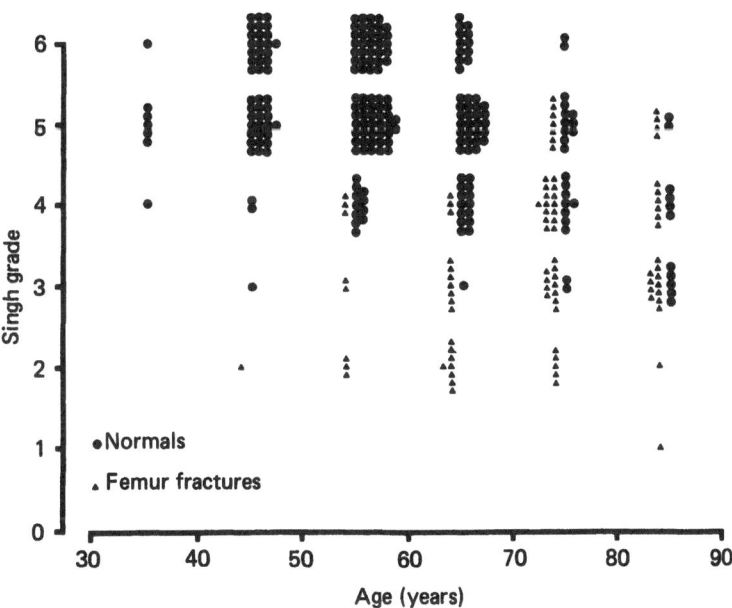

Fig. 17.4. Singh grade of the proximal femur in normal females and in females with femoral neck fractures.

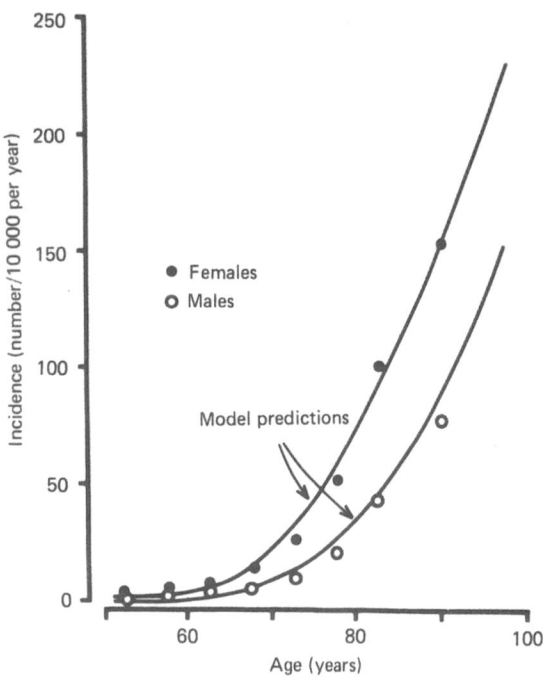

Fig. 17.5. Age-specific incidence of femoral neck fractures in Leeds. The curves are predictions of the stochastic model of age-related bone loss and fracture risk.

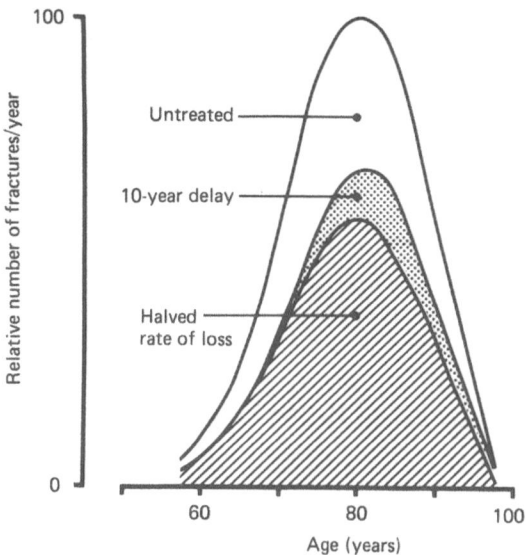

Fig. 17.6. Effect on fracture incidence of treating half the female population at random with therapy which either delays the age of onset of bone loss by 10 years or halves the rate of bone loss from the age of onset to the end of life.

incidences of femoral neck fracture can be closely matched in both sexes (Fig. 17.5). The only difference between the two simulations generating the male and female incidence curves in Fig. 17.5 was the value of the young adult amount of bone, implying that it is not *necessary* to invoke differences in the rate of bone loss between the sexes in order to explain the different fracture rates, as has previously been suggested (Nordin 1973).

The model has also been used to predict the effects on subsequent fracture risk of treatments designed to modify normal age-related bone loss; values of the model parameters affected by treatment are changed and the predicted incidence is recomputed. Figure 17.6 shows the effects of two different types of treatment on fracture incidence, mortality of the population as a whole having been taken into account; the areas under the curves are proportional to the total number of fractures. A treatment which delays the onset of bone loss in females is hormone replacement therapy (Horsman et al. 1977a), although at the lower doses now used to control menopausal symptoms the protective effect is reduced (see Fig. 17.2). There is some evidence that calcium supplementation can halve the rate of bone loss (Recker et al. 1977; Nordin et al. 1979). Whatever form treatment might take, delaying the onset

of bone loss by 10 years or halving the rate of bone loss from the age of onset to the end of life would have about the same effect on fracture incidence: if 50% of the population were treated at random, it would be reduced by 40%–50%.

The benefit of screening procedures, such as Singh grading and the other techniques described above, in optimizing the allocation of prophylactic therapies have also been evaluated using simulation techniques (A. Horsman and D. H. Marshall unpublished data 1985). If the whole population were to be screened in middle age to identify those individuals who comprised the lowest 25% of the distribution of amount of bone at the fracture site, then the model predicts that treatment of that 25% would have the same effect on fracture incidence as treating 50% of the population at random.

References

Adams P, Davies GT, Sweetnam PM (1969) Observer error and measurements of the metacarpal. Br J Radiol 42:192–197

Adams P, Davies GT, Sweetnam PM (1970) Osteoporosis and the effects of ageing on bone mass in elderly men and women. Q J Med 39:601–615

Armes FM, Horsman A, Bentley HB (1979) Effects of rotation

on radiographic dimensions of the metacarpals. Radiography 45:172–175

Barnett E, Nordin BEC (1960) The radiological diagnosis of osteoporosis. Clin Radiol 11:166–174

Cameron JR, Sorenson J (1963) Measurement of bone mineral in vivo: an improved method. Science 142:230–232

Christiansen C, Rødbro P (1977) Long-term reproducibility of bone mineral content measurements. Scand J Clin Lab Invest 37:321–323

Colbert C, Garrett C (1969) Photodensitometry of bone roentgenograms with an on-line computer. Clin Orthop 65:39–45

Cooper C, Barker DJP, Hall AJ (1985) Evaluation of the Singh index and femoral calcar width as epidemiological methods for measuring bone mass in the femoral neck. Clin Radiol 37:123–125

Currey JD, Horsman A (1981) Strength of the distal radius. In: Stokes AF (ed) Mechanical factors and the skeleton. Libbey, London, pp 91–97

Dequeker J (1972) Bone loss in normal and pathological conditions. University Press, Leuven

Garn SM (1970) The earlier gain and the later loss of cortical bone; in nutritional perspective. CC Thomas, Springfield (Illinois)

Garn SM, Rohmann CG, Wagner B (1967) Bone loss as a general phenomenon in man. Proc Fed Am Soc Exp Biol 26:1729–1736

Hall MC (1961) The trabecular patterns of the neck of the femur with particular reference to changes in osteoporosis. Can Med Assoc 85:1141–1144

Horsman A (1976a) Bone mass. In: Nordin BEC (ed) Calcium, phosphate and magnesium metabolism. Churchill Livingstone, Edinburgh, pp 357–404

Horsman A (1976b) Bone morphometry and densitometry. In: Nordin BEC (ed) Calcium, phosphate and magnesium metabolism. Churchill Livingstone, Edinburgh, pp 570–578

Horsman A, Kirby PA (1972) Geometric properties of the second metacarpal. Calcif Tissue Res 10:289–301

Horsman A, Simpson M (1975) The measurement of sequential changes in cortical bone geometry. Br J Radiol 48:471–476

Horsman A, Gallagher JC, Simpson M, Nordin BEC (1977a) Prospective trial of oestrogen and calcium in postmenopausal women. Br Med J ii:789–792

Horsman A, Reading DH, Connolly J, Bateman JE, Glasgow W, McLachlan MSF (1977b) Bone mass measurement using a xenon-filled multiwire proportional counter as detector. Phys Med Biol 22:1059–1072

Horsman A, Simpson M, Kirby PA, Nordin BEC (1977c) Nonlinear bone loss in oophorectomized women. Br J Radiol 50:504–507

Horsman A, Nordin BEC, Aaron J, Marshall DH (1981) Cortical and trabecular osteoporosis and their relation to fractures in the elderly. In: DeLuca HF (ed) Osteoporosis: recent advances in pathogenesis and treatment. University Park Press, Baltimore, pp 175–184

Horsman A, Nordin BEC, Simpson M, Speed R (1982) Cortical and trabecular bone status in elderly women with femoral neck fracture. Clin Orthop 166:143–151

Horsman A, Jones M, Francis R, Nordin BEC (1983) The effect of oestrogen dose on postmenopausal bone loss. N Engl J Med 309:1405–1407

Horsman A, Marshall DH, Peacock M (1985) A stochastic model of age-related bone loss and fractures. Clin Orthop 195:207–215

Horsman A, Armes FM, Simpson M (1986) Application of cusums to the analysis of sequential measurements of bones. Int J Math Model 7:981–990

Kleerekoper M, Parfitt AM, Ellis BI (1984) Measurement of vertebral fracture rates in osteoporosis. In: Christiansen C, Arnaud CD, Nordin BEC, Parfitt AM, Peck WA, Riggs BL (eds) Osteoporosis I. Glostrup Hospital (Department of Clinical Chemistry), Glostrup (Denmark), pp 255–262

Knowelden J, Buhr AJ, Dunbar O (1964) Incidence of fractures in persons over 35 years of age. A report to the MRC working party on fractures in the elderly. Br J Prev Soc Med 18:130–141

Koch JC (1917) The laws of bone architecture. Am J Anat 21:177–298

Mazess RB (1984) Advances in single- and dual-photon absorptiometry. In: Christiansen C, Arnaud CD, Nordin BEC, Parfitt AM, Peck WA, Riggs BL (eds) Osteoporosis I. Glostrup Hospital (Department of Clinical Chemistry), Glostrup (Denmark), pp 57–63

Meema HE, Meema S (1969) Cortical bone mineral density versus cortical thickness in the diagnosis of osteoporosis: a roentgenologic–densitometric study. J Am Geriat Soc 17:120–141

Meema HE, Schatz DL (1970) Simple radiologic demonstration of cortical bone loss in thyrotoxicosis. Radiology 97:9–15

Morgan DB (1973) Ageing and osteoporosis, in particular spinal osteoporosis. Clin Endocr Metab 2:187–201

Newton-John HF, Morgan DB (1968) Osteoporosis; disease or senescence? Lancet I:232

Nordin BEC (1973) Metabolic bone and stone disease. Churchill Livingstone, Edinburgh

Nordin BEC, Horsman A, Marshall DH, Simpson M, Waterhouse GM (1979) Calcium requirement and calcium therapy. Clin Orthop 140:216–239

Nordin BEC, Horsman A, Crilly RG, Marshall DH, Simpson M (1980) Treatment of spinal osteoporosis in postmenopausal women. Br Med J 280:451–454

Price WA (1901) The science of dental radiology. Dent Cadmos 43:483

Recker RR, Saville PD, Heaney RP (1977) Sex hormones or calcium supplements diminish postmenopausal bone loss. Nebr State Med J 62:42

Singh M, Nagrath AR, Maini PS (1970) Changes in trabecular pattern of the upper end of the femur as an index of osteoporosis. J Bone Jt Surg [Am] 52:457–467

Singh M, Riggs BL, Beabout JW, Jowsey J (1972) Femoral trabecular pattern index for evaluation of spinal osteoporosis. Ann Intern Med 77:63–67

Virtama P, Helela T (1969) Radiographic measurements of cortical bone. Variations in a normal population between 1–90 years of age. Acta Radiol [Suppl] (Stockh) 293

18 Photon Absorptiometry

P. Tothill

Introduction 251
X-ray (or Photon) Densitometry 251
   Technique 251
   Limitations 252
Single Photon Absorptiometry 252
   Technique 252
   Limitations 253
Dual Photon Absorptiometry 254
   Choice of Isotope 254
   Technique 254
   Limitations 255
   Clinical Studies 256
   Conclusions 257
References 257

Introduction

Most quantitative methods for assessing bone mineral rely on the absorption of X-rays or gamma-rays by the relatively dense and high atomic number constituents of the skeleton. The first to be introduced was "X-ray densitometry" using continuous-spectrum X-rays with appropriate means of calibration, film as the detecting medium and an optical densitometer to measure blackening. Later came techniques using gamma-radiation and a scintillation detector. The term "densitometry" was also applied to these techniques initially, but more recently they have been characterized as "absorptiometry", which more closely reflects the actual principles involved. Although the X-ray methods rely on many of the same principles and could be termed "radiographic absorptiometry", there has been a tendency to retain "densitometry" to describe them.

X-ray (or Photon) Densitometry

Technique

X-ray densitometry has the advantage that little special equipment is required for the initial acquisition of an image. The radiograph can be obtained with standard hospital apparatus. It is necessary to compensate for variations in kilovoltage, exposure, film characteristics and processing by including a reference wedge located next to the body part in the radiograph. The wedge should be of similar effective atomic number and specific gravity to that of bone. A variety of materials has been used, including animal bone, ivory, mineral salt solution and aluminium or its alloys. The metal wedges can be reproduced more accurately and uniformly. Variable thicknesses of soft tissue should be compensated for, preferably by immersion of the body part in water.

The simplest measurements are made at a single defined position or at a few sites. A photodensitometer is used to measure the optical density of the film at a selected site and also that of the wedge image, so that the mineral mass equivalent can be deduced. If the bone thickness can be established from an orthogonal radiograph, mineral concentration is obtained. Such spot measurements have been made in the radius, ulna, metacarpal, phalanx, femur and tibia.

Choice and reproduction of site selection set a limit on the precision of spot measurements and an improvement can be obtained at the expense of complexity by scanning a profile across the bone image. A scanning microdensitometer is needed. The optical density of each point is compared with that of the wedge to obtain the mineral equivalent profile. Manual processing is possible, but tedious, and a computer or microprocessor attached to the densitometer is highly desirable. A further development is for multiple scans to be performed, to give a mean mineral density over a defined area. Such area scanning simplifies site identification and aids precision, but increases the time of film density measurement substantially.

Limitations

Even when attention is paid to thickness equalization, wedge selection, and standardization of exposure and processing, possible problems of scattered radiation, beam hardening, and non-uniformity of field intensity and energy and film development remain, so X-ray densitometry has a lower precision than gamma-ray absorptiometry. It has become less popular since the introduction of the latter technqiue; nevertheless it has yielded valuable results in the study of metabolic bone diseases and their responses to treatment (Colbert and Bachtell 1981).

Single Photon Absorptiometry

Photon absorptiometry was introduced to overcome the problems associated with the use of X-rays and film. A single-energy gamma-ray source eliminates varying output and beam hardening and a scintillation detector scanning across the measurement site copes with scatter and non-uniform film sensitivity and development. The technique was first described by Cameron and Sorenson in 1963; since then there have been many developments and refinements and much equipment is available commercially.

Technique

The amount of bone mineral in the path of the beam is derived from the attenuation over bone-plus-soft-tissue relative to that over soft-tissue alone. It is a requirement of the theory that the overall thickness of bone-plus-soft-tissue should be constant. For measurements of the femur the thigh can be squeezed between parallel plates. For the forearm, water bags or water-equivalent mouldable material can be used with similar plates, but most operators obtain a greater precision by immersing the arm in

a water bath. Early apparatus used a horizontal scan with the palm of the hand downwards; more recently it has been recognized that a vertical scan, with the hand gripping a rod, avoids twisting the wrist and improves the precision of positioning. The source is coupled to the detector by a C-arm and the combination driven across the limb of interest by motor. Collimators are fitted to both source and detector to define a narrow beam of gamma radiation. Pulses from the scintillation detector are fed through an amplifier to a pulse-height analyser to select the appropriate energy and minimize scattered radiation and are then counted.

If the logarithm of detected intensity is plotted as a function of position across the bone (Fig. 18.1) the area between the curve and the soft tissue baseline is proportional to the bone mineral in the slice of bone traversed by the photon beam. This area can be determined manually or by off-line computer, but all commercial instruments now incorporate microprocessors or computers that lead to an automatic readout of bone mineral content.

The lower the energy of the radiation, the higher the contrast between bone and soft tissue, but the lower the intensity at the detector, so a compromise is needed; availability in practice of a suitable source has also to be considered. A number of studies have been made of the optimum energy, which depends on the thickness of bone and soft tissue at the site investigated. In practice, forearm measurements are usually carried out using ^{125}I. The K-characteristic X-rays and gamma-ray emitted, at about 30 keV, are close to the ideal energy, although the departure from true monoenergy gives rise to possible problems of slight beam hardening. The main inconvenience of the source is its relatively short half-life of 60 days, which results in it requiring replacement three or four times a year. The 60-keV radiation from ^{241}Am is near optimum for thicker tissues such as the thigh and it has been used for the forearm, when the lower costs associated with the 458 year half-life were more important than the loss of precision.

Other compromises have to be made between activity, collimator and source dimensions and scanning speed. A typical set of parameters for forearm scanning is: ^{125}I activity 4 GBq, beam diameter 2 mm, scanning speed 2 mm/s, 1-mm steps, time for six scans 5 minutes.

The result of the computation of bone mineral content may be in arbitrary units peculiar to the particular apparatus, but is better converted to the mass of a defined standard by experimental calibration. The width of the bone can also be obtained from the count-rate profile, and division by this factor gives a degree of normalization for body size.

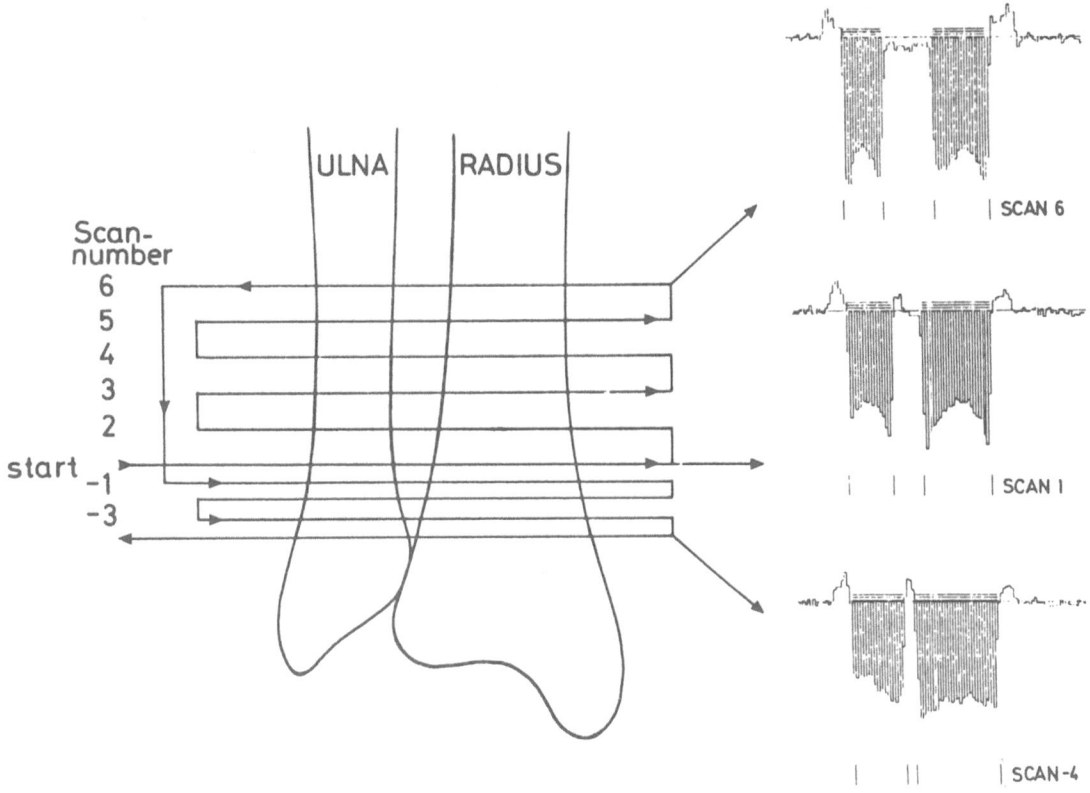

Fig. 18.1. Measurement set-up in forearm with examples of scan printouts. Fat correction is illustrated by horizontal lines moving baseline upwards. (From Nilas et al. 1985.)

Limitations

Because of the requirement for a constant, definable total tissue thickness, single photon absorptiometry is limited to the examination of the appendicular skeleton. By far the most attention has been paid to the forearm, but measurements have also been made of the femur, humerus, finger and calcaneus. A recent development has been the determination of bone mineral in the whole hand, necessitating a two-dimensional scan (Nicoll et al. 1985). Two-dimensional imaging of the wrist, allowing a retrospective selection of site of interest, has also been achieved by using a multi-wire proportional counter, avoiding any mechanical scanning (Horsman et al. 1977).

The theory of single photon absorptiometry requires that there be only two phases present: bone and homogeneous soft tissue. In many cases this is not true; fat has a lower attenuation than muscle and manifests itself as "negative bone". The effect is seen in Fig. 18.1, as a hump in the scan profile adjacent to the bone. The distribution of fat across

the wrist is far from uniform. Some equipment makes allowance for the error by measuring the negative excursion and programming the computer to give a correction, based on the assumption of a shell of fat of uniform thickness around the bone.

Probably the biggest limitation of precision, particularly in measurements of the forearm, is the reproducibility of the position of the scan. It was usual for this to be based on manual location of the radial or ulnar styloid, the scan being performed a defined distance proximal to this point. Accurate location is not easy, so there is a tendency to use a scan site where the bone mineral content is not changing greatly with position; sites one third or one half the bone length from the styloid tip have commonly been used. These positions are in the shafts and the bone almost entirely cortical.

As there is a desire to include more trabecular bone, more distal sites are to be preferred and more objective location required. Modern equipment makes this possible by automatically selecting the scan site from the scan itself, using the distance between the radius and ulna as the criterion

(Christiansen et al. 1975). Separations of 6 or 8 mm are common, and it is usual to perform six scans, 4 mm apart, proximal to this point. This repetition minimizes the repositioning error and improves the precision. However, in this area trabecular bone constitutes less than 25% of the total. Recently, Awbrey and colleagues (1984) and Nilas and others (1985) have extended the scan procedure by obtaining additional scans distal to the same starting point, making measurements where up to half the bone is trabecular (Fig. 18.1).

There is no doubt that commercial equipment currently available has eliminated the subjectivity of site selection. Automatic scan control and data processing have also made the apparatus easy to use.

Dual Photon Absorptiometry

In parts of the body such as the trunk it is impossible to achieve a constant thickness of soft tissue. Even if the external dimensions could be standardized, with a water bath for example, the amount of bowel gas remains unknown and variable. The simultaneous measurement of the transmission of gamma radiation of two different energies provides the basis of a method to compensate for different soft tissue thicknesses and permits the determination of bone mineral in the spine and hip. The technique was developed by Reed (1966), Roos and colleagues (1970) and Mazess and co-workers (1970). In areas where soft tissue thickness can be controlled, dual photon absorptiometry can be applied to determine another phase, for example fat, in addition to bone.

Choice of Isotope

There have been several theoretical studies of the optimum radiation energies required (Watt 1975; Smith et al. 1983). The optimum combination depends on the likely soft tissue thickness and amount of bone mineral; the calculations also predict the best ratio of beam intensities. For an average trunk thickness of 20 cm and bone mineral density of 1 g/cm^2, the optimum lower energy is about 40 keV; the higher energy is not very critical, as long as it is not less than 100 keV. The first measurements used ^{241}Am (60 keV) with ^{137}Cs (662 keV). This combination has the attraction of long half-life and relatively low cost. The former has

the concomitant disadvantage of low specific activity, self-absorption and the need for a relatively large source diameter if high activities are used, which leads to poor resolution. ^{137}Cs needs substantial shielding and the detecting crystal must be of a reasonable size to ensure good photo-peak efficiency.

^{153}Gd provides, in a single radionuclide, a combination of energies and abundances that is close to ideal. The electron capture process gives 44 keV characteristic X-rays and gamma-rays close to 100 keV. The half-life is rather short (240 days), though source size can therefore be small. Shielding and detector requirements are minimal. The use of ^{153}Gd leads to the theoretical coefficient of variation on statistical grounds being two thirds of that achieved with ^{241}Am/^{137}Cs. Its main disadvantage is the need to change sources every 12–18 months and the relatively high cost of doing so. At times there have been difficulties in the availability and radionuclide purity of ^{153}Gd, but these seem to have been largely overcome. All commercially available apparatus uses ^{153}Gd. Recently, however, dual-energy X-ray absorptiometry has been introduced. The two energies are obtained either by using K-edge filtration (Mazess et al. 1988) or by rapidly switching the tube potential (Wahner et al. 1988). Better precision and a shorter measurement time are claimed.

Technique

In early studies of the spine, Roos and colleagues (1970) used X-rays and an image intensifier to localize the vertebra of interest and then substituted their ^{241}Am/^{137}Cs source/detector combination to measure bone mineral. All subsequent workers have carried out a two-dimensional scan, formed a bone mineral image and then selected the area of interest from it (Fig. 18.2).

The mechanical requirements of coupling source and detector movement were readily met by modifying dual-headed radionuclide emission scanners, which were becoming redundant. Data were stored and processed off-line. Transmission scanning is more demanding on the nucleonics, in view of the high counting rates encountered, and there is no doubt that purpose-built apparatus, with on-line computing, has improved precision and simplified operation. Compromises of source activity, detector collimation, scanning speed and acceptable counting rates still have to be made, but these are largely chosen by the manufacturer. For measurements on the lumbar vertebrae a typical scanning time is 30 minutes.

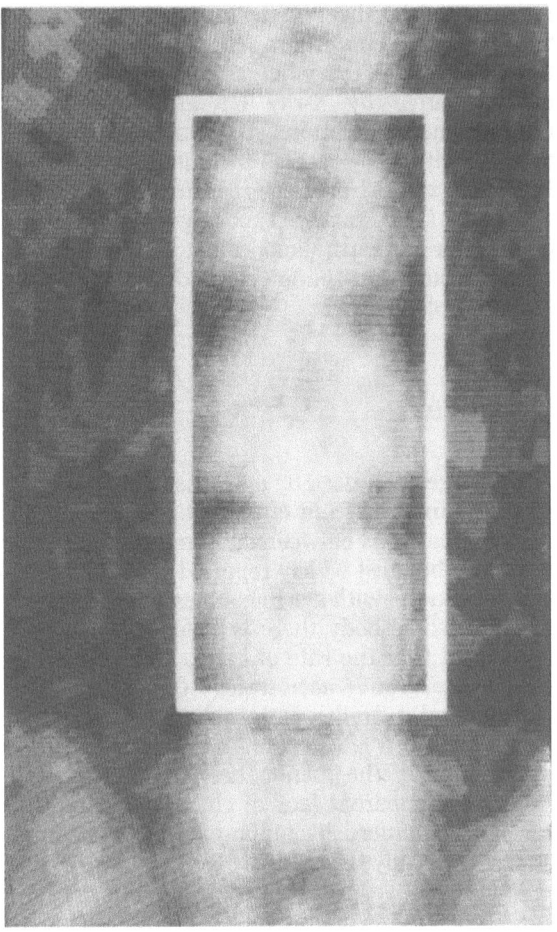

Fig. 18.2. Bone mineral image of lumbar vertebrae, with region of interest selected.

For each pixel of the scan the computer takes in the outputs from both energy channels, corrects for crossover and any dead-time losses, performs the attenuation calculations and produces a figure proportional to bone mineral, to be displayed on a TV screen and/or printed on paper. The operator then selects the area of interest; it is also necessary to select a soft tissue background area lateral to the bone above which bone mineral is determined. Such selection may be by the operator or automatically by the apparatus.

The total bone mineral is obtained either in arbitrary units or, with appropriate calibration, in grams of bone mineral. In the spine expression of total mineral in a number of lumbar vertebrae (commonly three) reduces problems due to compression fractures (Krølner and Pors Nielsen 1980), although identification and boundary selection are then much more difficult and there is no normalization for size. Division by the length considered gives a value in g/cm, providing some normalization and reducing the variation due to inappropriate site selection. If an image edge-detection system is available, the width of bone can be determined, leading to bone density in g/cm^2. This area density may be thought to give the most appropriate normalization, but the spinous processes complicate the determination of lateral borders, and the edge-detection routine may be dependent on source activity.

Limitations

The theory of dual-energy absorptiometry allows for variable soft tissue thicknesses, but not for differences of composition. Fat is a particular problem in spine measurements. Superficial fat may be reasonably uniform in thickness, and therefore modify only the background, but intraperitoneal fat is markedly non-uniform. Its effect can often be seen as a slope lateral to the vertebrae on a scan profile, but recognition does not suffice. Variable fat overlying the vertebral bodies, or contained within them, remains undetected. The presence of fat affects the accuracy of bone mineral determination, but may also influence the precision, as the soft tissue background may be more uncertain.

Dual-photon absorptiometry has mostly been applied to the spine, but is increasingly used for measurements of the neck of femur. Theoretically any part of the skeleton can be examined and there have been reports of the measurement of total bone mineral (Peppler and Mazess 1981). The technical problems become more difficult, as a wide range of counting rates is encountered, leading to dead-time problems. The biggest problem concerns fat; it is theoretically impossible using only two energies to characterize a three-phase system. The pragmatic solution is to program the computer to determine the average amount of fat in the "non-bone" area of the body and then assume that it is the same over the skeleton. Total body bone mineral measured by absorptiometry correlated highly with total body calcium measured by neutron activation analysis (Mazess et al. 1981), but the acceptability of the method in disease states remains unproven.

The theoretical solution to a multi-phase system is the use of additional gamma-ray energies. There have been a few experiments on these lines, but although accuracy may be improved, reproducibility is worsened. It may be that the use of semiconductor detectors, with their much better energy resolution, would offer an improvement, permitting the determination of other constituents than bone.

The absorbed radiation dose from absorptiometry procedures is acceptably low, around 0.1 mGy, to a relatively small volume of tissue. It is comparable to the dose from X-ray densitometry or morphometry and much less than that from the alternative bone mineral determination techniques of X-ray CT or neutron activation analysis. There is, therefore, no difficulty in justifying repeated measurements for longitudinal studies.

It is quite easy to establish the precision, or reproducibility, of absorptiometry by repeated measurements on individuals or groups. For measurements in the forearm, using automatic site selection, the coefficient of variation can be as good as 1% in normal subjects provided attention is paid to calibration. Precision may be worse with demineralized subjects. The quoted coefficients of variation of dual photon measurements of the spine in normal subjects have ranged from about 2% to 4%; osteoporosis or obesity can worsen the precision markedly.

It is not so easy to assess accuracy, or the concordance between what is measured and the true value. Experiments in which excised bones have been scanned and then ashed for a direct determination of mineral have shown a very high correlation with measured values. However, this does not necessarily demonstrate that the calibration figure used in vivo is correct. For longitudinal studies or comparisons between groups made using the same apparatus, precision is the important factor. Comparisons between centres demand accuracy and some apparent differences between normal populations suggest that more attention needs to be paid to calibration procedures.

Comparisons between results obtained at different parts of the skeleton and by different techniques are very important. Can relatively simple and cheap techniques such as forearm absorptiometry be used to predict spine or whole-skeleton status? The answer seems to be "not well enough". Several such comparisons have yielded a correlation coefficient between measurements on the two sites in normal subjects of about 0.6. The correlation is worse in osteoporotic subjects and the parameters of the regression equations differ between the disease groups. Although such correlations may be statistically highly significant, they lead to a 95% confidence interval for the prediction of lumbar spine density from radial density in an individual at about $\pm 25\%$ – no better than a prediction based on sex, size and age. The differences are biological, not a function of measurement techniques. If bone mineral in the spine is the parameter of interest it should be measured directly.

Better agreement is obtained when the same site is measured by different techniques. For example Sambrook and co-authors (1985) found a correlation coefficient of 0.8 when comparing spine densities measured by X-ray CT and dual photon absorptiometry. A more stringent comparison is between changes revealed in longitudinal studies. Few such studies have been reported, but Smith and colleagues (1981) showed good agreement between changes in forearm bone mineral measured by single photon absorptiometry and neutron activation analysis.

Clinical Studies

The changes produced by age, disease or treatment are often inferred from cross-sectional studies and here comparisons between sites and authors are of interest. The most widely reported variation is that of bone mineral with age in females. For the forearm and the whole body there is practically universal agreement that the rate of loss is small before the menopause, but accelerates thereafter. Most authors find a similar pattern for bone mineral in the spine, but a few report no acceleration of loss at the time of the menopause. In some of these studies the apparent lack of change of slope is an artefact introduced by inappropriate curve fitting procedures. Only the study by Riggs and colleagues (1981) demonstrated a more or less linear rate of loss from the age of about 30. The difference between their results and other authors is not understood (Smith and Tothill 1983).

For establishing changes with time, longitudinal studies are more satisfactory, though more time consuming and demanding high precision. Such studies have demonstrated a markedly increased rate of loss of spine bone mineral immediately after the menopause (Krølner and Pors Nielsen 1982).

From the point of view of individual subjects and for some group studies, the main value of bone mineral measurements is in predicting fracture risk. Many people have shown that osteoporotic subjects, as defined by vertebral crush fractures, have a mean bone mineral in various parts of the skeleton that is lower than that for age-matched control subjects. However, there is a great deal of overlap and such correlations do not reveal how well a particular measurement will predict the likelihood of a future fracture. There has been a dearth of the appropriate prospective studies, but recently Wasnich and colleagues (1985) have published the results of an investigation into the value of bone mineral measurements in predicting post-menopausal fracture risk. They found that the os calcis bone mineral content measurement was the best predictor of non-spinal fracture risk and, rather surprisingly, that it was also the best indicator of the risk of vertebral crush fracture. Such studies require a lot of effort over several years, but are important if a screening programme to identify subjects at greatest risk of sustaining a fracture is to be justified, so that preventive measures can be instituted.

Conclusions

Photon absorptiometry offers a precise method of measuring bone mineral in both the axial and appendicular skeleton. It has been used to study differences between groups, to deduce the effects of age or disease and to assess the results of treatment or prophylaxis. It is a low radiation dose, medium cost technique that lends itself to repeated measurements in longitudinal studies. Its value in measurements on individual subjects is not yet well established, but this aspect deserves further investigation. It seems likely that screening procedures may identify women with low peak bone mass as candidates for prophylactic measures such as hormone replacement therapy.

References

Awbrey BJ, Jacobson PC, Grubb SA, McCartney WH, Vincent LM, Talmage RV (1984) Bone density in women: a modified procedure for measurement of distal radial density. J Orthop Res 2:314–321

Cameron JR, Sorenson J (1963) Measurement of bone mineral in vivo: an improved method. Science 142:230–232

Christiansen C, Rödbro P, Jensen H (1975) Bone mineral content in the forearm measured by photon absorptiometry: principles and reliability. Scand J Clin Lab Invest 35:323–330

Colbert C, Bachtell RS (1981) Radiographic absorptiometry (photodensitometry). In: Cohn SH (ed) Non-invasive measurements of bone mass and their clinical application. CRC Press, Boca Raton, Florida, pp 51–84

Horsman A, Reading DH, Connolly J, Bateman E, Glasgow W, McLachlan MSF (1977) Bone mass measurement using a xenon-filled multiwire proportional counter as detector. Phys Med Biol 22:1059–1072

Krølner B, Pors Nielsen S (1980) Measurement of bone mineral content of the lumbar spine. I. Theory and application of a new two-dimensional dual-photon attenuation method. Scand J Clin Lab Invest 40:653–663

Krølner B, Pors Nielsen S (1982) Bone mineral content of the lumbar spine in normal and osteoporotic women: cross-sectional and longitudinal studies. Clin Sci 62:329–336

Mazess RB, Ort M, Judy P (1970) Absorptiometric bone mineral determination using 153Gd. In: Cameron JR (ed) Proceedings of bone measurement conference (Conference 700515). US Atomic Energy Commission, pp 308–312

Mazess RB, Peppler WW, Chesnut CH, Nelp WB, Cohn SH, Zanzi I (1981) Total body bone mineral and lean body mass by dual photon absorptiometry. II. Comparison with total body calcium by neutron activation analysis. Calcif Tissue Int 33:361–363

Mazess RB, Sorenson JA, Hanson JA, Collick BD (1988) Dual-photon X-ray absorptiometry. In: Ring EFJ, Evans WD, Dixon AS (eds). Proceedings of the Conference on Osteoporosis and Bone Mineral Measurement, Bath, April 1988. Institute of Physical Sciences in Medicine, York (in press)

Nicoll JJ, Smith MA, Tothill P, Reid D, Nuki G (1985) Single photon absorptiometry of the hand. Br J Radiol 58:823

Nilas L, Borg J, Gotfredsen A, Christiansen C (1985) Comparison of single and dual-photon absorptiometry in postmenopausal bone mineral loss. J Nucl Med 26:1257–1262

Peppler WW, Mazess RB (1981) Total body bone mineral and lean body mass by dual-photon absorptiometry. I. Theory and measurement procedure. Calcif Tissue Int 33:353–359

Reed GW (1966) The assessment of bone mineralization from the relative transmission of 241Am and 137Cs radiations. Phys Med Biol 11:174

Riggs BL, Wahner HW, Dunn WL, Mazess RB, Offord KP, Melton LJ (1981) Differential changes in bone mineral density of the appendicular and axial skeleton with aging. J Clin Invest 67:328–335

Roos B, Rosengren B, Skoldborn H (1970) Determination of bone mineral content in lumbar vertebrae by a double gamma-ray technique. In: Cameron JR (ed) Proceedings of bone measurement conference (Conference 700515). US Atomic Energy Commission, pp 243–253

Sambrook PN, Bartlett C, Evans R, Hesp R, Katz D, Reeve J (1985) Measurement of lumbar spine bone mineral: a comparison of dual photon absorptiometry and computed tomography. Br J Radiol 58:621–624

Smith MA, Tothill P (1983) Intra-laboratory variations using dual-photon absorptiometry. Phys Med Biol 28:748–750

Smith MA, Elton RA, Tothill P (1981) The comparison of neutron activation analysis and photon absorptiometry at the same part–body site. Clin Phys Physiol Meas 2:1–7

Smith MA, Sutton D, Tothill P (1983) Comparison between 153Gd and 241Am, 137Cs for dual-photon absorptiometry of the spine. Phys Med Biol 28:709–721

Wahner H, Morin R, Dunn W, Brown M, Riggs B (1988). Dual energy radiography for bone mineral analysis of the lumbar spine. J Nucl Med 29 (Supplement) 855

Wasnich RD, Ross PD, Heilbrun LK, Vogel JM (1985) Prediction of postmenopausal fracture risk with use of bone mineral measurements. Am J Obstet Gynaecol 153:745–751

Watt DE (1975) Optimum photon energies for the measurement of bone mineral and fat fractions. Br J Radiol 48:265–274

19 Quantitative Computed Tomography (QCT)

J.E. Adams

Introduction 259
Quantitative Computed Tomography (QCT) 261
    Technical Aspects 261
    Scanning Technique 263
    Precision, Accuracy and Radiation Dose and Comparison with Photon
      Absorptiometry 264
Clinical Applications 265
Future Developments 266
References 267

Introduction

Bone is a specialized form of connective tissue made up of organic (24%) and inorganic (76%) components. The organic component, or osteoid, is a collagen matrix containing non-collagenous proteins, and the inorganic or mineral component consists principally of calcium hydroxyapatite crystals. The adult skeleton is composed of two types of bone, compact bone (80%) and trabecular bone (20%). Compact bone forms the cortex of the bones and is found mainly in the shafts of the long bones. Trabecular or cancellous bone is found mainly in the bones of the axial skeleton (vertebral bodies and pelvis) and in the metaphyseal regions of long bones (proximal femur, distal radius). All the bones of the skeleton contain some compact and cancellous bone, although the amounts present vary with the anatomical site; both forms of bony tissue contribute to the strength of the bones. Bone tissue is continually being made and removed (bone turnover). During bone formation, osteoblasts lay down collagen fibres which then become mineralized: this process is influenced by various humoral, nutritional and physical factors. Bone is resorbed by osteoclasts which are stimulated by certain hormones (parathyroid and thyroid hormones), local humoral factors and by physical factors (immobilization). Bone resorption and bone formation are normally linked in an organized

sequence (Frost 1973), and both processes take place at bone surfaces (periosteal, endosteal and trabecular). Because of its more extensive surfaces relative to bone volume, trabecular bone is eight times more active in metabolic terms than cortical bone. This makes trabecular bone a more sensitive site for monitoring changes in bone mass.

Changes in bone mass can be divided into three phases (Parfitt 1983). During the growing period of life, there is a progressive accumulation of trabecular and cortical bone which accelerates during the adolescent growth spurt. Growth in length ends with epiphyseal fusion and at this stage 90% of the peak bone mass has been achieved. There then follows a period of consolidation of about 5 to 15 years during which the bony trabeculae become thickened and the cortical bone becomes less porous. Peak bone mass is achieved during the third decade, thereafter bone is lost progressively with advancing age. This age-related loss of bone occurs in two patterns and to varying extents in cortical and trabecular bone. In men and women there is a slow, continuous loss of bone which occurs at a rate of 0.3%–0.5% per annum, and begins at about the age of 40 years. At the menopause this loss of bone is accelerated and occurs at a rate of 2%–3% per annum: in some women this loss of bone may be as high as 10% ("fast" losers). Postmenopausal women become osteoporotic and on average lose about 35% of their cortical bone, and 50% of their trabecular bone during their lifetime (Riggs and

Melton 1986). As a result some develop the clinical syndrome of osteoporosis, where bone mass is reduced to an extent which causes mechanical failure of the skeleton and easy fracture. Whether the presence of fracture is a necessary criterion for the clinical diagnosis of osteoporosis is arbitrary, and some workers feel that a bone mass reduced below that expected for age and sex, irrespective of whether or not a fracture is present, is a more appropriate definition of osteoporosis in clinical practice (Stevenson and Whitehead 1982). Certainly the increased incidence of fractures which accompanies advancing age is related to other factors in addition to the reduced amount of bone, especially the propensity of the elderly to fall (Prudham and Evans 1981; Cummings et al. 1985; Ray et al. 1987; Kelsey and Hoffmann 1987).

Osteoporotic fractures occur predominantly in the vertebrae (wedge and crush fractures), femoral neck and distal radius, sites which are all rich in trabecular bone. The incidence of these fractures increases with advancing age and their combined incidence is 35%–40% in women over 65 years. In women the prevalence of vertebral wedge fractures has been estimated to be about 2.5% at the age of 50 years and 7.5% at 80 years of age (Nordin et al. 1980); these fractures lead to progressive dorsal kyphosis and loss of height. All these fractures, particularly those of the proximal femur, have important implications for the public health especially in relation to the cost of health services. The mortality following hip fractures has fallen with improved surgical management, but remains at between 15% and 20%; the incidence of fractures of the femoral neck is increasing at 6% per annum (Wallace 1983).

There is an increasing awareness among patients and doctors of the consequences of osteoporotic fractures not only to the patient, but to the community and health care system. Much effort has been channelled into identifying patients at risk, and the development of strategies for preventive therapy. It is now well established that oestrogens will prevent the rapid loss of bone which accompanies the menopause, and prevent or largely reduce the incidence of age-related osteoporotic fractures (Hutchinson et al. 1979; Weiss et al. 1980; Horsman et al. 1983; Ettinger et al. 1985; Cummings et al. 1985).

A precise, reproducible and sensitive non-invasive method of measuring cortical and trabecular bone mass is a desirable and necessary requirement for the study of age-related bone loss, the monitoring of treatment in osteoporosis and other metabolic bone diseases, and the identification of those at risk from developing osteoporotic frac-

ture. The established methods have been reviewed by Horsman (1976). *Precision* here means the longitudinal reproducibility in serial studies; *accuracy* means how closely the value measured by the technique reflects the actual bone mineral content, *sensitivity* indicates the capability of a measurement to separate an abnormal from a normal population or in longitudinal studies the ability to detect small changes in bone mass with time. The principal methods now in clinical use are radiogrammetry, photon absorptiometry and quantitative computed tomography. The anatomical site (cortical or trabecular, axial or appendicular), the technique used, the age of the patient and the predicted rate of change have important implications for the estimation of bone mass, and the minimum time interval necessary for longitudinal studies (Reinbold et al. 1986).

The measurement of cortical thickness in a peripheral skeletal site directly from radiographs (radiogrammetry) (Chap. 17) is simple, cheap and readily available; the most commonly measured site is the mid shaft of the second metacarpal. The method has provided useful population data in health and disease (Garn 1970), but the measurement reflects principally the effects of endosteal erosion in a peripheral cortical site only, and does not take into account intra-cortical porosity. The measurement is also subject to considerable observer variation (8%–11%) (Adams et al. 1969), which makes it relatively insensitive for measuring longitudinal changes among individual patients, except over very long periods of time. These peripheral cortical measurements also do not correlate closely with measurements of bone mass made in clinically more relevant areas, such as the spine.

Single photon absorptiometry (SPA) (Chap. 18) has been used for the measurement of cortical bone mass (midshaft of the radius), and for an integral measurement of cortical and trabecular bone mass combined (at the wrist). A large amount of normal data have been collected using this technique; the precision is 2%–3% and accuracy 6% (Cameron et al. 1968). As with radiogrammetry, the method is applicable only to peripheral skeletal sites. It measures principally cortical and integral bone, together with adjacent soft tissue. To overcome the inaccuracies introduced by marrow fat and overlying soft tissue, dual energy photon absorptiometry (DPA) was introduced (Chap. 18). This technique can be applied to the axial skeleton (spine, hip) and the whole body. The precision of the technique is 2%–3% and the accuracy 1%–2% with dipotassium hydrogen phosphate solutions and 4%–10% in vertebral specimens (Peppler and Mazess 1981). However, the inclusion of the cortical components

(35%) of the spine (neural arches, vertebral end plates), together with any adjacent mineral which lies in the path of the photon beam (aortic calcification, osteophytes and sclerotic apophyseal joints) introduces errors, and makes the method less sensitive to small changes in trabecular bone. Other techniques which have been applied to the measurement of bone mass include neutron activation analysis (Cohn and Dombrowski 1971), Compton scattering (Shukla et al. 1986), dual energy digital radiography (Fraser et al. 1986) and ultrasound (Langton et al. 1984), but these techniques are either not widely available, or their clinical relevance and applications are still being assessed.

The technique of quantitative digital radiography (QDR) which has recently been introduced may replace DPA in the near future (Sartoris et al. 1987). The method uses a polychromatic dual energy X-ray beam instead of an isotope source. Examination time is shorter (5 minutes compared with 20 minutes for DPA in the spine), spatial resolution is higher (2 mm vs 5 mm) and precision is improved (less than 1.0%). The limitations of the technique are, however, similar to DPA in that separate estimates of cortical and trabecular bone are not available and at present only an integral bone mineral measurement of a lumbar spine segment is possible.

Quantitative Computed Tomography (QCT)

Technical Aspects

With the introduction of computed tomography (CT) for imaging the brain, it became possible to demonstrate cross-sectional anatomy and to make precise measurements of the linear X-ray attenuation coefficients of small elements (voxels) of tissue in vivo, expressed as Hounsfield units (HU) (Hounsfield 1973). Substances with density differences as small as 1 in 1000 could be differentiated (Rutherford et al. 1976). This permitted identification of substances with specific attenuation characteristics, such as fat (-100 HU), water (± 10 HU), soft tissue ($+40$ HU to 55 HU) and others, offering important diagnostic information (Williams et al. 1980). The implications for quantitative measurement of bone mass were soon appreciated and the application of

one of the original EMI CT brain scanners to bone mass measurement in the forearm showed it to be a precise method, with a reproducibility of 0.2% in vitro and 2% in vivo (Isherwood et al. 1976).

The introduction of general purpose scanners in the mid 1970s allowed QCT to be applied to more clinically relevant sites in the axial skeleton (spine and femoral neck), and the use of QCT in bone mass measurement has expanded since that time, particularly over the past 8 years. Several hundred centres around the world, particularly in the United States, now offer this CT application, although the limited availability of CT scanners for this purpose in the United Kingdom restricts QCT bone mass measurements to only a few centres at the present time.

QCT is unique amongst the noninvasive methods of bone mass measurement, in that it provides a precise three-dimensional anatomical display, allows separate estimation of trabecular and cortical bone and can be applied to both axial (Cann and Genant 1980) and appendicular (Jensen et al. 1980; Ruegsegger et al. 1981; Sartoris et al. 1986) skeletal sites. QCT also provides a mineral density measurement per unit volume of bone, rather than the linear or area measurements of photon absorptiometry.

CT attenuation values are susceptible to a variety of errors, some of which may be energy dependent (Williams et al. 1980). Consideration of these potential sources of inaccuracies is obviously important when performing QCT, and efforts must be made to minimize their effects where possible. Some inaccuracies are inherent, either in the scanner (detector sensitivity, reconstruction algorithm, partial volume effect, field variability), or in the tissue being examined. Not all CT scanners are suited to QCT applications (Cann 1987a). The polychromaticity of the X-ray beam of commercial CT results in "beam hardening effects" – the lower energy photons being progressively absorbed as they pass through the body. To correct for this effect, and for any scanner instability, QCT examinations have to be performed with a calibration reference phantom containing various concentrations of material similar to that being measured. In QCT bone mass measurement these are solutions of dipotassium hydrogen phosphate (K_2HPO_4) which has similar X-ray attenuation characteristics to calcium hydroxyapatite. Several special-purpose, low dose CT scanners have been built in an effort to achieve a monoenergetic X-ray beam using an I^{125} source, but these are only applicable to the appendicular skeleton (Ruegsegger et al. 1981; Hangartner and Overton 1982; Hosie and Smith 1986). Unless a structure is homogeneous and completely fills the width of the CT slice, the attenuation value of a voxel or region of

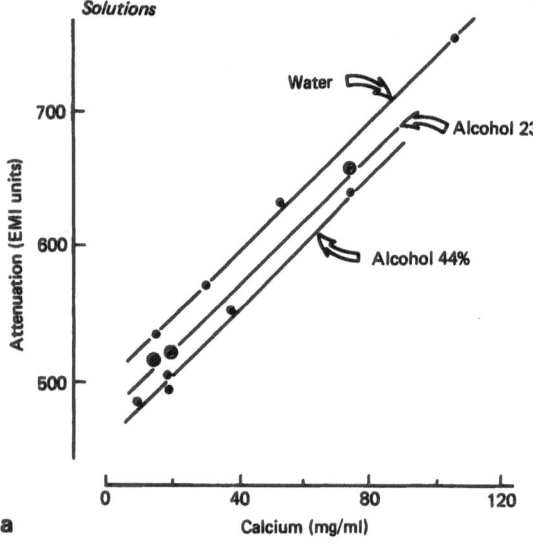

Fig. 19.1. a The relation between single energy QCT attenuation values (1 EMI unit = 2 HU) and calcium content showing that by increasing the proportion of ethyl alcohol (used to simulate fat) in an aqueous calcium chloride solution, the attenuation for each calcium concentration is reduced. **b** Relation between calcium concentration of trabecular bone of the distal femur (measured by chemical analysis) and single energy CT attenuation values and, **c**, the improved relation between calcium concentration and atomic number derived from a simultaneous dual energy QCT technique (Adams et al. 1982, reproduced from J Comput Assist Tomogr with permission).

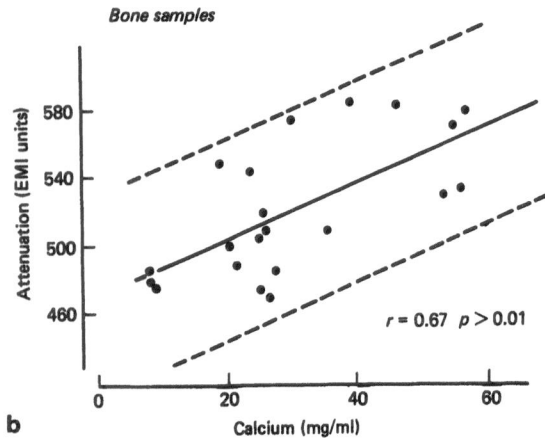

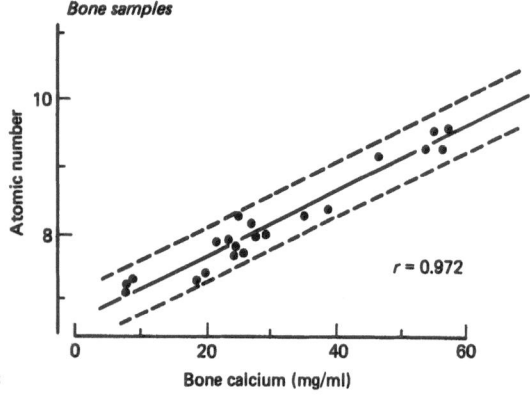

interest will be a mean value for all the components within that volume and will not reflect independently the individual constituents. This leads to another source of inaccuracy, the partial volume effect (Cann 1987b). In vitro studies have shown that there is a close and highly significant positive relation between CT attenuation values and the calcium concentration of compact bone (r = 0.994) (Posner and Griffiths 1977). This relationship is less strong for trabecular bone (r = 0.67) (Adams et al. 1982). This difference is explicable in terms of the differences in the composition of these two forms of bony tissue. Trabecular bone is heterogeneous and is composed of a mineralized collagenous matrix (bone), fat, water and other soft tissues. In whole bones fat is distributed in the medullary cavity and in between bony trabeculae. The amount of fat varies with age and, perhaps also, with the amount of bony tissue present (Dickerson 1962; Meunier et al. 1971). The presence of fat will reduce the CT attenuation value (Fig. 19.1a) and cause single energy QCT to underestimate the amount of trabecular bone mineral present (Adams et al. 1982; Cann 1987b). Theoretical considerations suggest, and experimental data confirm, that this problem can be reduced by scanning at two different energies – dual energy QCT (Genant and Boyd 1977). Dual energy scanning exploits the differential effects of X-ray attenuation by the photoelectric and Compton component by different substances, giving information on electron density and atomic number. With trabecular bone a much stronger correlation has been found between mineral concentration and atomic number derived from dual energy CT (r = 0.972) than between mineral concentration and single energy attenuation value (r = 0.67) (Adams et al. 1982) (Fig. 19.1b & c).

Dual energy CT can be performed by a variety of techniques, either simultaneously or by performing two separate scans at different energies (Ritchings and Pullen 1979; Rutt and Fenster 1980; Laval-Jeantet et al. 1984; Genant et al. 1987). The increased accuracy of dual energy CT is obtained at

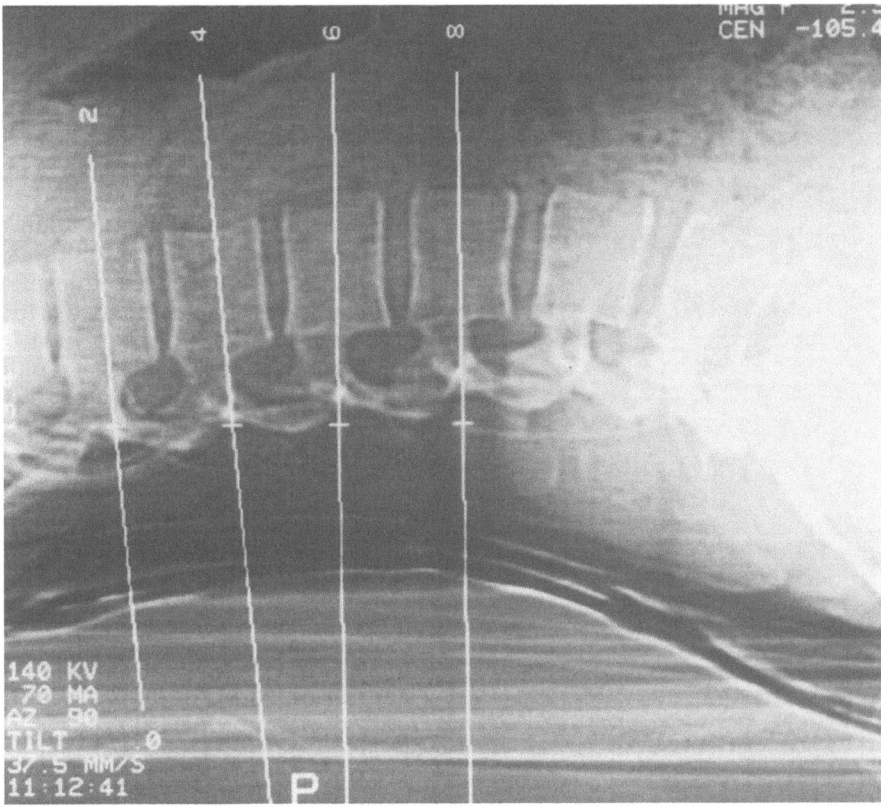

Fig. 19.2. Annotated lateral scanned projection radiograph indicating the plane of the scans obtained at QCT through the middle of each vertebral body from T_{12} to L_3.

the cost of some reduction in precision, increase in radiation dose and considerable technical effort, which may not be feasible except in a research setting. Attempts to overcome these difficulties have been made with the application of an age-related correction for vertebral trabecular fat based on the data of Dunnill et al. (1967). The majority of QCT bone mass measurements are therefore derived from a single energy technique which Genant believes to be adequate for longitudinal studies where precision is paramount (Genant 1985). The increased accuracy and qualitative information of dual energy CT may be more important in comparative studies between different patient groups.

Scanning Technique

Single Energy

The patient lies supine on the scan table with the phantom placed below and adjacent to the lumbar spine with an intervening small water pillow, so that the minimum of air lies adjacent to the phantom. The knees are flexed over a 90° supporting pillow to flatten the lumbar lordosis, and the feet are secured symmetrically in a foot rest. The arms are elevated out of the scanning field. Initially a lateral scanned projection radiograph is obtained and a cursor is placed to define the scanning plane through the mid-vertebral body, parallel to the end plate (Fig. 19.2). An antero-posterior projection radiograph may be obtained to check for any scoliosis which may cause end plates to be included in the CT section. A low dose technique for scanning can be used (80 kV, 70 mA, 2 s) and sections performed with appropriate gantry angulation through the midplane of four adjacent vertebrae, generally L_{1-4} or T_{12} to L_3. The scanning takes 10–15 minutes. The digital analysis is performed at the physicians' console and takes an additional 20 minutes. For each section the attenuation of the calibration solutions is measured (Fig. 19.3) and the regression line and intercept is plotted. A region of interest (ROI),

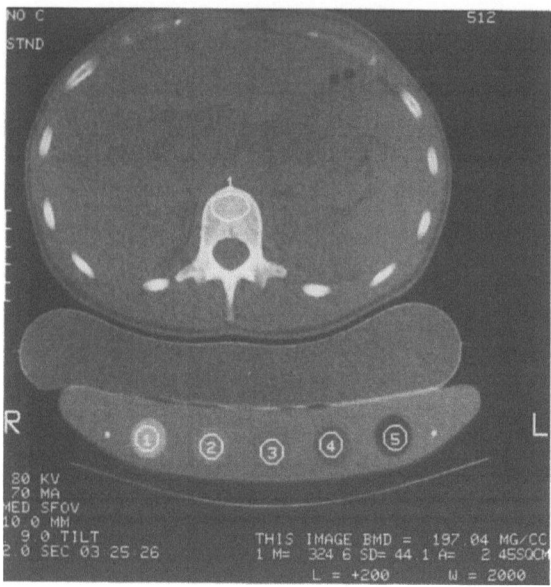

Fig. 19.3. CT scan through the midplane of a lumbar vertebra. The patient is lying on the crescentic calibration phantom containing a water reference and different concentrations of K_2HPO_4. Attenuation values are obtained from the trabecular bone of the vertebral body. A water bag is interposed between the patient and the phantom to eliminate air from this gap.

usually elliptical, is placed over the vertebral trabecular bone, avoiding any cortical bone and the entry of the basi-vertebral vein (Fig 19.3). An attenuation value is obtained and from the regression line of the calibration solutions, the attenuation value can be converted into a bone mineral density (BMD), expressed as bone mineral equivalents in mg/ml. The BMD is usually the mean value for the four vertebrae scanned. The BMD value measured is compared with the age-matched data from a normal population (Cann and Genant 1980) (Fig 19.4). Many of the steps in this analysis program have now been automated (and are commercially available), thus speeding up what otherwise can be a tedious and time consuming procedure. If vertebral wedge fractures are present, it may be necessary to perform narrower 5 mm slices, but even then the end plate may still be included in the section (Fig. 19.5) leading to a falsely high BMD value. Such data should be omitted from the digital analysis.

For consistent results it is important to keep the vertebra in the same position within the scan field (usually as close as possible to the centre) and to use an appropriate field size so that large patients do not extend outside the scanning field and influence the scanner reference detectors. Meticulous

attention to detail at all stages of the technique is imperative if the numerical measurements obtained are to be of any value.

Dual Energy

Several methods are available for dual energy scanning either using preprocessing (Rutt and Fenster 1980) or post-processing (Laval-Jeantet et al. 1984) techniques. The simplest method is to perform two single energy scans through the same plane, ensuring that the patient does not alter position and using different scanning parameters for each scan. A scanner which operates at different kVs is clearly essential. The data are analysed in the same way as with the single energy technique. The corrected BMD, where the effect of marrow fat is largely eliminated, is calculated using an appropriate formula (Laval-Jeantet et al. 1984).

Precision, Accuracy and Radiation Dose and Comparison with Photon Absorptiometry

Single energy QCT has a precision of 1%–3%, an accuracy of 1%–2% for K_2HPO_4 solutions and 5%–15% for human vertebrae (Genant 1985). Using the technique described, the radiation dose is 1.75–2.0 mG (175–200 mrem dose equivalent) per examination, about one tenth of the dose for a conventional CT examination of the spine. Even lower

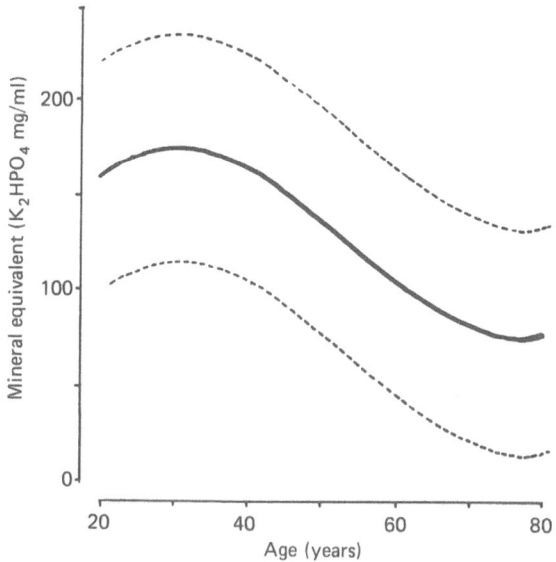

Fig. 19.4. Normal female vertebral trabecular bone mineral content expressed as mineral equivalents of K_2HPO_4 in mg/ml related to age (derived from the data of Cann and Genant 1980).

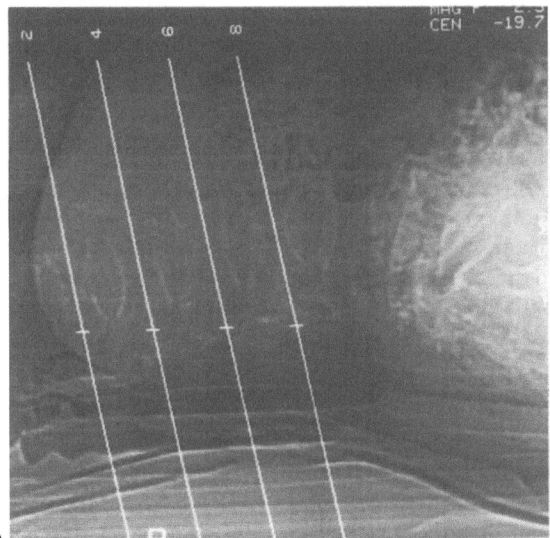
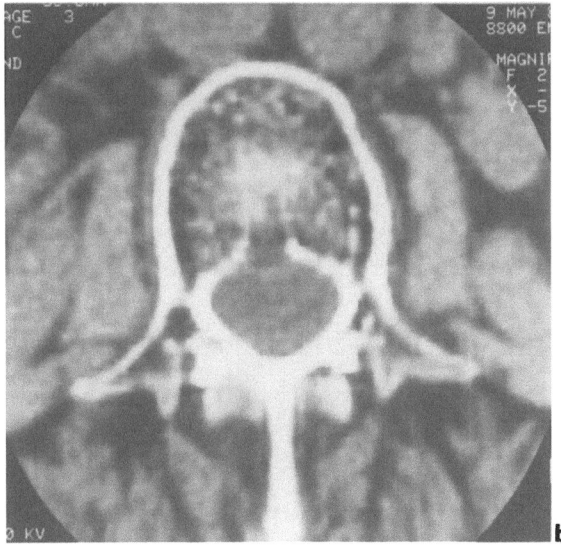

Fig. 19.5. a Annotated lateral scanned projection radiograph in a patient with severe osteoporosis and vertebral fractures. Thinner (5 mm) sections have to be used, but the vertebral end plate may still be included in the CT section. b There is increased attenuation of the central trabecular bone and consequent over-estimation of bone mineral. Such data must be excluded from the analysis.

doses are feasible and still yield useful quantitative data (Cann 1981). This is an important consideration in a measurement which is to be repeated at intervals over time.

Dual energy CT improves the accuracy of the technique to 3%–6% but with some loss of precision. There is also a doubling of radiation dose. With SPA the precision is 2%–4%, accuracy 1%–6% and an extremely low radiation dose equivalent of 2–5 mrem. DPA precision is 1%–3%, accuracy 1%–2% with K_2HPO_4 solutions and 4%–6% in vertebral phantoms; radiation dose equivalent 5–15 mrem. The cost of a QCT is estimated in the USA to be $150–300 and that of DPA $75–200. Certainly CT scanners (£250 000–£600 000) are more expensive than SPA (£20 000) or DPA (£60 000) equipment, but in its other applications CT is more versatile than single or dual energy photon absorptiometry, which can only be used for the measurement of bone mass. The three techniques are therefore similar in their precision and accuracy, but QCT has been shown to be the more sensitive technique for monitoring small changes in trabecular bone mass with time or in response to treatment (Genant et al. 1982; Reinbold et al. 1986; Ettinger et al. 1987). QCT carries a higher radiation dose but this can be minimized by using a low dose technique.

Clinical Applications

QCT has been widely applied to the measurement of bone mass in a variety of metabolic bone disorders, and has been shown to provide useful clinical information. QCT can detect age-related changes in vertebral trabecular bone in the normal population (decrements males −0.72% and females −1.2% per year) (Cann et al. 1985) and the accelerated loss in females at the menopause (up to −5.6% per year) (Firooznia et al. 1986). The data obtained by Cann and Genant (1980) (Fig. 19.4) are generally used as the reference for the normal age-matched BMD values. There is evidence to suggest, however, that this may not be appropriate for all populations, even those of similar ethnic backgrounds (Compston et al. 1988). QCT has demonstrated a reduction in bone mass in amenorrhoeic women (Cann et al. 1984) and a reversible loss of bone in women receiving a gonadotrophin releasing hormone agonist for endometriosis (Cann et al. 1987). As QCT permits the separate measurement of vertebral trabecular bone mass, it is the most sensitive technique available for monitoring changes in BMD at this site, either with time or therapeutic regimes (Genant et al. 1982; Reinbold et al. 1986).

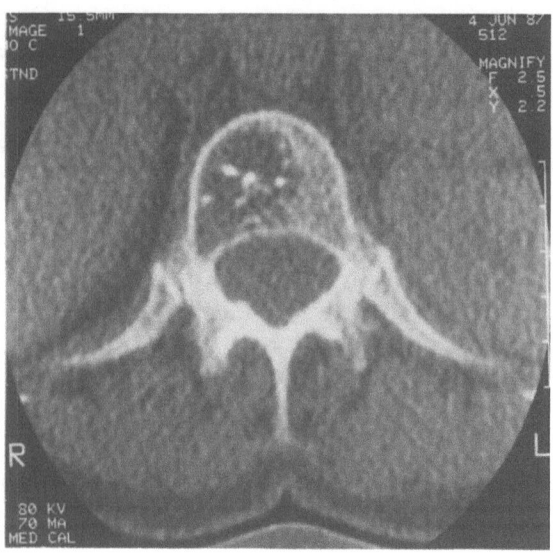

Fig. 19.6. CT section through a vertebral body with heterogenous distribution of trabecular bone. Study of this pattern of bone loss may contribute towards improvement in fracture prediction from QCT measurement.

The relation between fracture prevalence and vertebral trabecular mineral has been examined and there is a correlation of r = − 0.74, (Richardson et al. 1985); the incidence of fractures increases as the BMD falls progressively below 110 mg/ml and fractures are inevitable below 60–70 mg/ml, the so-called "fracture threshold" (Cann et al. 1985; Gallagher et al. 1985). However, in older women there is an overlap in the amount of bone between the normal population and those with osteoporotic fracture. This is perhaps to be expected since other factors apart from BMD are relevant in determining whether or not a fracture occurs, e.g. propensity to falls. A study to examine the relation between QCT vertebral BMD and compressive vertebral strength found only a weak correlation (r = 0.46) between these parameters (McBroom et al. 1985). This suggests that other factors, such as trabecular arrangement, may be relevant to determining bone strength.

There are many reports of the relationship of BMD measurements in both peripheral and central sites by the principal noninvasive methods of measurement. Although there is correlation between the different sites and methods (correlation coefficients between 0.3 and 0.9) the variability precludes the result from one measurement or site being used to predict that for another (Genant et al. 1987).

There has been recent discussion as to the value of population screening for osteoporosis (Ott 1986;

Hall 1987). Hall (1987) argues that since oestrogen therapy is claimed to be appropriate for many – perhaps most – postmenopausal women (Mac-Donald 1986) and that knowledge of age alone permits the prediction of bone mass in the spine and femoral neck to within ± 10% (Riggs and Melton 1986) widespread screening will contribute little to management, but the argument remains unresolved. A more selective use of BMD measurements would seem appropriate to identify those patients at particular risk of developing osteoporosis (Editorial Lancet 1985) and who would have most to gain from hormone replacement therapy. QCT also offers an effective and sensitive tool to study bone behaviour in general and in a variety of metabolic bone disorders.

Future Developments

The Cann and Genant calibration phantom is the one most widely used in QCT clinical studies, and a phantom and appropriate software of similar design is now available commercially (Arnold 1987). Several CT manufacturers have developed their own phantoms and bone mineral programs, and as the fluid K_2HPO_4 phantom has some limitations (accumulation of air in solutions with time) there has been a stimulus to develop solid but malleable hydroxyapatite phantom materials (International General Electric). However, data from one phantom cannot predict the results from another, and in longitudinal studies it is imperative always to examine the patient using the same phantom and technique. Although QCT results obtained on one scanner may be extrapolated to those obtained on another using the same scanning technique with a coefficient of variation of 3%–4% this may not always be the case (Genant 1985; Cann 1987a).

To increase further the precision of the technique, methods are being devised to automate the selection of not only the CT slice plane but also the region taken for analysis. More satisfactory techniques are being devised for examination of the hip by QCT (Gluer and Genant 1987), and image analysis techniques are being applied to look at the distribution of trabeculae from CT in addition to measuring the mineral content. The distribution of bone loss within the vertebrae may not be uniform (Fig. 19.6) and the identification of the pattern of this loss may provide additional predictive value of QCT to fracture risk (Dickie et al. 1987; Sandor et al. 1987).

References

Adams JE, Chen SZ, Adams PH, Isherwood I (1982) Measurement of trabecular bone mineral by dual energy computed tomography. J Comput Assist Tomogr 6:601–607

Adams PH, Davies GT, Sweetnam PM (1969) Observer error and measurements of the metacarpal. Br J Radiol 42:192–197

Arnold BA (1987) Automated software and Phantom improvements for bone mineral analysis by quantitative computed tomography. In:Genant HK (ed) Osteoporosis update. Radiology Research and Education Foundation, San Francisco, California, pp 197–202

Cameron JR, Mazess RB, Sorenson JA (1968) Precision and accuracy of bone mineral determination by direct photon absorptiometry. Invest Radiol 3:141–150

Cann CE (1981) Low dose CT scanning for quantitative spinal mineral analysis. Radiology 140:813–815

Cann CE (1987a) Quantitative CT applications: comparison of current scanners. Radiology 162:257–261

Cann CE (1987b) Quantitative computed tomography for bone mineral analysis: technical considerations. In Genant HK (ed) Osteoporosis update. Radiology Research and Education Foundation, San Francisco, California, pp 131–144

Cann CE, Genant HK (1980) Precise measurement of vertebral mineral content using computed tomography. J Comput Assist Tomogr 4:493–500

Cann CE, Martin MC, Genant HK, Jaffe RB (1984) Decreased spinal mineral content in amenorrheic women. JAMA 251:626–629

Cann CE, Genant HK, Kolb FO, Ettinger B (1985) Quantitative computed tomography for prediction of vertebral fracture risk. Metab Bone Dis Rel Res 6:1–7

Cann CE, Henzl M, Burry K et al. (1987) Reversible bone loss by GnRH agonist Nafarelin. In: Cohn DV, Martin TJ, Meunier PJ (eds) Calcium regulation and bone metabolism: basic and clinical aspects Vol 9, pp 123–127

Cohn SH, Dombrowski CS (1971) Measurement of total body calcium, sodium, chlorine, nitrogen and phosphorus in man by in vivo neutron activation analysis. J Nucl Med 12:499–505

Compston JE, Evans WD, Crawley EO, Evans C (1988) Bone mineral content in normal UK subjects. Br J Radiol 61:631–636

Cummings SR, Kelsey JL, Nevitt MC, O'Dowd KJ (1985) Epidemiology of osteoporosis and osteoporotic fractures. Epidemiol Rev 7:178–208

Dickerson JWT (1962) Changes in the composition of the human femur during growth. Biochem J 82:56–61

Dickie DL, Flynne MJ, Goldstein SA, Ge F (1987) The in-vitro multivariate correlation of vertebral regional bone mineral density measurements and compressive strength. In: Book of Abstracts of Sixth International Workshop on Bone and Soft Tissue Densitometry, 22–25 September 1987, Buxton, England, p 47

Dunnill MS, Anderson JA, Whitehead R (1967) Quantitative histological studies on age changes in bone. J Pathol Bacteriol 94:275–291

Ettinger B, Genant HK, Cann CE (1985) Long term estrogen replacement therapy prevents bone loss and fractures. Ann Int Med 102:319–324

Ettinger B, Genant HK, Cann CE (1987) Postmenopausal bone loss is prevented by treatment with low-dose oestrogen with calcium. Ann Int Med 106:40–45

Firooznia H, Rafii M, Golimbu C, Schwartz MS, Ort P (1986) Trabecular mineral content of the spine in women with hip fracture: CT measurement. Radiology 159:737–740

Fraser RG, Hickey NM, Niklason LT et al. (1986) Calcification in pulmonary nodules: detection with dual energy digital radiography. Radiology 160:595–601

Frost HM (1973) The origin and nature of transients in human bone remodelling dynamics. In: Frame B, Parfitt AM, Duncan H (eds) Clinical aspects of metabolic bone disease. Excerpta Medica, Amsterdam, pp 124–137

Gallagher C, Goldgar D, Mahoney P, McGill J (1985) Measurement of spine density in normal and osteoporotic subjects using computed tomography: relationship of spine density to fracture threshold and fracture index. J Comp Assist Tomogr 9:634–635

Garn SM (1970) The earlier gain and later loss of cortical bone. Nutritional perspectives. CC Thomas, Springfield, Illinois, pp 146

Genant HK (1985) Assessing osteoporosis: CT's quantitative advantage. Diagnostic Imaging 8:52–57

Genant HK, Boyd D (1977) Quantitative bone mineral analysis using dual energy computed tomography. Invest Radiol 12:545–551

Genant HK, Cann CE, Ettinger B, Gordan GS (1982) Quantitative computed tomography of vertebral spongiosa: A sensitive method for detecting early bone loss after oophorectomy. Ann Int Med 97:699–705

Genant HK, Block JE, Steiger P, Gluer CC (1987) Quantitative computed tomography in the assessment of osteoporosis. In: Genant HK (ed) Osteoporosis update. Radiology Research and Education Foundation, San Francisco, California, pp 49–71

Gluer CC, Genant HK (1987) Quantitative computed tomography of the hip. In: Genant HK (ed) Osteoporosis update. Radiology Research and Education Foundation, San Francisco, California, pp 187–195

Hall FM (1987) Bone-mineral screening for osteoporosis. AJR 149:120–122

Hangartner TN, Overton TR (1982) Quantitative measurement of bone density using gamma-ray computed tomography. J Comp Assist Tomogr 6:1156–1162

Horsman A (1976) Bone mass. In: Nordin BEC (ed) Calcium, phosphate and magnesium metabolism. Churchill Livingstone, Edinburgh, London, New York, pp 357–404

Horsman A, Jones M, Frances R, Nordin C (1983) The effect of oestrogen dose on postmenopausal bone loss. N Engl J Med 309:1405–1407

Hosie CJ, Smith DAS (1986) Precision of measurement of bone density with a special purpose computed tomography scanner. Br J Radiol 59:345–350

Hounsfield GM (1973) Computerised transverse axial scanning (tomography) I. Description of system. Br J Radiol 46:1016–1022

Hutchinson TA, Polansky SM, Feinstein AR (1979) Post menopausal oestrogens protect against fractures of hip and distal radius: a case-control study. Lancet II:705–709

Isherwood I, Rutherford RA, Pullan BR, Adams PH (1976) Bone mineral estimation by computer assisted transverse axial tomography. Lancet II:712–715

Jensen PS, Orphanoudakis SC, Rauschkolb EN, Baron R, Lang R, Rasmussen H (1980) Assessment of bone mass in the radius by computed tomography. Am J Radiol 134:285–292

Kelsey JL, Hoffmann S (1987) Risk factors for hip fracture. N Engl J Med 316:404–406

Lancet (Editorial) (1985) Risk factors in postmenopausal osteoporosis. I:1370–1372

Langton CM, Palmer SB, Porter RW (1984) The measurement of broadband ultrasonic attenuation in cancellous bone. Eng Med 13:89–91

Laval-Jeantet AM, Cann CE, Roger BM, Dallant P (1984) A post-processing dual energy technique for vertebral CT densitometry. J Comput Assist Tomogr 9:1164–1167

McBroom RJ, Hayes WC, Edwards WT, Goldberg RP, White AA (1985) Prediction of vertebral body compressive fracture using quantitative computed tomography. J Bone Joint Surg [Am] 67:1206–1214

MacDonald PC (1986) Estrogen plus progestin in postmenopausal women – act II. N Engl J Med 315:959–961

Meunier P, Aaron J, Edouard C, Vignon G (1971) Osteoporosis and the replacement of cell populations of the marrow by adipose tissue. A quantitative study of 84 iliac bone biopsies. Clin Orthop 80:147–154

Nordin BEC, Peacock M, Aaron J et al. (1980) Osteoporosis and osteomalacia. Clin Endocrinol Metab 9:177–205

Ott S (1986) Should women get screening bone mass measurements. (Editorial) Ann Intern Med 104:874–876

Parfitt AM (1983) Dietary risk factors for age-related bone loss and fractures. Lancet II:1181–1184

Peppler WW, Mazess RB (1981) Total body bone mineral and lean body mass by dual photon absorptiometry. I. Theory and measurement procedure. Calcif Tissue Int 33:353–359

Posner I, Griffiths HJ (1977) Comparison of CT scanning with photon absorptiometric measurement of bone mineral content in the appendicular skeleton. Invest Radiol 12:542–544

Prudham G, Evans JG (1981) Factors associated with falls in the elderly: a community study. Age Ageing 10:141–146

Ray WA, Griffin MR, Schaffner W, Baugh DK, Melton LJ III (1987) Psychotropic drug use and the risk of hip fracture. N Engl J Med 316:363–369

Reinbold WD, Genant HK, Reiser UJ, Harris ST, Ettinger B (1986) Bone mineral content in early-postmenopausal and postmenopausal osteoporotic women: comparison of measurement methods. Radiology 160:469–478

Richardson ML, Genant HK, Cann CE et al. (1985) Assessment of metabolic bone diseases by quantitative computed tomography. Clin Orthop 195:224–238

Riggs BL, Melton LJ III (1986) Involutional osteoporosis. N Engl J Med 314:1676–1686

Ritchings RT, Pullan BR (1979) A technique for simultaneous

dual energy scanning: a technical note. J Comput Assist Tomogr 3:842–846

Ruegsegger P, Anliker M, Dambacher M (1981) Quantification of trabecular bone with low dose computed tomography. J Comput Assist Tomogr 5:384–390

Rutherford RA, Pullan BR, Isherwood I (1976) Calibration and response of an EMI scanner. Neuroradiology 11:7–13

Rutt B, Fenster A (1980) Split-filter computed tomography: a simple technique for dual energy scanning. J Comput Assist Tomogr 4:501–509

Sandor T, Weissman B, Brown E (1987) Assessment of trabecular and cortical spinal mineral content using single and dual energy CT. In: Book of Abstracts of The Sixth International Workshop on Bone and Soft Tissue Densitometry, 22–25 September 1987. Buxton, England, p 69

Sartoris D, Andre M, Resnick C, Resnick D (1986) Trabecular bone density in the proximal femur: quantitative CT assessment. Radiology 160:707–712

Sartoris DJ, Stein JA, Ramos E et al. (1987) Quantitative dual energy digital radiography of the spine: comparison to dual photon absorptiometry and quantitative computed tomography. In: Book of Abstracts of Sixth International Workshop on Bone and Soft Tissue Densitometry, 22–25 September 1987, Buxton, England, p. 77

Shukla SS, Leichter I, Karellas A, Craven JD, Greenfield MA (1986) Trabecular bone mineral density measurement in vivo: use of the ratio of coherent to compton-scattered photons in the calcaneus. Radiology 158:695–697

Stevenson JC, Whitehead MI (1982) Postmenopausal osteoporosis. Br Med J 285:585–588

Wallace WA (1983) The increasing incidence of fractures of the proximal femur: an orthopaedic epidemic. Lancet I:1413–1414

Weiss NS, Ure CL, Ballard JH, Williams AR, Daling JR (1980) Decreased risk of fractures of the hip and lower forearm with post menopausal use of estrogen. N Engl J Med 303:1195–1198

Williams G, Bydder GM, Kreel L (1980) The validity and use of computed tomography attenuation values. Br Med Bull 36:279–287

Part 3:

Clinical Indications

20 Musculoskeletal Trauma

H. Stein

Spinal Injuries 272
    Cervical Spine 273
    Thoracic, Thoraco-Lumbar and Lumbar Spine 275
Trauma to the Hip Joint and Pelvic Ring 277
Other Injuries 281
    Fractures 281
    Soft Tissue Injuries 281
References 281

We are living in a mechanized age in which sophisticated, high-speed machinery is used for an ever increasing number of tasks. Many thousands are injured daily in this "Machine Age" and, from the medical point of view, the 1980s may be called "The Age of Trauma". Trauma is gradually becoming the commonest pathology in medical practice, producing a vast diversity of injuries some of which are unusual in their complexity and severity. The demanding task of managing such injuries, many of them complex and life threatening, needs resourceful and original thinking, sophisticated diagnostic techniques, and awareness of even minor clinical signs. Significant injuries to the musculoskeletal system usually result in radiographic abnormalities and, therefore, imaging is of paramount importance in evaluating such patients.

The best way to recognize an abnormality is to understand thoroughly what is normal (Cone 1984). Knowledge of normal appearances and relationships will allow identification of even subtle fractures and dislocations.

Until a few years ago, radiographic imaging of the musculoskeletal system could only demonstrate the presence of fractures, foreign bodies, and defects in calcified tissues. Recent advances in computer technologies and their application in medicine have added the ability to demonstrate the site and extent of soft tissue and organ injuries. The development and clinical use of computed tomography (CT), magnetic resonance imaging (MRI), sonography,

scintigraphy, and most recently, three-dimensional reconstructions from axial computed tomographs (3DCT) have provided the clinician with both fine detail and an improved understanding of the damaged tissues. A high proportion of accurate diagnoses can be attained, an achievement which was not possible only a few years ago (Mettler 1947; Pakusch 1982; Rosenberger and Bojzson 1986). Modern imaging techniques allow the clinical team to plan therapeutic management in detail thereby reducing surgical time, morbidity and complication rates.

The problems facing the trauma surgeon are often complex and unorthodox. Every patient needs to be investigated and assessed on an individual basis since bone and joint injuries are not identical although they may appear similar on routine radiographs. Protocols for the examination of trauma patients have evolved over the years, and vary from one hospital to another. In our institution, protocols consist of both careful clinical and conventional radiological examination, with provision for special imaging techniques in specific types of injury.

Upon arrival in the Accident and Emergency Department each patient has a comprehensive physical examination after removal of all clothes. All physical findings are recorded in detail, including a full neurological assessment. In instances of mass casualties, a medical secretary, who is responsible for recording the medical findings as dictated by the examining physician, works together with the admitting medical officer. In patients with spinal injuries, and for trauma to the pelvis and hip, with or without dislocation or fracture of the acetabulum, CT of the injured part immediately follows routine radiographic examination. This type of in-detail examination on admission allows a better assessment of the magnitude of the injury with minimal patient movement and enhances decision making.

Spinal Injuries

The level of injury has first to be identified by routine antero-posterior (AP) and cross table lateral views (CTLV). In the presence of a fracture, dislocation or fracture-dislocation, lateral films of the entire spine, from the cranio-vertebral to the lumbo-sacral junction are recommended. The latter are necessary to determine whether non-contiguous injuries have occurred. In a series of 710 spinal injury patients, Calenoff et al. (1978) found that 4.5% had multiple, non-contiguous vertebral injuries and that in 50% of them, the time from initial injury to the diagnosis of the second injury was 53 days.

High resolution CT is undoubtedly superior to other imaging modalities in assessing the extent and degree of injury sustained by the spinal column following trauma. It offers major advantages in the detection and localization of bone fragments within the spinal canal, and of posterior arch fractures. CT has, however, been found to be deficient in demonstrating the amount of anterior vertebral body compression (Keene et al. 1982; Keene 1984).

Most spinal fractures are not associated with loss of neurological function. Their immediate and accurate assessment is nevertheless mandatory for both planning treatment and prevention of further injury (Angtuaco and Binet 1984).

Plain radiographs may be normal even in the face of neurological deficit (Angtuaco and Binet 1984). In such instances, CT is indicated. Ten to twenty-three per cent of patients with a spinal fracture go on to develop some neurological deficit (Faerber et al. 1979), affecting multiple levels in 5%–20% (Calenoff et al. 1978; Post 1980). Radiological assessment of the entire spinal column is therefore necessary, supplemented by CT of suspicious areas.

Strong forces are necessary to fracture the thoracic and lumbar vertebrae. The commonest mechanism of injury is hyperflexion, the resultant injury

varying from a simple wedge fracture of the vertebral body to transverse fractures of the vertebral body with horizontal fractures of the pedicles, laminae and spinous processes (Chance type fracture). If the distraction component of the injury passes through the disc space, either a compression or a transverse fracture of the vertebral body may develop with rupture of the posterior ligamentous complex. The position of the body and its fixation (e.g. by a seat-belt) at the time of impact may influence the incidence associated intra-abdominal injuries.

During diagnostic evaluation, care must be taken to avoid further injury. The patient should be kept supine throughout all investigative procedures, since most unstable fractures are reduced in this position. The AP radiograph should be inspected for soft tissues injuries. The presence and location of a paraspinal haematoma usually points to the site of maximal injury. The degree of compression is usually best visualized on a lateral radiograph. Loss of posterior vertebral body height indicates a burst fracture, severe compression, and the possible presence of bone fragments within the spinal canal. At times, fracture dislocations reduce spontaneously.

Necropsy studies in post-traumatic patients have shown that while the bone lesions may reflect the area of forceful impact, extensive subarachnoid and extradural haemorrhage is common, and spinal cord lesions can be spread over many segments. The initial spinal radiographs, therefore, are often not a reliable guide to the severity and extent of spinal cord damage (Kakulas and Bedbrook 1976).

Assessment of damage to the posterior neural arch structures is difficult due to superimposed bony anatomy. Pitfalls in imaging spinal column structure and alignment by routine radiography frequently result from improper technique and/or difficult patient-positioning (Handel and Lee 1981). Overlying ribs, pedicles and transverse processes pose difficulties in the correct assessment of the thoracic spine on routine radiographs, which often underestimate the degree of injury to the spinal canal (Angtuaco and Binet 1984). These difficulties can be overcome by contrast-enhanced CT carried out with the patient in the supine position. The routine use of this imaging modality for problem cases has been advocated by various authors (Roub and Drayer 1979; O'Callaghan et al. 1980; Brant-Zawadzki et al. 1982; Post et al. 1982; Andersen 1983; Newton and Potts 1983). Myelography is not advocated in the first 12 hours following admission, although it has been suggested for delineation of spinal cord or cauda equina compression in acute spinal trauma (Angtuaco and Binet 1984). It is best carried out with the patient supine, via a lateral C1–

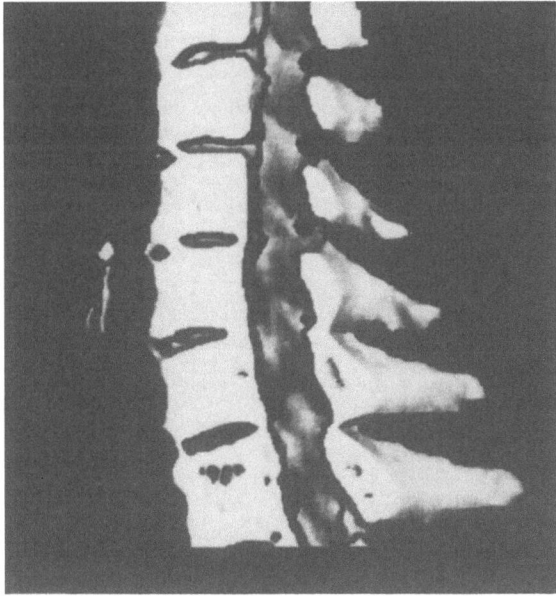

Fig. 20.1. 3-D tomography of a normal cervical spine.

Table 20.1. Cervical spine injuries

	Level of injury	Neurological impairment
1)	Fracture C4; C4–5 dislocation	None
2)	Fractured dens	None
3)	Fractured dens	None
4)	Fractured C6 – body and post elements	Quadriplegia
5)	C3–4 fracture; unilat facet dislocation	None
6)	Fractured dens; C1–2 dislocation	None
7)	C1 Fracture; C4–5 fracture dislocation	Quadriplegia on arrival Significant neurological recovery within 6 months
8)	C2 Fracture	Complete quadriplegia
9)	C4 burst fracture	None
10)	C3 burst fracture	None
11)	C7 burst fracture	None
12)	C2 fracture neural arch	None
13)	C3 fracture C6 fracture; C6–7 dislocation	Monoparesis (rt upper limb)
14)	C5 fracture; C5–6 subluxation	None
15)	C3 fracture; C3–4 subluxation	Paraplegia
16)	C3 fracture; C3–4 unilat facet dislocation	None
17)	C6 fracture; C6–7 dislocation	Paraplegia
18)	C7 burst fracture	None
19)	C7 burst fracture	Paraplegia
20)	C4–5 dislocation	Quadriplegia
21)	C3–4 dislocation	Quadriplegia
22)	C4–5 dislocation; C4 fracture	Quadriplegia (Neural canal severely compromised > 50%)
23)	C3 burst fracture; C3–4 dislocation	Quadriplegia
24)	C6 burst fracture; C6–7 subluxation	Monoparesis – lt upper arm
25)	C6 burst fracture	Quadriplegia on arrival; complete recovery within 10 months
26)	Blunt trauma; C3 haemomyelia	Central cord syndrome
27)	C3 fracture; C3–4 subluxation	None
28)	C2 fracture	None
29)	C3 fracture; C3–4 dislocation	Quadriplegia
30)	C3 fracture; C3–4 subluxation	None

2 puncture, using a low osmolality water-soluble contrast agent. In our experience, however, high resolution CT has provided all the necessary diagnostic data to assess spinal trauma shortly after admission, without exposing the patient either to delay or to the discomfort and danger of further damage inherent in change of posture and transfer to different examining tables. Moreover, CT also provides sufficient information for detailed assessment in combined spinal and intra-abdominal injuries (Rosenberger and Bojzsen 1986). It is both efficient and time saving in mass casualty situations. The ability of CT to demonstrate, within the spinal canal, cortical bone fragments 0.6 mm thick and cancellous bone fragments 1.2 mm thick, has proved of considerable benefit (Lindahl et al. 1983; Newton and Potts 1983). The resultant narrowing of the spinal canal can be exactly measured. The addition of 3DCT that requires neither additional radiation nor any change in the patient's position, has permitted direct visualization of fractures and dislocations, including Chance fractures and flexion and dislocation injuries which have been poorly demonstrated on routine CT (McAfee et al. 1983).

Cervical Spine

In patients with cerebral injuries, a complete investigation of the cervical spine must be carried out. Fractures and dislocations of the cervical spine may

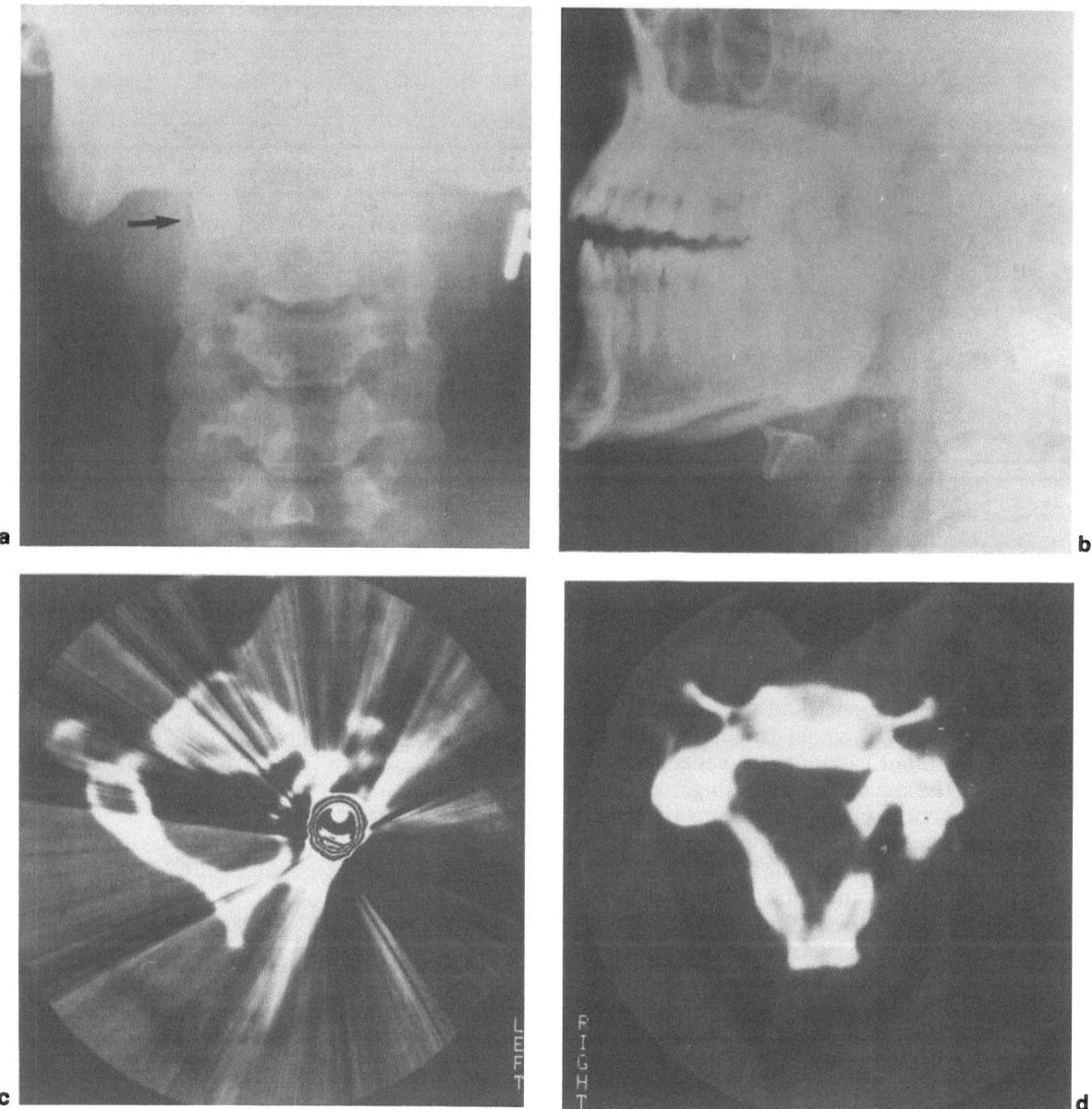

Fig. 20.2. a Antero-posterior view of a cervical gunshot wound injury. Bullet (*arrow*) located in C2. No neurological deficit. **b** Lateral view. **c** CT image of C2. Bullet located in the left side of neural arch. Small bone fragments in the spinal canal. **d** Bone loss in neural arch of C3.

be present without any clinical signs or symptoms, particularly in unconscious patients. Therefore, radiographic examination of the cervical spine must be carried out, on admission, in such patients. Routine views include a cross table lateral (CTLV), an AP and an open mouth AP view. They must demonstrate both structure and alignment of all cervical vertebrae – including C7 (Fig. 20.1). The accuracy of standard radiographs for detecting cervical spine injuries has recently been challenged, and CT recommended as the most useful imaging modality (Goldstein et al. 1982; Baker and Grubb 1983; Evans 1983; Streitwieser et al. 1983; Koyama et al. 1984; Lee et al. 1984; Yetkin et al. 1985; Kim et al. 1986; Edeiken-Monroe et al. 1986; Daffner et al. 1987).

Between January 1982 and December 1986, 30 consecutive patients with severe cervical spinal injuries were evaluated by this protocol. Fifteen had signs of neurological involvement which varied both in severity and extent. Data available from CT on each of these patients provided a better understanding of the magnitude of the damage (Fig. 20.2) and the development of neurological deficit (Table 20.1). Furthermore, the detailed anatomical visualization allowed a more precise assessment of stability at that level. Accurate assessment of the presence and extent of damage indicated how the stability had been impaired and treatment could be based on exact anatomical data.

The presence of foreign bodies in the spine can be exactly located (Fig. 20.2). Magnetic resonance imaging (MRI) complements the information provided by CT scans, and raises the level of diagnostic accuracy by improved contrast, but is not yet routinely available. Its use is best deferred for the investigation of soft tissue abnormalities.

3DCT (Fig. 20.1) conveys many details of the surface configuration of bone and joint structure. High-quality 3-D images can be obtained on some CT systems within minutes.

Thoracic, Thoraco-Lumbar and Lumbar Spine

The routine radiographic investigation of spinal trauma at the thoracic and lumbar levels utilizing AP and CTLV views does not demonstrate either the full extent of vertebral body damage in the presence of compression, the posterior element fractures, or the degree of spinal instability. Spinal alignment may be preserved. CT can demonstrate bone extruded into the canal, the midsagittal diameter of the spinal canal and posterior element fractures in some detail. Significant retropulsion of bony fragment can be detected inside the spinal canal in some quite innocent-looking compression fractures of the vertebral body (Fig. 20.3).

In our series of 35 consecutive patients who had sustained thoracic, thoraco-lumbar or lumbar injuries their routine clinical and radiographic examination was supplemented in the presence of neurological deficit, or a vertebral fracture with or without dislocation, by CT of the affected level. In 19 of these patients significant extrusion of bone into the spinal canal (Fig. 20.3) was demonstrated (Table 20.2). None of them, however, showed any neurological deficit. There was no correlation between the presence of bone spicules in the spinal canal or the degree of canal narrowing, and the

presence of neurological deficit. A better understanding of the pathomechanics of spinal trauma and the development of neurological deficit is needed. The significance of bone spicules in the spinal canal, physically narrowing the diameter of the latter, is not well understood (Figs 20.3, 20.4). It has been suggested that latent spinal stenosis will ensue, but our present knowledge is insufficient to confirm this hypothesis. Complete fracture dislocations of the thoracic spine without neurological deficit – a rare injury – have recently been described (Harryman 1986), whilst Trafton and Boyd (1984) have reported the development of neurological signs in 60% of patients with burst fractures whose spinal canal diameter was narrowed by at least half.

Standard radiographs are capable of delineating certain fractures and fracture dislocations of the spine, but do not demonstrate the neural arch, the facet joints, or the neural canal adequately and, therefore, are best augmented by CT. The advantages of CT are:

1. The ability to obtain detailed transverse axial sections of the spinal column and canal with the patient supine, in 10–20 minutes, visualizing both bone and surrounding soft tissues.

2. Detection of injuries to other organs without moving the patient.

3. The reformatting of data in alternative planes and the production of 3-D images with no further patient movement or irradiation.

4. Less total radiation than is required for conventional tomography (Keene 1984).

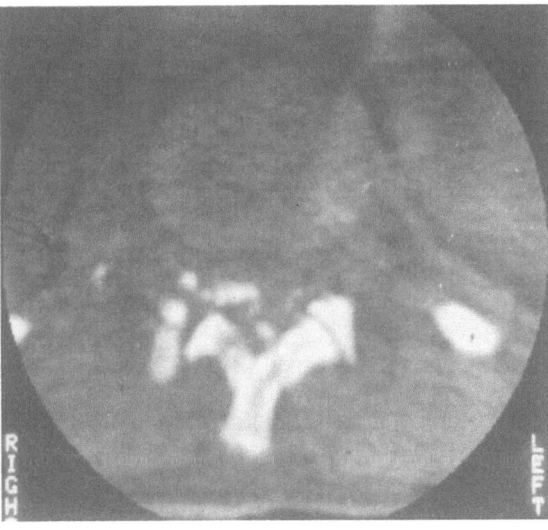

Fig. 20.3. Fracture of L2. Bone fragments in neural canal. No neurological deficit.

Table 20.2. Thoracic and lumbar spine injuries

	Level of injury	Neurological signs
1)	Burst fractures D12, L1, L2, L4; Bone fragments in neural canal	None
2)	Fracture L1; D12–L1 dislocation; 50% narrowing of neural canal	None
3)	Burst fractures D1, 2, 3, 4	Paraplegia D2-level
4)	Burst fractures D4, 5, 6; Bone fragments in neural canal at all levels	Paraplegia D6-level
5)	Burst fracture D12; Severe narrowing of spinal canal by bone fragments	None
6)	Fractures D10, D11 involving middle and posterior columns. Free bone fragments in neural canal	None
7)	Gunshot wound. Burst fracture L4	Paraplegia
8)	Gunshot wound. Burst fracture of posterior elements of L1	Paraplegia
9)	Burst fracture of L3. Free bone fragments in neural canal	None
10)	Burst fracture L5; L5–S1 subluxation	None
11)	Burst fracture L2 mimicking compression fracture. Bone fragments filling neural canal almost 50%	None
12)	Burst fracture L2 mimicking compression fracture. Many bone fragments in neural canal	None
13)	Fracture D11; Fractures L1, 2, 3, 4, 5	Paraparesis
14)	Gunshot wound – complete blowout – L2	Paraplegia
15)	Gunshot wound – compound retroperitoneal injury and D12 fracture	Paraplegia
16)	Compression fracture L2 with loss of posterior body height. Free fragments in neural canal	None
17)	Fracture D11, D12, L1; Dislocation D12–L1	Paraplegia
18)	Fracture D11. Bone fragments in neural canal	None
19)	Fracture D5; Fracture D6. Bone fragments in neural canal	None
20)	Burst fracture L2. Many bone fragments in neural canal	None

Table 20.2. (*continued*)

21)	Burst fracture of L1 mimicking compression fracture. Bone fragments in neural canal	None
22)	Fracture of bodies of D12, L1, L2. Many bone fragments in neural canal	None
23)	Fracture of L1; D12–L1 dislocation. Bone fragments in neural canal	None
24)	Fracture of both body and posterior elements L4 and L5. Traumatic spondylolisthesis L5–S1	Motor weakness L5 level
25)	Compressed fracture of L2 with many bone fragments in neural canal	Sphincter paralysis
26)	Fracture of L1; D12–L1 dislocation	None
27)	Burst fracture L4. 50% spinal canal stenosis due to bone spicules	None
28)	Fracture of L1 with complete disruption of the anterior column	None
29)	Gunshot wound – blow out fracture D2–D3	Paraplegia
30)	Gunshot wound – fracture D9	Paraplegia
31)	Burst fracture L1; D12–L1 dislocation. Spinal canal obliterated by bone spicules	Paraplegia
32)	Fracture of D12 with disruption of middle and posterior columns	None
33)	Burst fracture of L1. Bone spicules in neural canal	Paraplegia
34)	Fracture of D5; Dislocation D3–4. Bone spicules in spinal canal	Paraplegia
35)	Fracture of L1; Dislocation of D12–L1. Disruption of anterior and middle columns. Bone spicules in neural canal	Loss of right quadriceps function

CT has also been shown to be a valuable means of determining spinal stability following injury (McAfee et al. 1983; Denis 1984). It is strongly advocated, therefore, that CT should be a routine procedure in the initial study of acute spinal trauma patients in the assessment of cervical, thoracic or lumbar injury. Figure 20.5 suggests a plan for the radiological investigation of patients with spinal trauma.

Trauma to the Hip Joint and Pelvic Ring

In patients with multiple injuries or in mass casualty situations, attention may be diverted from the pelvis and hip. Head, chest and abdominal injuries,

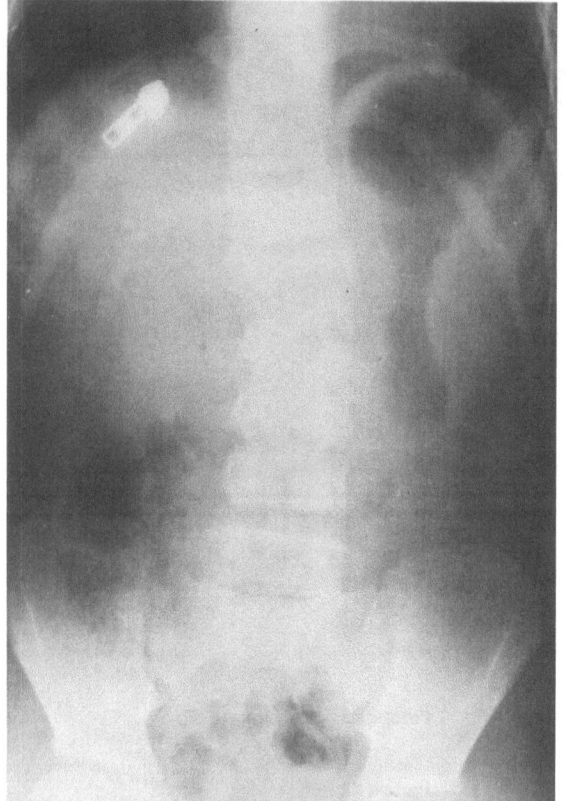

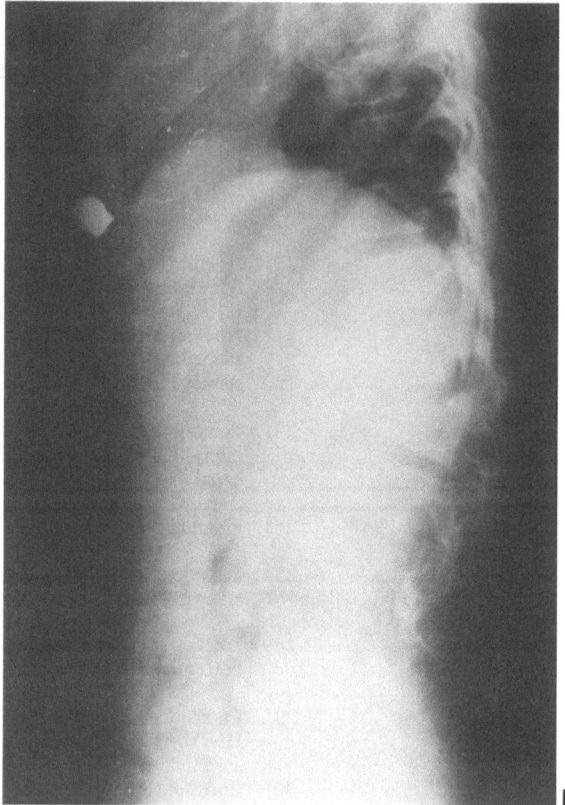

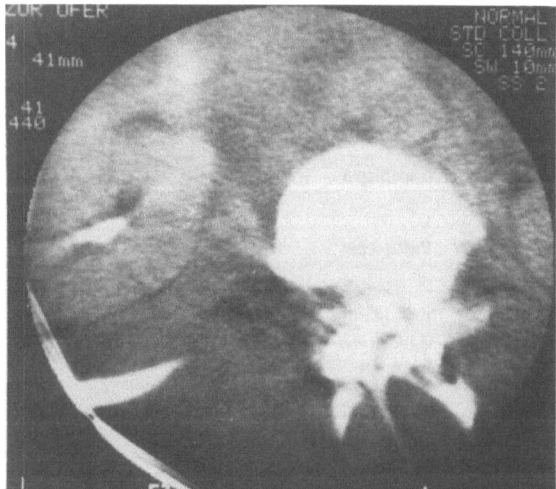

Fig. 20.4a–c. Fracture of L1, with D12–L1 dislocation. The patient was paraplegic on arrival. **a** AP radiograph. **b** CTLV radiograph. **c** CT scan showing almost complete obliteration of spinal canal.

together with open or closed long bone fractures, may obscure important clinical and diagnostic signs that suggest trauma to the hip joint. Contusion or laceration over the knee, or an adducted, abducted, slightly flexed or rotated femur, should alert the emergency physician.

Physical examination often yields insufficient information in the face of multiple injuries. Routine radiographs of the pelvis must be taken in all such patients, to avoid missing pelvic disruption or dislocation. Fractures and disruptions of the pelvic ring are most difficult to assess (Pennal et al. 1980; Tile and Pennal 1980; Tile 1984). Conventional radiography may produce views obscured by superimposed shadows and, in the presence of multiple injuries, positioning the patient for special views may be impossible. Traumatic dislocation of the hip is a very serious injury; it may be associated with fractures of the femoral head (Urist 1948), and requires early treatment (Epstein et al. 1984). The presence of a widened joint space on the AP radiograph raises the suspicion of loose fragments or soft tissue interposition in the joint. Persistent widening

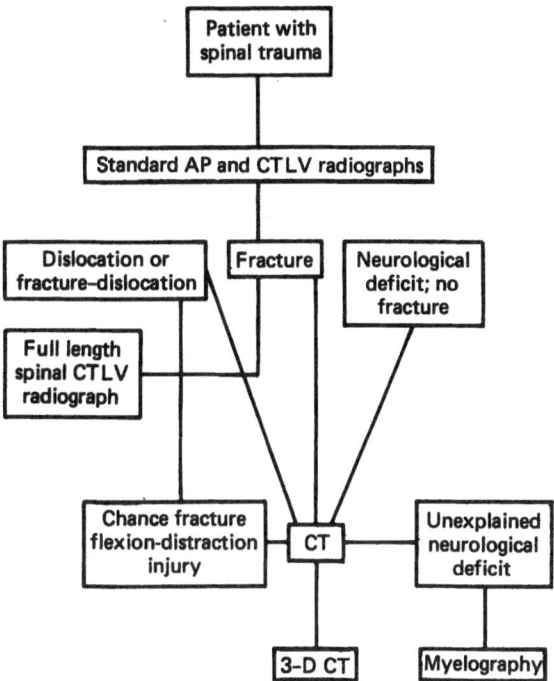

Fig. 20.5. Algorithm for the assessment of a patient with spinal trauma.

tures has resulted in the evolution of a new classification (Hoffmeyer et al. 1984; Gill and Bucholz 1984; St. Pierre et al. 1984). The degree of comminution, mainly of the superior articular surface of the acetabulum, can be visualized to an extent hitherto unknown, at the same time allowing an assessment of associated intra-abdominal lesions. Pre-operative planning has become both simpler and more accurate.

Dashboard injuries and other types of violent direct impact to the flexed knee, with the hip flexed and slightly abducted, may cause "slice fractures" of the femoral head, without dislocation of the hip joint. Osteochondral fragments are "shaved" off the femoral head by the acetabular rim, as the head executes a shearing type of movement against the acetabular rim. These osteo-cartilagenous fragments may be very small (Figs. 20.6, 20.7). They and the fracture bed on the femoral head are infrequently detected on routine radiographs since they are often located on the postero-medial aspect, or on the border between the posterior and superior aspects of the femoral head – the so-called radiological blind spots. Those affected complain of severe, persistent pain, limp, and are often labelled as "avascular necrosis of the femoral head", although both routine radiographs and scintigrams are negative.

We have treated 14 such patients, between 1980 and 1985. Twelve were young (age range 17–40 years) and two were 60 years old and 72 years old respectively. Twelve were injured in road traffic accidents, the other two in sport accidents. All complained of severe pain in the affected groin radiating to the ipsilateral knee, aggravated by movement of the affected hip. Routine AP and "frog" position

of the joint space has been described as an absolute indication for arthrotomy (Epstein 1973).

The introduction of CT into routine clinical practice has significantly improved the possibility of an exact assessment of injuries to the pelvis and hip (Lasda et al. 1978; Sauser et al. 1980; Lange and Alter 1980; Tile 1980; Stein 1983; Hoffmeyer et al. 1984). CT can be performed on admission, without further delay, with the patient in the supine position, and has become indispensible for detailed imaging of these anatomical areas. This is a most important development, since fractures which are slightly displaced, or associated with a dislocation, pose formidable imaging and diagnostic problems. With conventional radiological techniques, they often defy exact classification. Many different methods, including isotope scanning, have been tried for better definition (Pennal et al. 1980; Gertzbein and Chenoweth 1982). CT, however, allows both exact and immediate imaging and is crucial in determining the treatment most suited for the individual patient (Gilula et al. 1979; Lange and Alter 1980; Tile 1980; Tile and Pennal 1980; Hansen 1982; Mack et al. 1982; Tile 1984). The better definition of both pelvic ring and acetabular frac-

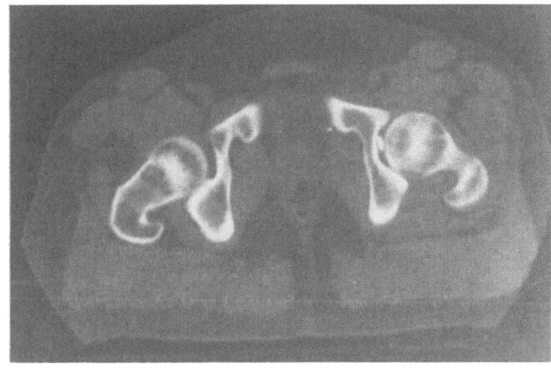

Fig. 20.6 CT scan demonstrating an intra-articular osteochondral fragment.

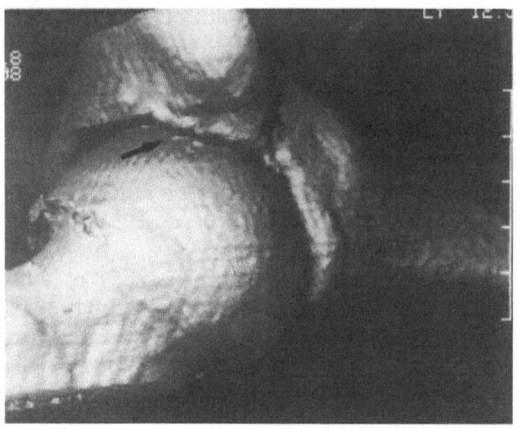 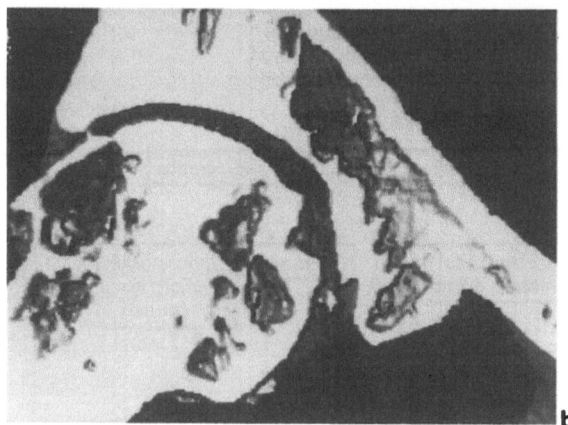

Fig. 20.7a,b. Fracture of the femoral head. a 3-D image of the postero-superior aspect of an affected hip joint. Arrow points towards the bed of a "slice fracture". b 3-D tomographic image demonstrating the presence of fine osteochondral fragments, free in the joint cavity.

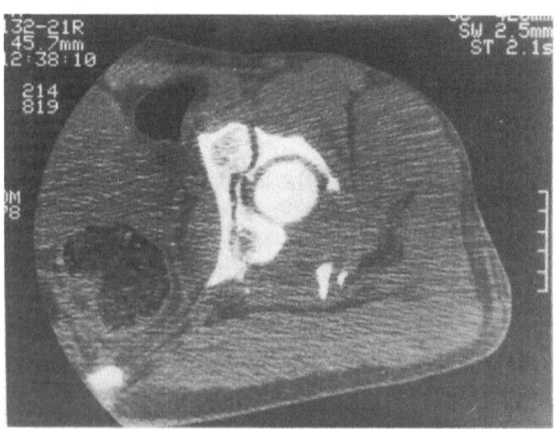

Fig. 20.8. CT scan showing the complex pattern of a transverse, yet extra-articular fracture of the acetabulum.

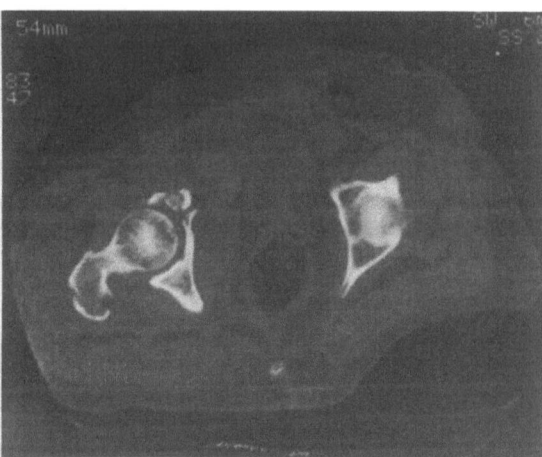

Fig. 20.9. CT scan demonstrating the presence of an intra-articular anterior column acetabular fracture.

radiographs of both hips were negative. Scintigrams showed no signs of avascular necrosis. On CT, loose osteochondral fragments were demonstrated in the joint cavity (Figs. 20.6, 20.7). The fracture bed and the size of the fragments could be measured on 3DCT. In three patients who were late referrals (1–2 years following injury) the fragments were localized in the posterior-inferior portion of the joint cavity, where they had gravitated over time. Walker and Burton (1982), Harley et al. (1982) and Mack et al. (1982) have reported similar findings.

CT allows a significantly better definition of fracture patterns in the pelvis and around the hip (Figs. 20.8, 20.9, 20.10, 20.11). The integrity of the weight-bearing acetabular dome can be directly visualized (Figs. 20.7, 20.9, 20.10, 20.11). Furthermore, the congruity of the joint surfaces, the presence of comminution, and the size and location of fracture fragments, can be fully assessed (Figs. 20.7–20.11).

During the past 5 years, every patient admitted to our service with an injury to the pelvis, and where routine radiographic examination showed distorted anatomy around the hip joint, has been further evaluated by CT. Fracture patterns could be precisely delineated on admission (Fig. 20.10), differentiating between intra-articular and extra-articular injury (Figs 20.9, 20.10, 20.11). Joint congruity and stability could be assessed, and surgical management planned shortly after admission.

We, therefore, recommend that all patients admitted with pelvic trauma and/or trauma around the hip, should be investigated by CT of the affected area.

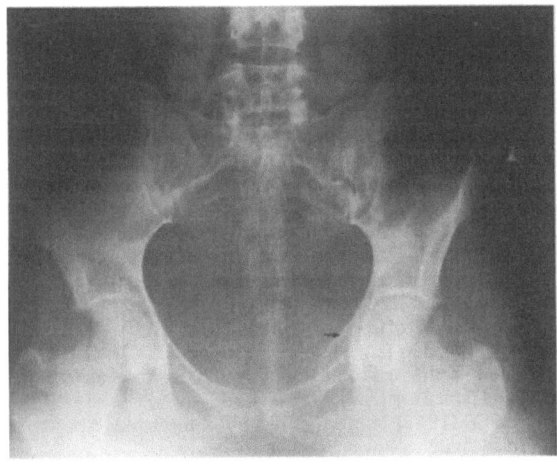
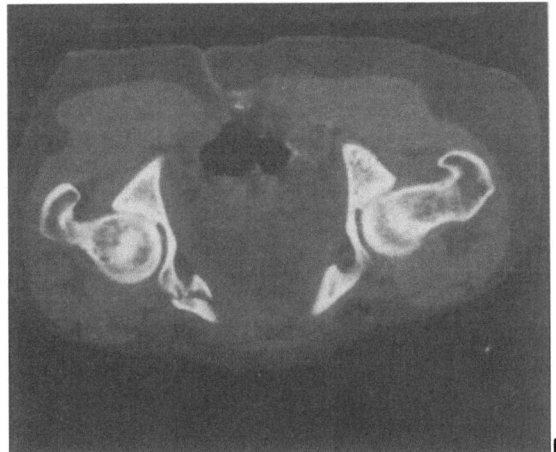

Fig. 20.10a,b. Acetabular fracture. **a** Routine antero-posterior pelvic radiograph of a 20-year-old patient injured in a road traffic accident. There is a probable acetabular fracture (*arrow*). **b** CT scan shows the presence of an extra-articular fracture.

Other Injuries

Fractures

For most other fractures plain radiographs suffice. Two radiographs must be taken and the joint above and below the fracture must be included. Post-manipulation films are required, whilst the patient is still anaesthetized, and internal fixation should be carried out with image intensification, or check radiographs taken before the anaesthetic is terminated.

Special views may be required, for example the subtalar view to demonstrate adequately an os calcis fracture. Occasionally tomograms may be needed, for example if there is doubt about a possible fracture of the femoral neck.

CT scanning may be indicated, particularly for fractures around joints. It is useful to define triplanar fractures of the distal tibial epiphysis and Dias et al. (1987) found CT scanning most helpful in classifying the type of fracture, evaluating the degree of communition and measuring displacement of tibial plateau fractures.

Soft Tissue Injuries

The diagnosis is usually clinical, but arthrography (Chap. 3), and ultrasound (Chap. 16) may be indicated.

References

Angtuaco EJ, Binet EF (1984) Radiology of thoracic and lumbar fractures. Clin Orthop 189:43–57

Andersen PE (1983) Sectional imaging methods. A comparison. University Park Press, Baltimore, p. 235

Baker RP, Grubb RL (jr) (1983) Complete fracture-dislocation of cervical spine without permanent neurological sequelae. J Neurosurg 58:760–762

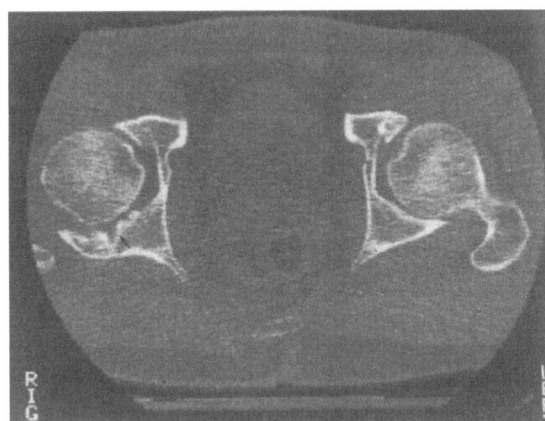

Fig. 20.11. CT scan of a 23-year-old male, injured in a road traffic accident. Routine pelvic radiographs were negative. Note the undisplaced crush fracture of the posterior acetabular wall (*arrow*).

Brant-Zawadzki M, Jeffrey RB (jr), Minagi H, Pitts LH (1982) High resolution CT of thoracolumbar facets. AJR 138:699–704

Calenoff L, Chessare JW, Rogers LF, Toerge J, Rosen JS (1978) Multiple level spinal injuries. Importance of early recognition. AJR 130:665–669

Cone RO (1984) Clues to the initial radiographic evaluation of skeletal trauma. Emerg Med Clin North Am 2:245–278

Daffner RH, Deeb ZL, Rothfus WE (1987) The posterior vertebral body line: importance in the detection of burst fractures. AJR 148:93–96

Denis F (1984) Spinal instability as defined by the three-column spine concept in acute spinal trauma. Clin Orthop 189:65–76

Dias JJ, Stirling AJ, Finlay DBL, Gregg PJ (1987) Computerised axial tomography for tibial plateau fractures. J Bone Joint Surg [Br] 69:84–88

Edeiken-Monroe B, Wagner LK, Harris JH (jr) (1986) Hyperextension dislocation of the cervical spine. AJR 146:803–808

Epstein HC (1973) Traumatic dislocation of the hip. Clin Orthop 92:116–142

Epstein HC, Wiss DA, Cozen L (1985) Posterior fracture dislocation of the hip with fractures of the femoral head. Clin Orthop 201:9–17

Evans DK (1983) Dislocation of the cervico-thoracic junction. J Bone Joint Surg [Br] 65:124–133

Faerber EN, Wolpert SM, Scott RM, Belkin SC, Carter BL (1979) Computed tomography of spinal fractures. J Comput Assist Tomogr 3:657–661

Gertzbein SD, Chenoweth DR (1977) Occult injuries of the pelvic ring. Clin Orthop 128:202–207

Gill K, Bucholz RW (1984) The role of computerized tomographic scanning in the evaluation of major pelvic fractures. J Bone Joint Surg [Am] 66:34–39

Gilula LA, Murphy WA, Tailor CC, Patel RB (1979) Computed tomography of the osseous pelvis. Radiology 132:107–114

Goldstein SJ, Woodring JH, Young AB (1982) Occipital condyle fracture associated with cervical spine injury. Surg Neurol 17:350–352

Handel SF, Lee YY (1981) Computed tomography of spinal fractures. Radiol Clin North Am 19:69–89

Hansen ST (jr) (1982) CT for pelvic fractures. AJR 138:592–593

Harley JD, Mack LA, Winquist RA (1982) CT of acetabular fractures: Comparison with conventional radiography. AJR 138:413–417

Harryman DT (1986) Complete fracture dislocation of the thoracic spine associated with spontaneous neurologic decompression. A case report. Clin Orthop 207:64–69

Hoffmeyer P, Seigne JM, Garcia J, Vasey H (1984) The value of computerized tomography in fractures of the pelvic ring. Int Orthop 8:1–8

Howie JL (1985) Computed tomography of the bony pelvis: A protocol for multiplanar imaging. Part II Trauma. J Can Ass Radiol 36:287–295

Kakulas BA, Bedbrook GM (1976) Pathology of injuries of the vertebral column In: Vinken PJ, Bruyn GW (eds) Handbook of clinical neurology, vol. 25, North Holland, Amsterdam, p. 27

Keene JS (1984) Radiographic evaluation of thoraco-lumbar fractures. Clin Orthop 189:58–64

Keene JS, Goletz TH, Lilleas R, Alter AJ, Sackett JF (1982) Diagnosis of vertebral fractures. A comparison of conventional radiography, conventional tomography and computed axial tomography. J Bone Joint Surg [Am] 64:586–595

Kim KS, Rogers LF, Regenbogen V (1986) Pitfalls in plain film diagnosis of cervical spine injuries: false positive interpretation. Surg Neurol 25:381–392

Koyama T, Uchibori M, Kubo Y, Handa J (1984) Diagnostic value of CT in atlanto-axial dislocation and the choice of treatment. No Shinkei Geka 12:1281–1290

Lange TA, Alter AJ (jr) (1980) Evaluation of complex acetabular fractures by computed tomography. J Comput Assist Tomogr 4:849–852

Lasda NA, Levinsohn EM, Yuan, HA, Burnell WP (1978) Computerized tomography in disorders of the hip. J Bone Joint Surg [Am] 60:1099–1102

Lee C, Rogers LF, Woodring JH, Goldstein SJ, Kim KS (1984) Fractures of the cranio-vertebral junction, associated with other fractures of the spine; overlooked entity. AJNR 5:775–781

Lindahl S, Willen J, Irstam L (1983) Computed tomography of bone fragments in the spinal canal. An experimental study. Spine 8:181–186

Mack LA, Harley JD, Winquist RA (1982) CT of acetabular fractures: analysis of fracture patterns. AJR 138:407–412

McAfee PC, Yuan HA, Fredrickson BE, Lubicky JP (1983) The value of computed tomography in thoraco-lumbar fractures. J Bone Joint Surg [Am] 65:461–473

Mettler CC (1947) Surgery in history of medicine. Blackistone, Philadelphia

Newton TH, Potts DG (1983) Computed tomography of the spine and spinal cord. In: Newton TH, Potts DG (eds.) Modern neuroradiology, vol. 1, San Anselmo, Clavadel

O'Callaghan JP, Ullrich CG, Yuan HA (1980) CT of facet distraction in flexion injuries of the thoraco-lumbar spine. The "NAKED" facet. AJR 134:563–568

Pakush RS (1982) Present concepts in diagnostic radiology. Proc. Latterman Arm Med Cent Congr San-Francisco

Pennal GF, Tile M, Waddell JP, Garside H (1980) Pelvic disruption. Assessment and classification. Clin Orthop 151:12–21

Post MJD (1980) Radiographic evaluation of the spine. Current advances with emphasis on computed tomography. Masson, New-York

Post MJ, Green BA, Quencer RM, Stokes NA, Callahan RA, Eismont FJ (1982) The value of computed tomography in spinal trauma. Spine 7:417–431

Rosenberger A, Bojzsen E (1986) Radiology in war. Acta Radiol [Diagn] Suppl 367

Roub LW, Drayer BP (1979) Spinal computed tomography. Limitations and applications. AJR 133:267–273

Sauser DD, Billimoria PE, Rouse GA, Mudge K (1980) CT evaluation of hip trauma. AJR 135:269–274

Stein H (1983) Computerized tomography for ascertaining osteocartilagenous intra-articular (slice) fractures of the femoral head. Isr J Med Sci 19:180–184

St Pierre RK, Oliver T, Somoygi J, Whitesides T, Fleming LL (1984) Computerized tomography in the evaluation and classification of fractures of the acetabulum. Clin Orthop 188:234–237

Streitwieser DR, Knopp R, Wales LR, Williams JL, Tonnemacher K (1983) Accuracy of standard radiographic views in detecting cervical spine fractures. Ann Emerg Med 12:538–542

Tile M (1980) Pelvic fractures: Operative versus nonoperative treatment. Orthop Clin North Am 11:423–464

Tile M, Pennal GF (1980) Pelvic disruption. Principles of management. Clin Orthop 151:56–64

Tile M (1984) Fractures of the pelvis and acetabulum. Williams & Wilkins, Baltimore, London

Trafton PG, Boyd CA (jr) (1984) Computed tomography of thoracic and lumbar spine injuries. J Trauma 24:506–514

Urist MR (1948) Fracture-dislocation of the hip joint: the nature of the traumatic lesion, treatment, late complications and end results. J Bone Joint Surg [Am] 30:669–727

Walker RH, Burton DS (1982) Computerized tomography in assessment of acetabular fractures. J Trauma 22:227–234

Yetkin Z, Osborn AG, Giles DS, Haughton VM (1985) Uncovertebral and facet joint dislocations in cervical articular pillar fractures; CT evaluation. AJNR 6:633–637

21 Primary Tumours of Bone and Soft Tissue

F.H. Sim, T.H. Berquist and R.A. McLeod

Introduction 283
Benign Bone Tumours 284
Malignant Bone Tumours 285
Soft Tissue Tumours 289
Summary 290
References 291

Introduction

The management of patients with musculoskeletal tumours remains one of the most challenging problems in oncology. These tumours continue to pose difficulties in terms of diagnosis and treatment. Although relatively rare they encompass a wide variety of lesions, many with different biological capabilities. Because these tumours are rare, few physicians encounter enough of them to feel comfortable with their diagnosis. In addition, the clinical presentation is often insidious, which makes early recognition difficult. Many patients present with symptoms that are attributed to various degenerative or inflammatory conditions, particularly when the neoplasm was not considered in the differential diagnosis. Moreover, many lesions are missed because the radiographs are of poor quality. Chondrosarcomas, for example, commonly occur along the inner wall of the acetabulum in elderly patients, where symptoms may be attributed to degenerative hip disease unless the possibility of neoplasm is considered and good-quality radiographs are obtained (Fig. 21.1).

The first hurdle in dealing with musculoskeletal tumours is recognizing the existence of the lesion. The evaluation of patients with these tumours is divided into four phases:

1. Discovery
2. Diagnosis
3. Pre-operative staging
4. Biopsy

Orthopaedic oncology requires teamwork with effective coordination among oncologists, orthopaedic surgeons, radiologists and pathologists to provide an accurate diagnosis and effective treatment. A systematic approach to the radiographic interpretation is essential because the integration of the clinical and the radiographic information will determine the further investigations required. If a benign lesion is suspected, a few simple diagnostic tests may be indicated before biopsy. However, if a malignant lesion is suspected, a sophisticated and extensive diagnostic staging strategy is necessary before biopsy. Even the decision to biopsy is based on the clinical and radiographic interpretation. For instance, if a typical fibrous cortical defect is diagnosed, observation alone may be indicated.

If a malignant lesion is suspected it should be staged pre-operatively. Careful evaluation is essential to determine the precise extent of local tumour involvement and whether distant metastases have developed. Additional studies such as skeletal scintigraphy, computed tomography (CT) of the lesion and lungs, magnetic resonance imaging (MRI), and digital subtraction angiography may be necessary to aid in the pre-operative planning (Figs 21.2, 21.3 and 21.4). Pre-operative imaging techniques should be completed before the biopsy, because changes induced by the biopsy will alter the critical staging studies. The pre-operative evaluation may be modified depending on the location of the tumour. With pelvic and spinal lesions, excretory urography or cystography may give information concerning the extent of deviation of the ureters and bladder, and

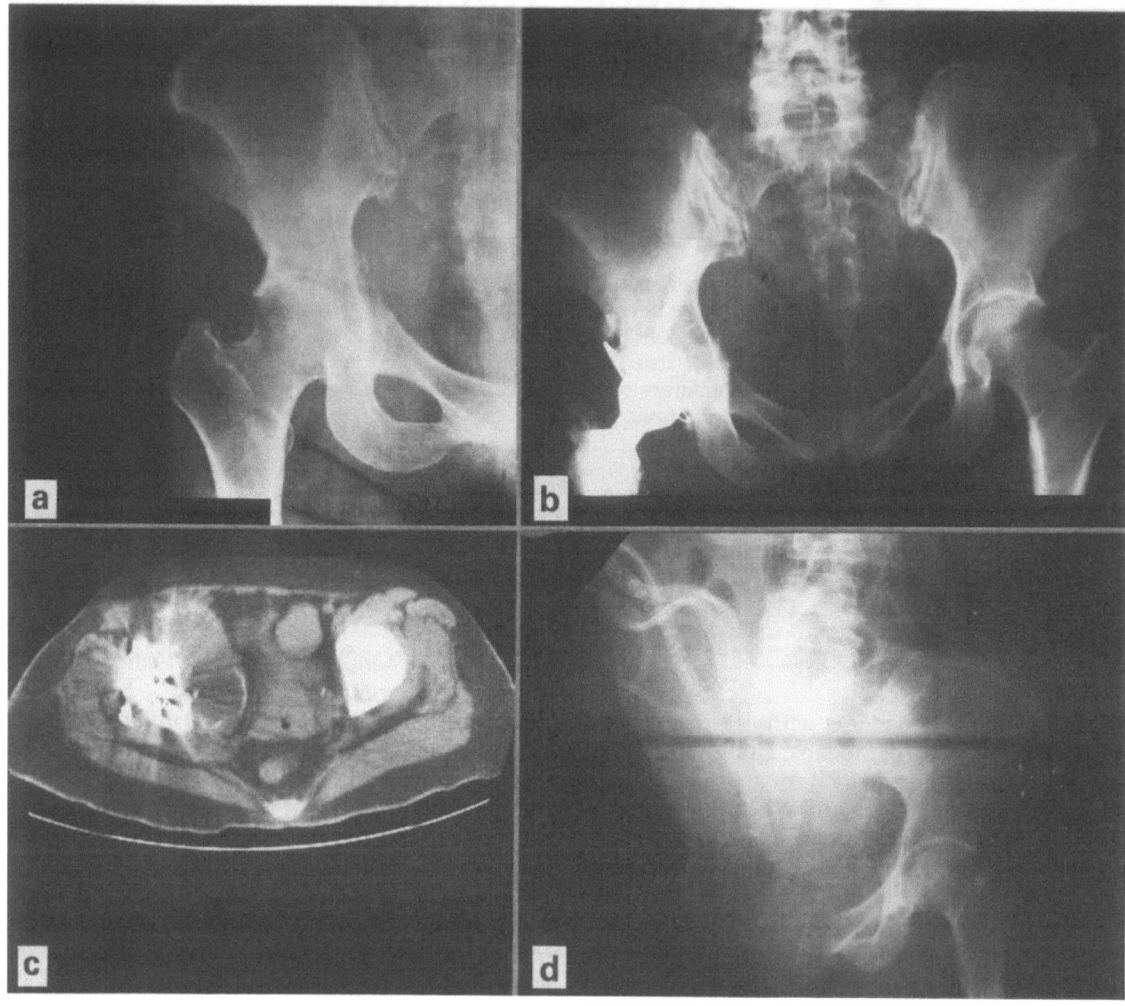

Fig. 21.1. a Antero-posterior view of the right hip shows a destructive lesion involving the acetabulum. b The patient had degenerative joint disease, and a total hip arthroplasty was performed. c CT scan of the pelvis shows a destructive lesion with large intrapelvic soft tissue extension. Biopsy revealed dedifferentiated chondrosarcoma. d Antero-posterior view of the pelvis after extended hemipelvectomy.

a barium enema will indicate the relationship of a pelvic tumour to the large bowel. In the spinal column, a myelogram is necessary to assess the relationship of the spinal tumour to the neural contents. A liver and spleen scan may be helpful in disseminated sarcoma or to determine the pattern of a lymphoma. The pre-operative evaluation of the patient with a musculoskeletal neoplasm, however, must be individualized, depending on the expected diagnosis.

Benign Bone Tumours

Patients with benign bone tumours usually present with local symptoms of pain or swelling or both. The

first goal of imaging is to detect or exclude the presence of a lesion. The symptoms serve as a guide to the proper site for radiographic studies. Most of these tumours are detected on plain radiographs (McLeod et al. 1978; Levine 1981; Lukens et al. 1982; Hudson et al. 1985). Small lesions such as osteoid osteoma, especially those located in anatomically complex areas such as the spinal column, shoulder girdle, hip girdle, hands and feet, may require conventional tomography, computed tomography or skeletal scintigraphy for demonstration (Hudson et al. 1985). Tumours arising superficially so that the bone is little altered, or those, such as sacral lesions, obscured by overlapping structures, may require CT or MRI for detection (McLeod et al. 1978; Zimmer et al. 1984). These techniques may also be useful in demonstrating small lesions located in trabecular bone or in an intramedullary location that may be undetected on plain radiographs.

After detection, a differential diagnosis must be developed, based primarily on the clinical findings and plain radiographs. Routine radiographs remain the most informative diagnostic modality (Hudson et al. 1985). On occasion, though, subtle changes may be seen earlier with isotope studies. Although not commonly used, thermography has also been employed for the detection of subtle lesions (Gershon-Cohen 1970). An area of increased temperature is detectable over the lesion, but the finding is non-specific. Conventional tomography may be indicated for intraosseous lesions that are small or obscured by overlapping structures or by reactive sclerosis (Halpern and Freiberger 1970). CT is occasionally useful in diagnosis, especially in lesions that are located centrally in sites difficult to evaluate radiographically. Tumour density, mineralization and composition are more accurately seen by CT, and this information may allow a more accurate diagnostic evaluation. CT is also useful in showing subtle destruction of cortical or cancellous bone, intramedullary tumour, or a soft tissue component not visible radiographically. MRI may be equally useful in this regard. Because of the relative lack of experience with MRI in benign neoplasms, most radiologists are more comfortable interpreting CT studies (Zimmer et al. 1984; Weekes et al. 1985a; Berquist 1987).

After plain radiographs have been interpreted, most benign bone lesions can be either observed or biopsied and the patient treated without further imaging being required. Occasionally, CT or MRI may be indicated for further localization. For example, an osteoid osteoma of the acetabulum can be a challenging surgical problem. Accurate localization may aid the surgeon in selecting the best approach for removal (Fig. 21.5). Generally, plain radiographs are adequate for follow-up of these patients after treatment.

In summary, plain radiography is the initial study of choice. When the radiographs are indicative of a benign lesion, additional imaging studies are not usually necessary, and the patient can either be observed or undergo surgery, whichever is indicated.

Malignant Bone Tumours

As with patients who have benign lesions of bone, the vast majority of patients with malignant lesions

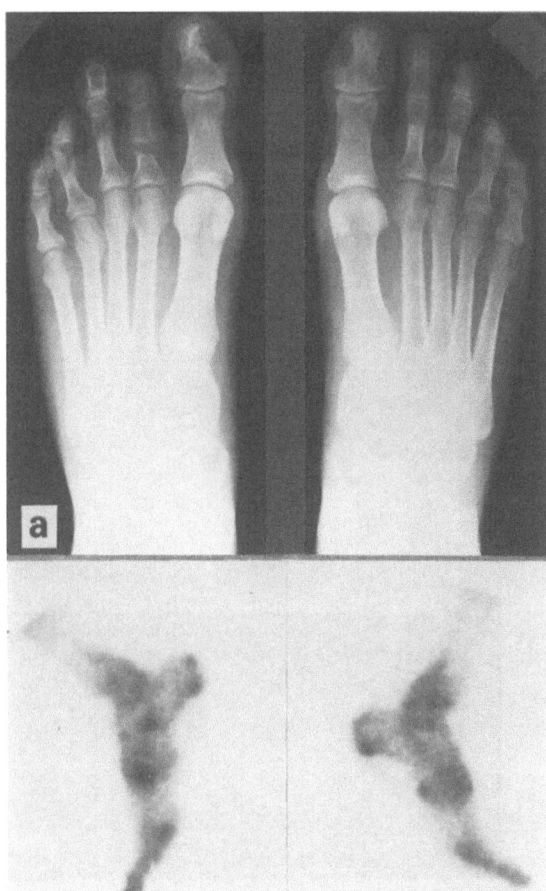

Fig. 21.2. a Antero-posterior view of both feet shows lytic destruction of the distal phalanx of the left great toe. b Skeletal scintigrams of both feet show increased uptake in the distal phalanx, as well as in the tarsal bones. Biopsy revealed angiosarcoma. Multiple lytic lesions in the angiographic area are common in angiosarcoma.

of bone present with local symptoms that direct the radiographic evaluation to the appropriate site. Again, conventional radiography is the initial study of choice (McLeod et al. 1978; Hudson et al. 1985; Berquist 1987). Radiographs will detect most lesions and provide valuable information regarding the aggressiveness of the tumour and the differential diagnosis. Other imaging modalities are sometimes helpful for detection and diagnosis in much the same fashion as was discussed for benign bone tumours.

When malignancy is suspected on the basis of conventional radiographs, additional imaging is almost invariably indicated (Halpern and Freiberger 1970; Levine et al. 1979). CT and MRI are the tech-

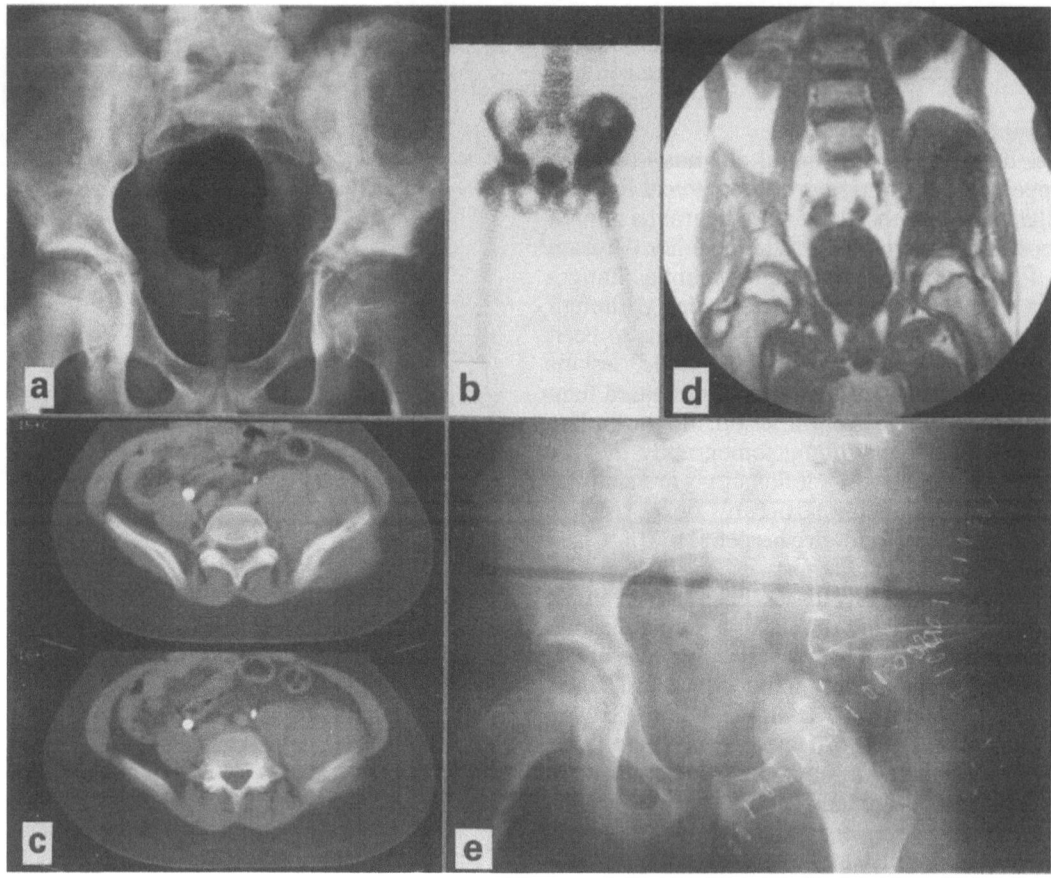

Fig. 21.3. a Antero-posterior view of the pelvis shows a large destructive lesion of the left hemipelvis with large Ewing's sarcoma. **b** Scintigram shows increased uptake in the left hemipelvis. **c** CT scan shows a large soft tissue mass extending both intrapelvically and extrapelvically. **d** MRI gives additional information on the extent of the lesion. **e** After en bloc resection and ischial femoral stabilization.

niques of choice in demonstrating tumour extent locally, regionally and systemically. This information profoundly influences patient management (Levine et al. 1979; Hudson et al. 1983; Zimmer et al. 1984; Aisen et al. 1986; Daffner et al. 1986; Berquist 1987).

Although CT is useful throughout the body, it is especially helpful in and near the trunk (McLeod et al. 1978; Levine et al. 1979; Levine 1981; Lukens et al. 1982; Kumpan et al. 1986). It is well suited to showing the extent of a malignant bone tumour with a soft tissue component because it demonstrates the pathological anatomy of both bone and soft tissue simultaneously.

The excellent density resolution and the cross-sectional display of CT allow an accurate assessment of tumour location and extent, as well as the effect on adjacent neurovascular structures and organs. A disadvantage of CT in this regard is the beam-

hardening artefact, which tends to obscure the juxtacortical soft tissues (Hudson et al. 1983; Berquist 1987). CT is also useful for demonstrating tumour spread within the medullary canal. The normal canal has a CT density similar to that of adjacent subcutaneous fat, but the presence of tumour will increase this density to near that of muscle. Cortical destruction is shown to good advantage, but it requires the use of very high window levels and wide window widths. In this situation many axial CT sections are required to examine a long bone, and direct sagittal and coronal imaging is not possible.

MRI has significant advantages in evaluating malignant bone lesions. Tissue contrast is superior to that of CT, allowing the extent of muscle, fat and neurovascular involvement to be more accurately assessed (Zimmer et al. 1984; Berquist 1987). Intravenous contrast material is not required to study the vascularity or vascular involvement of a

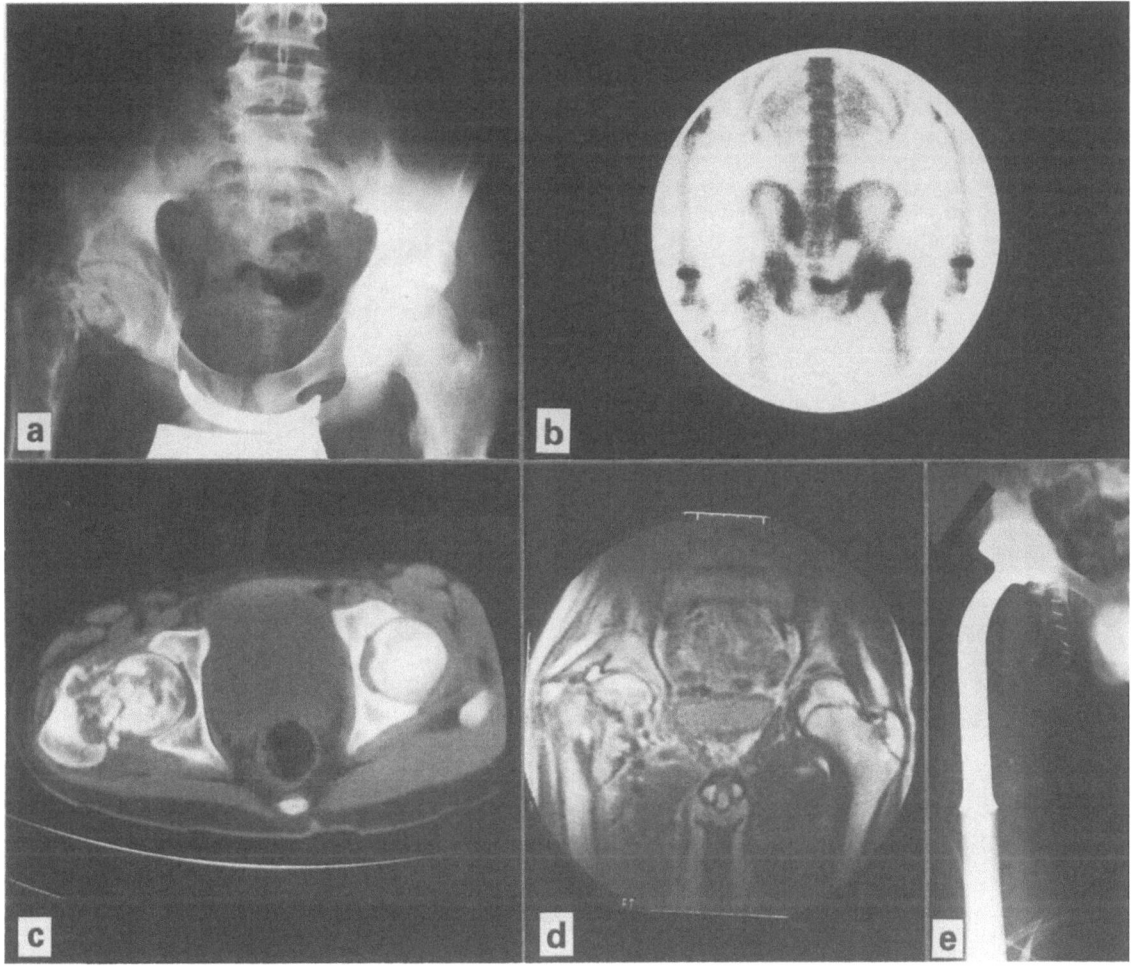

Fig. 21.4. a Antero-posterior view of the right hip shows a large osteosarcoma. Pathological fracture is present. b Scintigram shows increased uptake in the proximal femur. c CT scan shows bone destruction and tumour extending into the hip joint and surrounding soft tissues. d MRI confirms bone destruction and the extent of soft tissue involvement. e Antero-posterior view of the proximal femur after resection and prosthetic replacement. A portion of the acetabulum was removed with the specimen.

lesion. Additional advantages of MRI include direct coronal and sagittal imaging capabilities and no beam-hardening artefact from cortical bone (Hudson et al. 1983). Therefore, in a significant number of patients MRI is superior to CT in determining the extent of the lesion and planning limb-salvage surgery or radiation therapy portals. CT remains superior for the detection of subtle calcification. This finding is sometimes useful in predicting the histological pattern of the lesion (Zimmer et al. 1984).

CT may show regional or distant metastatic disease. The combination of a plain chest radiograph and a CT scan is the method of choice to search for pulmonary metastases in such cases. Currently, MRI is less effective than CT in evaluating pulmonary metastasis. Subtle lesions in the spinal column and pelvis may be detected with MRI or CT when radiographic or isotopic findings are negative, equivocal, or difficult to interpret (Berquist 1987). This is particularly true in older patients with osteoporosis or degenerative changes which can make the detection of myeloma or metastasis difficult. Sagittal MRI of the spinal column and coronal images of the pelvis can be performed quickly using partial saturation sequences (TE $\leq$ 25 ms, TR $\leq$ 500 ms). Well-defined areas of low intensity are seen in patients with myeloma or metastasis (Daffner et al. 1986; Berquist 1987).

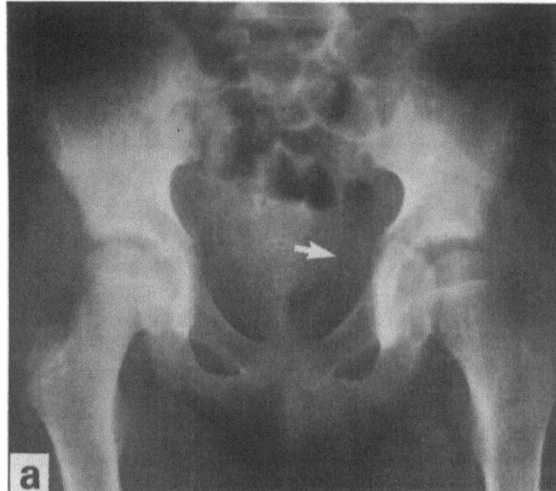

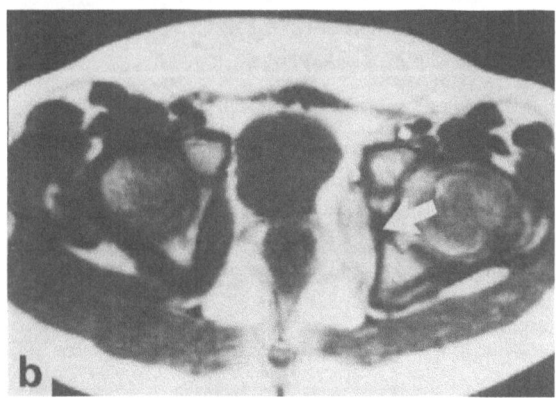

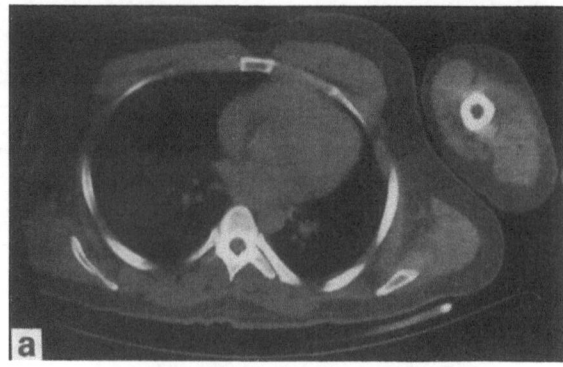

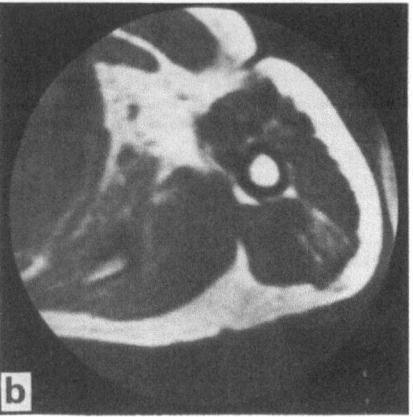

Fig. 21.6a,b. Patient with suspected recurrent desmoid tumour in the upper arm. a CT scan does not clearly demonstrate a lesion. b Axial MRI (TE 60 ms, TR 2000 ms) clearly shows recurrence in postero-lateral muscles.

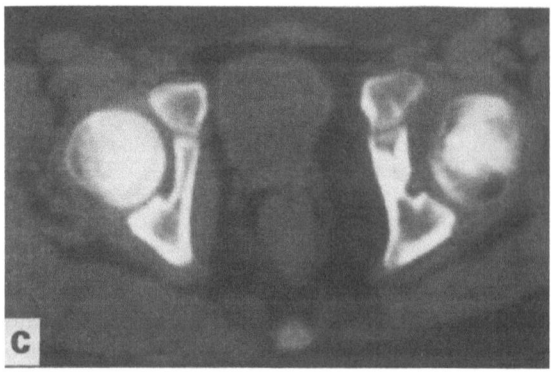

Fig. 21.5a–c. Teenage boy with acetabular osteoid osteoma who presented with chronic hip pain and synovitis. a Antero-posterior view of the pelvis shows widening of the joint space in the left hip with swelling of obturator internus (*arrow*). b Axial MR image (TE 26 ms, TR 2000 ms) shows a mass medial to the femoral head, with no signal (*arrow*) in the acetabulum. c CT scan on the same plane more clearly defines this as an osteoid osteoma.

Other studies are used less commonly. Skeletal scintigrams are useful in searching for additional lesions and in detecting the extent of bone involvement. However, MRI is more accurate (Gershon-Cohen 1970; Berquist 1987). Angiography may be useful in evaluating the soft tissue extent of tumour and defining the major feeding vessels, but this invasive technique usually is not necessary (Enneking 1985). Angiography may provide information regarding the response of the tumour to pre-operative chemotherapy (Kricun 1983).

Once a malignant tumour of bone has been resected, regular assessment for possible recurrence is usually required. Radiography, sometimes supplemented with conventional tomography, is the method of choice for detecting possible intraosseous recurrence. However, the recurrence may be in soft tissues, and chondrosarcomas and chordomas are particularly likely to recur. CT is an accurate method of detecting soft tissue recurrences but it is

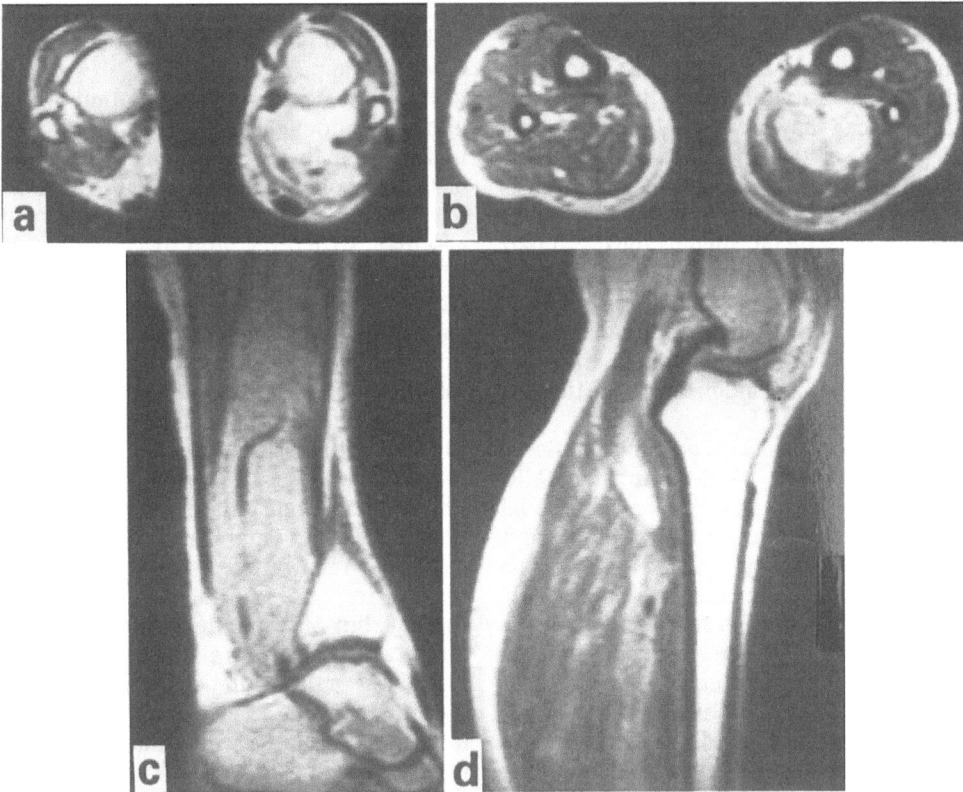

Fig. 21.7a–d. Malignant fibrous histiocytoma. **a** and **b** Axial MRI shows a high-intensity signal from a tumour in calf and ankle. **c** and **d** Sagittal images more clearly demonstrate the tremendous extent of the lesion. Note the vascular encasement in c.

not infallible, and false-positive, false-negative and indeterminate scans occur because of the inability to distinguish the CT appearance of early recurrence from that due to post-operative changes. Surgical clips and metal prostheses are sometimes present and may significantly degrade the CT image (Zimmer et al. 1984; Berquist 1987). Correlation of the CT findings with the clinical examination, and the use of serial examinations, will resolve the issue in most instances.

MRI may be particularly useful in detecting tumour recurrence. In patients with metal implants the degree of artefact is much less significant than with CT (Zimmer et al. 1984; Berquist 1987). In addition, T_2-weighted (TE $\geq$ 60 ms, TR $\geq$ 2000 ms) MRI sequences will show whether areas of high intensity due to tumour or inflammation are present. Scar tissue has low signal intensity on both T_1- and T_2-weighted sequences (Berquist 1987).

CT and MRI are both very useful in evaluating the response of a tumour to chemotherapy or radiation therapy.

Soft Tissue Tumours

In contrast to skeletal lesions, both routine radiographs and xeroradiographs have significant limitations in examining soft tissue lesions (McLeod and Stephens 1979; Bernardino et al. 1981). The information is seldom definitive, and a negative examination never excludes the possibility of a soft tissue mass (Bernardino et al. 1981).

Ultrasonography is the best modality for determining whether a mass is cystic or solid (Bernardino et al. 1981). However, in nearly all other aspects, CT and MRI have become the methods of choice for the evaluation of soft tissue neoplasms (Roach 1970; Levine 1981; Hudson et al. 1983; Dooms et al. 1985; Weekes et al. 1985b).

CT provides excellent anatomical detail of the soft tissues and soft tissue neoplasms. In nearly all cases, it will reliably detect or exclude the presence of a clinically suspected tumour. However, accurate CT evaluation of the soft tissues requires that adequate fat be present. Individual vessels, nerves, muscles and tumours are visualized because they are enveloped by low-density fat. When there is a paucity of fat the CT scan may be severely compromised. This problem may arise in patients who are thin, chronically ill and emaciated, and in infants. It is also a frequent problem when examining anatomical areas that have little fat, such as the distal part of the leg and the upper extremity (Fig. 21.6). The intravenous infusion of contrast material may be required to detect an isodense tumour within muscle, demonstrate tumour vessels or enhancement, or demonstrate the relationship of the tumour to the adjacent vessels.

Although CT is often useful in defining soft tissue masses, the superior soft tissue contrast of MRI allows lesions to be more clearly defined. Coronal and sagittal images provide more information about the extent of involvement. Also, no contrast medium is needed to evaluate neurovascular structures (Fig. 21.7). Therefore, in many cases MRI is now used in place of CT, especially in evaluating the peripheral extremities (Dooms et al. 1985; Weekes et al. 1985b; Aisen 1986; Berquist 1987).

CT and MRI often allow the distinction between benign and malignant neoplasms (Roach 1970; Berquist 1987). Benign lesions usually have sharply defined margins and a homogeneous density. Generally they do not involve multiple groups or compartments, nor do they alter the appearance of adjacent fat. Malignant tumours usually lack well-defined margins because the invasive tumour blends irregularly with the adjacent soft tissues. Areas of low density are common as a result of intralesional haemorrhage or necrosis or both. The presence of hazy blurring and increased density of adjacent fat favours a malignant process. Subtle soft tissue changes are more easily seen with MRI. Involvement of multiple muscle groups, bone invasion and irregular calcification also indicate a malignant process. Calcification is more easily noted with CT. Caution must be exercised when predicting the benign or malignant nature of a soft tissue tumour on the basis of the image appearance. All the previously mentioned findings are occasionally identified in both benign and malignant tumours. However, if these criteria are carefully applied, more than 80% of lesions can be correctly categorized as benign or malignant (Roach 1970).

With few exceptions the CT and MRI appearances of soft tissue tumours are not sufficiently characteristic to allow prediction of the histological diagnosis. A tumour composed entirely of fat can be reliably diagnosed as a benign lipoma, while one consisting primarily of blood vessels can be identified as a hae-

mangioma or an arteriovenous malformation. Malignant tumours do not have a pathognomonic CT or MRI appearance.

The most significant contribution of CT and MRI is in the anatomical demonstration of the size, shape and extent of these tumours before therapy. In most instances, both techniques will also demonstrate the relationship of the tumour to adjacent neurovascular structures and organs. Unfortunately, without an intervening plane of normal tissue, CT will not differentiate a structure that was simply displaced by and applied to the tumour pseudocapsule from one that was engulfed or invaded by tumour. Intravenous contrast material may be required to evaluate the status of adjacent vessels. MRI may be superior in these situations.

In selected cases CT is useful in searching for possible regional or distant metastasis. As with skeletal lesions, CT is a valuable modality for the detection of tumour recurrence. It is also useful in assessing tumour response to radiation therapy or chemotherapy, but MRI may be more useful in differentiating recurrence from post-operative change. Scar tissue has a low intensity on both T_1- and T_2-weighted MRI sequences. In contrast the signal intensity of tumour or inflammation is significantly increased owing to longer T_2 relaxation times, so these areas have a high intensity on T_2-weighted images.

Summary

The improved outcome of treatment of musculoskeletal tumours is due, in part, to the better assessment of the lesion. Better diagnostic techniques and earlier diagnosis have an impact on survival irrespective of contemporary therapeutic regimens. Advances in pre-operative investigative measures have improved the detection of systemic occult metastatic disease and have defined more clearly the nature and local extent of the primary lesion. The latter information is needed before a decision between amputation and limb-saving resection can be made. Current imaging techniques approach 90% accuracy in clinical staging (Enneking 1985).

Bone tumours are challenging problems that require a high index of suspicion. Once the lesion is discovered, a systematic approach to pre-operative evaluation is mandatory in order to provide effective management of the patient.

References

Aisen AM, Martel W, Braunstein EM, McMillin KI, Phillips WA, Kling TF (1986) MRI and CT evaluation of primary bone and soft-tissue tumors. AJR 146:749–756

Bernardino ME, Jing B-S, Thomas JL, Lindell MM Jr, Zornoza J (1981) The extremity soft-tissue lesion: a comparative study of ultrasound, computed tomography, and xeroradiography. Radiology 139:53–59

Berquist TH (1987) The musculoskeletal system. In: Higgins CB, Hricak H (eds) Magnetic resonance imaging of the body. Raven Press, New York, pp 469–489

Daffner RH, Lupetin AR, Dash N, Deeb ZL, Sefczek RJ, Schapiro RL (1986) MRI in the detection of malignant infiltration of bone marrow. AJR 146:353–358

Dooms GC, Hricak H, Sollitto RA, Higgins CB (1985) Lipomatous tumors and tumors with fatty component: MR imaging potential and comparison of MR and CT results. Radiology 157:479–483

Enneking WF (1985) Preoperative staging of sarcomas. Cancer Treat Symp 3:67–70

Gershon-Cohen J (1970) Thermography and panography in diagnosis of bone disease. Radiol Clin North Am 8:241–249

Halpern M, Freiberger RH (1970) Arteriography as a diagnostic procedure in bone disease. Radiol Clin North Am 8:277–288

Hudson TM, Schiebler M, Springfield DS, Hawkins IF Jr, Enneking WF, Spanier SS (1983) Radiologic imaging of osteosarcoma: role in planning surgical treatment. Skeletal Radiol 10:137–146

Hudson TM, Hamlin DJ, Enneking WF, Pettersson H (1985) Magnetic resonance imaging of bone and soft tissue tumors: early experience in 31 patients compared with computed tomography. Skeletal Radiol 13:134–146

Kricun ME (1983) Radiographic evaluation of solitary bone lesions. Orthop Clin North Am 14:39–64

Kumpan W, Lechner G, Wittich GR et al. (1986) The angiographic response of osteosarcoma following pre-operative chemotherapy. Skeletal Radiol 15:96–102

Levine E (1981) Computed tomography of musculoskeletal tumors. CRC Crit Rev Diagn Imaging 16:279–309

Levine E, Lee KR, Neff JR, Maklad NF, Robinson RG, Preston DF (1979) Comparison of computed tomography and other imaging modalities in the evaluation of musculoskeletal tumors. Radiology 131:431–437

Lukens JA, McLeod RA, Sim FH (1982) Computed tomographic evaluation of primary osseous malignant neoplasms. AJR 139:45–48

McLeod RA, Stephens DH (1979) Computed tomography of pelvic musculoskeletal neoplasms. Contemp Orthop 1:36–41

McLeod RA, Gisvold JJ, Stephens DH, Beabout JW, Sheedy PF (1978) Computed tomography of soft tissues and breast. Semin Roentgenol 13:267–275

Roach JF (1970) Xeroradiography. Radiol Clin North Am 8:271–275

Weekes RG, Berquist TH, McLeod RA, Zimmer WD (1985a) Magnetic resonance imaging of soft-tissue tumors: comparison with computed tomography. Magn Reson Imaging 3:345–352

Weekes RG, McLeod RA, Reiman HM, Pritchard DJ (1985b) CT of soft-tissue neoplasms. AJR 144:355–360

Zimmer WD, Berquist TH, Sim RH et al. (1984) Magnetic resonance imaging of aneurysmal bone cyst. Mayo Clin Proc 59:633–636

22 Metastatic Tumours

C.S.B. Galasko and I. Isherwood

Diagnosis of a Symptomatic Lesion 293
  Clinical Features 293
  Radiographs 295
  Scintigraphy 297
  Computed Tomography 298
  Biopsy 300
Assessment of Extent of Dissemination 300
  General Dissemination 300
  Evaluation of Local Dissemination 301
  Tumour Localizing Isotopes 302
Staging of Cancer 302
  Clinical, Biochemical and Radiographic Features 302
  Skeletal Scintigraphy 302
Response to Treatment 303
  Clinical and Biochemical Assessment 303
  Radiological Assessment 303
  Skeletal Scintigraphy 304
  Irradiation 304
  Other Methods of Assessment 305
Conclusions 305
References 305

The detection of skeletal metastases may be important under three circumstances.

1. The diagnosis of a painful lesion in a patient who may, or may not, be known to have cancer.
2. The assessment of the extent of dissemination in a patient with metastatic cancer.
3. The assessment of a patient with apparently "early" cancer in an attempt to stage the disease before starting treatment.

Diagnosis of a Symptomatic Lesion

Clinical Features

Pain

Pain in a middle-aged or elderly patient is the commonest presenting symptom, but is not always present. Review of 86 patients with advanced mammary carcinoma, all of whom had skeletal metastases evident on plain radiography, showed that only 65% complained of pain (Galasko 1972). When present it was related to some, but not all of their metastases. Mettler and Guiberteau (1983) reported that 30%–50% of patients with skeletal metastases did not have bone pain, particularly patients with disseminated prostatic carcinoma, and Front et al. (1979) found that 32% of patients with skeletal metastases from mammary carcinoma had no bone pain.

Bone pain is not specific and may be due to other causes. Galasko and Sylvester (1978) found that only 66% of patients who presented with back pain and had a previous history of malignancy, had skeletal metastases. In the other patients a benign cause was found for their pain. Winchester et al. (1979) reported that only 60% of their patients with bone pain proved to have skeletal metastases.

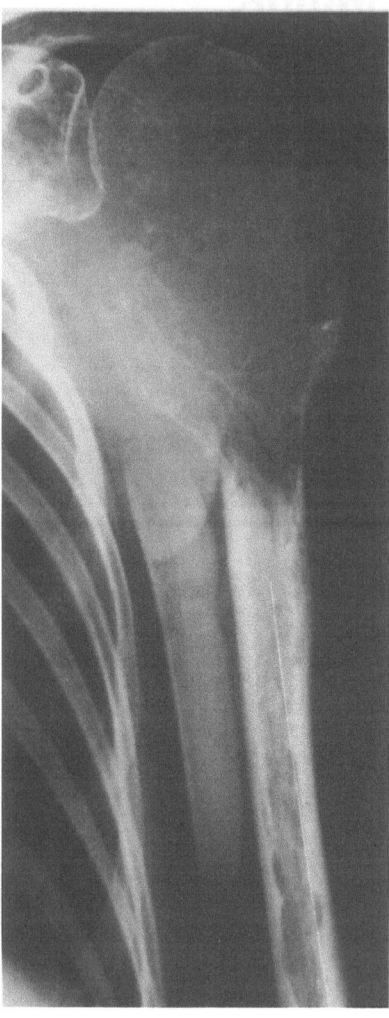

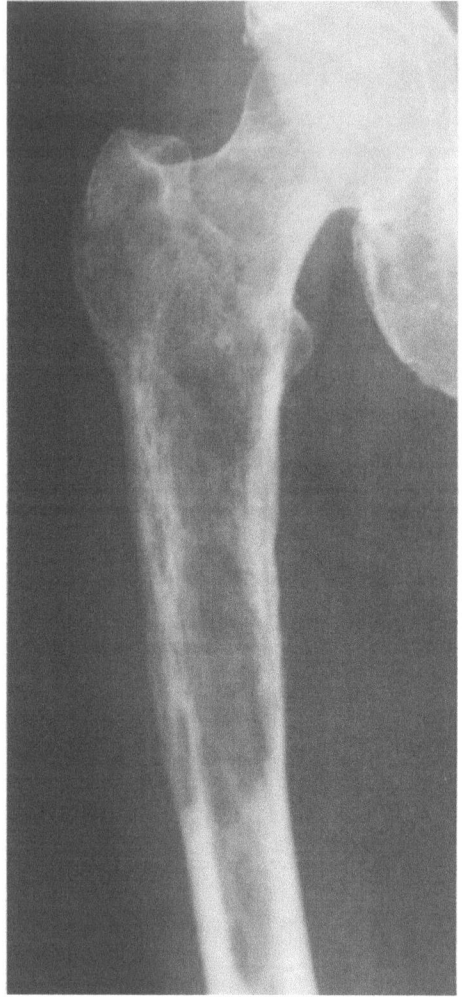

Fig. 22.1. Geographic metastasis. Lytic deposit from a primary renal carcinoma. A geographic pattern of bone destruction with associated cortical expansion. Metastases from breast and thyroid tumours may give similar appearances. Disease is also present in the humeral shaft. Reproduced from Adams and Isherwood (1983).

Fig. 22.2. Moth-eaten metastasis. Lytic deposit in right femur from breast carcinoma. A moth-eaten pattern of bone destruction with ill-defined margins and cortical destruction. Reproduced from Adams and Isherwood (1983).

Swelling

A skeletal metastasis may sometimes present as a tender mass, particularly if a subcutaneous bone such as the clavicle or a phalanx is affected. Such a tender swelling may mimic an infection.

Tenderness

Tenderness is uncommon and was only elicited in 16% of patients with radiographic evidence of skeletal metastases (Galasko 1972).

Biochemical Parameters

The biochemical parameters currently available lack specificity and are inaccurate. Galasko (1972) found that the alkaline phosphatase level was the most sensitive of biochemical parameters evaluated, but was raised in only 66% of patients with radiographically proven skeletal metastases from mammary carcinoma. There is a high incidence of false positives and negatives (Bishop et al. 1985). The urinary hydroxyproline level and the hydroxyproline/creatinine ratio are slightly more sensitive indi-

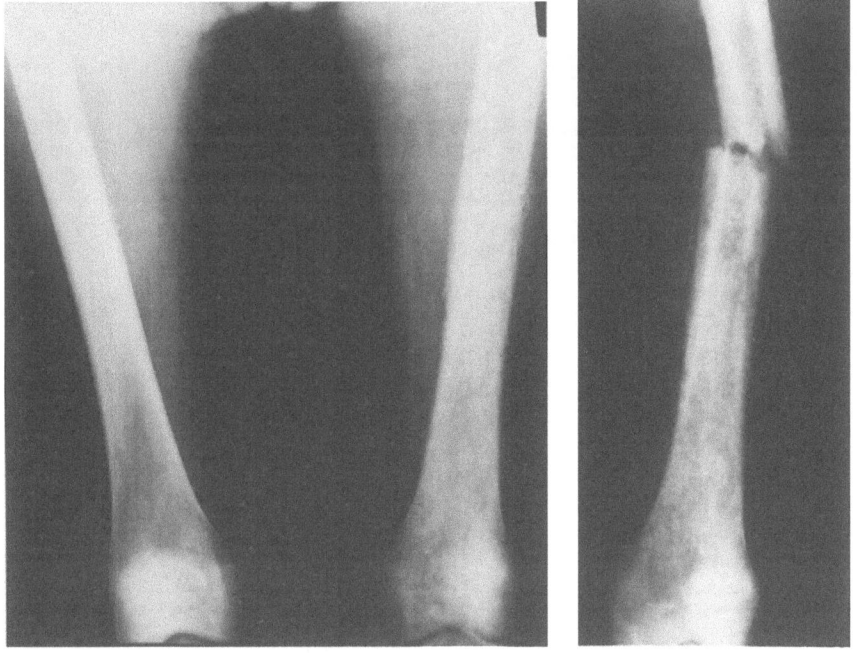

Fig. 22.3a,b. Patient with rectal carcinoma. **a** There are multiple permeative metastases throughout the left femur. Patient was advised to have a prophylactic stabilization of his femur. He decided to think about surgery during the weekend. **b** He was admitted as an emergency two days later with a pathological fracture through the affected femur.

cators than the alkaline phosphatase level, but are still associated with a high false-negative rate that varies with different methods of estimation (Cuschieri et al. 1978).

Radiographs

Skeletal metastases are usually multiple, but isolated lesions do occur. They may be lytic, sclerotic or mixed. Sclerotic metastases are most commonly from prostatic carcinoma, but also occur with mammary, gastrointestinal and bladder cancers. Lytic metastases occur with every type of primary tumour, and mixed lesions most commonly arise from mammary cancer.

Unlike Paget's disease the cortex is not thickened in sclerotic metastases nor is the trabecular pattern disorganized.

There are three types of lytic lesion (Adams and Isherwood 1983).

1. *Geographic.* These are large, solitary, well-defined lytic areas, more than one centimetre in diameter and usually with a sharply demarcated edge (Fig. 22.1)

2. *Moth-eaten.* There are multiple, smaller lytic areas (2–5 mm) which may coalesce to form larger confluent areas (Fig. 22.2). Their margins are usually ill-defined

3. *Permeative.* There are multiple tiny lytic areas (usually 1 mm or less) seen principally in cortical bone (Fig 22.3).

Geographic destruction is usually found in the slowest developing metastases, whereas permeative destruction occurs in the most aggressive lesions. A patient with multiple metastases usually shows one of the three principle patterns. Pathological fracture is a major complication of skeletal metastases. It usually occurs with lytic metastases and the risk of this complication occurring is related to the amount of cortical bone destruction (Fidler 1981). Pathological fractures may also occur with moth-eaten or permeative metastases.

Radiographic examination is insensitive. Edelstyn et al. (1967) found that at least 50% of the bone must be destroyed in the beam axis of the X-ray before the lesion could be seen radiographically. Most skeletal metastases develop in the medulla and

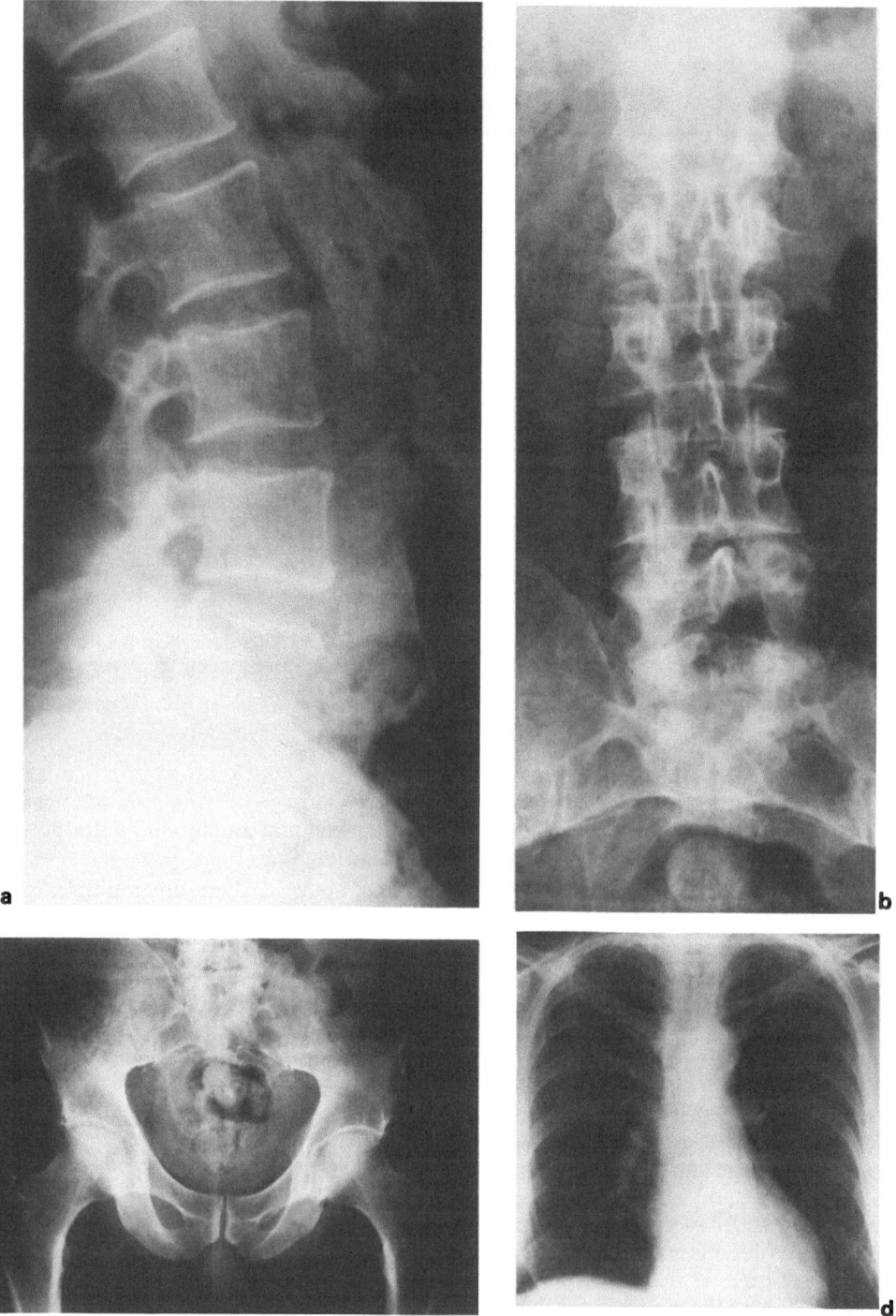

Fig. 22.4a–e. Patient with prostatic carcinoma who presented with back pain. **a,b,c,d** Radiographs of lumbar spine, pelvis and chest show no radiographic evidence of skeletal metastases. **e** ^{99m}-Tc-MDP skeletal scintigram shows multiple areas of increased uptake in his spine, pelvis and rib cage (next page).

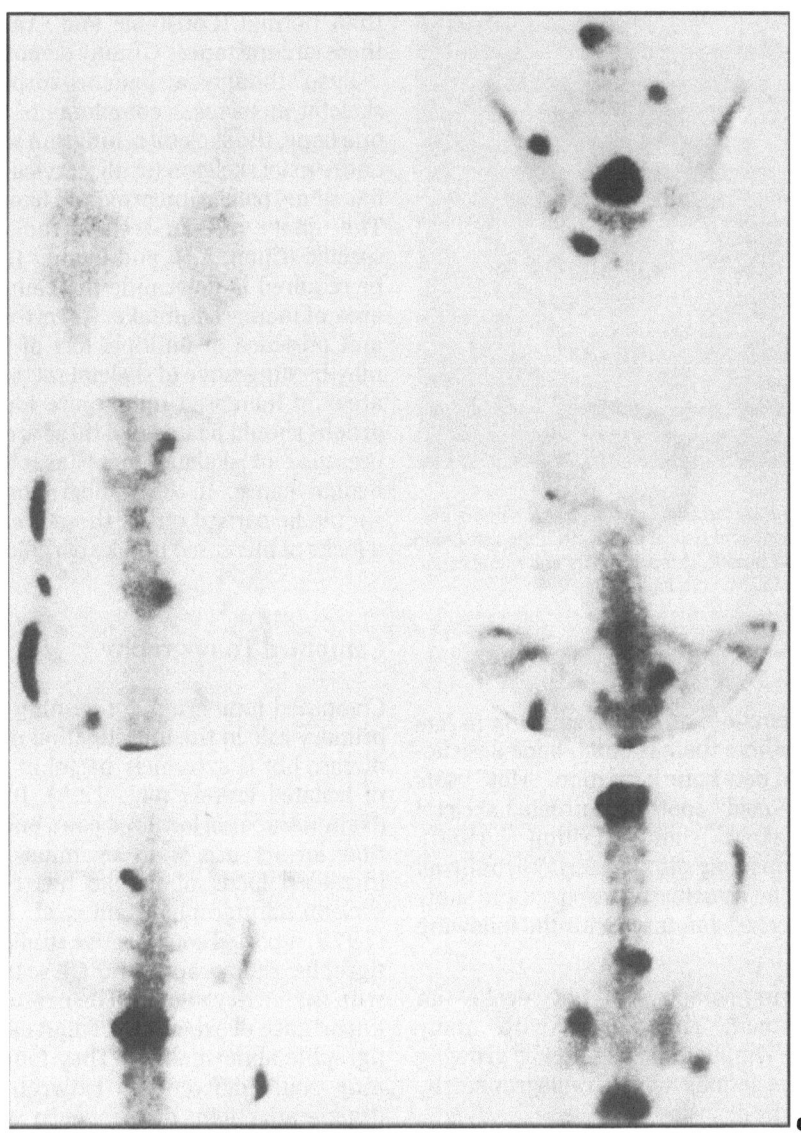

Fig. 22.4e. See caption on previous page.

only involve the cortex late. In contrast, lesions which primarily involve the cortex can be detected when very much smaller.

Loss of a pedicle may be the first radiographic sign of skeletal metastases, and an avulsion fracture of the lesser trochanter, in the absence of trauma, has also been described as the first sign of dissemination (Bertin et al. 1984).

Scintigraphy

Much evidence has now accumulated that skeletal scintigraphy is more sensitive than radiography for the detection of skeletal metastases (Galasko 1984a, Chap. 13, Fig. 22.4). Skeletal metastases are usually seen as localized areas of increased uptake. Occasionally they may appear as areas of diminished

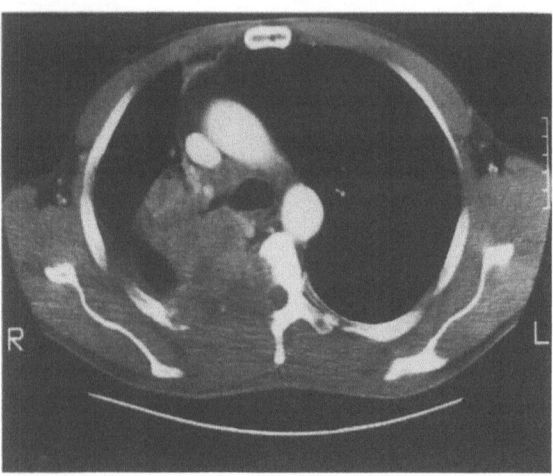

Fig. 22.5. CT scan of a metastasis. Lytic deposit involving posterior rib, vertebral body and neural arch with large soft tissue component in adjacent muscle, thoracic cavity and spinal canal. Primary bronchial neoplasm with lobar collapse.

than normal (Constable and Crannage 1981). In these circumstances CT may demonstrate the lesion.

Even though a patient suspected of having skeletal metastases complains of pain localized to one bone, the skeletal scintigram should include the entire axial skeleton (skull, cervical, dorsal and lumbar spine, pelvis and proximal femora and humeri). The uptake of bone-seeking radionuclides is non-specific (Chap. 13), and further investigation may be required to determine the cause of the localized area of increased uptake. Nevertheless, the pattern and presence of multiple foci of increased uptake may be suggestive of skeletal metastases. If multiple areas of increased uptake are found, plain radiographs should be taken of these areas to confirm the presence of skeletal metastases or to exclude a benign cause. If the radiographs are normal CT should be carried out of those areas where there is a focus of increased uptake of radionuclide.

uptake due to infarction, or more frequently in late lytic metastases where there is much bone destruction with minimal new bone formation. "Hot" spots may progress to "cold" spots in untreated skeletal metastases (Makoha and Britton 1980). "Doughnut" lesions may also be seen. Virtually all metastases evoke an osteoblastic response and show up as areas of increased uptake, with the following exceptions.

1. Those tumours which do not evoke an osteoblastic response. This occurs with many myelomata, some lymphomata and rapidly growing highly destructive lesions which radiographically appear as large lytic deposits.

2. Small deposits. Very small lesions are likely to be missed. With emission isotopic tomographic scintigraphy it is possible that lesions 2 mm in diameter may be detected (Ell et al. 1980). This probably explains why post-operative serial scintigrams show an increase in incidence of skeletal metastases.

In patients with widespread metastatic disease, the skeletal scintigram may be misinterpreted as normal, when the uptake is symmetrical and there are no localized areas of increased concentration – instead there is an overall markedly increased uptake (the so-called "superscan"). Sy et al. (1975) suggested that under these circumstances there may be a reduction in urinary excretion of isotope and faint or absent renal uptake may indicate generalized symmetrical disease. Quantitation may indicate a local bone uptake significantly greater

Computed Tomography

Computed tomographic scanning does not have a primary role in the investigation of metastatic bone disease but is extremely useful in the confirmation of isolated lesions (Fig. 22.5). It can be used to examine areas of localized pain, but the main indication for its use is to examine areas where an increased focus of uptake has been detected on skeletal scintigraphs (Rafii et al. 1986). Best et al. (1979) reported comparative studies of skeletal scintigraphs, radiographs and CT scans in 30 patients with mammary cancer. Their results confirmed the importance of excluding benign causes for the scintigraphic abnormalities. They found that CT scanning could differentiate between metastases and degenerative joint disease, even when the two co-existed and that degenerative arthritis of the spinal facet joints was a common cause of increased radionuclide uptake, although not always apparent on conventional radiographs. The extent of soft-tissue involvement is well demonstrated by CT.

CT is not organ-specific and may reveal associated or causative disease not evident on conventional imaging (Adams and Isherwood 1983).

Fig. 22.6a–d. Patient who presented with back pain. There was no history of an underlying carcinoma. **a,b** Radiographs of the spine showed an enlarged pedicle of D10. **c** ^{99m}-Tc-MDP scintigram showing multiple areas of increased uptake in the spine, particularly D10, and rib cage. **d** A needle biopsy was carried out under radiographic control. Histology revealed a small cell undifferentiated metastasis.

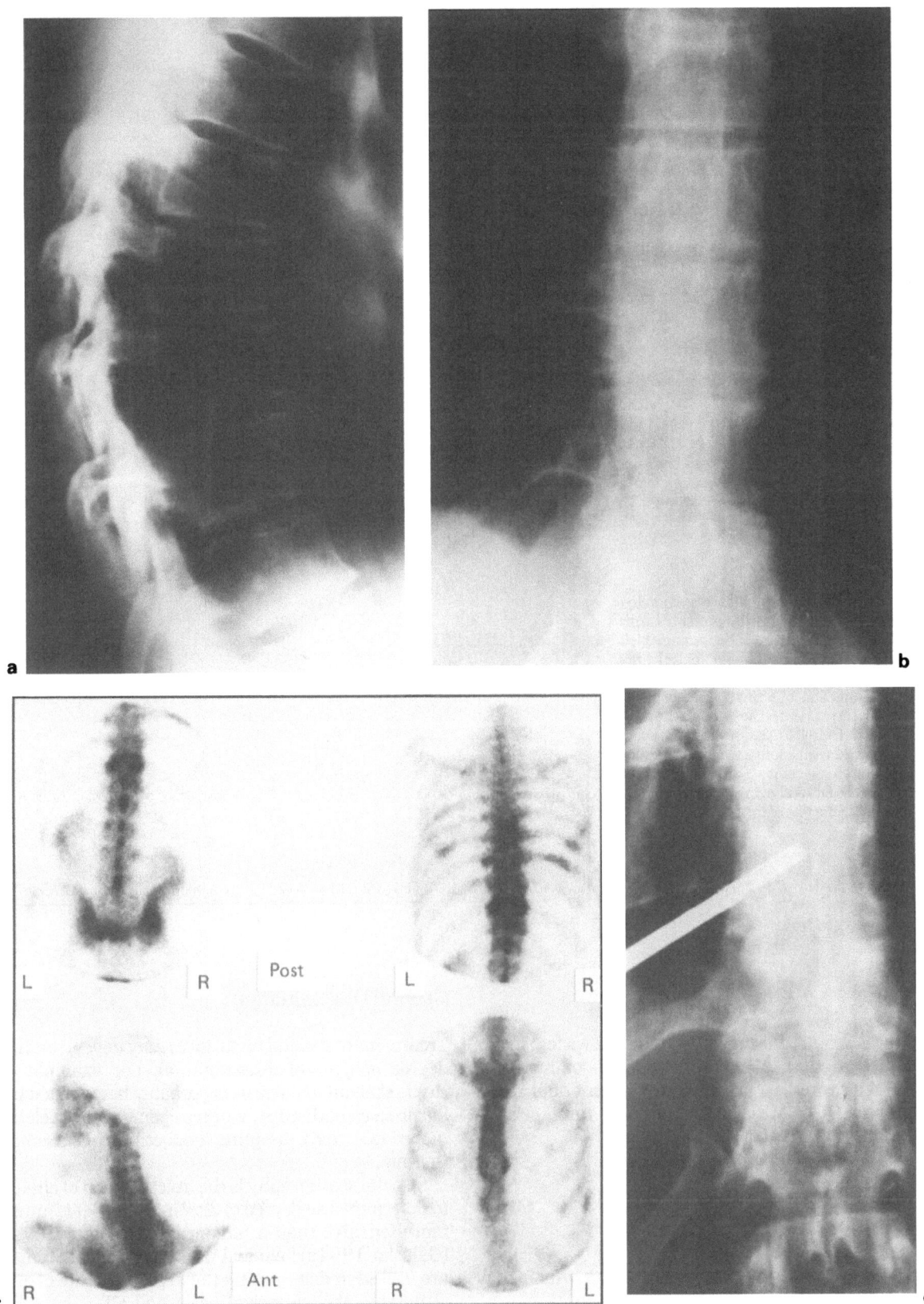

a

b

c

Post

Ant

d

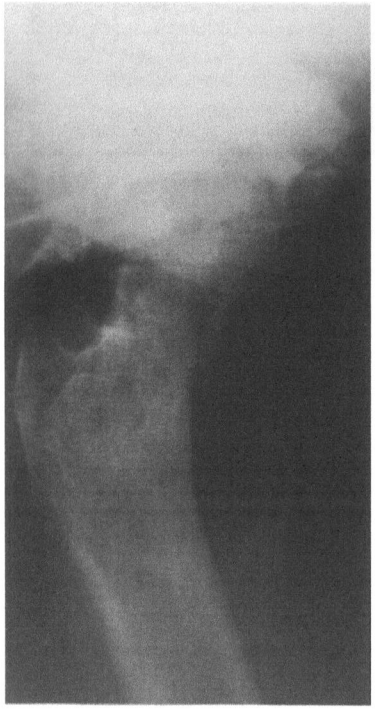

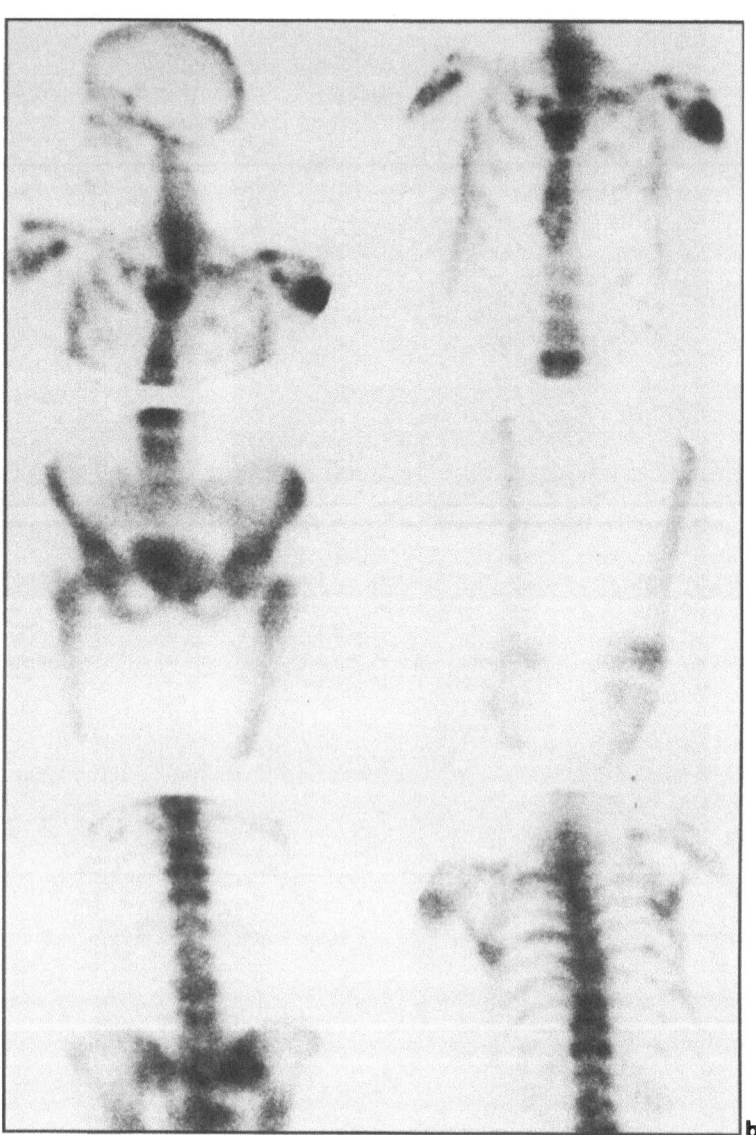

Fig. 22.7a,b. Patient with disseminated mammary carcinoma who presented with a pathological fracture of her proximal left femur. a Transcervical pathological fracture of left femur. b ^{99m}-Tc-MDP skeletal scintigram. She has multiple metastases. There is increased uptake through the shaft of the left femur. Therefore, the metastasis was treated with a long-stemmed Charnley total hip replacement arthroplasty, the stem of the femoral component being used to stabilize the rest of the femur.

Biopsy

This is required if the scintigraph shows few foci of increased uptake and other causes of increased uptake cannot be excluded by conventional radiography, CT or MRI, or if the primary tumour is not known (Fig. 22.6).

Assessment of Extent of Dissemination

There are two types of dissemination which may require elucidation.

General Dissemination

Treatment of skeletal metastases may depend on the degree of general dissemination. For example, a single skeletal metastasis is probably best treated by localized radiotherapy, whereas generalized skeletal metastases may require endocrine or chemotherapy.

Skeletal scintigraphy is the investigation of choice to determine the degree of dissemination. It is much more sensitive than a radiographic skeletal survey (Galasko 1984a); clinical and biochemical studies are useless in determining the degree and site of disseminated skeletal metastases; and CT cannot be used to screen the entire axial skeleton. However, plain radiographs, tomographs or CT may need to be undertaken of areas with foci of increased uptake to confirm that these are due to multiple skeletal metastases.

Evaluation of Local Dissemination

Treatment of a single metastasis depends on the degree of spread, and the amount of bone destruction. As indicated above, irradiation is the treatment of choice for a localized painful skeletal metastasis. It is important that the edges of the radiotherapy field do not inadvertently cross asymptomatic metastases, which may subsequently require treatment (Galasko et al. 1982). Scintigraphy is often used before the field is planned, since it is more accurate than radiographs in establishing the full extent of the lesion requiring radiotherapy, as well as the presence of neighbouring lesions. CT can be used as an alternative. Internal stabilization may be required for large lytic metastases, pathological fractures and spinal instability. The implant should also stabilize adjacent metastases, which otherwise may lead to pathological fracture or spinal instability (Fig. 22.7). The treatment of a pathological fracture or spinal instability adjacent to a pre-existing implant is much more difficult than if this lesion had been stabilized at the time of primary surgery. Skeletal scintigraphy should be carried out prior to surgical stabilization, to determine the length of implant required to stabilize adjacent metastases.

Scintigraphy cannot be used to demonstrate the amount of bone destruction or its soft tissue extent and these features may be particularly important in planning spinal stabilization. CT myelography, or in some circumstances CT alone, can be used to demonstrate the extension of tumour into the spinal canal, assess spinal cord or cauda equina compression, and the degree and site of decompression required (Figs. 22.8, 22.9). Myelography is frequently used without CT scanning, to detect spinal epidural metastases in patients with symptoms or signs of spinal cord or cauda equina compression (Fig. 22.8, Calkins et al. 1986; Rodichok et al. 1986).

MRI, particularly after intravenous administration of Gd-DTPA, can be of value in the detection of spinal metastases (Fig. 22.10). Sagittal and transverse sections may reveal the extent of bone involvement, the degree of intracanal spread and spinal cord or cauda equina compression. The role of MRI in metastatic bone disease has not yet been evaluated fully.

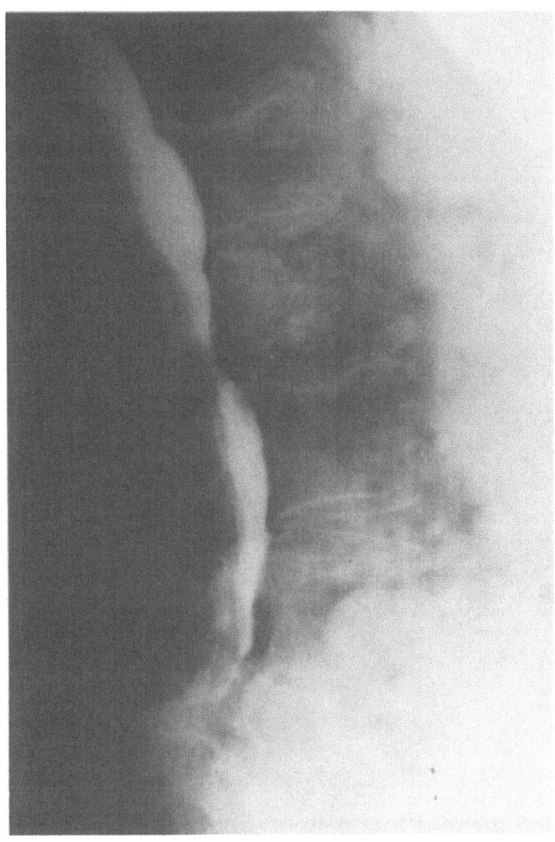

Fig. 22.8. Patient with disseminated mammary carcinoma who presented with spinal instability and weakness affecting her left thigh. Myelogram shows destruction of L3 with compression of the cauda equina at that level. She was treated by simultaneous decompression and stabilization, followed by hormonal therapy. She made a full neurological recovery and four and a half years later is alive, well, free from pain and still on her hormonal therapy.

The evaluation of pelvic metastases can be difficult. Lesions in the pubis and ischium may be missed on the scintigraph (Galasko and Doyle 1972b). Bone-seeking radionuclides are excreted in the urine and their concentration in the bladder tends to mask the pubis. If a lesion is suspected in the pubis, the patient may have to be catheterized before images of the pelvis are obtained. With many techniques of scintigraphy the ischium and sacrum are clearly visualized. A lateral projection of the sacrum may be helpful (Epstein and Stern 1977), but where metastases are suspected in the pelvis CT scanning or, if there is still doubt about the diagnosis, a bone biopsy may be required.

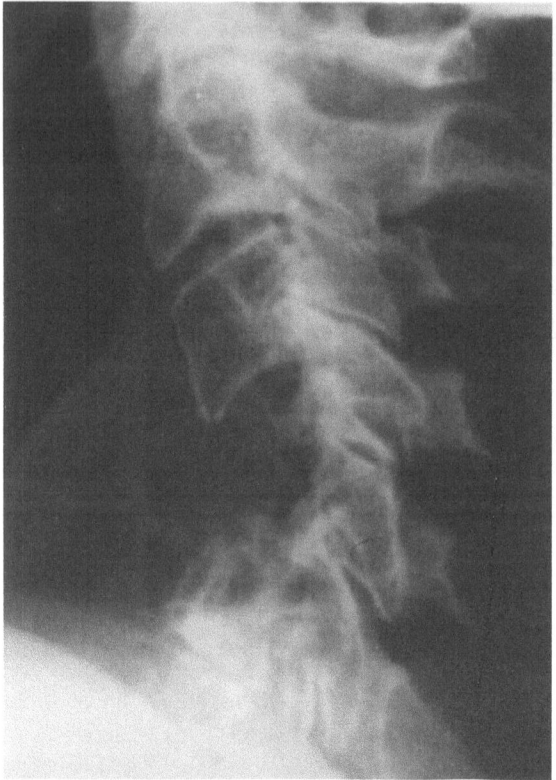

a

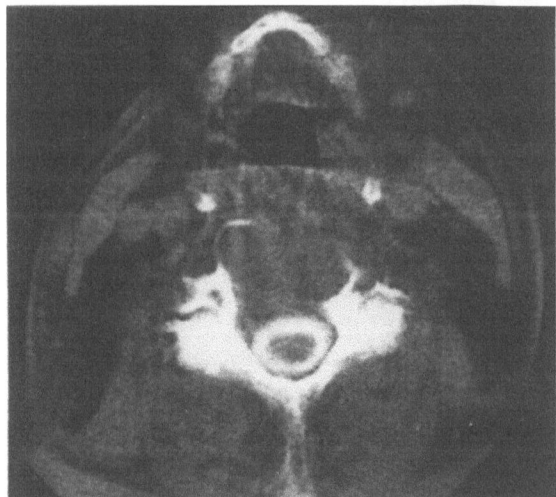

b

Fig. 22.9a,b. Patient with disseminated chondrosarcoma. One year previously the primary tumour was resected from his chest wall. He presented with severe neck pain which had not responded to radiotherapy. **a** Lateral radiograph of the cervical spine shows complete destruction of the bodies of C4 and 5. **b** CT myelogram shows destruction of the body of C4 with no cord compression. He was treated by surgical stabilization of his neck with relief of pain.

Tumour Localizing Isotopes

The development of a radiopharmaceutical which would be concentrated in the primary neoplasm, soft tissue metastases and skeletal metastases has attracted much research. This would make the assessment of malignant tumours more accurate. Several tumour localizing isotopes have been developed. They tend to be accurate in the diagnosis of large lesions that are evident clinically or radiographically, but the results obtained in the detection of small lesions and skeletal metastases have been disappointing.

It is possible that polyclonal or monoclonal antibodies may become useful in this context.

Staging of Cancer

Clinical, Biochemical and Radiographic Features

A history of bone pain is important and radiographs or CT scans should be obtained of any painful area. Chest radiographs are usually carried out, but skeletal surveys are probably of little value. Routine CT or MRI is of no value, but radiography or CT must be obtained of areas with foci of increased radionuclide uptake. Raised alkaline phosphatase, acid phosphatase or urinary hydroxyproline are suspicious but not specific, and less sensitive than skeletal scintigraphy.

Skeletal Scintigraphy

There is no disagreement about the use of skeletal scintigraphy for the detection of painful lesions, or in assessing the extent of skeletal involvement in a patient with advanced carcinoma. The use of scintigraphy in patients with apparently "early" carcinoma in order to stage the disease before starting treatment, however, is more controversial. Skeletal scintigraphy has been evaluated in a number of primary tumours (Galasko 1986), but the majority of studies have been carried out in patients with mammary carcinoma. The detection rate of skeletal metastases in patients with otherwise apparently "early" mammary carcinoma has ranged from 2%–28%. The accuracy of detection is dependent on the isotope chosen (^{99m}Tc-diphosphonates, particularly MDP, are more sensitive than ^{99m}Tc-phosphates), the choice of detecting apparatus (the gamma

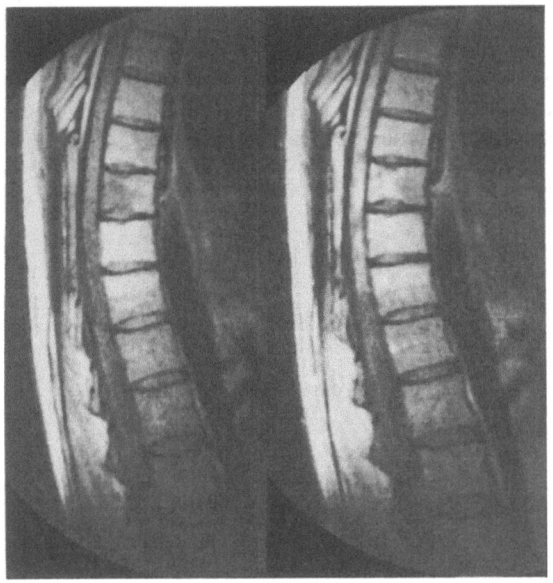

Fig. 22.10. MRI of spine showing metastases. T_1 weighted sequences (a) Pre Gd-DTPA demonstrating lytic deposit in T_{10} vertebral body. (b) Post Gd-DTPA demonstrating increased signal in bony deposit and also in spinal cord due to intramedullary disease. Note increased signal from lower thoracic vertebral bodies generally due to effects of radiation therapy (fat replacement of haemopoietic marrow).

camera is more sensitive than a whole-body scanner), the technical qualities of the scintigram (Merrick 1973) and probably the behaviour of the tumour. There may be a significant difference in tumour populations (e.g. size, invasiveness) between different series which may explain some of the differences in reported results. Whatever the explanation for this variation in detection rate, it cannot be denied that in any group of patients with apparently "early" cancer, there are two populations: those who have a normal scintigram and a better prognosis and those with a positive scintigram and a poorer prognosis. Whether skeletal scintigraphy should be used to evaluate patients prior to treatment for apparently localized carcinoma, will probably depend on the perceived cost effectiveness of the technique and the results obtained in that particular laboratory. If additional lesions are detected the patient requires treatment for disseminated carcinoma, and unnecessary major surgery may be avoided. Turner and Haggith (1981) investigated 57 patients thought to have an operable bronchial cancer and found that scintigraphy saved three patients from thoracotomy.

Response to Treatment

Response to a particular form of treatment should be assessed objectively, and as early as possible, so that if the patient has failed to respond, the treatment can be altered.

Clinical and Biochemical Assessment

The relief of pain is important, but the clinical assessment of the response of skeletal metastases may be unreliable (Galasko and Doyle 1972a). The patient may minimize the severity of the pain, or it may be controlled by analgesics without affecting the underlying lesions. Nevertheless, relief of pain following irradiation, endocrine or chemotherapy is often indicative of an objective response.

Serial biochemical changes may be useful, but frequently do not reflect the response of skeletal metastases. Serial changes in the alkaline phosphatase level were only useful in assessing the response in 53 of 92 patients with advanced mammary carcinoma (57.6%) (Galasko 1972). Measurement of the isoenzymes of alkaline phosphatase allowed for greater precision in the monitoring of skeletal metastases (Parbhoo 1985) and serial measurements of the urine hydroxyproline level may be useful (Gielen et al. 1976; Powles et al. 1975), although the changes are not always reliable (Roberts and Baum 1975; Niell et al. 1981). Changes in urinary calcium excretion may be a useful marker of response to treatment in patients with skeletal metastases (Williams et al. 1984; Grainger et al. 1984).

Radiological Assessment

It is sometimes difficult to interpret the radiographic changes. The development of new lytic lesions, or the enlargement of existing ones, indicates progression of the disease. In patients with sclerotic metastases progression of disease is associated with the enlargement of existing metastases and the appearance of new lesions. With remission of disease, bones with lytic metastases may regain a normal radiographic appearance, or the lytic areas may become sclerotic. Occasionally "new" sclerotic metastases may develop and it may be impossible then to differentiate those sclerotic lesions due to progression of disease from those due to healing of lytic lesions which were not apparent on the initial radiographs (Galasko and Doyle 1972a).

Such is the difficulty of evaluating serial changes radiographically, that the International Union Against Cancer (UICC) specifically excluded mixed and sclerotic lesions in their assessment of response, but made some allowance for changes in lytic metastases (Hayward et al. 1977). They defined complete objective regression as calcification of all osteolytic lesions, if present, and an absence of new lesions on the radiograph.

Skeletal Scintigraphy

Serial scintigrams are more accurate than serial radiographs in assessing response to treatment (Galasko and Doyle 1972a; Hammond et al. 1978; Citrin et al. 1981; Coombes et al. 1983).

Skeletal metastases which respond to treatment lose their increased avidity for bone-seeking isotopes, irrespective of their radiographic appearance; whereas increased uptake can be anticipated in those metastases which do not respond to treatment. Patients who do not respond to treatment usually develop further metastases. Very advanced metastases may have a normal, or even diminished, uptake and serial scintigrams, therefore, must not be read in isolation. Serial radiographs of relevant areas may be required and if there is still doubt, CT scans may be necessary.

A successful response to therapy may be associated with an early increase in uptake of the radionuclide. This initial "flare" may be seen on a repeat scintigraph obtained within 4 to 8 weeks of starting treatment, but if treatment is successful, later scintigrams will show a decrease in uptake. It is possible that the initial "flare" is due to active mineralization during the early healing phase (Greenburg et al. 1972; Gillespie et al. 1975). If the second scintigram is delayed for 3 to 4 months, this "flare" phenomenon may not be seen. Alexander et al. (1976) could not correlate a transient "flare" with response and treatment should not be influenced by its presence or absence.

Similar changes occur with metastases from prostatic carcinoma, even though they are radiographically sclerotic. Successful treatment results in a significantly decreased uptake, the scintigrams returning completely to normal in some, whereas with failure of treatment the serial scintigrams may show more foci of increased uptake (Langhammer et al. 1978, 1981; Pollen and Shlaer 1979; Stone et al. 1980; Levenson et al. 1981). Similar changes have been reported in patients with skeletal metastases from adenocarcinoma of the colon (De Luca et al. 1983).

Irradiation

Skeletal metastases are often treated by radiotherapy which may affect the underlying bone and its scintigraphic appearance.

The Effect on Normal Bone

There probably are three phases to the changes that occur in normal bone after irradiation (Galasko 1984a).

1. In the few days immediately following exposure to radiation, a hyperaemic phase occurs, associated with increased uptake of isotope seen on the blood pool image.

2. During the ensuing few months there is an increased uptake associated with new bone formation. This phase is dependent on the dose and schedule of irradiation.

3. This is followed by a reduction in bone formation associated with prolonged decreased vascularity and decreased isotope uptake. This phase may last many years, but the uptake may eventually revert to normal.

Although the common appearance of irradiated bone is decreased uptake with loss of anatomical detail, there may be foci of increased uptake at the margin of the irradiated area (Galasko 1984a) which must not be mistaken for new metastases.

Replacement of haemopoietic marrow by fat in vertebral bodies following radiotherapy gives rise to an increase in signal on both T_1 and T_2 weighted with images (Fig. 22.10).

Avascular Necrosis

Irradiation may cause avascular necrosis. In the early stage of pure avascularity both the blood pool and skeletal images show diminished uptake. In the second phase new vessels grow into the avascular area and new bone is laid down, usually on trabeculae of necrotic lamellar bone. There is some concomitant resorption of necrotic bone and during this phase there is an increased uptake of bone-seeking radionuclide. Radiographs may appear normal until the changes are very advanced.

Other Methods of Assessment

The results of serial bone marrow biopsies are not sufficiently reliable for routine evaluation of the response to treatment (Hortobagyi et al. 1984).

Serial CT of selected skeletal lesions in patients with multiple skeletal metastases, or all the lesions in patients with a few metastases, may be very sensitive, particularly quantitative CT (Golimbu et al. 1986).

Conclusions

There is no ideal method for detecting skeletal metastases. Currently skeletal scintigraphy is the most sensitive technique available, but the uptake of bone-seeking radionuclide is not specific. Radiography or CT may be required of areas where there is a focus of increased uptake, particularly if such a focus is solitary.

Serial scintigraphy appears to be the most sensitive and accurate method of assessing the response of skeletal metastases to treatment, but serial examinations should not be read in isolation. CT or MRI may prove to be more sensitive.

References

Adams JE, Isherwood I (1983) Conventional and new techniques in radiological diagnosis. In: Stoll BA, Parbhoo S (eds.) Bone metastasis, monitoring and treatment. Raven Press, New York, pp. 107–148

Alexander JL, Gillespie PJ, Edelstyn GA (1976) Serial bone scanning using technetium-99m diphosphonate in patients undergoing clinical combination chemotherapy for advanced breast cancer. Clin Nucl Med 1:13–17

Bertin KC, Horstman J, Coleman SS (1984) Isolated fracture of the lesser trochanter in adults: an initial manifestation of metastatic malignant disease. J Bone Joint Surg [Am] 66:770–773

Best JJK, Forbes WStC, Adam NM, Isherwood I (1979) Computed tomographic scanning and radioisotope bone scanning: a comparison. In: Gerhardt P, van Kaick G (eds) Total body computed tomography. George Thieme Publishers, Stuttgart, pp 216–221

Bishop MC, Hardy JG, Taylor MC, Wastie ML, Lemberger RJ (1985) Bone imaging and serum phosphatases in prostatic carcinoma. Br J Urol 57:317–324

Calkins AR, Olson MA, Ellis JH (1986) Impact of myelography on the radiotherapeutic management of malignant spinal cord compression. Neurosurgery 19:614–616

Citrin DL, Hougen C, Zweibel, W, et al. (1981) The use of serial bone scans in assessing response of bone metastases to systemic treatment. Cancer 47:680–685

Constable AR, Cranage RW (1981) Recognition of the superscan in prostatic bone scintigraphy. Br J Radiol 54:122–125

Coombes RC, Dady P, Parsons C et al. (1983) Assessment of response of bone metastases to systemic treatment in patients with breast cancer. Cancer 52:610–614

Cuschieri A, Jarvie R, Taylor WH, Cant E, Furnival CM, Blumgart LH (1978) Three-centre study on urinary hydroxyproline excretion in cancer of the breast. Br J Cancer 37:1002–1005

De Luca SA, Castronovo FP, Rhea JT (1983) The effects of chemotherapy on bony metastases as measured by quantitative skeletal imaging. Clin Nucl Med 8:11–13

Edelstyn GA, Gillespie PJ, Grebbel FS (1967) the radiological demonstration of osseous metastases. Experimental observations. Clin Radiol 18:158–162

Ell PJ, Dixon JH, Abdullah AZ (1980) Unusual spread of juxta cortical osteosarcoma. J Nucl Med 21:190–191

Epstein DA, Stern H (1977) The lateral view in radionuclide imaging of the sacrum. Radiology 123:704

Fidler M (1981) Incidence of fracture through metastases in long bones. Acta Orthop Scand 52:623–627

Front D, Schenck SO, Frankel A, Robinson E (1979) Bone metastases and bone pain in breast cancer. Are they closely associated? JAMA 242:1747–1748

Galasko CSB (1972) Skeletal metastases and mammary cancer. Ann R Coll Surg Engl 50:3–28

Galasko CSB (1973) Skeletal scintigraphy. In: Gilliland I, Peden M (eds) The scientific basis of medicine annual reviews 1973. Athlone Press, London, pp 187–202

Galasko CSB (1975) The significance of occult skeletal metastases, detected by skeletal scintigraphy, in patients with otherwise apparently "early" mammary carcinoma. Br J Surg 62:694–696

Galasko CSB (1984a) Irradiated bone. In: Galasko CSB, Weber DA (eds) Radionuclide scintigraphy in orthopaedics. Churchill Livingstone, Edinburgh, pp 210–214

Galasko CSB (1984b) Tumours. In: Galasko CSB, Weber DA (eds) Radionuclide scintigraphy in orthopaedics. Churchill Livingstone, Edinburgh, pp 65–109

Galasko CSB (1986) Skeletal metastases. Butterworths, London

Galasko CSB, Doyle FG (1972a) The response to therapy of skeletal metastases from mammary cancer. Assessment by scintigraphy. Br J Surg 59:85–88

Galasko CSB, Doyle FH (1972b) The detection of skeletal metastases from mammary cancer. A regional comparison between radiology and scintigraphy. Clin Radiol 23:295–297

Galasko CSB, Sylvester BS (1978) Back pain in patients treated for malignant tumours. Clin Oncol 4:273–283

Galasko CSB, Bush H, Sutton ML (1982) Tumours of bone, cartilage and synovium. In: Halnan KE (ed) Treatment of cancer. Chapman and Hall Ltd, London, pp 623–651

Gielen F, Dequeker J, Drochmans A, Wildiers J, Merlevde M (1976) Relevance of hydroxyproline excretion to bone metastasis in breast cancer. Br J Cancer 34:279–285

Gillespie PJ, Alexander JL, Edelstyn GA (1975) Changes in ^{87m}Sr concentrations in skeletal metastases in patients responding to cyclical combination chemotherapy for advanced breast cancer. J Nucl Med 16:191–193

Golimbu M, Golimbu C, Firooznia H, Rafii M, Al-Askari S, Morales P (1986) Spongious bone density determination for staging and follow-up of patients with prostatic cancer. Urology 28:534–539

Grainger R, Reda M, Fitzpatrick JM (1984) Calcium excretion in metastatic prostatic carcinoma. Br J Urol 56:687–689

Greenburg EJ, Chu FCH, Dwyer AJ, Ziminski EM, Dimich AB, Laughlin JS (1972) Effects of radiation therapy on bone lesions as measured by 47-Ca and 85-Sr local kinetics. J Nucl Med 13:747–751

Hammond N, Jones SE, Salmon SE, Patton D, Woolfenden J (1978) Predictive value of bone scans in an adjuvant breast cancer programme. Cancer 41:138–142

Hayward JL, Carbone PP, Heuson J-C, Kumaoka S, Segaloff A, Rubens RD (1977) Assessment of response to therapy in advanced breast cancer. A project of the programme on clinical oncology of the International Union against Cancer. Cancer 39:1289–1294

Hortobagyi GN, Libshitz HI, Seabold JE (1984) Osseous metastases of breast cancer. Clinical, biochemical, radiographic and scintigraphic evaluation of response to therapy. Cancer 53:577–582

Langhammer H, Sintermann R, Hor G, Pabst HW (1978) Serial bone scintigraphy for assessing the effectiveness of treatment of osseous metastases from prostatic cancer. Nuklearmedizin 17:87–91

Langhammer H, Sintermann R, Hör G, Pabst HW (1978) Serial results of serial bone scintigraphy in prostatic cancer. Nucl Med Commun 2:110

Levenson RM Jr, Sauerbrunn BJ, Ihde DC, Bunn PA Jr, Cohen MH, Minna JD (1981) Small cell lung cancer: radionuclide bone scans for assessment of tumour extent and response. AJR 137:31–35

Makoha FW, Britton KE (1980) Reversion of a "hot" spot to a "cold" spot in untreated metastatic bone disease – a case report. Nucl Med Comm 1:233–238

Merrick MV (1973) Detection of skeletal metastases. A comparison of three radioisotopic techniques using ^{18}F and radiology. Br J Radiol 46:968–971

Mettler FA Jr, Guiberteau MJ (1983) Essentials of nuclear medicine imaging. Grune and Stratton, Orlando, Florida.

Niell HB, Palmieri GM, Neely CL, McDonald MW (1981) Postabsorptive urinary hydroxyproline test in patients with metastatic bone disease from breast cancer. Arch Intern Med 141:1471–1473

Parbhoo SP (1985) Usefulness of current techniques in detecting and monitoring bone metastases from breast cancer. J R Soc Med 78 [suppl 9]:7–10

Pollen JJ, Shlaer WJ (1979) Osteoblastic response to successful treatment of metastatic cancer of the prostate. AJR 132:927–931

Powles TJ, Leese CL, Bondy PK (1975) Hydroxyproline excretion in patients with breast cancer and response to treatment. Br Med J 2:164–166

Rafii M, Firooznia H, Golimbu C, Beranbaum E (1986) CT of skeletal metastasis. Sem Ultrasound CT MR 7:371–379

Roberts JG, Baum M (1975) Predictive value of hydroxyproline creatinine ratio in advanced breast cancer. Br Med J 2:559

Rodichok LD, Ruckdeschel JC, Harper GR, et al. (1986) Early detection and treatment of spinal epidural metastasis: the role of myelography. Ann Neurol 20:696–702

Stone AR, Merrick MV, Chisholm GD (1980) The bone scan as a monitor of prostatic cancer. Clin Oncol 6:349–360

Sy WM, Patel D, Faunce H (1975) Significance of absent or faint kidney sign on bone scan. J Nucl Med 16:454–456

Turner P, Haggith JW (1981) Preoperative radionuclide scanning in bronchogenic carcinoma. Br J Dis Chest 75:291–294

Williams MR, Morris AH, Woolfson A, Campbell FC, Blamey RW (1984) Urinary calcium excretion as a marker of response to treatment in bone metastases from carcinoma of the breast. Paper presented to Surgical Research Society Meeting

Winchester DP, Sener SF, Khandekar JD et al. (1979) Symptomatology as an indicator of recurrent or metastatic breast cancer. Cancer 43:956–960

23 Infection

D.R.A. Davies

Osteomyelitis 307
    Radiographs 307
    Scintigraphy 307
Subacute Osteomyelitis 308
Chronic Osteomyelitis 309
Septic Arthritis 309
Infected Implants 309
Tuberculosis 310
References 310

Osteomyelitis

Radiographs

Classical acute haematogenous osteomyelitis presents with a febrile child with toxicity, marked bone pain and tenderness, a polymorphonuclear leucocytosis and a raised erythrocyte sedimentation rate (ESR). In these children there usually is little doubt about the diagnosis and the site of infection, and unnecessary investigations should not delay prompt, effective treatment with intravenous antibiotics and possible surgical drainage. Radiographs should always be taken as, although initially normal, they provide a valuable baseline and sometimes reveal some unexpected abnormality. One of our cases, a 2-year-old boy, was admitted at night with a painful swollen ankle and a pyrexia; not unnaturally a diagnosis of osteomyelitis was made. The next day he came out in the typical rash of chickenpox and a radiograph of the ankle showed a juxta-epiphyseal fracture of the tibia.

Bone changes are not seen on radiographs for 10–14 days. The earliest signs are those of soft tissue swelling, loss of well-defined muscle planes, and a diffuse hazy appearance. Rarefaction is the first change seen in the bone and it represents demineralization caused by inflammation and hyperaemia. Periosteal new bone formation and bone lysis tend to occur at about the same time although their appearance may be delayed or even suppressed by prompt effective antibiotic treatment.

Once the diagnosis has been made, antibiotic treatment must be continued for 6 weeks; the lack of typical radiographic changes developing at 2 weeks should not be a cause for revising the diagnosis and stopping antibiotics. Such a course can result in the development of chronic osteomyelitis.

Scintigraphy

Scintigrams with ^{99m}Tc-labelled diphosphonates can be performed relatively quickly and cheaply and are readily available. The diphosphonates accumulate at sites of immature new bone formation or increased blood flow but are not specific for infection (see Chap. 13). However, they have proved very useful in evaluating patients with musculoskeletal sepsis.

Skeletal scintigrams will detect acute osteomyelitis before any radiographic changes are present (Duszynski et al. 1975; Majd and Frankel 1976; Galasko 1984). Early diagnosis is important, as prompt effective treatment will lessen the risk of serious complications. In the first 24 hours after the onset of infection the scintigram may be negative, but the majority are positive within 48 hours. It is most important that the finding of a normal scintigram is not allowed to interfere with good clinical judgement and the instigation of effective treatment. This point of view has been forcefully expressed by Nade (1983): "I am amazed that, often, skilled clinicians doubt their own experience and pay homage to a typewritten report provided by a department with a new machine. The scan should not be used as an excuse for poor clinical examination."

It is important that clinicians receive copies of the scintigram so that they may become familiar with normal and abnormal appearances. Just as a clinician will discuss the radiographic appearances of a problemetical case with a consultant radiologist, so he must be able to discuss similar problems in nuclear medicine. Skeletal scintigraphy may be particularly helpful in patients with less acute osteomyelitis, who are afebrile, whose white cell count may be normal although their ESR is usually raised, and who present with low-grade bone pain and tenderness.

A cold (photopaenic) area on the scan is not inconsistent with acute osteomyelitis – increased intramedullary pressure and thrombosis of vessels may result in ischaemia (Garnett et al. 1977; Teates and Williamson 1977; Jones and Cady 1981) – but is indicative of extensive disease with a subperiosteal abscess that requires urgent surgical treatment (Howie et al. 1983). The uptake of isotope from these areas changes over a period of a few days from low to high; it is possible that this change represents an increase in vascularity because of a decrease in pressure resulting from spontaneous or surgical drainage of intraosseous or subperiosteal pus. Acute osteomyelitis is only one cause of cold areas on a skeletal scintigram; they can also occur in metastases, sickle-cell crises, Perthes' disease and aseptic necrosis.

^{67}Ga- and ^{111}In-labelled leucocyte scintigrams take several days to obtain and their spatial resolution is inferior to that of skeletal scintigrams, so they are not useful in acute osteomyelitis, except possibly in those cases without overt clinical symptoms and with equivocal ^{99m}Tc-labelled diphosphonate scintigrams. Even then it may be preferable to repeat the skeletal scintigram after 48 hours.

On occasion it may be difficult to differentiate cellulitis from acute osteomyelitis and combining the early and late phases of the skeletal scintigram can be helpful (Howie et al. 1983). Such differentiation is important because of the subsequent bearing on treatment. In cellulitis there is a diffuse increased uptake in the early or blood-pool image without a focal increased uptake in bone in the delayed image (Fig. 13.16). In osteomyelitis there is a diffuse increase uptake in the blood-pool image and a focal increased uptake in bone in the delayed image (Fig. 13.14).

Osteomyelitis in deep sites such as the pelvis can be notoriously difficult to diagnose on clinical grounds alone and in such cases skeletal scintigraphy is especially useful. Pelvic osteomyelitis is uncommon and is often confused with an acute abdomen, septic arthritis of the hip, or with osteomyelitis of the proximal femur. The initial radiographs are frequently normal but the scintigram is usually positive (Highland and LaMont 1983). Following early diagnosis most patients respond to medical treatment with antibiotics and do not require surgical drainage.

In neonates under 40 days of age the diagnosis of osteomyelitis can be exceptionally difficult because of the lack of physical signs. One would expect skeletal scintigraphy to be most helpful in confirming the diagnosis and the site of infection, but according to Ash and Gilday (1980) this is unfortunately not the case. Bressler and Conway (1983), however, have reported more favourable results.

Subacute Osteomyelitis

The radiographic features of subacute osteomyelitis in children can be classified into two main groups (Ross and Cole 1985), although more extensive classifications have been suggested (Roberts et al. 1982).

One group presents with radiographic (as well as clinical and haematological) features that are highly suggestive of a primary malignant bone tumour, especially a Ewing's sarcoma. The lesions may be in the diaphysis or metaphysis and show onion skin periosteal new bone formation and bone erosion. These children require urgent pre-biopsy investigation, including a skeletal scintigram and computed tomographic (CT) scans of the lesion and of the chest. The scintigram should detect lesions in other bones, as well as any skip lesions in the affected bone. The CT scan of the lesion will help determine its extent and the presence of any soft tissue component. CT has proved invaluable in the detection of small pulmonary metastases. The investigations required in a suspected primary malignant bone tumour are discussed more thoroughly in Chap. 21. Whilst these are useful in the pre-operative investigation of a possible primary malignant bone tumour they are rarely diagnosticaly helpful in these cases of subacute osteomyelitis with an aggressive radiographic appearance. Biopsy usually reveals both the diagnosis and the causative organism.

The other group of children have cavities in the metaphysis or epiphysis that are radiographically typical of subacute osteomyelitis. The metaphyseal cavities are eccentrically situated and either oval or elongated in shape. They have a well-defined margin which is usually somewhat sclerotic. The cavities frequently cross the growth plate into the epiphysis. Those cavities that occur solely in the epiphysis are again eccentrically placed and are either circular or oval with a well-defined thin sclerotic margin or a margin of normal bone. Skeletal scintigrams and CT are not usually of any further diagnostic help in these patients. After treatment, radiographic signs of healing are usually apparent over a 6–12-month period. Serial skeletal scintigrams may be useful in assessing the response to treatment, especially in those treated by antibiotics alone.

Chronic Osteomyelitis

There are two common clinical problems in dealing with chronic osteomyelitis: identification of possible sequestra prior to surgery; and assessment of whether the infection is quiescent or an acute flare-up is present.

Radiography, tomography and CT are all useful in the identification of sequestra and *sinography* can also be helpful in planning surgery.

Radiography is of little value in the assessment of a possible flare-up of infection and in these cases *skeletal scintigraphy* is important in both the diagnosis and the assessment of response to treatment. The scan can be repeated at intervals of several months. The usefulness of *gallium scintigraphy* in the detection of exacerbation of chronic osteomyelitis has been shown by Deysine and colleagues (1975) and the greater accuracy of [111]*In-labelled leucocyte imaging* over sequential [99m]Tc–[67]Ga scintigraphy demonstrated by Merkel and co-authors (1985).

Septic Arthritis

Although uncommon, septic arthritis is important because of the effect of suppuration in causing destruction of articular cartilage and possible subluxation or dislocation. It most commonly affects the hip or knee. In neonates the diagnosis is especially difficult and the effects of infection on the joint more severe.

Radiographs should always be taken. They may be normal initially or show distension of the joint capsule, widening of the apparent joint space, and sometimes subluxation of the joint even in an early

case. Morrey and colleagues (1976) placed little value on soft tissue changes seen on radiographs of the hip and pointed out that the interpretation of radiographic changes in the hip in the young child was difficult. If the septic arthritis is secondary to osteomyelitis then the radiographic features of bone infection may be present.

In late cases of septic arthritis of the hip Wientroub and others (1981) have shown that damage to the triradiate cartilage of the acetabulum is a reliable indication of severe damage to the femoral head.

Skeletal scintigraphy is rarely indicated in septic arthritis and in suspected cases treatment should not await such investigations. Prompt effective treatment comprises diagnostic aspiration followed by surgical drainage of the affected joint and appropriate systemic antibiotic therapy. It is only in those patients in whom the diagnosis remains in doubt after aspiration that scintigraphy should be carried out. A photopaenic area surrounding the joint on the early blood-pool image indicates an effusion and is due to compression of blood vessels by the tension of fluid in the joint. The delayed image shows an increased uptake on both sides of the joint, although in some cases this may not be very marked and gallium or indium scans should be considered.

Infected Implants

The differentiation of aseptic loosening of a prosthetic joint component from low-grade sepsis around the prosthesis is a common clinical problem. Three to six months may elapse before the radiographic signs of infection appear, and even then the signs of aseptic loosening and of infection are similar: a radiolucent zone at the bone/cement interface; scalloping of the endosteal cortex; and a periosteal reaction giving a laminated appearance.

Despite the number of diagnostic imaging techniques available for the assessment of the possibly infected joint prosthesis, the simple investigations of ESR and *serial plain radiographs* give the most useful information. The ESR is nearly always elevated above 30 mm in the first hour in cases of infection (Salvati et al. 1982), although a normal ESR does not entirely exclude infection. Benson and Hughes (1975) advised caution in the interpretation of a raised ESR in patients with active rheumatoid arthritis.

Arthrography or *subtraction arthrography* can be helpful in showing that loosening has occurred but give no real information on the possible presence of infection, although they do permit aspiration and culture to be performed at the same time. It is also doubtful whether they give much more evidence of loosening than do good plain radiographs.

Computed tomography has not yet proved useful in the diagnosis of infected implants because the metal of the implant produces artefacts that interfere with the image.

Skeletal scintigrams show increased uptake for about 6–12 months after any total joint replacement and they lack specificity for infection. A strongly positive scan suggests the presence of infection and a mildly positive one suggests aseptic loosening (Gristina and Kolkin 1983), but many have an indeterminate appearance between these extremes.

The initial results of sequential ^{99m}Tc–^{67}Ga scintigraphy in distinguishing infection from other pathological processes were encouraging (Handmaker and Giammona 1976; Handmaker and Leonards 1976) and one study reported only one false negative scan in 79 patients, of whom 19 had true positive scintigrams (Reing et al. 1979). The criteria of infection are a lack of spatial congruity of the uptake of technetium and of gallium, or spatial congruity with a relatively more intense uptake of gallium than of technetium. Spatial congruity with a similar intensity of uptake is equivocal, and congruity with a less intense gallium uptake is indicative of a negative scan.

A prospective study comparing ^{111}In-labelled leucocyte imaging with sequential ^{99m}Tc–^{67}Ga scintigraphy (Merkel et al. 1985) has shown 94% accuracy for ^{111}In-labelled leucocyte scintigrams compared with 75% for sequential ^{99m}Tc–^{67}Ga scintigraphy in patients with a prosthesis. It is possible that this technique will replace the sequential ^{99m}Tc–^{67}Ga scintigram. In addition to being cheaper it is a single test that can be performed in 24 hours compared with 2–3 days for ^{99m}Tc–^{67}Ga scintigraphy.

Tuberculosis

Skeletal scintigrams are accurate in determining the site and extent of disease and can give more information than *radiographs*, although sometimes false negative scintigrams can occur. They are of value in assessing recurrent activation of disease but of no use in differentiating tuberculosis from other forms of infection.

Alexander (1981) considered *CT scanning* the procedure of choice in the investigation of psoas abscesses.

In tuberculous spondylitis the diagnosis can be difficult and neurological impairment can occur without demonstrable bone lesions. *CT scanning* is helpful in assessing the extent of disease and the bony integrity of the spine, especially in the upper cervical spine. Lifeso and colleagues (1985) found CT scanning of value in planning surgical approaches to the spine and also in disease of the upper cervical spine to determine whether the arch of the atlas was intact; if it was intact they fused C1 and C2, if it was not the occiput was fused to C2 and C3.

References

Alexander CJ (1981) CT scanning in orthopaedic surgery. J Bone Joint Surg [Br] 63:467

Ash JM, Gilday DL (1980) The futility of bone scanning in neonatal osteomyelitis: concise communication. J Nucl Med 21:417–420

Benson MKD, Hughes SPF (1975) Infection following total hip replacement in a general hospital without special orthopaedic facilities. Acta Orthop Scand 46:968–978

Bressler EL, Conway JJ (1983) Bone scintigraphy in neonatal osteomyelitis. Radiology 149:35 (abstract)

Deysine M, Rafkin H, Teicher I (1975) Diagnosis of chronic and postoperative osteomyelitis with gallium-67 citrate scans. Am J Surg 129:632–635

Duszynski DO, Kuhn JP, Afshani E, Riddlesberger MMJ (1975) Early radionuclide diagnosis of acute osteomyelitis. Radiology 117:337–340

Galasko CSB (1984) Infection. In: Galasko CSB, Weber DA (eds) Radionuclide scintigraphy in orthopaedics. Churchill Livingstone, Edinburgh, pp 134–162

Garnett ES, Cockshott WP, Jacobs J (1977) Classical acute osteomyelitis with a negative bone scan. Br J Radiol 50:757–760

Gristina AG, Kolkin J (1983) Current concepts review: total joint replacement and sepsis. J Bone Joint Sug [Am] 65:128–134

Handmaker H, Giammona ST (1976) The "hot joint" – increased diagnostic accuracy using combined ^{99m}Tc-phosphate and ^{67}Ga-cirtrate imaging in pediatrics. J Nucl Med 17:554 (abstract)

Handmaker H, Leonards R (1976) The bone scan in inflammatory osseous disease. Semin Nucl Med 6:96–105

Highland Tr, LaMont RL (1983) Osteomyelitis of the pelvis in children. J Bone Joint Surg [Am] 65:230–234

Howie DW, Savage JP, Wilson TG, Paterson D (1983) The technetium phosphate bone scan in the diagnosis of osteomyelitis in childhood. J Bone Joint Surg [Am] 65:431–437

Jones DC, Cady RB (1981) "Cold" bone scans in acute osteomyelitis. J Bone Joint Surg [Br] 63:376–378

Lifeso RM, Weaver P, Harder EH (1985) Tuberculous spondylitis in adults. J Bone Joint Surg [Am] 67: 1405–1413

Majd M, Frankel RS (1976) Radionuclide imaging in skeletal inflammatory and ischaemic disease in children. AJR 126:832–841

Merkel KD, Brown ML, Dewanjee MK, Fitzgerald Jr RH (1985) Comparison of indium-labelled-leucocyte imaging with sequential technetium–gallium scanning in the diagnosis of low grade musculoskeletal sepsis. J Bone Joint Surg [Am] 67: 465–476

Morrey BF, Bianco AJ, Rhodes KH (1976) Suppurative arthritis of the hip in children. J Bone Joint Surg [Am] 58:388–392

Nade S (1983) Acute haematogenous osteomyelitis in infancy and childhood. J Bone Surg [Br] 65:109–119

Roberts JM, Drummond DS, Breed AL, Chesney J (1982) Subacute haematogenous osteomyelitis in children: a retrospective study. J Paediatr Orthop 2:249–254

Reing CM, Richin PF, Kenmore PI (1979) Differential bone-scanning in the evaluation of a painful total joint replacement. J Bone Joint Surg [Am] 61:933–936

Ross ERS, Cole WG (1985) Treatment of subacute osteomyelitis in childhood. J Bone Joint Surg [Br] 67:443–448

Salvati EA, Chekofsky KM, Brause BD, Wilson PD Jr (1982) Reimplantation in infecton: a 12-year experience. Clin Orthop 170:62–75

Teates CD, Williamson BRJ (1977) "Hot and cold" bone lesions in acute osteomyelitis. AJR 129:517–518

Wientroub S, Lloyd-Roberts GC, Fraser M (1981) The prognostic significance of the triradiate cartilage in suppurative arthritis of the hip in infancy and early childhood. J Bone Joint Surg [Br] 63:190–193

24 Skeletal Dysplasias

J.F. Crossan

Introduction 313
Classification 313
Diagnosis 314
    Pre-natal Diagnosis 314
    Post-natal Diagnosis 314
Hip Joints 315
Lower Limb Malalignment 317
Dorsolumbar Spine 319
Cervical Spine 320
    Normal Appearances in the Child 320
    Abnormal Appearances in Developmental Disorders 321
Disorders of Decreased Bone Density 322
    In Infancy 322
    In Childhood and Adolescence 322
Summary 322
References 322

Introduction

Many developmental disorders are encountered only rarely by the orthopaedic surgeon. They can be considered in the following groups, in many of which the musculoskeletal system is extensively involved:

1. The *chromosomal abnormalities* often produce serious defects and in many instances the infant is stillborn. The most common chromosomal abnormality which comes to the attention of the orthopaedic surgeon is Down's syndrome.

2. *The skeletal dysplasias* are single-gene conditions with a simple pattern of inheritance which is commonly autosomal dominant or recessive. These are generalized disorders of bone and cartilage and, although rare, they confront the orthopaedic surgeon with difficult diagnostic and management problems.

3. *The malformation syndromes* are disorders with skeletal involvement alone or in combination with visceral involvement. Most cases are sporadic but some may show a pattern of inheritance. The majority of isolated localized limb defects are sporadic.

4. *Disorders of multifactorial inheritance* are conditions with a wide range of clinical severity and are much commoner within the population. In these disorders environmental factors are essential to "trigger" the defect. Such disorders include congenital talipes equinovarus, congenital dislocation of the hip, idiopathic scoliosis, spondylolisthesis and slipped upper femoral epiphysis.

5. Finally a number of *non-genetic disorders* are encountered in orthopaedic practice, the commonest of which is Perthes' disease.

In this chapter greatest consideration will be given to the role of imaging techniques in the diagnosis and management of the first three categories, as the latter conditions are considered elsewhere.

Classification

There are more than 100 different types of skeletal dysplasia and it is likely that as many as 10 000 people suffer from these disorders in the United Kingdom, although many of this number will be affected only mildly (Wynne-Davies and Gormley 1985).

Table 24.1. Simplified working classification of the skeletal dysplasias

1. *Epiphyseal disorders*
   Multiple epiphyseal dysplasia

2. *Spondyloepiphyseal disorders*
   Spondyloepiphyseal dysplasia tarda
   Spondyloepiphyseal dysplasia congenita

3. *Short limbs, normal trunk*
   Achondroplasia
   Hypochondroplasia
   Dyschondrosteosis
   Metaphyseal chondrodysplasias
   Mesomelic dwarfism

4. *Short limbs and trunk*
   Pseudoachondroplasia
   Diastrophic dwarfism
   Metatropic dwarfism
   Kniest disease

5. *Storage diseases*
   Mucopolysaccharidoses (esp. Morquio's syndrome)

6. *Decreased bone density*
   Osteogenesis imperfecta

7. *Increased bone density*
   Osteopetrosis

The European Society of Radiologists established a classification of the skeletal dysplasias in 1969. This is known as the Paris Nomenclature and has been revised periodically to include new syndromes as they arise. The list of conditions is exhaustive (Paris Nomenclature 1983) and many of them do not come to the attention of the orthopaedic surgeon, either because the infants die in the perinatal period, or because the skeletal manifestations do not affect the limbs or spine. A simpler and more useful classification for the orthopaedic surgeon is shown in Table 24.1 which describes the conditions most commonly encountered in orthopaedic practice.

Diagnosis

In reaching a diagnosis it is most important to establish whether the patient is proportionate or disproportionate. This is done by measurement of the patient's height, span, and head to pubis/pubis to heel ratio.

Subsequently, the basis of a firm diagnosis is reached by interpretation of selected radiographs. A complete skeletal survey is unnecessary, and the diagnosis can be reached by performing the following standard radiographic views:

Lateral skull
Antero-posterior and lateral spine (T1 to S1 on one film)
Chest (include shoulders)
Pelvis (include hips)
Antero-posterior knee
Antero-posterior forearm
Postero-anterior hand and wrist

When these data are available a suitable atlas of skeletal dysplasias should be consulted if the diagnosis is still in doubt. The classic work of Fairbank (1951) has largely been superseded by the work of Wynne-Davies and colleagues (1985).

Pre-natal Diagnosis

Recent advances in ultrasonography have made the detection of foetal anomalies more reliable; thus the dangers of direct inspection by foetoscopy can be avoided.

The disorders which may be most readily identified are those in which there is congenital shortening of the lower limbs or congenital malformations of the upper limbs such as polydactyly or absence of the radius or ulna. Severe disorders such as achondrogenesis may be detected before the twentieth week of gestation whereas less severe conditions such as achondroplasia cannot be diagnosed reliably before the twenty-second week. Of particular interest to the orthopaedic surgeon is the ability to diagnose not only many of the disorders of short-limbed dwarfism, but also the severe form of osteogenesis imperfecta with multiple fractures. Congenital vertebral and limb anomalies such as "absence" defects and severe hypoplasia may also be detected.

The recent developments in this field of investigation have been well reviewed (Campbell and Pearce 1983).

Post-natal Diagnosis

The ages at which the commoner dysplasias are manifest are described in Table 24.2. The com-

Table 24.2. Clinical appearances and age at diagnosis in skeletal dysplasias

Conditions recognizable pre-natally
Lethal forms of short-limbed dwarfism
Osteogenesis imperfecta (severe form)

Short-limbed dwarfism recognizable in the first year of life
Achondroplasia
Diastrophic dwarfism
Metatropic dwarfism
Mesomelic dwarfism
Osteogenesis imperfecta
Metaphyseal chondrodysplasia type McKusick

Short-trunked dwarfism recognizable in the first year of life
Spondyloepiphyseal dysplasia congenita
Kniest disease

Short-limbed dwarfism in childhood
Hypochondroplasia
Pseudoachondroplasia
Metaphyseal chondrodysplasia type Schmid
Multiple epiphyseal dysplasia
Dyschondrosteosis
Osteogenesis imperfecta

Short-trunked dwarfism in childhood
Spondyloepiphyseal dysplasia tarda

monest dysplasia to be noted at birth is achondroplasia. The severe form of osteogenesis imperfecta may also be apparent and associated with a high perinatal mortality.

The non-lethal cases of osteogenesis imperfecta occur in two common forms. The more usual is characterized by blue sclerae and has an autosomal dominant inheritance. In the second type, pale blue or white sclerae are present, and are associated with severe progressive shortness of stature and deformity. These two types cannot always be identified with certainty until the age of 3 years (Wynne-Davies and Gormley 1981). In the post-natal period, accurate diagnosis of the condition may be facilitated by a whole body radiograph of the infant (Fig. 24.1).

The features of these disorders are well described and illustrated elsewhere (Wynne-Davies et al. 1985). In the present review of the subject, attention will be directed towards the value of radiographic techniques as applied to the hips, lower limb malalignment, the dorsolumbar spine, the cervical spine, limb deformities and to disorders of decreased bone density.

Hip Joints

The important skeletal dysplasias which affect the developing hip joint are:

Multiple epiphyseal dysplasia
Spondyloepiphyseal dysplasia tarda
Pseudoachondroplasia
Spondyloepiphyseal dysplasia congenita
Metatropic dwarfism
Diastrophic dysplasia
Morquio's syndrome

The features of the hip joint in each of these disorders are illustrated schematically in Fig. 24.2.

The commonest condition in this group is *multiple epiphyseal dysplasia*, the clinical features of which frequently occur in early childhood with hip pain. In early childhood there is delay in maturation of

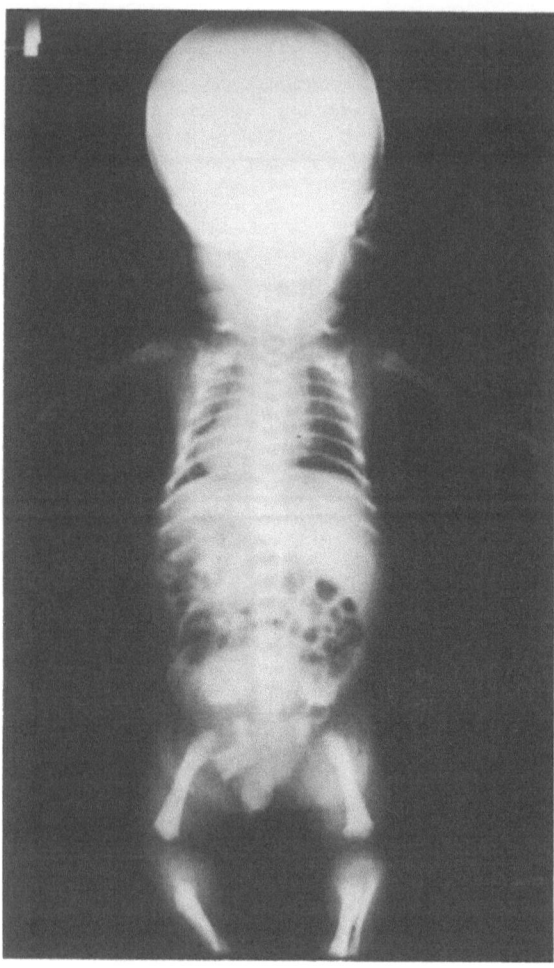

Fig. 24.1. Whole body radiograph of an infant with achondroplasia.

The remaining conditions are much more severe disorders and present in infancy or early childhood. *Pseudoachondroplasia* is associated with severe abnormalities in both the pelvis and the hip joints. The triradiate cartilage is characteristically wide and the acetabula poorly formed. The capital femoral epiphyses are small and round and fail to mature with age.

Spondyloepiphyseal dysplasia congenita has a mild and severe form (Wynne-Davies and Hall 1982). There is gross disorganization of the bony pelvis with poorly formed acetabula. The capital femoral epiphyses are extremely small and coxa vara may be severe or mild.

The most striking features of *metatropic dwarfism* are the delayed appearance of the capital femoral epiphyses and the great expansion of the intertrochanteric area. In *diastrophic dysplasia* mild coxa vara is characteristic, and although the radiographic features are less severe than in the previous condition, progressive contractures of the joints produce a crippling disability.

Finally, in *Morquio's syndrome* the capital femoral epiphyses are initially larger than normal, due to the accumulation of mucopolysaccharide, but between the ages of 5 and 10 years they collapse progressively and often disappear completely.

Following skeletal maturity it may be impossible to reach a diagnosis in most of these conditions on the basis of hip radiographs alone, and other evidence must be sought – for example the appearances of the spine. Spondyloepiphyseal dysplasia congenita does, however, retain a very characteristic appearance with evidence of coxa vara (Crossan et al. 1983).

In most clinical situations standard radiography of the hip joints provides sufficient information for both diagnosis and management of the condition. On occasions, however, arthrography (Chap. 3) of the joint may provide useful information. This is particularly true in spondyloepiphyseal dysplasia congenita, where it is important to define the anatomy of the hips when surgery in the form of corrective osteotomy is considered. It may also have some value in assessing the state of the hip joint in multiple epiphyseal dysplasia when the capital femoral epiphysis appears to be uncovered laterally (Fig. 24.3).

Intertrochanteric osteotomy may be required to correct the severe flexion contractures in diastrophic dysplasia and it is important in this disorder to assess the degree of pelvic deformity at the lumbosacral junction by means of a lateral radiograph prior to correction of contractures, lest an unacceptable lordosis is produced.

the capital femoral epiphyses. Subsequently they become flat and often appear to arise from multiple ossific centres. The appearances can superficially resemble those encountered in Perthes' disease; they can be distinguished by their homogeneous texture, their symmetry of involvement and the absence of cystic changes in the metaphysis (Crossan et al. 1983).

The radiolographic appearances in *spondyloepiphyseal dysplasia tarda* are very similar, but this disorder becomes clinically apparent at a later age, usually at the pre-pubertal stage. Radiographically platyspondyly is the most useful distinguishing feature; this is not present in multiple epiphyseal dysplasia.

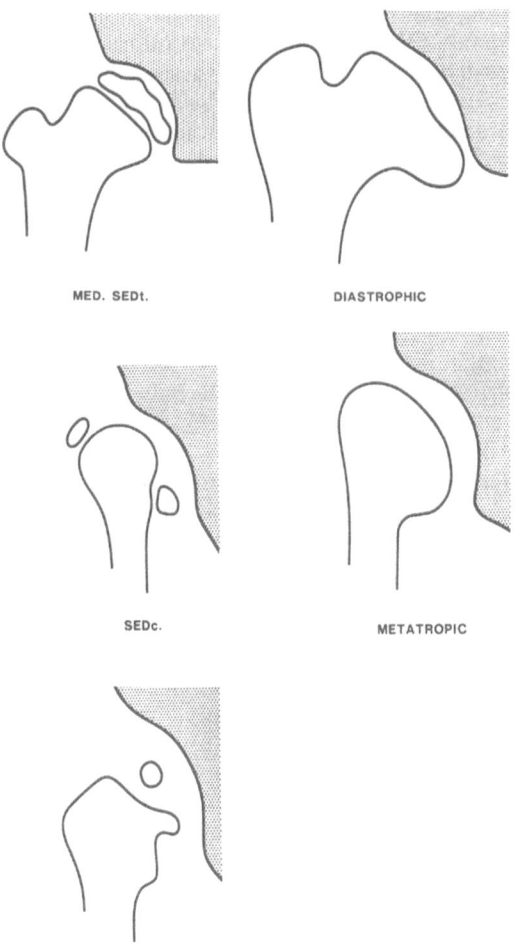

MED. SEDt.

DIASTROPHIC

SEDc.

METATROPIC

PSEUDOACH.

Fig. 24.2. Diagnostic appearances of the hip joint in epiphyseal dysplasias – multiple epiphyseal dysplasia and spondylo-epiphyseal dysplasia tarda, spondyloepiphyseal dysplasia congenita, pseudoachondroplasia, diastrophic dwarfism, metatropic dwarfism.

Lower Limb Malalignment

Malalignment of the knee joint may occur in almost any of the developmental disorders. In many conditions, severe disturbances in the metaphyseal or epiphyseal regions produce deformities which may be complicated by the presence of ligamentous laxity (Fig. 24.4). Malalignment is characteristically severe in the following conditions:

Multiple epiphyseal dysplasia
Achondroplasia
Pseudoachondroplasia
Morquio's syndrome
Metaphyseal chondrodysplasia

In *multiple epiphyseal dysplasia*, varus or valgus deformities of the knee result from partial failure of development of one or more of the tibial or femoral condyles. A deformity of sufficient severity to merit

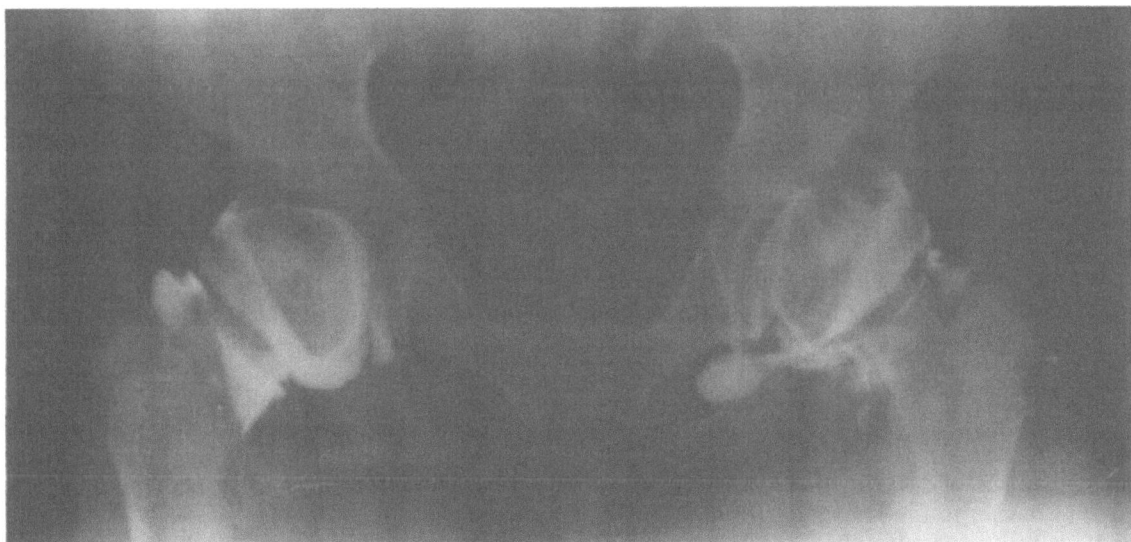

Fig. 24.3. Radiograph of the hip joint in an 8-year old with multiple epiphyseal dysplasia. Arthrogram shows the cartilaginous cap in the upper femoral epiphysis with congruity of the joint.

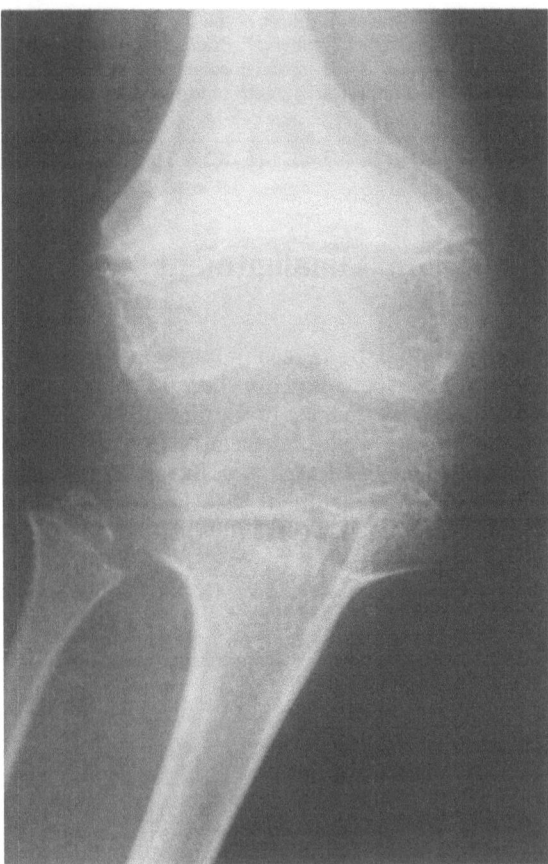

Fig. 24.4. Failure of normal development of the epiphyses in the knee of a child with Morquio's syndrome, producing a gross valgus deformity.

the calcaneus can occur.

Some of the most severe deformities may occur in *pseudoachondroplasia*, and these develop rapidly once weightbearing has begun. One of the most characteristic deformities is "windswept" knees. These are difficult to control, even by repeated osteotomies, due to severe failure of maturation in the epiphyses combined with considerable ligamentous laxity.

In *Morquio's syndrome* the characteristic deformity of genu valgum occurs by the age of 4 years, and is often disabling by the age of 10 years. Severe ligamentous laxity makes surgical correction difficult, but good permanent results have been obtained by corrective osteotomies performed at about the age of 10 years.

The genu varum deformity of *metaphyseal chondrodysplasia* is slowly progressive, in contrast to the rate of development of deformities in the previous conditions, and it occurs in half the patients. Although the deformities are much less severe, corrective osteotomies are often beneficial.

In the assessment of lower limb malalignment, standard radiographs do not provide sufficient information for planning surgery, and full-length weightbearing radiographs, to include the hips, knees and ankles, should be obtained. On occasion, especially in pseudoachondroplasia, the patient may be unable to cooperate in obtaining these films, and full-length stress films may be helpful. In addition, arthrography of the hips, knees and ankles may yield considerable information regarding the cartilaginous development of the joints, and this may also influence the planning of corrective surgery.

Achondroplasts are particularly suitable candidates for femoral lengthening as the redundant soft tissues in the thigh allow greater gains in length to be obtained than in normal patients. The morbidity of this procedure has been reduced by the introduction of more sophisticated external fixators and its popularity is increasing. In assessing and managing these patients it is important to perform leg length radiographs with a suitable scale lying parallel to the length of the limb.

Other disorders which present with different leg alignment problems are diastrophic dwarfism and dyschondrosteosis. In the former condition the primary flexion and adduction contracture of the hip joint frequently produces a flexion deformity in the knee, and radiography is of assistance in planning corrective osteotomy. In the latter condition disparity of growth between the tibia and fibula may lead to deformity at the hip or knee. This deformity should be sought radiographically in all patients presenting with Madelung's deformity of the wrist.

corrective osteotomy occurs in at least 10% of patients and in this condition there is no undue ligamentous laxity.

Achondroplasia is the commonest condition in which leg malalignment occurs, and the characteristic varus deformity of the knee, which develops soon after the child begins to walk, is complicated by ligamentous laxity which decreases over the years and which corrects spontaneously. In a recent review (Kopits 1976) half of these patients had straight legs; one quarter had tibial bowing but good alignment between hip, knee and ankle; and a further quarter had tibial bowing associated with poor alignment of the lower limb joints, with forces passing medial to the knee joint or lateral to the ankle joint. In some instances bowing is maximal in the lower tibia, and when this deformity is severe impingement of the tip of the lateral malleolus with

Dorsolumbar Spine

The dorsolumbar spine is commonly involved in the developmental disorders, with scoliosis being a frequent and expected physical finding even in the milder conditions. In multiple epiphyseal dysplasia, for example, it occurs in 15% of patients. Lateral radiographs of the dorsolumbar spine are often extremely useful in purely diagnostic terms as the vertebrae may assume characteristic shapes in different conditions (Fig. 24.5). In certain developmental disorders, spinal abnormalities are characteristically severe and may cause pain, deformity and paralysis.

The more common conditions with severe spinal involvement are:

Achondroplasia

Spondyloepiphyseal dysplasia congenita

Metatropic dwarfism

Diastrophic dwarfism

Morquio's syndrome

The spinal abnormalities in *achondroplasia* have been well documented (Bailey 1970; Bethem et al. 1981). In infancy a mild dorsolumbar kyphosis is often present. When the child begins to walk, a lumbar lordosis occurs, and in two thirds of patients a scoliosis is also present. The scoliosis rarely requires treatment.

One of the danger signs in achondroplasia is the development of a persistent thoracolumbar kyphosis, and this may occur in one third of patients. Its severity is exaggerated if it is associated with wedging or hypoplasia of the vertebra. Patients with such deformities are at risk of developing neurological complications.

The achondroplastic spine is particularly sensitive to these complications because of the diminished size of the spinal canal. This is caused by a decrease in the interpedicular distance in the lower lumbar spine, where the cross-sectional area of the spinal canal may be reduced by up to one third (Lutter et al. 1977).

In three other disorders, namely *spondyloepiphyseal dysplasia congenita, metatropic dwarfism* and *Morquio's syndrome*, a kyphosis occurs in the dorsolumbar region due to the wedging of the vertebral bodies. The kyphosis is often accompanied by a severe scoliosis producing a "corkscrew" deformity of the spinal canal, and frequently causes spinal cord compression (Fig. 24.6). On the other hand, although a structural scoliosis may occur in early childhood in diastrophic dwarfism, these

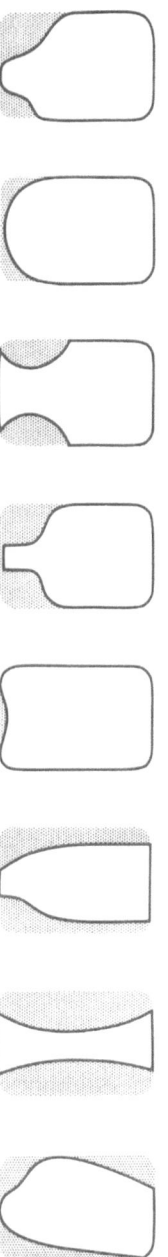

Fig. 24.5. Characteristic appearances of vertebral bodies in lateral radiographs from above: achondroplasia, spondyloepiphyseal dysplasia congenita, spondyloepiphyseal dysplasia tarda, pseudoachondroplasia, diastrophic dwarfism, spondylometaphyseal dysplasia, osteogenesis imperfecta and Morquio's syndrome.

curves rarely progress and spinal stenosis has not been documented.

The presence of early neurological signs, which commonly take the form of weakness or spinal

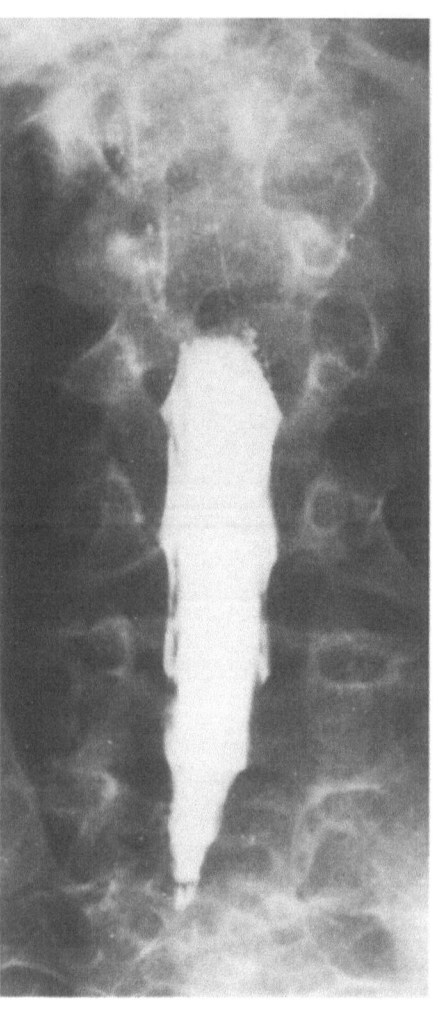

Fig. 24.6. Radiculogram of a paraparetic adult with spondylo-epiphyseal dysplasia congenita. There is complete block of the spinal canal at the dorsolumbar junction.

claudication, demands further investigation. This should initially be in the form of radiculography (Chap. 5), as the neurological signs may be due to associated disorders such as a prolapsed intervertebral disc, hypertrophy of the facet joints or vertebral instability. Computed tomography of the spine (Chap. 10), particularly when combined with radiculography, may yield much useful information.

Cervical Spine

One of the most serious complications in the developmental disorders is the presence of structural abnormalities and instability of the cervical spine, as these may produce not only quadriplegia but also sudden death in a small proportion of children. The disorders which are associated with these anomalies are:

Achondroplasia
Morquio's syndrome
Spondyloepiphyseal dysplasia congenita
Pseudoachondroplasia
Diastrophic dwarfism
Metatropic dwarfism
Kniest syndrome
Down's syndrome

A major difficulty in interpreting radiographs of a child's cervical spine is a failure to appreciate the range of normal appearances. In the developmental disorders problems arise from two causes: firstly *hypoplasia or absence of the odontoid process*, and secondly *instability at the atlanto-axial joint or the atlanto-occipital joint*.

Normal Appearances in the Child

Odontoid Process

The first cervical vertebra develops from three primary ossification centres – one for the body and two for the neural arches. The centre for the body appears during the first year of life and fuses with the neural arch centres at the age of 7.

The second cervical vertebra causes particular difficulties in radiographic interpretation. It has four primary ossification centres which are all present at birth. There is one centre for the odontoid process, one for the body and two for the neural arches, fusion occurring between the ages of 3 and 6 years. There also is a secondary ossification centre at the apex of the dens which appears at the age of 4 years and fuses at the age of 12 years (Bailey 1952).

Movement

It is well established that anterior displacement of the second cervical vertebra is much greater than might be expected and the unusual appearances have been described as "pseudosubluxation" (Cattell and Filtzer 1965). Before the age of 8 years, 50% of children have anterior displacement of 3 mm or more in flexion. In addition, posterior displacement of the second on the third cervical vertebra is observed in one child in six.

In children under the age of 7 years there is apparent widening of the space between the odontoid process and the arch of the atlas during flexion, and in 20% this distance exceeds 3 mm. In extension, apparent overriding of the anterior arch of the atlas on the odontoid process is also present in 20%.

Finally, absence of the normal cervical lordosis, which might be interpreted as indicating muscle spasm perhaps caused by early instability, is a normal finding in one child in six.

Further difficulties of interpretation of radiolographic appearances in children are often created by the inability of the child to cooperate in obtaining true lateral radiographs, and in performing full flexion and extension of the cervical spine.

Abnormal Appearances in Developmental Disorders

Achondroplasia is unusual in producing an abnormality in the upper cervical spine that is not encountered in any other disorder. These patients may have occipitalization of the first cervical vertebra associated with a reduction in the size of the foramen magnum (Bethem et al. 1981). The initial clinical manifestation may be a spastic quadriparesis. It is well recognized that the commonest cause of a spastic paresis in the lower limbs is spinal stenosis in the lumbar region, and it is therefore important in this clinical situation to assess any abnormalities at the level of the foramen magnum by radiography and computed tomography (Chap. 10).

Odontoid hypoplasia or aplasia is a common feature in *spondyloepiphyseal dysplasia congenita, pseudoachondroplasia, Morquio's syndrome, metatropic dwarfism* and *Kniest syndrome*. The presence of this abnormality does not necessarily indicate instability at the atlanto-axial level, confirmation of which must be obtained by lateral flexion–extension radiographs of the upper cervical spine (Fig. 24.7). Often difficulties in visualizing the odontoid process may be overcome by performing tomography of the atlanto-axial region.

Atlanto-axial dislocation has been recognized for some time to occur in *Down's syndrome* (Semine et al. 1978). As many as one child in five with the condition has abnormalities of the atlanto-axial articulation. Most children have subluxation alone and a smaller number have associated abnormalities of the odontoid process. Recently the presence of coexisting atlanto-occipital dislocation, an abnormality noted previously only in association with trauma and rheumatoid arthritis, has been demonstrated

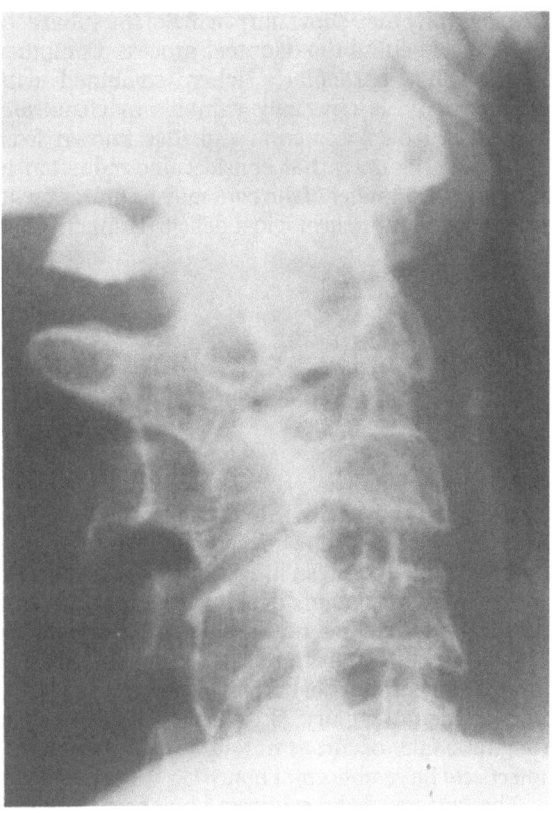

Fig. 24.7. Absence of the odontoid process in spondyloepiphyseal dysplasia congenita. Atlanto-axial instability is present in flexion, but there is no neurological deficit.

(Hungerford et al. 1981). Despite the presence of radiologically confirmed instability very few children develop neurological symptoms.

Diastrophic dwarfism has unique cervical spine abnormalities. Anomalies in the atlanto-axial region have not been recorded, but this disorder is characterized by a severe cervical kyphosis caused by hypoplasia of a vertebral body. The deformity is often so severe as to cause the odontoid process to lie parallel to the foramen magnum (Bethem et al. 1981).

The pattern of neurological signs in children with cervical instability is often bizarre and delay in diagnosis is common. For this reason, all children with the developmental abnormalities under discussion, or other unusual abnormalities, should be screened radiographically for abnormalities of the cervical spine; the views should include lateral flexion–extension radiographs of the cervical spine.

At the earliest sign of neurological involvement further investigations should be carried out.

Myelography may show narrowing of the subarachnoid space behind the odontoid process. Computed tomography, particularly when combined with myelography, is especially valuable in visualizing spinal cord displacements, and it is known from such investigations that considerable reduction in the sagittal diameter of the cord may be present with only a minimal neurological deficit (Hungerford et al. 1981).

Disorders of Decreased Bone Density

In Infancy

Many infants born with the deformities and multiple fractures of severe osteogenesis imperfecta die at or soon after birth, and such cases are not considered further here. The main difficulty of diagnosis in later infancy is to exclude non-accidental injury due to *child abuse* – the "battered baby" syndrome. The clinical appearances of bruising and neglect suggest non-accidental injury. Problems in radiological diagnosis may occur, as not all cases of *osteogenesis imperfecta* have abnormal bone.

The battered baby syndrome has been well described (Cameron and Rae 1975), as has its distinction from osteogenesis imperfecta (Paterson 1977). The main distinguishing features are that the fractures in osteogenesis imperfecta commonly occur in the diaphysis of long bones, and the bone is commonly osteoporotic. In the battered baby syndrome fractures tend to occur in the epiphyseal region, with characteristic avulsion of the metaphyses. New bone forms around the fracture site producing a "bucket-handle" appearance of new bone 7–10 days following injury. Long bone fractures, when they occur, are often in differing stages of healing. Fractures of the skull and multiple fractures occur commonly.

Other less common disorders must also be considered in the differential diagnosis. *Scurvy* produces radiographic appearances similar to those observed in the battered baby syndrome, with subperiosteal haematomas and subsequent calcification. Generalized disorders associated with porotic bones due to existing disease such as spina bifida cystica must also be borne in mind.

In Childhood and Adolescence

Osteogenesis imperfecta is by far the commonest cause of osteoporosis and fracture in childhood and adolescence. Other conditions which must be considered in the differential diagnosis include *idiopathic juvenile osteoporosis*, *Turner's syndrome*, *adrenocortical tumour* and *leukaemia*. Idiopathic juvenile osteoporosis produces characteristic rarified metaphyseal areas in long bones in addition to progressive vertebral collapse.

Two unusual features occur in osteogenesis imperfecta and lead to difficulty in diagnosis. The first is the presence of cystic change in long bones – easily mistaken for polyostotic fibrous dysplasia. The latter is usually unilateral. The second is the development of hyperplastic callus following a fracture. The radiographic appearances may be indistinguishable from those of osteosarcoma, and biopsy of the lesion is often necessary to establish the diagnosis. Other rare causes of hyperplastic callus may have to be considered such as scurvy, congenital syphilis, Caffey's disease and disorders producing generalized porosis of bone, examples of which are spina bifida cystica and chronic osteomyelitis.

A useful review of brittle bone disease has been produced by Smith et al. (1983).

Summary

The use of imaging techniques in the diagnosis of developmental disorders is largely confined to conventional radiography in the form of a modified skeletal survey. Refinements in ultrasonography give hope of earlier pre-natal diagnosis in disorders with spinal and limb malformations. More sophisticated techniques, such as arthrography, may be useful in planning limb surgery. Radiculography, especially when combined with computed tomography, is valuable in the investigation of neurological complications.

References

Bailey DK (1952) The normal cervical spine in infants and children. Radiology 59:712–719

Bailey JA (1970) Orthopaedic aspects of achondroplasia. J Bone Joint Surg [Am] 52:1285–1301

Bethem D, Winter RB, Lutter L et al. (1981) Spinal disorders of dwarfism. J Bone Joint Surg [Am] 63:1412–1425

Cameron JM, Rae LJ (1975) Atlas of the battered child syndrome. Churchill Livingstone, Edinburgh

Campbell S, Pearce JM (1983) Ultrasound visualization of congenital malformations. Br Med Bull 39:322–331

Cattell HS, Filtzer DL (1965) Pseudosubluxation and other normal variations in the cervical spine in children: a study of 160 children. J Bone Joint Surg [Am] 47:1295–1309

Crossan JF, Wynne-Davies R, Fulford GE (1983) Bilateral failure of the capital femoral epiphysis. J Pediatr Orthop 3:297–301

Fairbank T (1951) An atlas of general affections of the skeleton. Livingstone, Edinburgh

Hungerford GD, Akkaraju V, Rawe SE, Young GF (1981) Atlanto-occipital and atlanto-axial dislocations with spinal cord compression in Down's syndrome: a case report and review of the literature. Br J Radiol 54:758–761

Kopits SE (1976) Orthopaedic complications of dwarfism. Clin Orthop 114:153–179

Lutter LD, Lonstein JE, Winter RB, Langer LO (1977) Anatomy of the achondroplastic lumbar canal. Clin Orthop 126: 139–142

Paris Nomenclature (1983) Society of Paediatric Radiology, international nomenclature of constitutional disorders of bone. Ann Radiol (Paris) 26:457–462

Paterson CR (1977) Osteogenesis imperfecta in the differential diagnosis of child abuse. Arch Dis Child 52:808

Semine AA, Ertel AW, Goldberg MJ, Bull MJ (1978) Cervical spine instability in children with Down's syndrome (Trisomy 21). J Bone Joint Surg [Am] 60:649–652

Smith R, Francis MJO, Houghton GR (1983) The brittle bone syndrome. Butterworth, London

Wynne-Davies R, Gormley J (1981) Clinical and genetic patterns in osteogenesis imperfecta. Clin Orthop 159:26–35

Wynne-Davies R, Gormley J (1985) The prevalence of skeletal dysplasias: an estimate of their minimum frequency and the number of patients requiring orthopaedic care. J Bone Joint Surg [Br] 67:133–137

Wynne-Davies R, Hall C (1982) Two clinical developments of spondyloepiphyseal dysplasia congenita. J Bone Joint Surg [Br] 64:435–441

Wynne-Davies R, Hall C, Apley AG (1985) An atlas of skeletal dysplasias. Churchill Livingstone, Edinburgh

25 Back Pain

R.C. Mulholland

Introduction 325
Importance of Spinal Anatomy 325
Strategies in the Management of Back Pain 326
Specific Diagnostic Groups 326
    Spondylolysis and Spondylolisthesis 326
    Acute Back Pain or Lumbago 327
    Prolapsed Intervertebral Disc 327
    Spinal Stenosis 329
    Identification of Single Segment Failure 330
    The Problem Back 331
    The Multi-Operated Back 331
    Infection 332
    Spinal Neoplasm 333
References 334

Introduction

The great variety of imaging techniques now available necessitates careful selection to avoid wasting time and money (Steiner 1982) and subjecting patients to unnecessary investigation. The radiologist should be involved early in the diagnostic process to give advice on appropriate investigations and the order in which they should be carried out.

The demonstration of pathology in the spine is not necessarily of clinical significance. Many patients have marked degenerative change, disc space narrowing and deformity and are either asymptomatic or the symptoms they have are unrelated to obvious radiological abnormalities. It is clear that the relevance of anatomical or pathological changes to the patient's symptoms cannot be established by imaging techniques alone. A full clinical appraisal is essential.

The relevant imaging techniques are not only of value in diagnosis, but also allow evaluation of the efficacy of treatment. They may be of particular value in the planning of surgical exploration and extirpation, or in less invasive procedures such as needle biopsy.

Importance of Spinal Anatomy

Certain features of spinal anatomy make imaging difficult. The fact that the cancellous bone, which may be the key to the nature of the clinical disorder (tumour, infection, metabolic change), is surrounded by a shell of fairly radio-opaque cortical bone which is unaffected, prevents plain radiography from detecting changes in the cancellous bone until a late stage. This disparity between cortex and cancellous bone is least in the pedicles, and therefore a destructive process will affect the cortical shell of the pedicle at a much earlier stage than the shell of the body of a vertebra, and hence loss of a single pedicle on the antero-posterior plain film may be the earliest evidence of a destructive lesion in the spine.

The three-dimensional complexity of the vertebrae, spinous processes, laminae, facet joints, mammillary processes, transverse processes, and the presence of a canal within the bone creates considerable difficulty in detecting pathological change. The centring of the film may distort disc width. Hence oblique and coned films are often required as well as antero-posterior and lateral views. Perhaps the greatest impact of the newer imaging techniques,

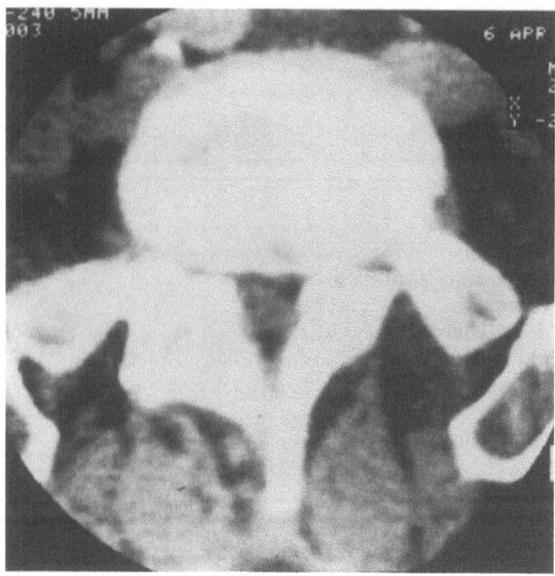

Fig. 25.1. CT scan. The spinal canal is narrow, due to enlargement of both facet joints. There is a particularly large facet joint on the right. The patient had bilateral radicular symptoms due to subarticular entrapment.

such as CT and MRI, is their ability to define the shape and size of the neural canal (Fig. 25.1) including the root canals (Bolender et al. 1985). Distortion and abnormality of the nerve tissues themselves are still best demonstrated using contrast radiography, although it is probable that in the near future the more sophisticated MRI may rival contrast radiography.

Strategies in the Management of Back Pain

Back pain is a symptom, it may be mild and yet of sinister import; it may be severe, and yet be due to a benign self-limiting disorder.

The history and physical examination may establish that the disorder is such that a precise diagnosis is not required, either because recovery is likely with the passage of time alone, or combined with a period of rest, analgesia, reassurance, and occasionally various physiotherapeutic manoeuvres; or a more precise diagnosis will not affect management and the physician is confident of the essentially benign

nature of the pain. However, back pain occurring for the first time in the over 60-year-old, or back pain in the lumbodorsal or dorsal area at any age, even if mild and considered clinically to be a benign mechanical disorder should have the benefit of plain radiographs. Back pain at these sites, in these circumstances, is somewhat uncommon and more likely to be due to a bony or retroperitoneal disorder.

Specific Diagnostic Groups

Back pain may be due to a disorder in which specific therapy is indicated, the choice of which will depend on the diagnosis. It is appropriate, therefore, to discuss the investigation of a series of specific disorders which may present with back pain.

Spondylolysis and Spondylolisthesis

Low back pain is unusual in adolescence and when it occurs the diagnosis of a spondylolysis or spondylolisthesis must be considered.

Spondylolysis is not diagnosable clinically, indeed clinical detection of a first degree spondylolisthesis is often not possible at the lumbosacral level. However, careful examination of plain lateral radiographs, in most cases, will reveal a lysis if one be present; if there is doubt oblique films will show it more precisely (Fig. 25.2). Even when seen on the lateral film, it is wise to have oblique films to exclude the possibility of a unilateral spondylolysis. Occasionally tomography may be necessary to resolve any ambiguity. Particular attention should be paid to the presence of spina bifida occulta, or obvious dysplasia of the posterior elements in association with a spina bifida, as this is indicative of the dysplastic variety of spondylolisthesis, in which progressive slip is more likely, and hence the indication for fusion is greater.

Spondylolysis is not present at birth but is present in some 5% of the population at the age of 7 years, increasing to 7% in the post-pubertal population. It behaves like a stress fracture, but its onset is usually painless, and in most people it remains asymptomatic throughout life, and therefore is not of clinical significance. On occasion, however, its development is sudden and painful. In this situation rest and support may encourage healing, and the ability to diagnose such a stress fracture is important. The acute nature of the spondylolysis can be established by scintigraphy which will reveal a localized area of increased uptake at the site of the defect. Occasionally tomography may be required to confirm the presence of a defect whose presence is suspected on the scintigram. Tomography may reveal the presence of callus. However, even if healing does not occur the spondylolysis may become asymptomatic, and cause no longterm problem. Progression to a spondylolisthesis is unusual but if this occurs it is almost always within the first year after the development of the lysis. Hence repeat radiographic examination of patients throughout their growing period is not indicated, especially if they are asymptomatic (Fredrickson et al. 1984).

Spondylolytic spondylolisthesis at the L4/5 level does progressively slip. It develops in the late second or early third decade and may progress to a 30% slip (Jackson et al. 1978). If recognized before any slip has occurred, surgical repair or segmental fusion is indicated. The choice is dependent on the underlying disc, as clearly if this is degenerate, segmental fusion is necessary, L4 to L5. Discography is an appropriate investigation to establish the morphology of the disc. More recently it has been shown that MRI examination of the discs is equally effective, but non-invasive.

Although spondylolytic spondylolisthesis of all three varieties (dysplastic, spondylolytic at the L5/S1 and at the L4/5 level) may present with root compromise, it is the L4/5 listhesis that most commonly does so, and in this group a coincident disc protrusion may be present. A CT scan may produce sufficient information, but as interest is directed towards the degree of root distortion, especially by the soft tissues around the lysis, radiculography is superior. However, routine radiculography is not necessary in the above types of spondylolysis and spondylolisthesis in the absence of radicular signs or symptoms.

Degenerative spondylolisthesis is a disorder of middle life, more common in women, in which there is a progressive slip forward of one vertebra upon another (almost always L4/5), to at most a 30% slip (Rosenberg 1975). It may present with backache, but it is the neurological complications that are of greater importance. It may produce a root entrapment or a spinal stenosis syndrome. Radiculography and/or a CT scan are necessary to establish the degree of bony distortion of the canal, and the degree of root distortion. Accurate knowledge of the anatomical distortion, obtained with these techniques, allows surgical decompression to be localized and effective.

Acute Back Pain or Lumbago

Acute lumbago is a term used to describe acute low back pain due to a soft tissue lesion, or mechanical derangement of the lumbar spine. Radiology has no role in the management of this disorder except to exclude, when the clinical picture suggests it, the possibility of sepsis, tumour, or bony collapse.

Prolapsed Intervertebral Disc

The initial symptom in a patient subsequently shown to have a prolapsed intervertebral disc is most commonly acute lumbago, but it is the nature and severity of the various syndromes produced by a prolapsed intervertebral disc that dictate treatment. The majority of patients recover with the passage of time aided by rest, reassurance,

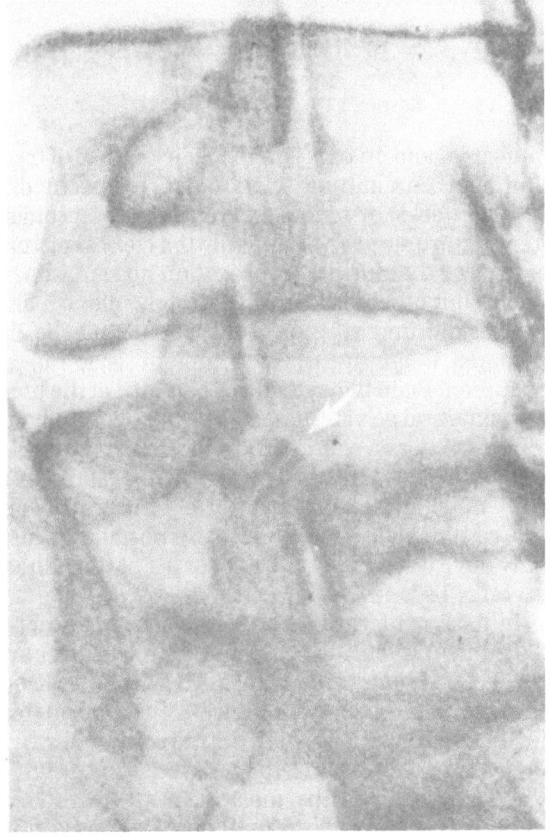

Fig. 25.2. Oblique X-rays of the lumbar spine. Note the pars articularis defect (*arrowed*).

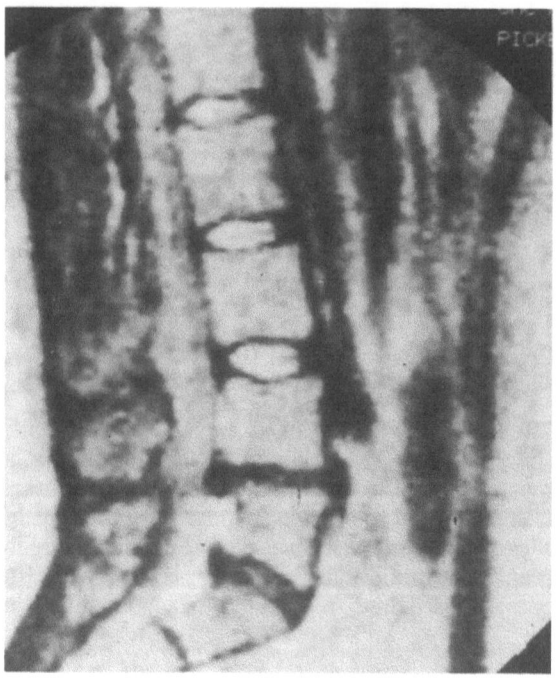

Fig. 25.3. Magnetic resonance image showing a protrusion of the L4/L5 disc.

analgesia, and on occasion the judicious use of traction; but unremitting sciatic pain, recurrent disabling attacks, or serious neurological compromise may require surgery. Commonly the clinical picture is so clear that further investigation appears superfluous, but other disorders may closely mimic a disc protrusion, and surgeon and patient may be ill-prepared if an unsuspected tumour is found at operation. Plain films should be obtained of the lumbar spine and pelvis. These films will exclude a bony abnormality as a cause of root entrapment, in either spine or pelvis. If disc-space narrowing is present it does not indicate the level of a disc protrusion. Indeed, the plain films are usually normal, or may only have a so-called sciatic tilt or list at the lumbosacral or L4/5 level.

In most patients it is the severe sciatic pain produced by root entrapment, that they wish to have relieved. Although the clinical story may indicate the root involved, and the clinical signs confirm this, further investigation is necessary to confirm the root distortion (Bell et al. 1984; Wiesel et al. 1984). Radiculography is the most accurate method of demonstrating this distortion, but the cause of the distortion is best shown by CT scanning. Demonstration of a disc protrusion in isolation is not of

value, as this may be entirely asymptomatic, and has been shown to be present in some 30% of patients undergoing radiculography for a cervical problem, and who had no symptoms referable to their lower lumbar spine (Hitselberger and Witen 1968). Different clinical situations may require one or both investigations. In the young person with normal plain films, no previous history of a disc protrusion and a clinical history and physical findings giving a clear indication of the root involved, demonstration of a disc protrusion at the appropriate level is a sufficient investigation, and either a CT or MRI examination (Fig. 25.3) is sufficient. However, in a patient with a previous history of lumbago or sciatica, and a root other than S1 involved, confirmation of the root abnormality is desirable, and radiculography is of greater value. In the older person with degenerative changes in the lower spine, where bony entrapment may be significant, one not only needs to confirm the root involved, but also the nature of the compressive lesion, and whether this is a combination of both bone and disc. In this situation a combination of radiculography and CT scanning is appropriate. On some occasions the non-invasive nature of a CT examination may be important. When a number of roots are involved, or there clearly is a cauda equina lesion, radiculography is necessary. In the presence of a complete block to the flow of contrast, a CT examination provides valuable information concerning the canal below the block. In patients with a history of sensitivity to iodine, a CT scan is indicated. The non-ionic water-soluble contrast media used for radiculography now produce such a clear demonstration of root pathology that venography is no longer a valid alternative as it used to be with the older oil-based media.

With the use of surface coils, magnetic resonance imaging (Chap. 12) is now producing satisfactory images of both disc protrusions, and nerve root amputations (Modic et al. 1983).

Epidurography (Chap. 6) demonstrates extradural defects, is somewhat less invasive than an intradural investigation and has a lower morbidity. Like venography it requires a radiologist who is used to the technique and uses it often enough to be skilled in interpretation, and a clinician who only wishes to know the fact that there is an extradural lesion, and is himself confident about its nature.

Chymopapaine Chemonucleolysis

Recently the reduction of the bulk of a disc protrusion has been achieved by means of intradiscal injection of a proteolytic enzyme, chymopapaine

(McCulloch 1980). This requires the precise placement of the drug within the nucleus pulposus, using a fine needle under radiographic control. This type of procedure requires close clinical and radiological collaboration. A proportion of such patients do not respond to injection, and require additional surgical intervention.

Spinal Stenosis

Lateral Spinal Stenosis

Root compression due to bony entrapment causes dermatomal pain, which may be severe but absent at rest, and the straight leg raising test may be normal. Radiographic evidence of root compression must be sought. The compression in lateral spinal stenosis is laterally placed, either beneath the facet joint or at the exit foramen. Plain films may show a narrow interpedicular distance, suggesting a narrow lateral recess. The facet joints may be close to the mid-line, and degenerate. The disc space itself may be narrowed, suggesting the possibility of foraminal stenosis. Asymmetry of the posterior elements is sometimes associated with lateral recess stenosis. Radiculography may show root cut off, but not infrequently the entrapment is too lateral to be demonstrated clearly by a radiculogram. CT is the method of choice in this situation (Fig. 25.4), even revealing the specific osteophytes causing the compression. MRI cannot easily demonstrate the cortical bony outlines which are causative of lateral canal stenosis, but it can detect loss of fat in the lateral recess, produced by the existence of compression. Increased sophistication of MRI suggests that it will be used to detect the consequences of compression, rather than the anatomical fact. This is of importance, as the anatomical appearances may be the same on either side yet the symptoms present on one side only (Crawshaw et al. 1984).

Central Spinal Stenosis

The great majority of patients with this disorder have a canal which though small initially, with the passage of time is encroached upon further by redundant ligamentum flavum and annular bulge, due to narrowing of disc spaces, and degenerating joints. The patient presents with diffuse multi-radicular symptoms in the lower limbs. Weakness on activity, fatigue, and a feeling of numbness are common, but pain is not a feature as it is of lateral

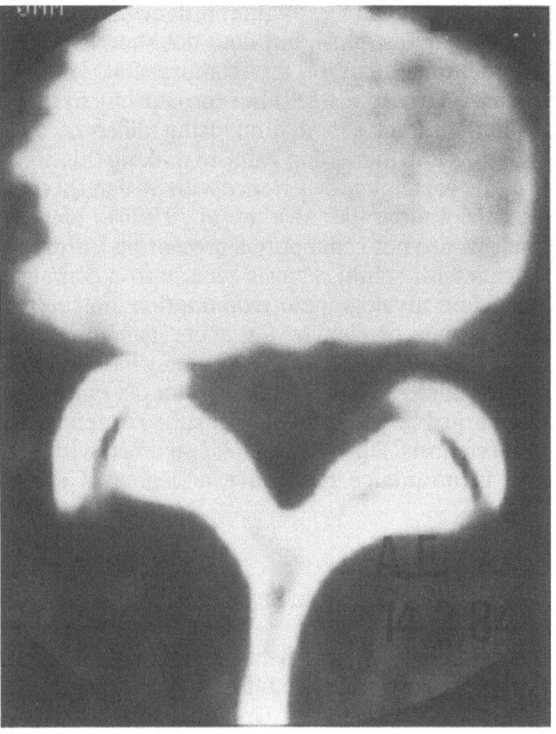

Fig. 25.4. CT scan of the lumbar spine showing unilateral subarticular entrapment on the right.

canal stenosis. The patient may observe that the symptoms disappear on stooping. In the stooped and sitting position the spine is flexed and the spinal canal space thereby increased.

Coincident vascular disease is not uncommon, and as the symptoms can be confused with vascular disease, demonstration of canal narrowing or stenosis is necessary. Although the condition may be suspected from plain films much of the loss of spinal diameter can be due to soft tissues within the canal. Short pedicles and a narrow interpedicular distance make the diagnosis likely, but radiculographic examination will localize the principal site of stenosis, or even block. It is of value to get contrast beyond any obstruction to determine whether a stenosis extends over a number of segments. Because of the marked effect of posture on the spinal canal diameters, flexion and extension views of the lumbar spine, with intrathecal contrast present are valuable. This can often reveal a complete block in extension, and free flow on flexion, reflecting the predominance of symptoms when standing, or walking downhill.

CT scanning is of less value; it demonstrates the fact of a narrow canal, but does not show well the longitudinal extent of the compression without detailed reformations. MRI has the capacity to show the longitudinal extent, and using different spin sequences is of increasing value in making this diagnosis. As yet clinical experience with MRI in this disorder is limited (McAfee et al. 1986). Bladder problems are not commonly a presenting feature in patients with spinal stenosis even with a complete block, but myelographic examination in such a patient may precipitate an acute cauda equina lesion, and urgent decompression may be required.

An apparent acute retention in an old man with an enlarged prostate, may in part be related to his spinal stenosis. Equally some older women with urinary incontinence may have a degree of spinal stenosis.

Identification of Single Segment Failure

Disc failure may lead to disturbances in spinal function, producing such disability that surgical intervention is considered. On occasion, there is associated significant root entrapment and precise definition of this is necessary. But combined with this may be a disturbance of the function of the spine as a supporting structure, and the spine will be described as feeling unstable by the patient. Such instability is a feature of a mobile back, and is seen in the 20 to 40-year-old age group, more frequently in women. If such disc failure is restricted to a single lumbar disc, local fusion may be appropriate.

There may be evidence on the plain films of segmental failure with local disc space narrowing and osteophytes restricted to a single level. In a younger person, under 30 years of age, with a one to two-year history of back pain, this is likely to be the source of the pain; but in an older patient with a longer history such changes may represent a previous problem, which has now stabilized, and the current problem may be from an adjacent segment. If the spine is fairly mobile, local anaesthetic blocks of the associated facet joints may relieve the discomfort experienced on hyperextension, thus identifying the painful segment. It is important that such a block is done under radiographic control, and the quantity of anaesthetic injected is only a few millilitres, preferably into the joint, so that the area anaesthetized is restricted to the joints suspected.

If the suspected segment is normal on plain films, a number of techniques may be used to identify an abnormal disc. Lateral films of the lumbar spine in flexion and extension may be taken. Rarely these show an actual forward translocation, but a more common abnormality is a discontinuity in the normal smooth curve of the lumbar flexion. Because the above method is imprecise, discography (Chap. 8) of the abnormal segment, and of adjacent segments is perhaps the most established method of showing disc abnormality or normality (McCulloch and Waddell 1978). The normal nucleus presents a bilobed structure. In the abnormal disc, this appearance is lost, with irregular extensions posteriorly and laterally. Injection into the inner annulus rather than the nucleus can produce an image that suggests an abnormal disc, and such artefacts must be recognized. Injection into the annulus may be painful, but is not significant. The more severe pain produced occasionally in an intact but degenerate disc, and mimicking the pain of presentation is presumed to be due to disc bulging with compression of adjacent nerve or inflamed anterior dura. The annulus of an acute protrusion in commonly very sensitive. The injection of local anaesthetic into the disc may relieve the patient's pain, to such a degree that with some confidence the painful segment is identified. Pain reproduction in the lumbar spine is not considered as valuable an investigation as in the cervical spine.

The other joint in the spinal segment is the facet joint. It is a synovial joint, and may develop degenerative change. Clearly it is a potential source of pain. The locked back may be a mechanical dysfunction of the segmental joint, especially those very short-lived yet exquisitely painful locked backs cured by a brief pull or manipulation. The facet joints can be investigated as a pain source, by injecting a small quantity of anaesthetic into the joint, under radiographic control (Chap. 9). On occasion longterm relief can be obtained by injecting steroid into the joint. A successful result from local anaesthetic injection, with or without steroid, can be used as a guide to the likely success of rhizolysis, or radiofrequency destruction of the small nerves to the posterior facet joints, carried out with a probe inserted on the lateral side of the joint. However the greatest value of anaesthetic block of a joint is to assist in the identification of a painful segment and in the assessment of suitability for segmental fusion.

MRI has the ability to detect changes in the disc, and correlates almost completely with discographic changes. At present its greatest value in the investigation of segmental failure is its ability to detect normality and abnormality. Unfortunately, there is a spectrum of abnormality, and demonstration of abnormality does not indicate that that particular disc is the symptomatic one.

On occasion radiculography may be of value, even in the absence of radicular pain, as marked disc bulging demonstrated on a lateral film in hyperextension can indicate a failing disc. It is the combination of abnormalities, all of which point to one level disc failure and exonerate adjacent discs, that will guide the clinician in his decision as to whether fusion may play a role, and which level is most appropriate to fuse.

In the middle-aged patient, mechanical low back pain is less likely to be due to a single segmental failure. Pain sources are likely to be multiple, so that single segment fusion is less often indicated. In the older patient investigations are commonly directed to exclude the possibility of tumour (primary or secondary), infection, or root entrapment, especially bony.

The Problem Back

Back pain not infrequently presents as a clinical problem, because one is dealing with a subjective complaint, and trying to relate it to an identifiable and causative pathology. The only measure of pain is the effect or disability it produces, and this is dependent as much on the nature of the patient as on the pain (Waddell et al. 1984). The aim of investigation is not merely the demonstration of pathology, but a sufficiently precise delineation of its nature to permit accurate correlation with symptoms and signs. At the same time other pathology which may be contributing to the patient's disability must be identified, and normality of other structures and tissues confirmed. On occasion the disability is much greater than the pathology discovered would lead one to expect. There, therefore, is great pressure to find causative pathology appropriate to the degree of disability and such patients are easily overinvestigated. A careful balance has to be achieved between sufficient investigation to reassure both patient and doctor that there is no serious undiscovered problem, and excessive investigation either producing iatrogenic disorder, or identifying asymptomatic pathology. In such patients non-invasive investigations are of most value, and a careful collaboration between radiologist and treating physician is essential.

The Multi-operated Back

Patients with a disabling low back problem may have back pain alone, back pain with leg pain, or leg pain alone. Unfortunately, not all such patients are curable surgically, yet because surgeons (and patients) are optimists, repeated operations may have been carried out. Although the likely cure after a third back operation is less than 10%, many patients have many more operations than this (Waddell et al. 1979). Because, on occasion, causative pathology is missed at operation, or alternatively previous operations may have caused disabling pathology, such multi-operated patients may require a very comprehensive series of investigations before deciding whether a further operation should be done, or the patient be persuaded to pursue non-surgical solutions to their problem (Calder et al. 1984).

Persisting radicular pain is much more likely to have a remediable cause. If a single root is suspected then a root block, using contrast to confirm that the needle is in the dural sleeve, is appropriate. Radiculography is not often of value, because previous surgery has usually produced scarring which obscures the root and dural outline. MRI with surface coils has demonstrated a distinction between scar and disc protrusion and may have greater application in the future. CT scanning will clearly demonstrate the anatomy of the root canal, revealing sites of possible compression. But observed abnormality must correlate with the clinical picture, confirmed if possible by root blocks; operation on a CT scan abnormality alone is inappropriate.

Persistent back pain in the multi-operated back is much less rewarding to investigate. The clinical problem can be divided into two groups; either the pain has never been cured (that is, it has persisted, with perhaps a few weeks of relief only, since the operation), or else there has been a substantial time interval between operation and onset of the pain. In the former situation, one has to review the indications for the first operation, and review the investigations. The wrong level may have been operated upon, and particular attention must be paid to errors of segmentation in the lumbar spine, as these may lead to operations at the wrong level. If the first operation has been a fusion, this may have failed. Plain films including obliques may show a failed fusion, as indeed may flexion and extension films, but if movement is present, it is very minimal. Discography of a disc space deep to a suspected failed fusion may be possible, and if this produces pain, then the fusion is not solid. Unfortunately, the commonly performed intertransverse fusion makes discography at such a level difficult. Tomography in both planes may show a fusion is not solid. However, there are as many cured patients amongst those whose fusion is not solid, so that demonstration of a failed fusion does not prove that that failure is the cause of the persistent pain (DePalma and Rothman 1968).

Pain recurring after a substantial interval may be due to new pathology. Localization of pain in the spine is poor, and pain sources from the 12th thoracic to the lumbosacral level may produce low back pain. A spondylolisthesis or lysis may develop above a fusion, especially if this has been accompanied by a decompression operation in which the pars inter-articularis was unduly thinned. A central disc protrusion may occur deep to a fusion, even if that is solid. Disc protrusion may occur above the fusion. Abutment of the fusion mass on the vertebra above may occur. Investigation of these patients must always include a review of previous investigations, and an awareness that the new pain may be due to entirely new pathology. It must be appreciated that previous surgery will always have produced abnormality of the anatomy of the area, and therefore results of investigations and their relevance to the symptomatology must be interpreted with care. As with all back pain problems the psychogenic element must always be borne in mind (Waddell et al. 1980).

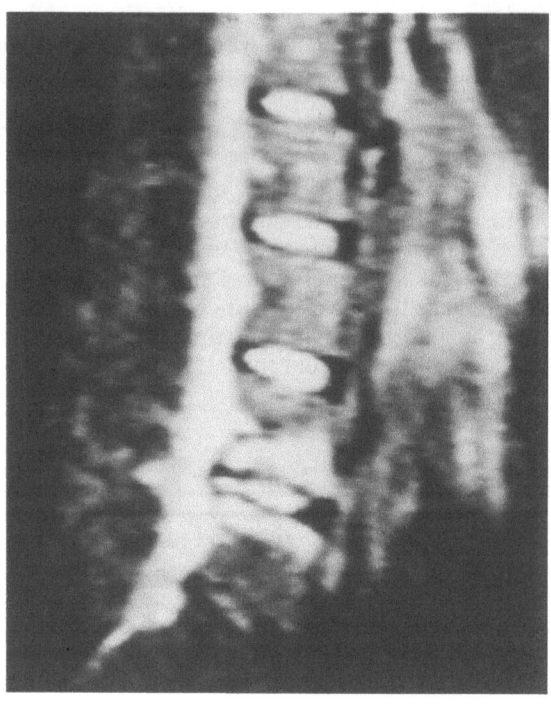

Fig. 25.5. Acute discitis (STIR TR1100 and TI100 ms).

Infection

Acute Spinal Infection

The outstanding feature of acute spinal infection is the severity of the pain and the stiffness of the spine. The infection may be of the bone or of the disc space. As with *osteomyelitis* elsewhere in children and the younger adult the fever and pain suggest infection. Whereas in most spinal disorders, local tenderness is not of great value, in patients with infection palpation of the spinous process of the affected vertebra is usually exquisitely painful. Abnormalities are not present initially on the plain radiographs but at a later stage the disc space appears narrowed. This is due to the disc sinking into the soft bone of the infected vertebra, and is not due to primary destruction of the disc, although once sunk into the vertebra it becomes infected. In the early stages, before changes are apparent on a plain radiograph, a skeletal scintigram is invaluable, and usually reveals an obvious "hot spot", coincident with the site of maximal spinal tenderness (Merkel et al. 1985; Chap 13).

Acute disc infection (discitis) is an uncommon disorder. It occurs in children, but its precise pathogenesis is debated. The disc narrows, the child has back pain and a stiff back. It is not like an acute infection, but is thought to have an infective basis. Needle biopsy of the disc space may be carried out in an attempt to find an organism, but one is seldom grown. In adults discitis is usually secondary to some invasive procedure. The increasing use of discography and chemonucleolysis has led to a number of cases. It can follow surgical treatment of a prolapsed disc. The patient will have severe pain, but may be apyrexial. The disc narrows when the infection involves the end plate, but this does not always occur, so that disc space narrowing is not an inevitable sequel of disc infection. In the early stages a skeletal scintigram may be negative. MRI may identify disc infection even when this is still restricted to the disc, and the scintigram is negative (Fig. 25.5).

Chronic Spinal Infection

This involves and produces destruction of bone. Because the infection is at the bony end plate, narrowing of the disc space usually occurs, the disc sinking into the bone. The adjacent vertebra becomes involved, producing the typical picture on plain films of two partially collapsed adjacent vertebrae, with no disc space between them. In the dorsal spine wedging or anterior collapse of the vertebrae occurs for mechanical reasons. Tuberculosis is the commonest cause, but needle biopsy is essential to confirm the diagnosis and obtain an organism (Fyfe et al. 1983). Occasionally staphylococcal infection can present as a chronic problem, producing either a sclerotic cavity in the vertebra, or less commonly a diffuse area of sclerosis, occasionally involving more than one vertebra. Preliminary tomography to localize the lesion is of value, and then the needle can be precisely directed. Spinal infection may follow surgical instrumentation of the genitourinary system, and in these patients, who may be infirm and in ill-health, the bone destruction can be so marked, and restricted to one vertebral body, without apparent disc space narrowing, that tumour may be suspected. Because of this, it is essential that even in a patient with a known primary, tissue confirmation of a spinal metastasis should be sought before starting treatment unless there are multiple metastases, or a previous skeletal metastasis has been identified.

Skeletal scintigraphy is of less value in the diagnosis of chronic infection. It cannot differentiate tuberculous from pyogenic infection, nor infection from degenerative changes; but it is extremely useful in assessing the response to treatment and particularly recurrence of infection. Tomography may reveal areas of bone destruction hidden by the sclerosis indicating an infective cause; and help accurate placement of a biopsy needle. Using a variety of spin sequences MRI has the capacity to distinguish between disc space narrowing due to infection (Fig. 25.6) and that due to degenerative change alone. This is of some importance in the elderly, when the infective process may be very insidious, and radiographically difficult to distinguish from degenerative change. In infection there will be a strong signal, whereas in degenerative disc space narrowing, the signal is low.

Needle Biopsy. Biopsy specimens can be obtained by needling at any spinal level with the possible exception of T2 and T3. It is preferable if the core diameter of the specimen is at least 2 mm, as this frequently will allow a tissue diagnosis to be made. The Harlow Wood needle has a 2-mm core diameter, and is safe and easy to use. It has a thin guide pin which can be safely and exactly placed using biplaner image intensification, or plain films in two planes and over this dilators are passed once the correct position is established. Down the dilator is then passed the biopsy needle. Slight suction is required using a syringe on the end of the biopsy needle to ensure the specimen is not lost.

Spinal Neoplasm

The commonest spinal neoplasms are *metastases*. The patient may present with back pain before the

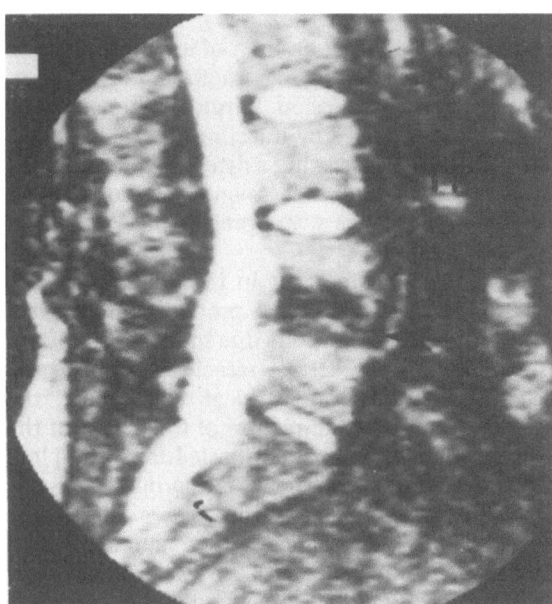

Fig. 25.6. Chronic healed disc infection with fatty replacement of the bone adjacent to the disc (STIR TR1100 and TI 100 ms).

primary tumour is detected. It is essential that a tissue diagnosis is made, and the clinician must decide whether to make this diagnosis by finding the primary, or by biopsy of a metastasis. Clearly if a relatively non-invasive procedure will produce a diagnosis it is preferable. The history and examination may incriminate the primary site, and a chest radiograph, IVP, or prostatic biopsy may be indicated. Blood tests include the serum proteins to exclude myeloma, and a serum acid phosphatase although it can remain normal in the presence of spinal metastases from a prostatic carcinoma. Before spinal biopsy a skeletal scintigram and radiographs or CT scans of areas of increased uptake (Chap. 22) are indicated. These may reveal multiple lesions and an easier site for biopsy.

Multiple myeloma presents a fairly typical radiographic appearance. The associated blood abnormalities usually confirm the diagnosis, and biopsy is not required. However, solitary plasmacytoma is not uncommon in the spine, and the serum proteins may be normal. Since tissue is readily accessible diagnosis by needle biopsy is most useful.

Osteoblastoma occurs in the spine (Pettine and Klassen 1986). This tumour arises more frequently in the laminae, transverse processes, and pedicles, than in the bodies, and may easily be missed on plain films. It commonly produces a scoliosis, which unlike the usual adolescent scoliosis is painful and may be anywhere in the spine. The skeletal scintigram usually shows an area of intense uptake at the apex of the curve, and tomography or CT scanning will reveal the lesion. Surgical removal of the tumour can be aided by injecting the radionuclide prior to surgery, and using a detecting probe during surgery to localize the lesion, and confirm its removal. This allows a very precise and local resection of the lesion.

Giant cell tumours occur in the vertebral bodies (Larsson 1979), and may produce catastrophic neurological complications due to local expansion, and bone collapse. Hence resection is necessary. Before embarking on surgical extirpation, the surgeon requires a full picture of the extent of the lesion. Its nature will be suspected from the plain radiographs but needle biopsy is appropriate to confirm this. An exception is in those cases where there is spinal cord compromise and emergency cord decompression is indicated. A CT scan is the most valuable investigation, and if surgery is urgently required the CT should be done as an emergency. When there is neurological compromise, myelography or MRI are necessary adjuncts to clarify the extent of the lesion in the sagittal plane, and the degree of cord distortion. On occasion the neurological picture may be worsened by a myelogram, and this should only be carried out, therefore, at a time and place where urgent surgical intervention can be carried out.

Paget's disease of the spine may be asymptomatic, it may produce deformity, or it may produce a spinal stenotic syndrome. Rarely a *sarcoma* may develop. The clinical feature is the onset of severe pain which is unusual in Paget's disease. The alkaline phosphatase is very high. Plain films and tomograms will show areas of bone destruction as well as the characteristic features of Paget's disease.

Intradural tumours may present to the orthopaedic surgeon because they produce back pain, and usually a stiff back, if they occur in a mobile segment of the spine. Neurological changes may be late in occurring, and may be minimal. Myelography and CT give characteristic appearances, but MRI is likely to achieve a more important role in primary diagnosis with technological improvements.

References

Bell GR, Rothman RH, Booth RE et al. (1984) A study of computer assisted tomography: comparison of metrizamide myelography and computer tomography in the diagnosis of herniated lumbar disc and spinal stenosis. Spine 9:552–556

Bolender NF, Schonstrom N, Spengler DM (1985) Role of computed tomography and myelography in the diagnosis of central spinal stenosis. J Bone Joint Surg [Am] 67:240–246

Calder TJ, Dawson EG, Bassett LW (1984) The role of tomography in the evaluation of the post operative spinal fusion. Spine 9:686–689

Crawshaw C, Kean DM, Mulholland RC et al. (1984) The use of nuclear magnetic resonance in the diagnosis of lateral canal entrapment. J Bone Joint Surg [Br] 66:711–715

DePalma AF, Rothman RH (1968) The nature of pseudarthrosis. Clin Orthop 59:113–118

Fredrickson BE, Baker D, McHolick WJ, Lubicky JP (1984) The natural history of spondylolysis and spondylolisthesis. J Bone Joint Surg [Am] 66:699–707

Fyfe IS, Henry APJ, Mulholland RC (1983) Closed vertebral biopsy. J Bone Joint Surg [Br] 65:140–143

Hitselberger WE, Witen RM (1968) Abnormal myelograms in asymptomatic patients. J Neurosurg 28:204–206

Jackson AM, Kirwan EOG, Sullivan MF (1978) Lytic spondylolisthesis above the lumbo-sacral level. J Bone Joint Surg [Br] 60:439–440

Larsson S (1979) Removal of the third thoracic vertebra and partial lung resection for a radio resistant giant cell tumour of the spine. J Bone Joint Surg [Br] 61:489–493

McAfee PC, Bohlman HH, Han JS, Salvagno RT (1986) Comparison of nuclear magnetic resonance imaging and computed tomography in the diagnosis of upper cervical spinal cord compression. Spine 11:295–304

McCulloch JA (1980) Chemonucleolysis. Clin Orthop 146:128–135

McCulloch JA, Waddell G (1978) Lateral lumbar discography. Br J Radiol 51:498–502

Merkel KD, Brown ML, Piwanjee N, Fitzgerald R (1985) Comparison of Indium-labelled leukocyte imaging with sequential Technetium-Gallium scanning in the diagnosis of low-grade musculo-skeletal sepsis. J Bone Joint Surg [Am] 67:465–476

Modic MT, Weinstein MA, Pavlicek W, Starnes DL, Duchesneau PM, Boumphrey F, Hardy RJ (1983) Nuclear magnetic resonance imaging of the spine. Radiology 148:757–762

Pettine KA, Klassen RA (1986) Osteoid osteoma and osteoblastoma of the spine. J Bone Joint Surg [Am] 68:355–361

Rosenberg NJ (1975) Degenerative spondylolisthesis. Predisposing factors. J Bone Joint Surg [Am] 57:467–477

Steiner RE (1982) New imaging techniques: their relation to conventional radiology. Br Med J 284:1590–1592

Waddell G, Kummel EG, Lott WN, Graham JD, Hall H, McCulloch JA (1979) Failed lumbar disc surgery and repeat surgery following industrial injuries. J Bone Joint Surg [Am] 61:201–207

Waddell G, McCulloch JA, Kummel EG, Venner RM (1980) Non organic physical signs in low back pain. Spine 5:117–125

Waddell G, Main CJ, Morris EW, Di Paola M, Gray KM (1984) Chronic low back pain. Psychological distress and illness behaviour. Spine 9:209–213

Wiesel SW, Tsourmas N, Feffer HL, Citrin CM, Patronas H (1984) A study of computer assisted tomography: the incidence of positive CAT scans in an asymptomatic group of patients. Spine 9:549–551

26 Spinal Deformity

J.E. Lonstein

Routine Evaluation 335
  Erect Views 335
  Bone Detail 336
  Evaluation for Treatment 337
  Large Curves 337
  Fusion Evaluation 337
Adults 337
  Curve Evaluation 337
  Pain Evaluation 337
Neuromuscular Deformities 338
Congenital Deformities 338
  Routine Evaluation 338
  Computed Tomography 338
  Tomography 339
Bone Tumours 339
  Conventional Techniques 339
  Skeletal Scintigraphy 340
  Computed Tomography 340
Spinal Cord Lesions 340
  Conventional Radiography 341
  Myelography 341
  Computed Tomography 341
  Magnetic Resonance Imaging 341
Vascular Studies 341
Painful Scoliosis 341
  Conventional Radiography 342
  Skeletal Scintigraphy 342
  CT Myelography 342
  Magnetic Resonance Imaging 342
Spinal Cord Compression 343
  Kyphosis Only 343
  Kyphosis plus Scoliosis 343
References 343

Routine Evaluation

The routine evaluation of spinal deformity (Binstadt et al. 1982; Board 1967; Bradford et al. 1988; Young et al. 1970) involves accurate assessment of the deformity, its aetiology and magnitude, and an appreciation of bone detail during both the initial and follow-up examinations.

Erect Views

In the initial assessment an erect radiograph is all that is usually necessary to make the diagnosis and plan treatment. Erect films are taken in the standing position, with sitting films used only in those unable to stand (e.g. neuromuscular scoliosis, small children). They are taken at a standard 6-foot (2-metre)

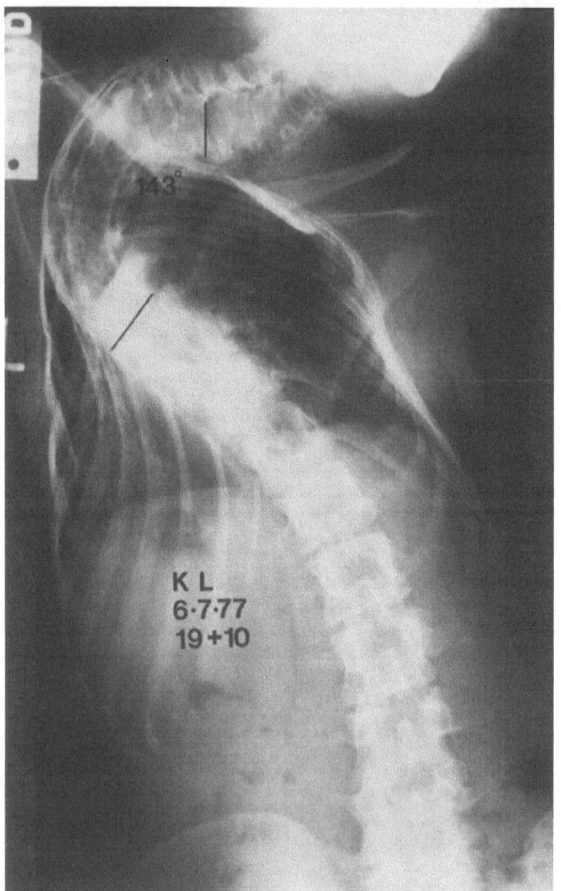
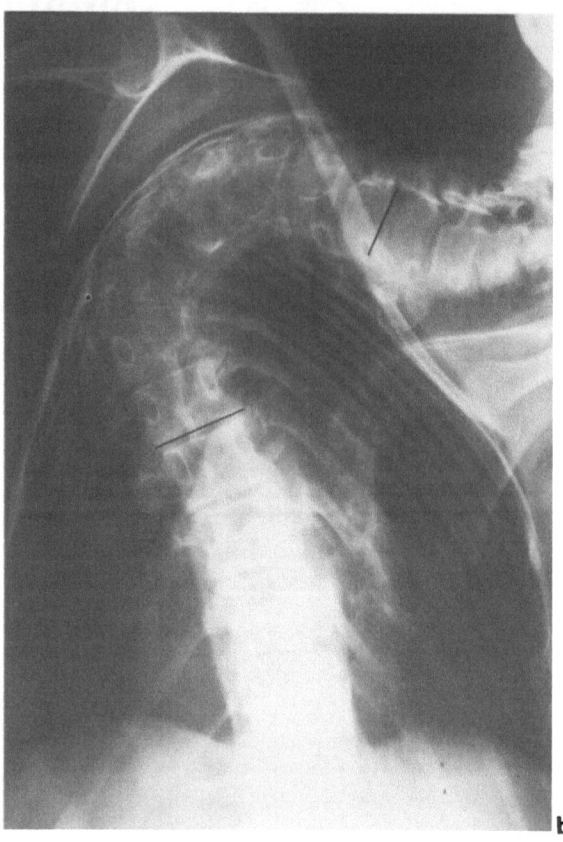

Fig. 26.1. a Standing postero-anterior view of spine shows a 143 degree upper left thoracic curve. The vertebral anatomy is not visible. b Derotated view shows the vertebral anatomy. There is a hemivertebra on the convexity of the curve with fusion of the vertebral bodies (*arrow*). (Reprinted with permission from Bradford DS, Lonstein JE, Ogilvie JW, Winter RB (1987) Moe's textbook of scoliosis and other spinal deformities. W.B. Saunders, Philadelphia, PA)

distance using 14 × 36 inch (36 × 91 cm) film which allows a complete assessment of the whole spine on a single radiograph. When this longer film is not available, or in small children, 14 × 17 inch (36 × 43 cm) film is used. The smaller film is positioned with the lower end of the film at the level of the anterior superior iliac spines, thereby allowing most of the spine to be viewed on a single radiograph.

To help decrease radiation exposure, and to make the radiographic density of the vertebral column uniform, an aluminium filter is used to screen out portions of the X-ray (Hopkins et al. 1984). Additional techniques used to minimize radiation include use of the postero-anterior position to reduce breast and thyroid dosage, use of fast exposure film, rare earth intensifying screens, collimation of the X-ray

beam, antiscatter grids and gonadal shielding (Gregg 1977; Nash et al 1979; DeSmet et al. 1981; Andersen et al. 1982; Gray et al. 1983).

Bone Detail

When additional bone detail is necessary (e.g. in congenital deformities, neurofibromatosis, spine infections) supine films are taken at 40-inch (102 cm) distance, using slower X-ray film. A more accurate appreciation of bone anatomy can be obtained where necessary by tomography or computed tomography (CT).

Special projections aid in the assessment of the anatomy in certain areas of the spine e.g. supine oblique views to visualize the pars interarticularis and the Ferguson view to demonstrate the anatomy of the lumbosacral articulation.

Evaluation for Treatment

Once the diagnosis has been made and active treatment (non-operative or operative) decided upon, additional views may be necessary to evaluate specific features.

Flexibility

Projections to assess the flexibility of the spinal curves are taken in the supine position. These consist of active flexion for scoliosis, hyperextension for kyphosis and flexion for lordosis. As these radiographs all involve active muscle power, they are not applicable in neuromuscular deformities or in the very young. In these cases, a traction film is used to assess flexibility of the spinal deformity.

Maturity

In growing children, an assessment of bone maturity plays a role in the decision-making process. This usually includes assessment of the iliac apophyses (Risser 1958) and carpal bones for comparison with accepted standards (Greulich and Pyle 1959).

Rib Hump View

When radiographic visualization and assessment of the rotational prominence in the thoracic area is deemed necessary, a special rib hump view is obtained. Pre- and post-operative comparison views are then possible.

Large Curves

In the asessment of larger spinal curves, the above techniques are sometimes inadequate in visualizing and appreciating the true deformity. The lateral deviation in these cases is accompanied by rotation and an apparent kyphosis – the "kyphosing scoliosis" of Stagnara (1974). To see the vertebral anatomy, a derotated view is used – the "plan d'election" of Stagnara (1974; Fig. 26.1). In some cases, tomography in these large curves is necessary to appreciate the detailed anatomy (congenital, tuberculosis, neurofibromatosis).

The flexion films to demonstrate flexibility are inaccurate in larger curves, where a traction view may be more appropriate.

Fusion Evaluation

Accurate visualization of the bony detail of a fusion mass is essential in post-operative follow-up and is achieved by oblique views. Tomograms may be indicated, especially in patients where there is a significant amount of instrumentation or, following an anterior fusion, to demonstrate the bone incorporation and continuity of osseous trabeculae across the disc space. In some areas (e.g. lumbosacral region) flexion views are sometimes helpful in evaluating the integrity of a fusion.

Scintigraphy may demonstrate a pseudarthrosis.

Adults

The above techniques are generally applicable in the assessment of spinal deformity in adults but, in addition, an assessment of the accompanying pain is sometimes necessary (see below).

Curve Evaluation

The radiographic techniques required to evaluate an adult with a spinal deformity depend on the type of deformity, and whether prior surgery has been performed. Because of the presence of larger curvatures, a derotated view and a lateral view are important to obtain a three-dimensional appreciation of the deformity. Careful technique is necessary to visualize bony detail in osteopaenic adults.

Pain Evaluation (Chap. 25)

As part of the assessment of an adult with a painful deformity, additional radiographic techniques may be necessary. To help assess the source of pain in the lumbar area, discography can be used. The radiographic appearance of the disc is not necessarily important, but rather whether, on injection of contrast medium, pain is produced which matches

Fig. 26.2. a Antero-posterior view of a 5+6 year-old-girl with myelodysplasia. The widened interpedicular distance in the lumbar area is seen. A thoracolumbar bony spur of a diastematomyelia is well seen. b CT cut of the spur shows the bifid spinal canal and cord. (Reprinted with permission from Bradford DS, Lonstein JE, Ogilvie JW, Winter RB (1987) Moe's textbook of scoliosis and other spinal deformities, 2nd Edn. W.B. Saunders, Philadelphia, PA)

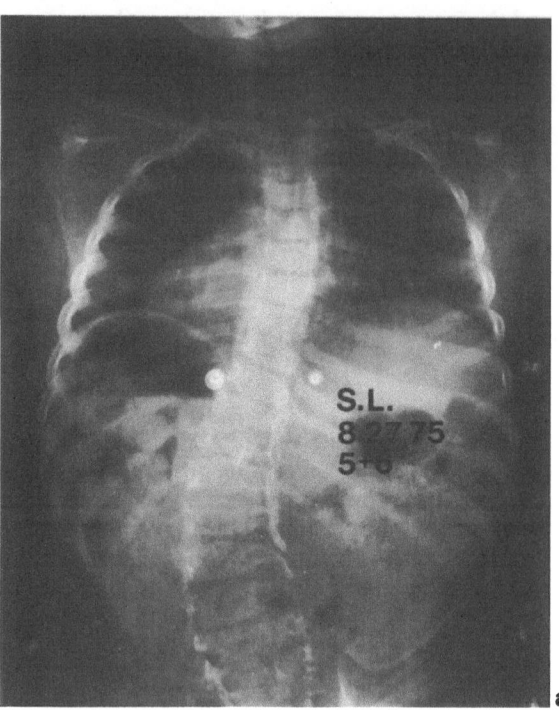

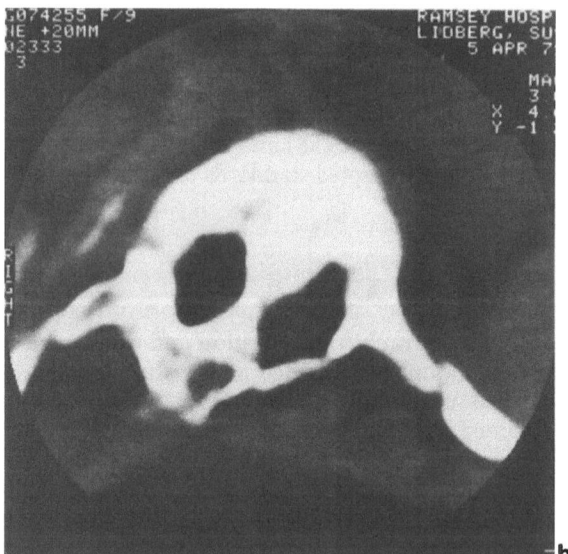

the presenting pain pattern. If on injection of contrast medium, pain occurs with the same character, site and radiation as the patient's symptoms, then that disc is the likely source of those symptoms.

In cases with radicular pain, water-soluble myelography, combined in some cases with CT, is essential in the assessment of the pain problem.

Neuromuscular Deformities

In neuromuscular deformities, alteration in the routine evaluation described above is necessary. Sitting upright films are obtained where unsupported standing is not possible. The sitting film must be unsupported so that the true curvature is visualized, minimal support being given where unsupported sitting is impossible. Due to the lack of muscle power in these patients active flexibility evaluation is impossible, and traction films are used. A useful method is with a traction frame (Cotrel/Risser) where careful positioning in traction is possible, allowing an assessment of the curve's flexibility.

Congenital Deformities

Routine Evaluation

In the routine evaluation of congenital deformities, good bone detail is necessary. Supine views are used when this detail is not visible on the erect examination, a derotated view being used when rotation obscures the anatomy. In the very young, the presence of cartilage in the vertebra makes an appreciation of the anatomy difficult. Careful assessment of the pedicles and disc space height will give clues about the nature of the congenital anomaly; namely failure of formation or failure of segmentation.

Computed Tomography

CT is the most useful technique to demonstrate complex three-dimensional spinal anatomy (Figs. 26.2, 26.3). Reformatting of thin trans-axial sections in alternative planes can be invaluable.

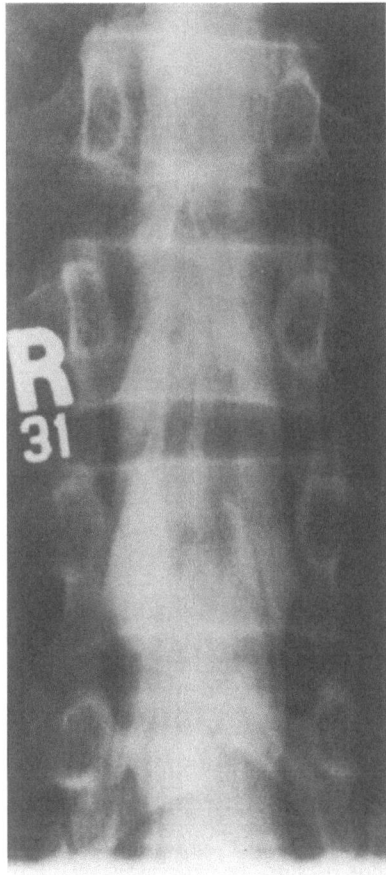

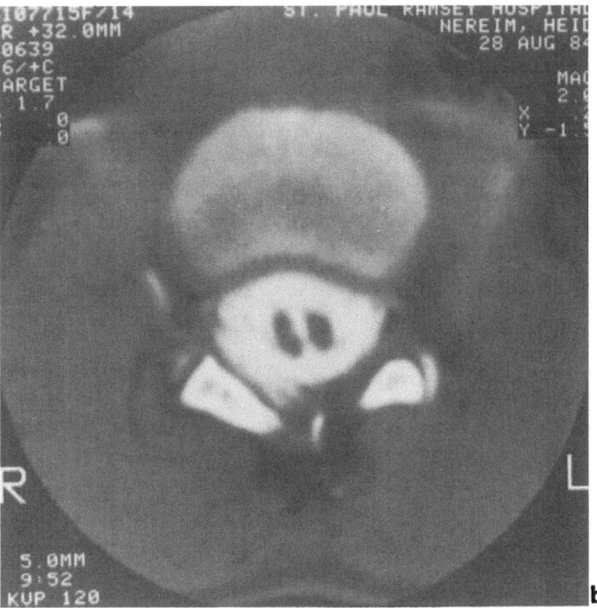

Fig. 26.3. a A metrizamide myelogram in another patient with diastematomyelia shows the mid-line spur and split cord. **b** CT cut with metrizamide shows the mid-line septum splitting the spinal cord. (Reprinted with permission from Bradford DS, Lonstein JE, Ogilvie JW, Winter RB (1987) Moe's textbook of scoliosis and other spinal deformities, 2nd Edn. W.B. Saunders, Philadelphia, PA)

Tomography

Tomography can be used when CT is unavailable to visualize the exact nature of congenital spine anomalies (Fig. 26.4). Coronal sections are used with scoliosis and sagittal sections with kyphosis, both being necessary for more complex deformities in order to appreciate the three-dimensional problem.

Spinal Dysraphism

Spinal dysraphism including embryonic tumours may be suspected when routine views show normal pedicles but with localized widening of the interpedicular distance compared to published standards (Hinck et al. 1966). In addition, the related disc spaces are often narrower than the adjacent spaces. A central bony spur i.e. diastematomyelia may be visible on routine views (Fig. 26.2). To demonstrate the dysraphism fully additional techniques are

necessary. Myelography may show a central filling defect and when combined with CT reveal a bony or a fibrous septum and/or a tethered cord. CT or MRI are essential to demonstrate the nature (e.g. lipoma) of any associated embryonic tumours. MRI may come to replace myelography in the future evaluation of this problem.

Bone Tumours (Chap. 25)

Bone tumours often present as painful scoliosis, with a "spasm" curve related to the bony tumour. The tumour is usually situated at the apex of the concavity of the lateral curve.

Conventional Techniques

Standing postero-anterior films are the first to be obtained in a patient with scoliosis. In every case,

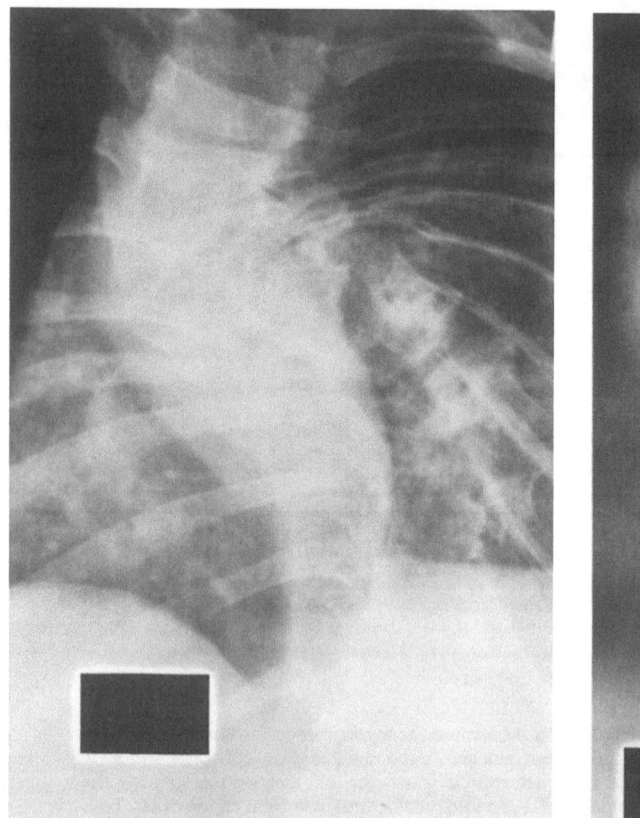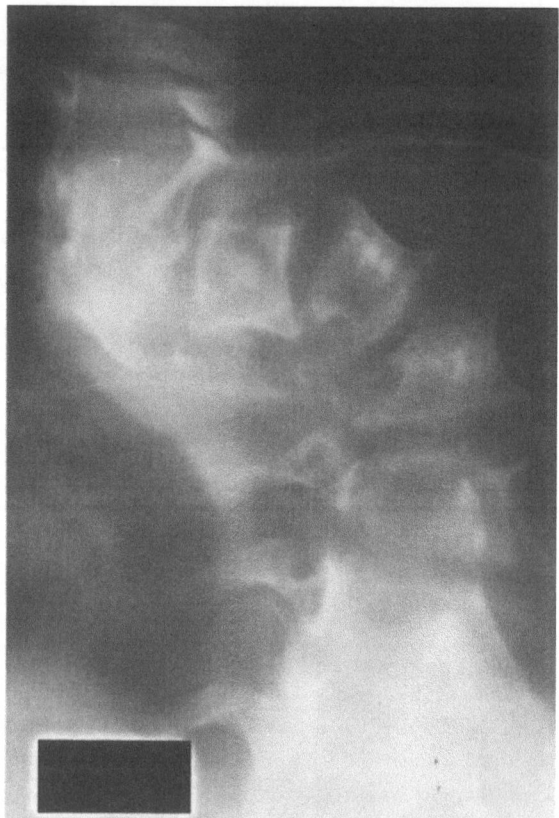

Fig. 26.4. a Antero-posterior spine radiograph in a case of neurofibromatosis poorly visualizes the vertebral anatomy. **b** Tomogram in the antero-posterior plane shows the severe vertebral dysplasia present. (Reprinted with permission from Bradford DS, Lonstein JE, Ogilvie JW, Winter RB (1987) Moe's textbook of scoliosis and other spinal deformities, 2nd Edn. W.B. Saunders, Philadelphia, PA)

the bone anatomy is evaluated, with or without the symptom of pain as not all bone tumours present with pain. The concavity of the curve apex is carefully examined for an area of sclerosis, osteopaenia or loss of the normal bony architecture. This may be in the body, posterior elements, pedicle, transverse process or adjacent rib. Oblique views help in accurate visualization when any suspicious area is seen.

Skeletal Scintigraphy

When suspicion of an osseous lesion is high, a scintigram is obtained. Using a pin-hole technique, accurate localization to the level, side and even segment of a vertebra is often possible.

Computed Tomography

For accurate visualization and localization of tumour, CT has replaced conventional tomography. A localized area for CT is possible as the level of pathology is known from a combination of the conventional radiographs and scintigram. CT will show the precise area of pathology allowing an accurate surgical plan to be formulated (Donavan-Post 1980).

Spinal Cord Lesions

Spinal cord lesions can present as either scoliosis alone, painful scoliosis or a neurological deficit. A high index of suspicion is necessary with *any* spinal curvature to allow early, prompt diagnosis of a spinal cord lesion. Any left thoracic, or non-typical curvature, should be viewed with suspicion and a neurological basis sought, using if necessary all the modalities of evaluation below.

Conventional Radiography

Routine radiographs are carefully evaluated. The interpedicular distance is noted (Fig. 26.5) and any localized widening evaluated further. Normal values are available for both children and adults. An area often overlooked is the cervical spine which is frequently not included in a routine scoliosis examination. For a complete spine evaluation, a separate antero-posterior cervical view may be necessary. Thinning or erosion of pedicles indicates an intraspinal lesion.

Myelography

Myelography still plays an important role in many centres in the evaluation of spinal cord lesions. Oil-based contrasts and air have been replaced by low osmolality water-soluble contrast materials. In the cervical spine, the examination is aided by the use of CT (Devkota et al. 1982). Where there is significant scoliosis, MRI may be difficult.

Computed Tomography

Computed tomography is often used in spinal cord lesions as an adjunct to myelography (Pettersson et al. 1982) to depict the extent of a spinal cord lesion. By careful windowing of the grey scale it is possible to differentiate a fatty from a cystic lesion. CT can be of particular value in the cervical spine where water-soluble contrast may be diluted. Where a syringomyelia is suspected, delayed images may demonstrate filling of the syrinx with contrast.

Magnetic Resonance Imaging

MRI, where available, is largely replacing myelography and to some extent CT in the evaluation of the spinal canal (Figs. 26.6, 26.7). MRI is particularly applicable when there is no or only slight scoliosis present. In larger curves, myelography may still be the examination of choice.

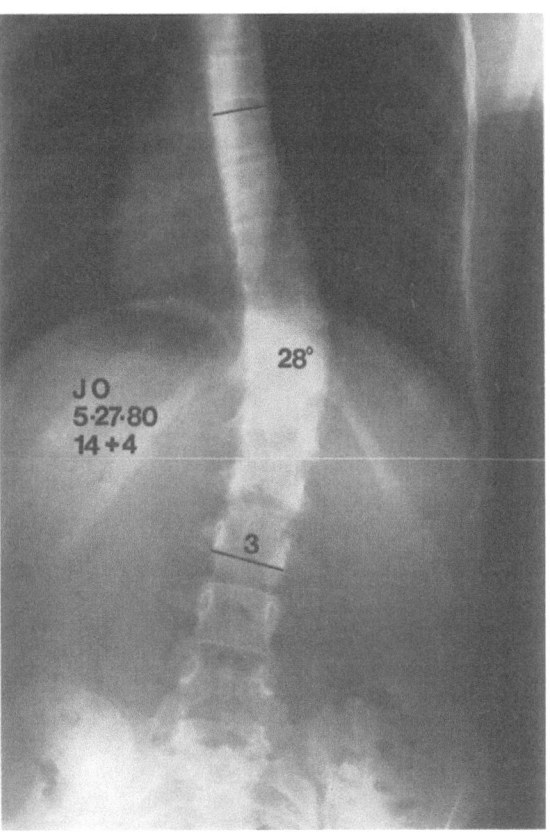

Fig. 26.5. This 14 + 4 year-old female presented with severe back pain. A postero-anterior view shows a widened interpediculate distance in the lumbar area with thinning of the pedicles. Exploration revealed a large ependymoma of the whole filum terminale.

Vascular Studies (Chap. 7)

An arteriogram is obtained in vascular intraspinal lesions (AV malformations, vascular metastatic lesions, e.g. renal) where a knowledge of the vasculature is essential for surgical treatment. At the same time, embolization of the main feeders of the lesion may be performed. Surgical removal follows immediately in an effort to minimize the possible intraoperative blood loss.

Painful Scoliosis

Scoliosis in the child and adolescent is painless. Pain in the adult may be due to facet arthritis or disc

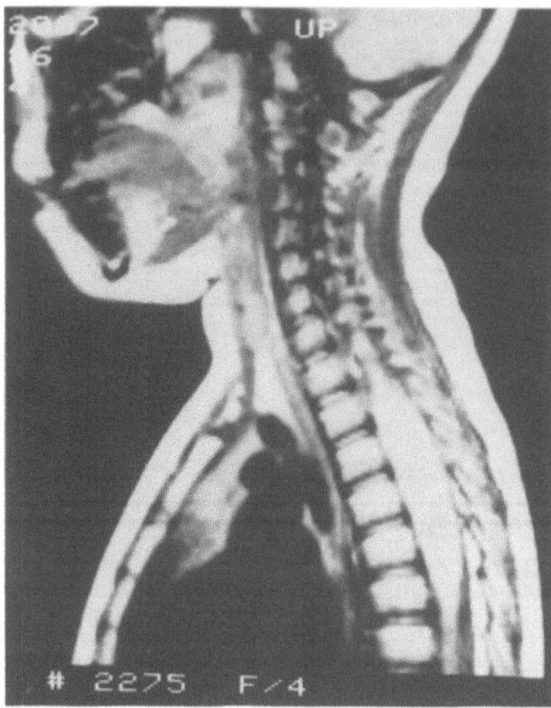

degeneration and protrusion. In the child and adolescent *every* painful scoliosis should be viewed with suspicion and evaluated fully. This also applies to the adult with atypical pain.

Conventional Radiography

The conventional radiographs are carefully examined for evidence of an abnormal curve pattern or "spasm curve", areas of bone sclerosis or erosion, bone tumours, widening of the interpedicular distance or pedicle erosion. This evaluation is essential as it may indicate the need for further investigation for other lesions e.g. bone tumours or spinal cord lesions as above. If the conventional radiographs are normal, further evaluation is still necessary.

Skeletal Scintigraphy

The next test in a painful scoliosis is a scintigram. The whole spine is evaluated with pin-hole collimated views of any area of increased uptake. In a positive test, a bone tumour is diagnosed and further evaluation follows the plan described above.

CT Myelography

The next test depends on the area of pain and differential diagnosis. If a protruded disc is suspected, CT or myelography may be appropriate. If there is significant scoliosis a myelogram followed by CT is indicated.

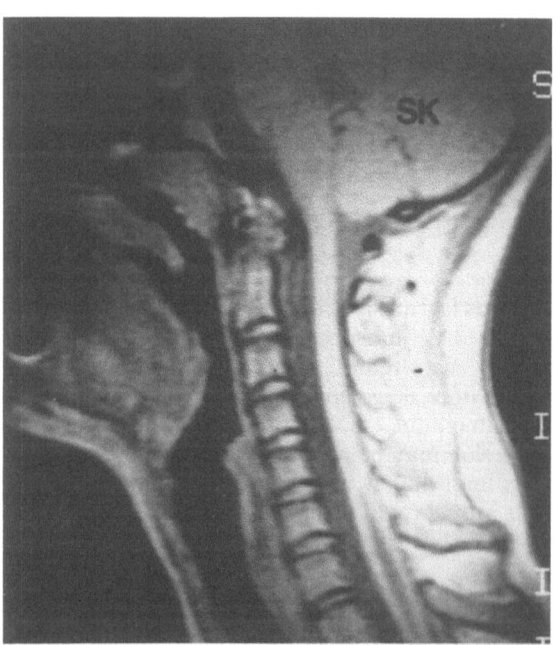

Fig. 26.7. This 13-year-old female presented with a left thoracic scoliosis. Neurological examination was normal. A MRI scan was obtained due to the presence of a *left* thoracic curve. The scan showed syringomyelia of the lower cervical spinal cord.

Magnetic Resonance Imaging

If there is minimal scoliosis with pain not in the lumbar area, MRI is the examination of choice. As this is non-invasive, it may be more readily used and allow earlier diagnosis of spinal cord tumours with painful scoliosis.

Spinal Cord Compression

Spinal cord compression can occur as a result of an untreated spinal deformity (Lonstein et al. 1980). The evaluation plan will depend on whether the deformity is pure kyphosis or a combination of kyphosis plus scoliosis.

Kyphosis Only

In cases of spinal cord compression due to kyphosis an evaluation of the spinal canal is essential. The technique used depends on the equipment available.

CT Myelography

Myelography is used to delineate the extent of the compression, the examination being augmented by CT with sagittal reconstruction of the digital data. This will give both an appreciation of the cord compression and accurate localization of the longitudinal extent of the compression. With this information, surgical decompression can be planned and, in addition, any intraspinal pathology present, diagnosed.

Magnetic Resonance Imaging

Where available, MRI can provide the same information as CT myelography in a non-invasive way. In the future, as this technique becomes more available, it may replace both myelography and CT.

Kyphosis plus Scoliosis

When spinal cord compression is related to kyphosis and scoliosis the examination of choice is CT myelography. This examination will differentiate cord compression due to deformity from that due to an intraspinal lesion. When due to spinal curvature, CT demonstrates the compressing anatomy e.g. vertebral body, pedicle, rib head. A careful surgical plan can thus be arranged, the extent of the compression and anatomical cause having already been diagnosed.

References

Andersen PE, Andersen PE, Van Der Kooy P (1982) Dose reduction in radiography of the spine in scoliosis. Acta Radiol [Diagn] 23:251–253

Binstadt DH, Lonstein JE, Winter RB (1978) Radiographic evaluation of the scoliotic patient. Minn Med 61:474–478

Board RF (1967) Radiography of the scoliotic spine. Radiol Technol 38:219–224

Bradford DS, Lonstein JE, Ogilvie JW, Winter RB (1988) Moe's Textbook on Scoliosis and Other Spinal Deformities. 2nd Edition. WB Saunders Co, Philadelphia

DeSmet A, Fritz SL, Asher MA (1981) A method for minimizing the radiation exposure from scoliosis radiographs. J Bone Joint Surg [Am] 63:156–158

Devkota J, El-Gammal T, Lucke JF (1982) Measurement of the normal cervical cord by metrizamide myelography. South Med J 75:1363–1365

Donavan-Post MJ (1980) Radiographic evaluation of the spine – Current advances with emphasis on computed tomography. Masson Publishers, NY

Gray JE, Hoffman AD, Peterson HA (1983) Reduction of radiation exposure during radiography for scoliosis. J Bone Joint Surg [Am] 65:5–12

Gregg EC (1977) Radiation risks with diagnostic x-rays. Radiology 123:447–453

Greulich WW, Pyle SI (1959) Radiographic atlas of skeletal development of the hand and wrist, 2nd edn. Stanford University Press, Stanford, CA

Hinck VC, Clark WM, Hopkins CE (1966) Normal interpediculate distances (minimum and maximum) in children and adults. AJR 97:141–153

Hopkins R, Grundy M, Serry-Mehl M (1984) X-ray filters in scoliosis x-rays. Orthop Trans 8:148

Lonstein JE, Winter RB, Moe JH, Bradford DS, Chou SN, Pinto WC (1980) Neurologic deficits secondary to spinal deformity. A review of the literature and report of 43 cases. Spine 5:331–335

Nash CL, Gregg EC, Brown RH, Pillai K (1979) Risk of exposure to x-rays in patients undergoing long term treatment for scoliosis. J Bone Joint Surg [Am] 61:371–380

Pettersson H, Harwood-Nash DCF, Fitz CR, Chuang HS, Armstrong E (1982) Conventional metrizamide myelography (MM) and computed tomographic metrizamide myelography (CTMM) in scoliosis. Radiology 142:111–114

Risser JC (1958) The iliac apophysis: an invaluable sign in the management of scoliosis. Clin. Orthop. 11:111

Stagnara P (1974) Examen du scoliotique, in deviations laterales du rachis: Scolioses. Encyclopedia Mediocochirurgicale (Paris) Appareil Locomoteur, 7

Young LW, Oestreich AE, Goldstein LA (1970) Roentgenology in scoliosis: Contribution to evaluation and management. AJR 108:778–795

27 Disorders in Childhood

C.S.B. Galasko

Hip Disorders 345
    Congenital Dislocation of the Hip 345
    Perthes' Disease 348
    Slipped Upper Femoral Epiphysis 350
    Irritable Hip (Transient Synovitis) 350
Fractures 352
    Child Abuse 352
    Physeal Injuries 352
    Injuries Around the Elbow 355
    Other Injuries 356
Tumours 356
    Bone Tumours 356
    Soft Tissue Tumours 357
Neuromuscular Disease 358
Back Pain 359
Deformity 360
    Limb Length 360
    Scoliosis 360
    Dysplasias 360
Infection 361
    Acute Infection 361
    Chronic Osteomyelitis 361
    Sinuses 361
    Tuberculosis 361
Miscellaneous Conditions 361
References 362

The conditions that occur in childhood often are completely different to those that are seen in adults. Even when the symptoms are similar, the underlying causes are frequently different. Therefore, the investigations required frequently differ.

In reaching a diagnosis it is essential to take a careful history. In young children this should be taken from the parents. A careful clinical examination is essential. The child must be relaxed, otherwise the findings may be fallacious. It is sometimes preferable to examine a young child whilst he is sitting on his mother's lap rather than on a hospital couch.

In many instances further investigations are not required, but the commonest investigation indicated for disorders of the locomotor system is plain radiography. The correct views must be requested (see below). For example, if a slipped upper femoral epiphysis is suspected, a lateral radiograph of the hip is essential. A normal antero-posterior radiograph does not exclude the diagnosis. In small children pin-hole collimator views are frequently necessary if skeletal scintigraphy is to provide maximum information.

Hip Disorders

Congenital Dislocation of the Hip

Early Congenital Dislocation of the Hip

The neonatal diagnosis of congenital dislocation of the hip is a clinical one. It is based on careful clinical

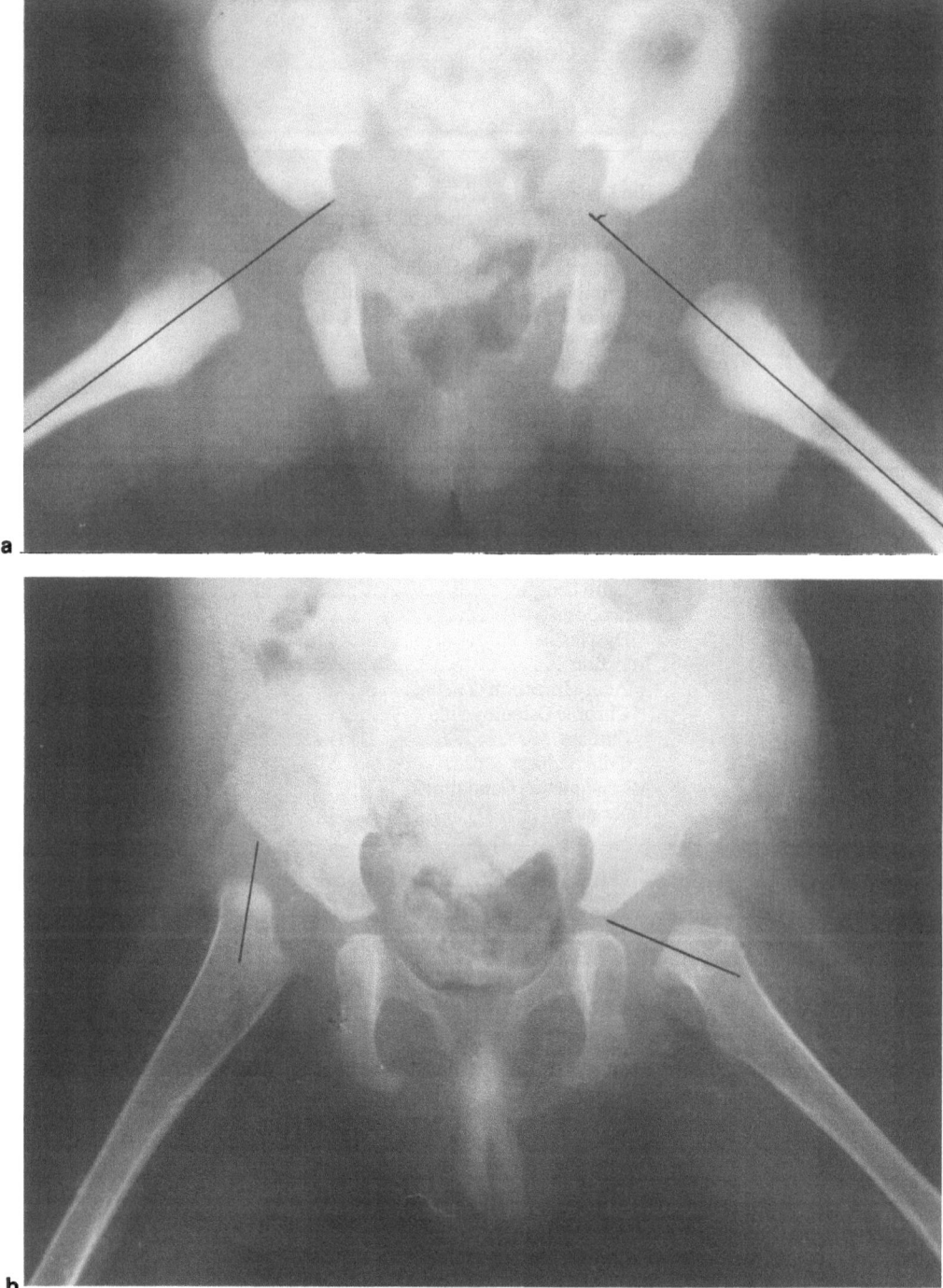

Fig. 27.1a,b. Diagnosis of early congenital dislocation of the hip. a Neonate suspected of having a congenital dislocation of her right hip. Radiograph with the legs abducted 45°. This suggests that both hips are in joint. Line drawn along neck of the femur enters the acetabulum. b Dislocated right hip.

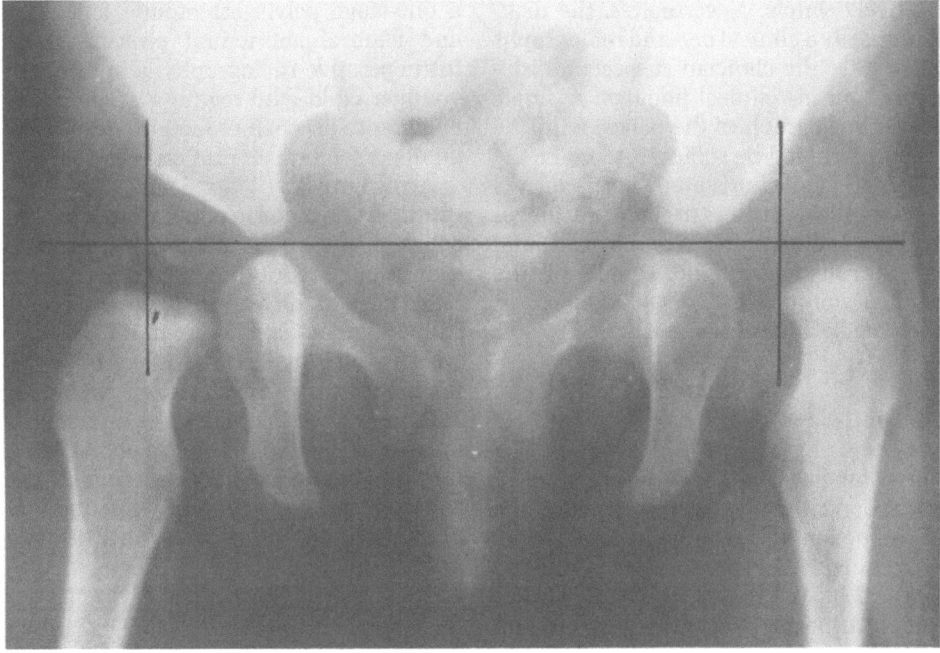

Fig. 27.2. Late congenital dislocation of the hip. Dislocation of the left hip. The ossification centre in the capital epiphysis has not yet appeared, whereas it is present on the right. The acetabular roof is sloping. If a horizontal line is drawn through the triradiate cartilage, and verticals drawn through this line to cross the acetabulum at its outer border, the capital epiphysis normally sits in the inferomedial quadrant, as can be seen on the normal right side.

examination of the neonate's hips. Routine radiographic investigation of all neonates is not indicated. The treatment depends on the clinical diagnosis. Thus an irreducible dislocation should either be treated with a Pavlik harness, or left until the child is older; a reducible dislocation should be treated with an abduction splint (e.g. a von Rosen splint) or a Pavlik harness; and a dislocatable hip, which remains dislocatable after 7–10 days, should also be treated in abduction. Plain radiographs are not used to confirm the diagnosis in the neonate, but should be taken after application of an abduction splint to check that the hip is reduced in the splint.

Recent studies have suggested that ultrasound may be useful in confirming the diagnosis (Berman and Klenerman 1986; Suzuki et al. 1987b). Whether routine ultrasound of all children's hips as a screening procedure shortly after birth will ever become practical is questionable, but the main indication is likely to be in children with an unstable hip in an attempt to determine whether immobilization in abduction is required. The latter should not be embarked upon lightly because of the potential, albeit minor, risk of avascular necrosis. This risk,

however, outweighs the complications of a persistent dislocation.

During the first few months of life, the diagnosis is primarily a clinical one, but radiographs become more reliable. The capital epiphysis does not appear until the child is 3–6 months of age and, until the capital epiphysis does appear, radiographic diagnosis may be difficult. It is based on measurement of the acetabular angle and the position of the femoral neck (Fig. 27.1).

Late Congenital Dislocation

There is no agreement about the definition of "late" congenital dislocation of the hip, some authors confining this definition to children who have started to walk, whereas others have used it to describe a dislocation of the hip in children older than 6 months, 3 months, or only 6 weeks. For the purposes of this chapter, a late dislocation will be used to describe a dislocation that is diagnosed after the capital epiphysis has appeared. Once the capital epiphysis has appeared the radiographic diagnosis becomes relatively simple. Nevertheless, the diagnosis is still primarily a clinical one and radiographs are only taken after the clinician suspects a dislocated hip, based on his clinical findings. A single antero-posterior radiograph of the pelvis, with the legs held together, should be sufficient to make the diagnosis (Fig. 27.2). A horizontal line is drawn across the pelvis through the triradiate cartilages and a vertical line is drawn at 90° to the horizontal line, passing through the outer angle of the acetabulum. In a normal hip the capital epiphysis is in the infero-medial quarter.

After-Treatment

Following treatment, regular antero-posterior radiographs are required to assess initially the adequacy of reduction, the maintenance of reduction, and subsequently the development of the hip joint. If a child is being treated in an abduction frame a radiograph on the frame must be taken to ensure that the hip has been reduced. There is no point in immobilizing a hip in abduction if it is still dislocated. If the hip is treated by traction, a radiograph should be taken on traction to ensure that the femoral head is coming down to the level of the acetabulum, before abduction is commenced. Following open reduction, the hip is immobilized in a plaster of Paris hip spica and a radiograph taken to ensure that the hip is reduced, before the anaesthetic is terminated. On all these occasions a single antero-posterior radiograph is all that is required. The frequency of subsequent X-ray procedures depends on the age at which the hip was treated, and the development of the acetabulum. Following the cessation of treatment, the hip should be radiographed at 3 months, 6 months, 12 months, 2 years, and then at 2-yearly intervals, unless there is a clinical indication to take further films. On each occasion a single antero-posterior radiograph with the legs held together is sufficient. During each X-ray examination the gonads should be protected, but the radiographer must take care with the placement of the shield so that it does not obscure the hip joints. Radiographs may be required at more frequent intervals should the child develop complications such as avascular necrosis of the femoral head, over-growth of the greater trochanter, recurrent and progressive subluxation of the hip, or valgus femoral neck with uncovering of the femoral head.

Intraoperative radiographs are not required in children undergoing primary open reduction during the first few years of life but X-ray screening, using an image intensifier, may be necessary following previously failed surgery, or in older children where a one-stage pelvic osteotomy, femoral osteotomy and femoral shortening procedure is indicated. Intraoperative radiography is not necessary in the younger child who requires a Salter osteotomy, in addition to an open reduction, nor is it required for an upper femoral derotation osteotomy.

Arthrography (Chap. 3; Wilkinson 1980) is not routinely indicated in patients with congenital dislocation of the hip. It is indicated, however, if there is any doubt about the position of the femoral head. Since most of the femoral head and acetabulum are still cartilaginous, it is sometimes difficult to assess whether a reduction is satisfactory, or whether the hip is starting to sublux on plain radiographs. Although some surgeons recommend its use preoperatively to assess the contents of the acetabulum, the investigation is only occasionally helpful. The cause of the obstruction to reduction will be found at surgery, and in most instances arthrography is not required.

Perthes' Disease

The diagnosis is suspected from the history. In the early stages a clinical examination may be entirely normal. The diagnosis is usually confirmed by plain radiographs. Antero-posterior and lateral films are essential and both hips should be radiographed. The progress of the disease is monitored by serial radiographs, initially 3-monthly, and subsequently at longer intervals.

In its earliest phase, the plain radiographs may be normal, but the skeletal scintigram may show diminished uptake in the femoral head (particularly on pin-hole collimated views) suggestive of avascularity (Fig. 27.3). Occasionally, arthrography may be required to outline the femoral head and acetabulum prior to osteotomy, to assess whether osteotomy is likely to give full cover to the femoral head, but usually this can be assessed by a plain antero-posterior radiograph taken with the hip in abduction. The latter should be taken with the limbs in neutral and in internal rotation. If the latter shows better femoral head cover, the varus osteotomy should be combined with a derotation osteotomy.

Plain radiographs can be used to help assess the prognosis. If the following radiological signs are present the femoral head is at risk and is likely to worsen rapidly (Catterall 1971):

1. Calcification lateral to epiphysis
2. Diffuse metaphyseal reaction
3. Metaphyseal lucency

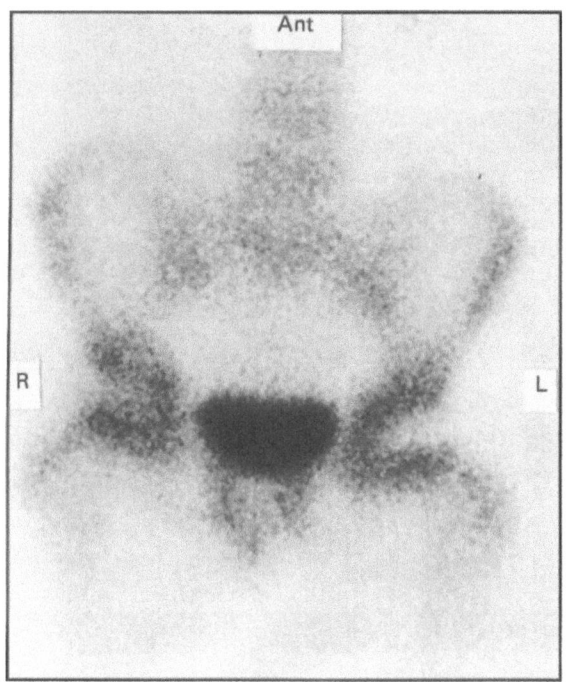

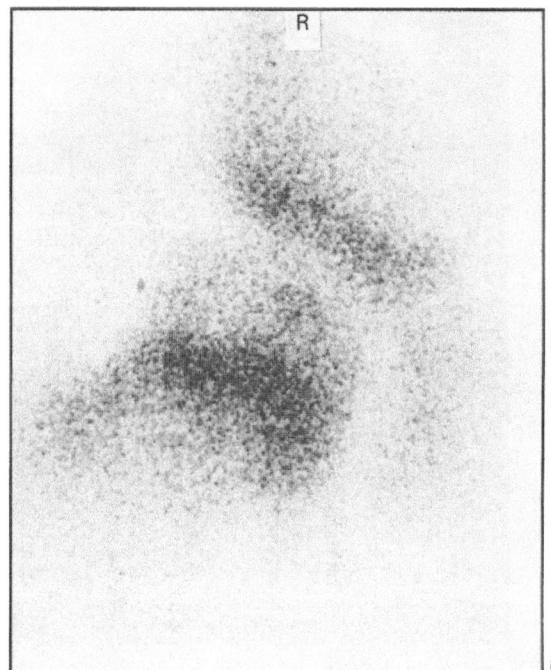

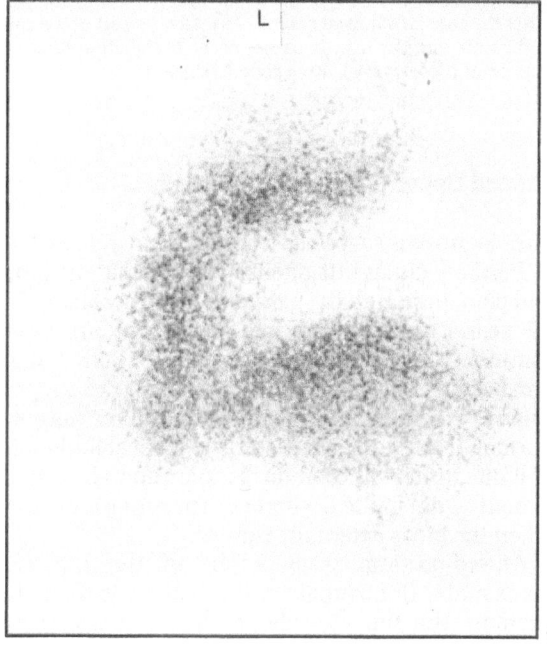

4. Lateral subluxation

5. Horizontal growth plate

Plain radiographs can also be used to group disease. The group indicates the amount of head that has been involved (Catterall 1971):

Group 1.   Less than the anterior 50% necrotic; no collapse; no sequestration.

Group 2.   More than anterior 50% necrotic; possible collapse; sequestration.

Group 3.   Posterior 33% viable; collapse; bulging.

Group 4.   Entire epiphysis necrotic; severe collapse; bulging.

The prognosis is good if the patient is less than 5 years old, the radiographs show Group 1 involvement and there are no "head at risk" signs; whereas it is poor if the child is 5 years old or more and the radiographs show Group 4 involvement, or "head at risk" signs.

Ultrasound may be useful in assessing Perthes' disease (Suzuki et al. 1987a). The changes of Perthes' disease are well seen on MRI. Areas of avascular necrosis are better demonstrated than on plain radiographs (Bassett et al. 1987). At present MRI is under evaluation, but in the future may become the technique of choice both for diagnosis and progress assessment.

Fig. 27.3a–c. Early Perthes' disease. The initial radiographs were normal, but the scintigram showed diminished uptake of the left femoral head. Subsequent radiographs showed the development of Perthes' disease. a ^{99m}Tc-MDP scintigram of the pelvis. Note the decreased uptake in the left femoral head. b Pin-hole collimator view of the right hip joint. The hip joint appears normal. The increased uptake is in the capital physis. c Pin-hole collimator view of the left femoral head. Note the diminished uptake of the capital epiphysis.

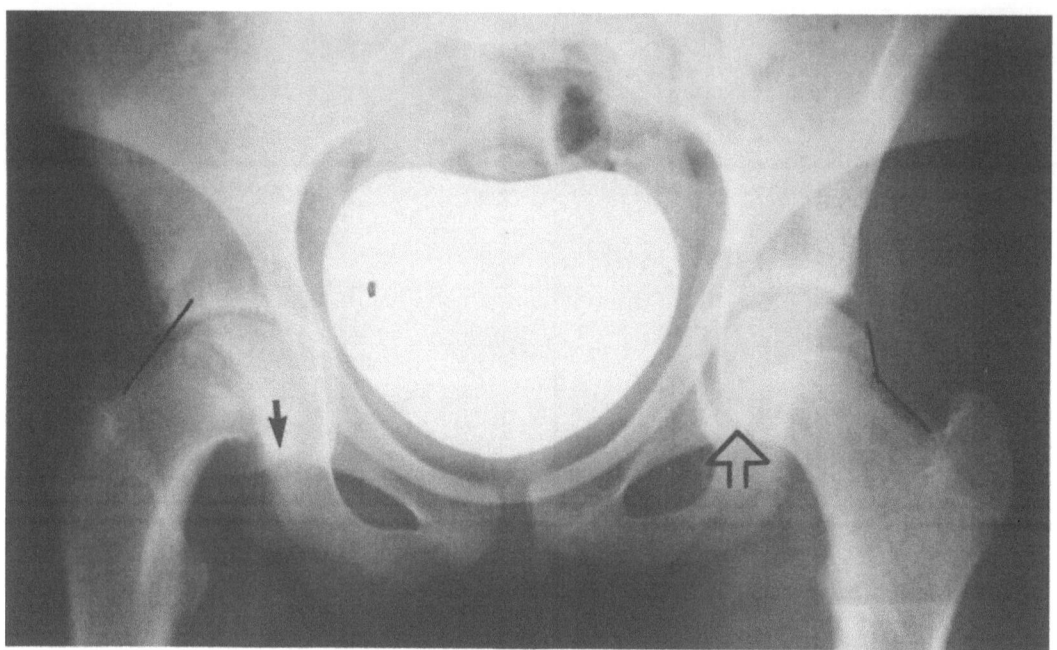

Fig. 27.4. Slipped upper femoral epiphysis. AP radiograph. Right slipped upper femoral epiphysis. A straight line drawn along the upper border of the neck of the femur usually crosses the capital epiphysis (left) but, in the presence of a slipped epiphysis, this is not the case (Trethowan's sign). Normally, no part of the capital epiphysis impinges between the medial corner of the metaphysis of the neck and the inferior corner of the acetabulum (*open arrow*) but, in the presence of a slipped upper femoral epiphysis, this does occur (*closed arrow*). (Note gonadal shield.)

Slipped Upper Femoral Epiphysis

The diagnosis is suspected from the history. Like that of Perthes' disease, it often is of intermittent limp and pain, although the patient is usually older (10–17 years), whereas Perthes' disease occurs most commonly in the 3–10-year age group. Both conditions occur more commonly in boys. If the slipped epiphysis is mild the clinical examination may be normal, if gross the characteristic clinical finding is of limited internal rotation. Flexion and abduction in neutral are limited, whereas their range is greater when the hip is externally rotated.

Antero-posterior radiographs of the hip are inadequate. Unfortunately, if a request is made to examine the hip by radiography most radiology departments will only carry out a single antero-posterior film and the diagnosis may be missed for months, during which time the slip progressively worsens. It is essential to obtain a lateral image. The capital epiphysis slips off the neck in a postero-medial direction. If it is marked, the diagnosis is obvious, but if early can be made by Trethowan's sign, or by noting that part of the femoral head lies between the inner metaphysis and the lower angle of the acetabulum (Fig. 27.4).

Irritable Hip (Transient Synovitis)

The diagnosis is one of exclusion. The child presents with a history of pain, limp, and sometimes inability to bear weight, usually of a few hours' or days' duration. Movements of the hip are restricted, particularly abduction and internal rotation. The differential diagnosis includes Perthes' disease, septic arthritis, and sickling crisis. Established Perthes' disease can be excluded by antero-posterior radiographs; acute septic arthritis by a normal pulse, temperature, white cell count and ESR; and a sickling crisis by normal haemoglobins. These investigations, however, do not exclude the presence of early Perthes' disease, nor of a subacute septic arthritis, although in the latter the ESR is usually slightly raised. Skeletal scintigraphy with pinhole collimator views of both hips, is of value in excluding these conditions (Fig. 27.3).

In transient synovitis the skeletal scintigram is normal, the symptoms settle after a few days bed rest with bilateral skin traction, and it is extremely rare for the disease to recur. In very early Perthes' disease an area of diminished uptake may be seen in the femoral head. Once there has been some new bone formation, initially at the edges of the

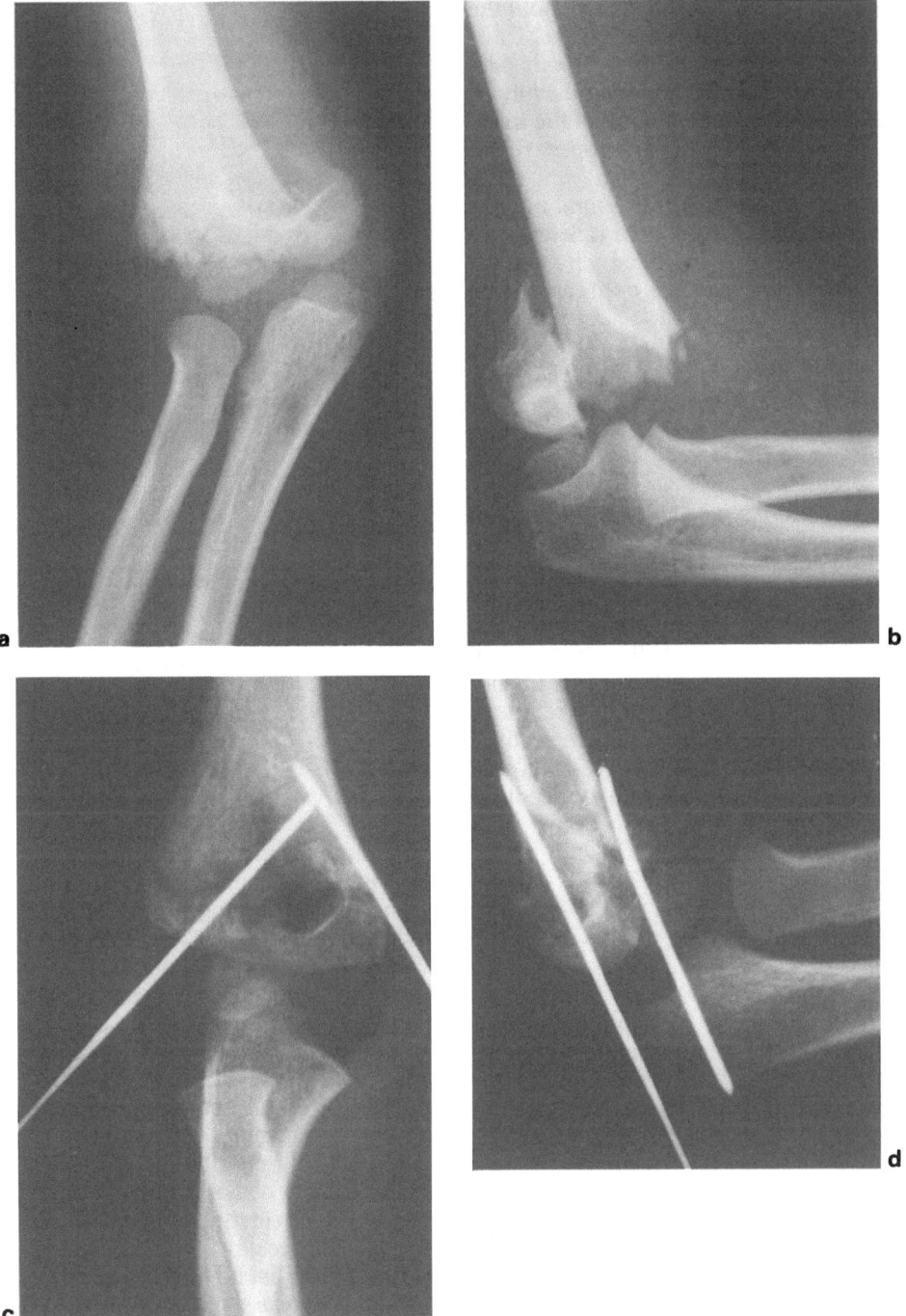

Fig. 27.5a–d. Supracondylar fracture of the humerus. **a,b** AP and lateral radiographs showing the supracondylar fracture. It was not possible to reduce the fracture by manipulation. **c,d** Therefore, an open reduction was carried out with Kirschner wire fixation. Intra-operative radiographs were taken, following the insertion of the Kirschner wires, to check the position.

avascular region, and subsequently throughout the avascular segment, there is increased uptake.

There is also increased uptake, but on both sides of the joint, in septic arthritis. This can usually be seen within 24–48 hours of the onset of the infection (Chap. 13). If septic arthritis is suspected, the hip should be aspirated.

There is some evidence that ultrasound may be of value (Wilson et al. 1984). If fluid is detected in the hip joint, aspiration is indicated whether the fluid is due to a transient synovitis, or to early septic arthritis.

Fractures

Antero-posterior and lateral films are required to make the diagnosis, and serial radiographs are needed to assess the efficacy of treatment and healing of the fracture. If a fracture requires manipulation under anaesthesia, post-manipulation films must be taken before the anaesthetic is terminated, and if the position is not satisfactory, a further reduction carried out. If internal fixation is required, it is best to obtain intraoperative radiographs once the fracture has been stabilized (Fig. 27.5), and only if the position is satisfactory, complete the definitive fixation of the fracture.

There are certain fractures in children which require special mention.

Child Abuse

Unfortunately, this seems to be increasing in incidence. A careful history is required and if the mechanism described does not fit the pattern of the fracture, this condition should be suspected and further investigations carried out. For example, a long spiral fracture is due to a twisting injury, whereas a transverse or short oblique fracture is usually due to a direct blow. It is difficult to explain a spiral fracture of the shaft of the femur in a 6-month-old child by a fall resulting in a direct blow on the thigh.

When child abuse is suspected, a radiographic skeletal survey is indicated looking for other fractures. Multiple fractures, at different stages of healing, are suspicious.

The fractures classically occur in the metaphyseal region of the long bones, or at the metaphyseal-epiphyseal junction (Kempe et al. 1962; Silverman 1972; O'Neill et al. 1973; Kogutt et al. 1974). Beaking of the metaphyseal region, suggestive of a healed fracture, is suspicious. Fractures of the shafts of long

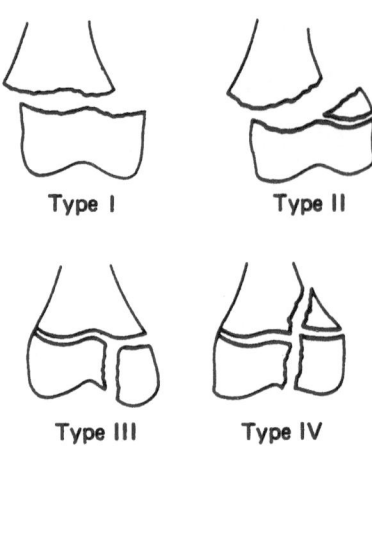

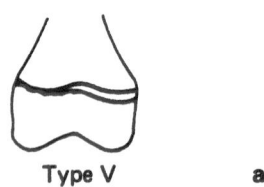

Fig. 27.6a (*see caption next page*).

bones are not uncommon and abundant subperiosteal new bone formation, consequent upon subperiosteal haemorrhage, is characteristic (Akbarnia and Akbarnia 1976). Fractures of the skull and widening of the sutures may occur. A skull radiograph is essential. The presence of Wormian bones suggest that the diagnosis is osteogenesis imperfecta, rather than child abuse. Radiographs of the spine may show narrowing of the disc spaces, anterior vertebral notching at the thoracolumbar junction and compression fractures.

Scintigraphy may be more sensitive than plain radiographs in demonstrating skeletal trauma and may be the screening method of choice when child abuse is suspected (Sty and Starshak 1983), but radiographs must be taken of all areas where there are foci of increased uptake. Nevertheless, skull fractures may be missed when the scintigram remains normal (Haase et al. 1980).

Physeal Injuries

Fractures affecting the growth plate are usually classified by the Salter–Harris classification (Fig. 27.6a).

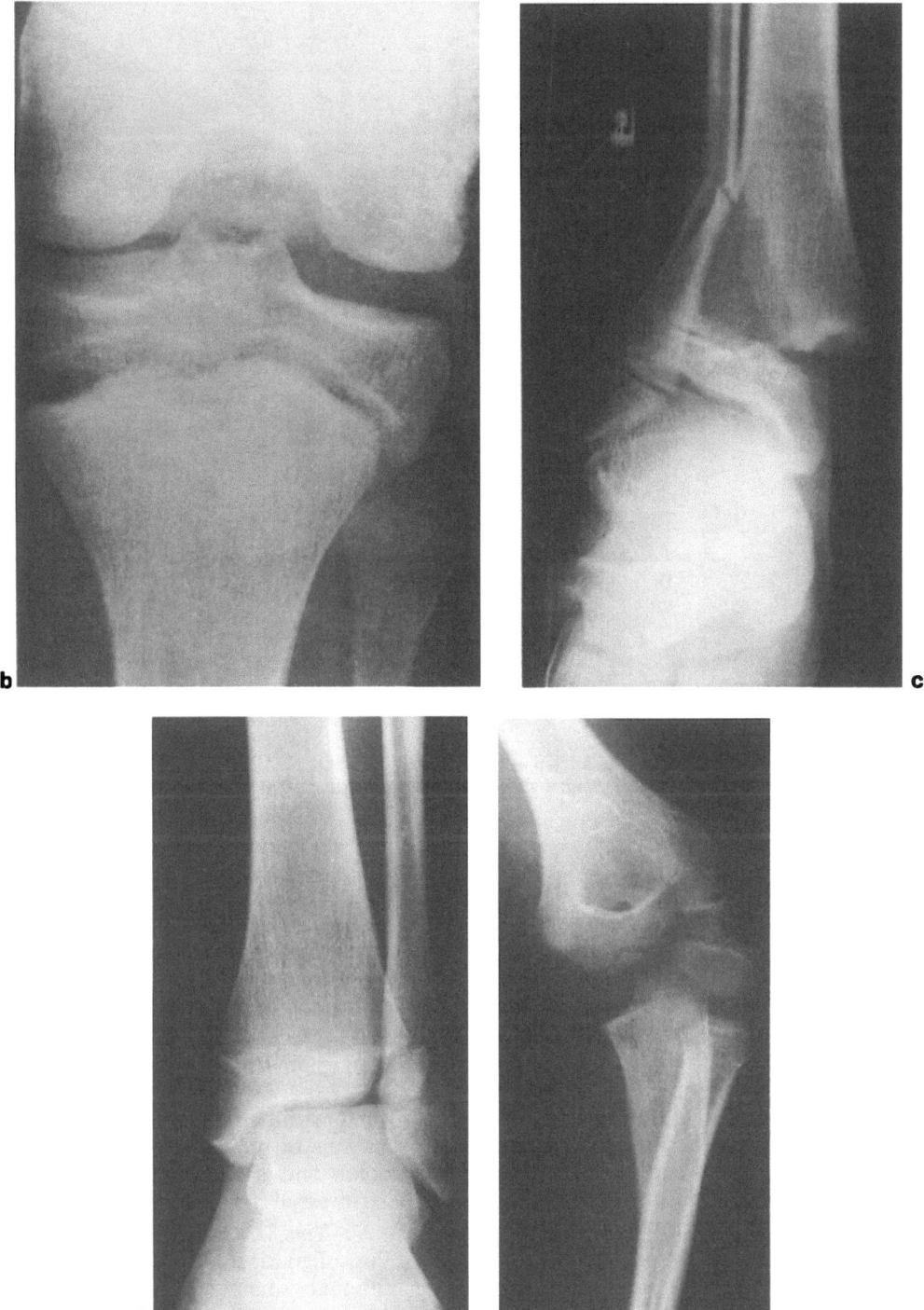

Fig. 27.6a–e. Physeal injuries. **a** Classification (after Salter and Harris 1963). **b** Type I separation of the proximal tibial epiphysis. **c** Type II fracture separation of distal tibial epiphysis. **d** Type III fracture of distal tibial epiphysis. The fracture crosses both the physis and epiphysis and involves the articular surface. **e** Type IV physeal injury, the fracture crossing the metaphysis, physis and epiphysis, and involving the articular surface.

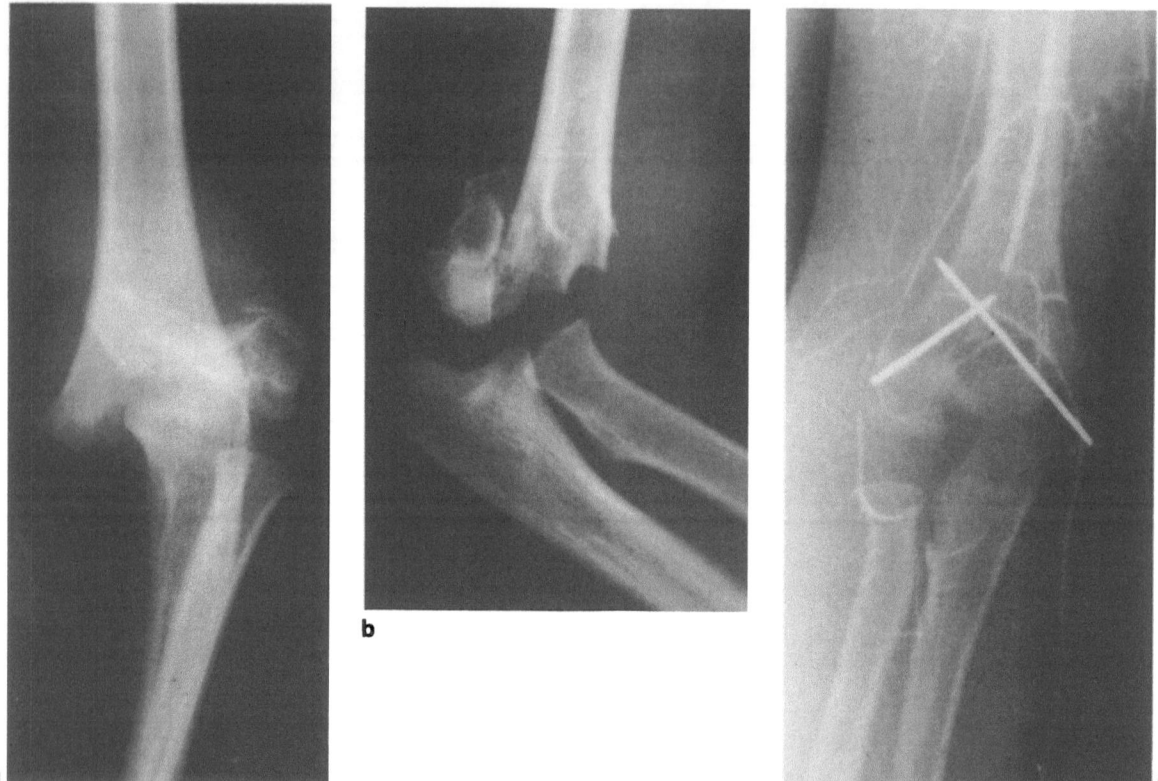

Fig. 27.7a–c. Supracondylar humeral fracture, associated with vascular impairment. a,b AP and lateral radiographs demonstrating the fracture. c The fracture has been fixed with Kirschner wires. The arteriogram shows that the brachial artery is occluded.

Type I. The fracture occurs on the metaphyseal side of the physis (Fig. 27.6b), through the zone of hypertrophic or degenerating cartilage and does not affect the germinative layer. A closed reduction is required and the injury usually does not affect growth.

Type II. A smaller or larger fragment of metaphysis remains attached to the epiphysis, the rest of the fracture line occurring through the hypertrophic or degenerative cartilage zone (Fig. 27.6c). The treatment is by closed or open reduction, and growth disturbance is rare.

Type III. The fracture runs across the metaphyseal side of the growth plate, crosses the physis and epiphysis and involves the articular surface (Fig. 27.6d). Thus both the growth plate and the articular surface are involved. Anatomical reduction with internal fixation is required. Despite anatomical reduction, premature fusion may occur at the site of physeal injury leading to growth abnormality. The patient must be kept under review for at least 2–3 years after the fracture has healed, and serial X-ray examinations are required to determine whether a growth abnormality is developing. If so, further serial radiographs may be required to monitor its progress and subsequent treatment.

Type IV. The fracture crosses the metaphysis, physis and epiphysis and involves the articular surface (Fig. 27.6e). As with Type III injuries, anatomical reduction and internal fixation is required. The complications of premature growth arrest at the fracture line and articular irregularity can only be excluded by serial radiographs.

Type V. This is a crush injury of the growth plate. Very often the initial radiographs appear normal, although sometimes the growth plate may appear narrowed. This injury is usually complicated by premature growth arrest and is diagnosed retrospectively.

The subsequent development of any deformity should be monitored by serial X-ray studies (see below).

In the older child the diagnosis of a physeal injury

is usually easily made from the radiographs. In a younger child, however, the diagnosis may be difficult and it often is necessary to obtain radiographs of the contralateral limb so that the anatomy of the secondary centres of ossification can be compared. Probably the most difficult of these injuries to diagnose is a Type III or Type IV physeal fracture of the lateral humeral condyle in the young patient (Fig. 27.6e).

Injuries Around the Elbow

The elbow is one of the commonest sites of injury in children and injury here may be difficult to diagnose.

Pulled Elbow

There is a partial subluxation of the radial head, usually produced by traction. Most commonly the mother is holding the child by the hand and the child pulls away, thereafter crying, complaining bitterly of pain and inability to use the elbow. The forearm is often pronated. The antero-posterior radiograph is taken with the elbow extended and the forearm supinated, and in so doing, the radiographer usually reduces the subluxation, so that the appearances may be normal.

Supracondylar Fractures

The fracture involves the humeral metaphysis and is diagnosed on antero-posterior and lateral radiographs. There may be associated damage to the brachial artery and if this is suspected, an arteriogram may be required (Fig. 27.7). Another complication is the development of a compartment syndrome. The diagnosis is a clinical one and radiographic investigations are of no value.

Fracture of the Medial Epicondyle

The medial epicondyle is avulsed. Occasionally this is associated with a dislocation of the elbow and the epicondyle may be trapped in the elbow joint. Usually, X-ray studies of the opposite elbow are required to compare the anatomy.

Fracture of the Lateral Condyle

This is usually a Type IV physeal injury (see above).

Monteggia Fracture Dislocation

It is essential to see the joint above and below a fracture (Fig. 27.8). Not infrequently, radiographs of the forearm do not include the elbow and the association of a dislocated radial head with a fracture of the ulna shaft is missed. If the elbow or wrist are not included in the X-ray examination of a forearm, irrespective of whether one or both bones are fractured, further images must be obtained. Occasionally a radial head may be dislocated in the presence of fractures of the shafts of both the radius and ulna.

Fractures of the Radial Neck

These are diagnosed on antero-posterior and lateral radiographs of the elbow. The treatment depends on

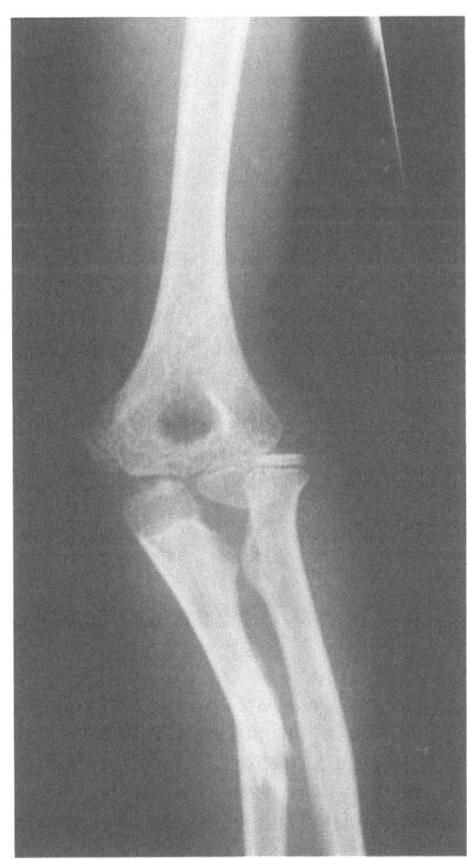

Fig. 27.8. Monteggia fracture dislocation. The shaft of the ulnar is fractured and the radial head is dislocated. This examination is not adequate. There may be a further injury of the distal radius or ulna and X-ray examination of the full length of both forearm bones should be undertaken.

the degree of angulation. If the displacement is unacceptable, reduction and possibly Kirschner wire fixation is required.

In many fractures around the elbow, percutaneous Kirschner wire fixation, under image intensification control, may be successful.

Other Injuries

CT scanning is occasionally indicated in children with fractures. Major fractures of the spine and pelvis (Chap. 20) are rare, but if there is any suggestion that a spinal fracture may be associated with retropulsion of bone fragments into the canal, or there is a pelvic fracture, CT scans may be necessary to delineate the fracture (Chap. 20).

The triplanar fracture is a Type III physeal injury of the distal tibia epiphysis, the fracture occurring both in the coronal and sagittal plane. It often is impossible to delineate the nature of this fracture without a CT scan (Spiegel et al. 1984).

Tumours

The finite diagnosis can only be made by histological examination of the tumour. Radiological investigation is essential to localize the tumour, is often helpful in suggesting the site of biopsy, may differentiate between a benign or malignant lesion, and may help make the diagnosis, particularly of a tumour-like lesion rather than a neoplasm.

Bone Tumours

Benign Tumours and Tumour-like Conditions

Benign lesions, such as cortical fibrous dysplasia and simple bone cysts, are usually diagnosed radiologically. No further treatment is indicated.

Cartilage capped exostoses (osteochondromata) can also be diagnosed radiologically, but malignant change may be difficult to detect. If such a lesion is found incidentally, surgery is probably not indicated. If the lesion is symptomatic because of its size or position, is enlarging, or is painful, it must be excised and submitted for histological examination. Osteomas and enchondromas can usually be diagnosed radiologically.

In general, benign lesions tend to thin and expand the cortex and rarely breach it. Their outline is usually smooth, frequently with an overlying intact shell of new bone. Occasionally a crack fracture through the expanded shell may produce subperiosteal new bone formation. The pattern of bone destruction consists of a well-defined area of radiolucency characterized by a sharp zone of transition between it and the normal bone. Course trabeculation results from irregular ridging of the host bone as often seen in chondromyxoid fibroma, or a simple bone cyst.

Osteoid osteomas occurring in the medulla are not usually associated with much bone reaction, but those arising in the cortex frequently stimulate a marked reaction. There is a small lucent area (which may only be seen on tomograms) surrounded by an extensive zone of cortical thickening. However, they may not be obvious on plain radiographs. They usually present with pain, and if the diagnosis is suspected, but radiology is normal, a skeletal scintigram is indicated. There is intense uptake of bone-seeking radionuclide (Fig. 13.12). In the spine, CT scans of the area of increased uptake of radionuclide are indicated to more carefully delineate the site of the lesion (Fig. 13.12). Surgical removal may be helped by using a sterilizable probe (gamma counter) during surgery, the patient having been given the radionuclide 2–3 hours previously and the bone with maximum uptake being excised (Szypryt et al. 1987).

Serial skeletal scintigraphy has been suggested in patients with diaphyseal aclasis. In this condition there is a definite risk that one of the osteochondromata may undergo malignant change. If, on serial scintigrams, any lesion shows increased uptake, it should be excised and examined histologically.

Scintigraphy and CT scanning may be required in patients with multiple enchondromatosis, particularly affecting the spine or pelvis, if there is associated pain, in an attempt to determine whether one of the lesions is undergoing a malignant change (Fig. 27.9).

Malignant Tumours

Malignant tumours of bone occur most commonly in adolescence, probably associated with the adolescent growth spurt. The radiographic appearance may suggest the diagnosis, but biopsy and histological examination are mandatory. A lesion with a large soft tissue component, including irregular areas of calcification is suggestive of a chondrosarcoma; a tumour with moth-eaten areas of

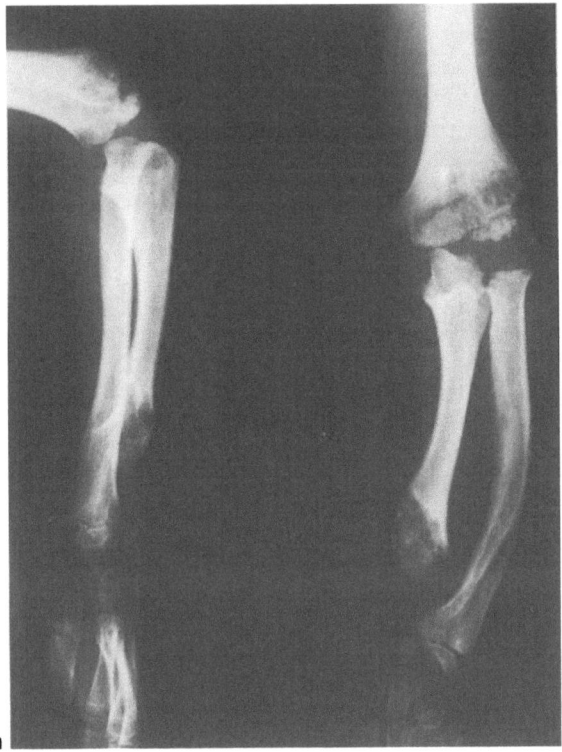

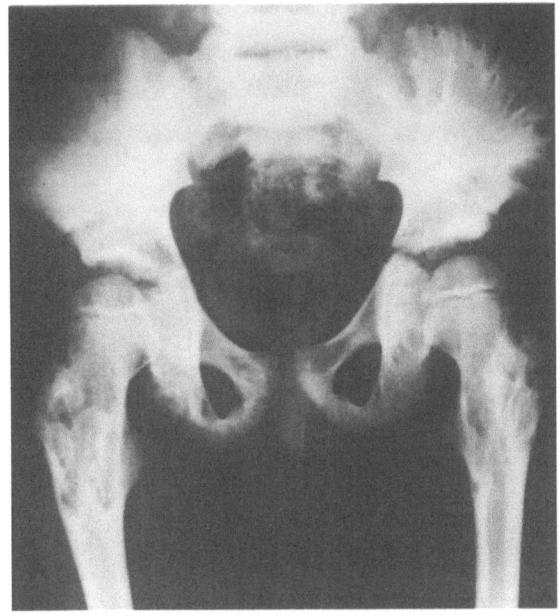

Fig. 27.9a,b. Radiographs of the forearms and pelvis of a patient with multiple enchondromatosis. This is associated with deformity. The patient complained of pain in his left buttock. The plain films do not demonstrate whether one of the enchondromata is undergoing a malignant change. CT or MRI is required.

bone destruction, and associated with sunray spiculation and a Codman's triangle, is suggestive of an osteosarcoma; layered periosteal new bone formation (onion skin appearance) is suggestive of an Ewing's sarcoma and a pure lytic lesion is suggestive of a fibrosarcoma. In a parosteal sarcoma there is dense new bone formation surrounding the metaphysis, without any involvement of the underlying bone.

Although the diagnosis of a malignant tumour is dependent on histological examination, imaging techniques are essential to diagnose the extent of the tumour and determine the treatment.

Skeletal scintigraphy is useful in assessing the extent of skeletal involvement, but in osteosarcoma the area of increased uptake may extend beyond the confines of the tumour, possibly due to an inflammatory response. It is useful in indicating skip lesions in the affected bone and may demonstrate distant metastases in lymph nodes, liver or lung. CT scanning is particularly helpful in detecting pulmonary metastases and is useful in demonstrating the soft tissue component of the tumour. MRI demonstrates the intramedullary extension of the tumour more accurately than CT scanning or scintigraphy, including skip lesions, as well as the soft

tissue extraskeletal component, but does not demonstrate the cortex as well as CT. It also is superior to CT in assessing involvement of the growth plate, joint space, adjacent soft tissues and the relationship to the neurovascular bundle.

The past 10–15 years has seen a dramatic change in the treatment of malignant bone tumours (Chap. 21) with the introduction of chemotherapy and localized resection with prosthetic replacement. The latter procedure can only be carried out if the tumour is localized and modern imaging techniques are essential to determine whether this is the case.

With the development of CT scanning and particularly MRI, pre-operative arteriography is no longer required to delineate the extent of the tumour.

Soft Tissue Tumours

Plain films are of little value. Ultrasound (Chap. 16) is valuable. It will differentiate between a solid and cystic mass and is useful in defining the edge of the tumour, suggesting whether the lesion is invasive or not. Computed tomography (Chap. 10) is also useful in determining the site of the tumour, but

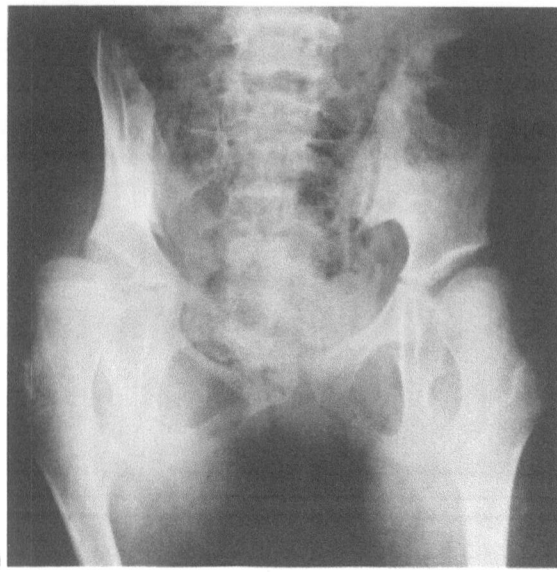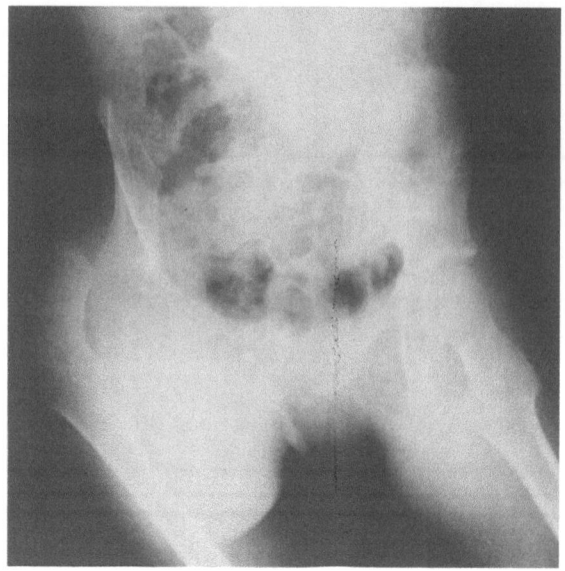

Fig. 27.10a,b. Severely affected patient with cerebral palsy. **a** AP radiograph of the pelvis indicating subluxation of the right hip. Surgery was advised, but refused. **b** The patient subsequently developed a painful right dislocated hip.

probably the investigation of choice at the moment is MRI. It is more sensitive in demonstrating the extent of the tumour and the involvement of adjacent structures, particularly the neurovascular bundle [Chap. 12]. CT cannot readily distinguish between engulfment and displacement of the neurovascular bundle, even with the use of an intravenous contrast agent, but demonstrates periosteal new bone formation more accurately. This is particularly important with soft tissue tumours that may involve bone.

CT is able to determine the site, size and configuration of tumours arising from bone with a high degree of accuracy, to assess the extraosseous spread of bone tumours, and the degree of bone involvement by soft tissue tumours, but cannot characterize tissue. MRI defines the extent of both bone and soft tissue tumours more clearly. Maximum contrast between tumour and fat (including marrow) is shown on the T1-weighted sequences and between tumour and muscle on T2-weighted sequences (Chap. 12).

Neuromuscular Disease

The diagnosis is made from the clinical findings, EMG and particularly muscle biopsy, including

histochemical staining. Imaging techniques, however, are sometimes useful in detecting abnormal muscle, and in assessing the severity of muscle involvement. Ultrasound offers a non-invasive method for detecting abnormal muscle and has been used in muscle dystrophy, spinal muscle atrophy, congenital dystrophy and in the "floppy baby" (Chap. 16). CT scanning probably delineates the degree of muscle damage accurately (Bulcke and Baert 1982) together with the amount of muscle replacement, but with MRI the limb musculature can be imaged in any plane and very early fatty infiltration detected. Where available, MRI is probably the modality of choice to determine early muscle involvement.

Neuromuscular disease is associated with secondary skeletal deformities (Galasko 1987). These can be detected on plain radiographs though in many patients serial examinations are necessary. For example, most patients with Duchenne muscular dystrophy develop a progressive collapsing scoliosis once they become wheelchair-bound. The development and progression of this complication can easily be monitored by serial radiographs. The timing of surgery depends more on the patient's general condition than on the severity of the curve and, therefore, X-ray studies cannot be relied upon to indicate when surgical stabilization is necessary.

Dislocation of the hip is an important complication in cerebral palsy. Antero-posterior radiographs

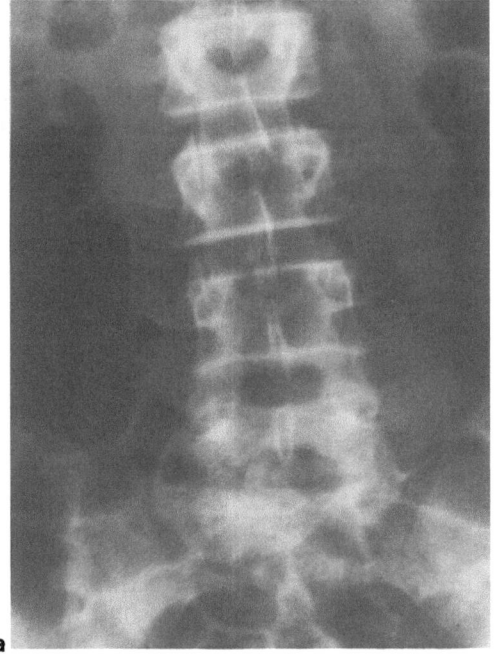 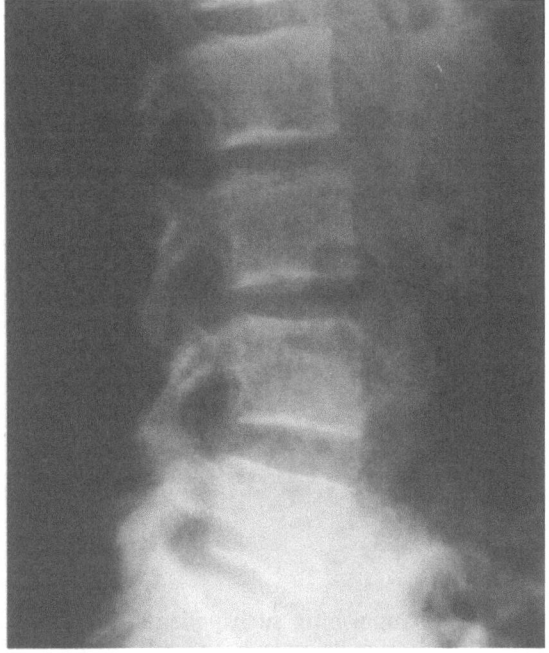

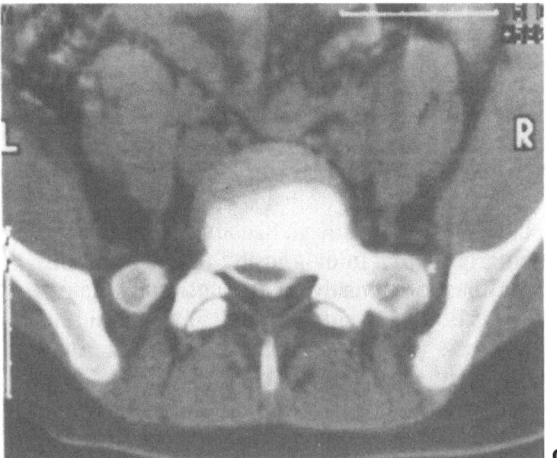

Fig. 27.11a–c. A prolapsed intravertebral disc in a 14-year-old male who presented with back pain, limitation of spinal movement and limited straight leg raising. a AP radiograph of the lumbosacral spine shows a list to the right. b Lateral radiograph of the lumbosacral spine. There is some narrowing of the L5–S1 disc space. c CT scan showing a slipped proximal sacral end plate. Following surgery, he made an uncomplicated recovery and obtained full relief of pain, with restoration of spinal movement and straight leg raising.

of the pelvis may indicate which hip is at risk and which should be considered for surgery, depending on the general condition of the patient (Fig. 27.10).

The development of other muscular skeletal deformities, such as equinus, equinovarus, flexion contracture of the knee etc. depend on regular and careful clinical examination. Pre-operative X-ray examination is important to show secondary deformation of the underlying bone, or subluxation of the joint.

Back Pain

Back pain occurs much less commonly in children, or adolescents, than in adults, but the proportion of those with pain who have a serious underlying disorder is much higher and a variety of imaging techniques may be required (Fitz 1985). Analysis of 61 children (Turner et al., in press) showed that clinical findings were sometimes

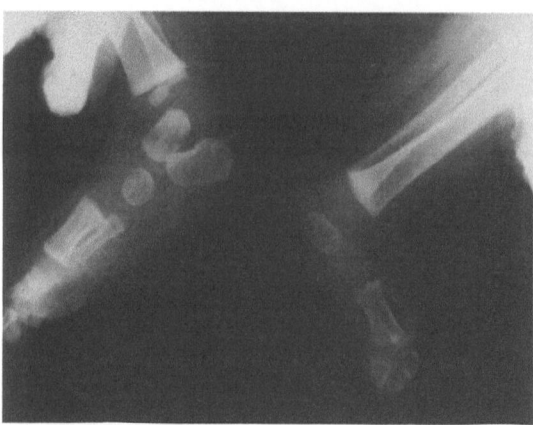

Fig. 27.12. Congenital deformity of the left foot. The os calcis is missing and there are many other congenital abnormalities of the tarsus, metatarsus and phalanges.

unreliable in distinguishing such patients. Thirty-two patients had a significant spinal disorder including tumours, infection, spondylolysis, spondylolisthesis, and juvenile osteoporotic vertebral collapse. Plain radiographs were of value in diagnosing spondylolisthesis. If a spondylolysis is suspected, oblique films of the lumbosacral spine are indicated, but these should not be carried out as routine. Very early cases of infection, or sterile discitis, may not be seen and the disease only detected when changes are slightly more advanced. Skeletal scintigraphy is particularly helpful in diagnosing these conditions. MRI may be more sensitive than scintigraphy for the early detection of discitis (Chap. 25). Skeletal scintigraphy was also particularly useful in the diagnosis of bony tumours, especially osteoid osteoma (Fig. 13.12).

Probably the most difficult diagnostic category is an intraspinal canal lesion such as a prolapsed disc or tumour. The presence of sciatica, limited straight leg raising, and limited spinal movements warrant radiculography. Two patients in this series, referred to our clinic with a provisional diagnosis of a typical Scheuermann's disease, were found to have cord tumours. A prolapse of the S1 end plate in a 14-year-old male with a 3-year history of back pain was shown by combined radiculography and CT scanning (Fig. 27.11). Radiculography should be carried out in combination with CT scanning as the lesion, particularly if low or very lateral, may be missed on the radiculogram. CT myelography is a most sensitive method of examining the spine and cord (Pettersson and Harwood-Nash 1982), but MRI is likely to be preferred in the future (Gibson et al. 1987; Chap. 25).

Deformity

The diagnosis is a clinical one, but plain radiographs are required to assess the position and shape of the underlying bones (Fig. 27.12), e.g. in congenital talipes equinovarus, adolescent hallus valgus, congenital vertical talus etc. Occasionally special views are required. For example CT may be required in some types of tarsal condition (Marchisello 1987). The amount of radiation is probably less with CT than with other radiographic methods for the assessment of femoral anteversion.

Limb Length

The diagnosis is a clinical one, as is the assessment of progression of the discrepancy. X-ray examination is required when the patient is first seen, and prior to surgical correction.

Either "spot" films centred on the hips, the knees, and the ankles, and incorporating a measuring device; or 3-foot standing films of the entire lower limbs, again incorporating a ruler on the film, can be used accurately to measure the limb lengths. Antero-posterior and lateral radiographs are required of the femur, tibia and fibula, and foot to determine whether there is any congenital anomaly associated with the discrepancy.

Scoliosis

On the first visit an erect antero-posterior radiograph is required, on which the severity and extent of the curve can be measured (Chap. 26), as well as lateral radiographs to determine whether there is any skeletal abnormality. The two examinations must be at 90° to each other. There is some argument as to whether the X-ray beam should be truly antero-posterior with respect to the patient or to the apical vertebra. In most centres, the antero-posterior and lateral films are aligned in relation to the body rather then the curve. In the presence of a congenital abnormality, including spina bifida, a CT myelogram is essential prior to surgical correction to exclude intraspinal pathology, such as a diastematomyelia which may not be evident on plain films (Chap. 26).

Dysplasias

A modified skeletal survey (Chap. 24) is required. The diagnosis is made from the clinical and radiographic features of the condition. Other imaging techniques may occasionally be required, for example arthrography of the hips prior to surgical correction of subluxation.

Infection

Acute Infection

Acute osteomyelitis and septic arthritis occur most commonly in childhood. The diagnosis of infection is made on clinical grounds associated with a raised ESR and white cell count (Chap. 23). Unfortunately, in younger children it may not be possible to localize the infection. Plain radiographs are usually of little help, although changes in the soft tissue plain films may indicate the site of infection. In the case of a septic arthritis the joint space may appear widened.

In contrast, skeletal scintigraphy is extremely useful in localizing acute osteomyelitis and septic arthritis, except in the neonate (Chap. 13). Often it is not possible to obtain this investigation at night or weekends, and if the child is extremely toxic and has not responded within a few hours to high dosage intravenous antibiotics, the infection must be surgically drained even if this requires a wider exposure. Scintigraphy is unreliable in detecting infection in children under the age of 3 months. The reasons for this are not fully understood and treatment usually has to be based purely on clinical findings. In very early cases ^{87}Gallium or ^{111}In-tagged white cell scintigrams may be more sensitive.

If septic arthritis of the hip is suspected, ultrasound may indicate the presence of fluid. If the condition is suspected, the hip should be aspirated irrespective of the radiographic findings.

Chronic Osteomyelitis

Once radiographic changes of periosteal new bone formation, bone necrosis, sequestrum formation etc. appear, the osteomyelitis is chronic. The diagnosis is made on straight radiographs. Tomograms may be required if a sequestrum is thought to be responsible for a continuing infection, and is not well seen on the plain films. CT is also extremely useful in localizing sequestra prior to surgical removal. Plain radiographs do not indicate whether the chronic osteomyelitis is "active" or not. Under these circumstances skeletal scintigraphy may be extremely useful (Chap. 13). If the chronic osteomyelitis is quiescent, the scintigram will tend to be normal, but if active will show increased uptake on both the vascular and skeletal phases.

Sinuses

Plain radiographs may indicate whether the underlying bone is infected, but do not indicate whether a sinus communicates with the underlying bone, and if it does, how much of the bone is involved. A sinogram – injection of radio-opaque contrast medium into the sinus under sterile conditions – will outline the sinus tract, show how far it extends, and whether the underlying bone or joint is involved.

Tuberculosis

Skeletal tuberculosis is uncommon in the developed world, but does occur. The commonest site is the spine, although any bone or joint may be affected. The diagnosis is made on plain radiographs which usually show destruction of a disc and adjacent vertebrae (to a greater or lesser degree), and a paraspinal abscess best seen on the antero-posterior view. However, tuberculosis cannot be differentiated from other chronic infections of the spine and a needle biopsy may be required to find the causative organism. This is usually carried out under X-ray control. Scintigraphy is of little value in making the diagnosis, but is most helpful in diagnosing a recurrence of infection. CT myelography is indicated if there is any suspicion of cord or cauda equina compression.

Miscellaneous Conditions

A variety of miscellaneous radiographic examinations may be required in children or adolescents.

Deep vein thrombosis is not confined to adults and if suspected, venography may be required.

Tumours, particularly of the spine and which may be highly vascular, should have their vascularity assessed by arteriography prior to surgery. If they are found to be highly vascular, embolization of the major feeding vessels may be required.

Needle biopsy of the spine may be indicated for infection or possible tumour. This should be carried out under X-ray control

Imaging techniques play little role in the treatment of an haemarthrosis in haemophilia, but X-ray examination is essential in the assessment of haemophiliac arthropathy and ultrasound may be most helpful in soft tissue lesions (Wilson et al. 1987).

References

Akbarnia BA, Akbarnia NO (1976) The role of the orthopedist in child abuse and neglect. Orthop Clin North Am 7:733–742

Bassett LW, Gold RH, Reicher M, Bennett LR, Tooke SM (1987) Magnetic resonance imaging in the early diagnosis of ischemic necrosis of the femoral head. Preliminary reults. Clin Orthop 214:237–248

Berman L, Klenerman L (1986) Ultrasound screening for hip abnormalities: preliminary findings in 1001 neonates. Br Med J 293:719–722

Bulcke JAL, Baert AL (1982) Clinical and radiological aspects of myopathies. CT scanning. EMG. Radioisotopes. Springer-Verlag, Berlin, Heidelberg, New York

Catterall A (1971) The natural history of Perthes' disease. J Bone Joint Surg [Br] 53:37–53

Fitz CR (1985) Diagnostic imaging in children with spinal disorders. Pediatr Clin North Am 32:1537–1558

Galasko CSB (1987) The orthopaedic management of the dystrophies, myopathies and atrophies, neuropathies and ataxias. In: Galasko CSB (ed), Neuromuscular problems in orthopaedics. Blackwell, Oxford, pp 83–105

Gibson MJ, Szypryt EP, Buckley JH, Worthington BS, Mulholland RC (1987) Magnetic resonance imaging of adolescent disc herniation. J Bone Joint Surg [Br] 69:699–703

Graf R, Schuler P (1986) Sonography of the infant hip: an atlas (translated by Telger T). VCH Verlagsgesellschaft, Weinheim, pp 1–276

Haase GM, Ortiz VN, Sfakianakis GN, Morse TS (1980) The value of radionuclide bone scanning in the early recognition of deliberate child abuse. J Trauma 20:873–875

Kempe CH, Silverman FN, Steele BF, Droegemueller W, Silver HK (1962) The battered-child syndrome. JAMA 181:17–24

Kogutt MS, Swischuk LE, Fagan CJ (1974) Patterns of injury and significance of uncommon fractures in the battered-child syndrome. AJR 121:143–149

Marchisello PJ (1987) The use of computerized axial tomography for the evaluation of talocalcaneal coalition. J Bone Joint Surg [Am] 69:609–611

O'Neill JA Jr, Meacham WF, Griffin JP, Sawyers JL (1973) Patterns of injury in the battered-child syndrome. J Trauma 13:332–339

Pettersson H, Harwood-Nash DCF (1982) CT and myelography of the spine and cord. Springer-Verlag, Berlin, Heidelberg, New York

Salter RB, Harris WR (1963) Injuries involving the epiphyseal plate. J Bone Joint Surg [Am] 45:587–622

Silverman FN (1972) Unrecognized trauma in infants, the battered-child syndrome and the syndrome of Ambroise Tardieu. Radiology 104:337–353

Spiegel PG, Mast JW, Cooperman DR, Laros GS (1984) Triplane fractures of the distal tibial epiphysis. Clin Orthop 188:74–89

Sty JR, Starshak RJ (1983) The role of bone scintigraphy in the evaluation of the suspected abused child. Radiology 146:369–375

Suzuki S, Awaya G, Okada Y, Ikeda T, Tada H (1987a) Examination by ultrasound of Legg-Calve-Perthes' disease. Clin Orthop 220:130–136

Suzuki S, Awaya G, Wakita S, Maekawa M, Ikeda T (1987b) Diagnosis by ultrasound of congenital dislocation of the hip joint. Clin Orthop 217:171–178

Szypryt EP, Colton CL, Hardy JG (1987) Intra-operative bone scanning in orthopaedics. In: Noble J, Galasko CSB (eds), Recent developments in orthopaedic surgery. Manchester University Press, Manchester, pp 62–65

Turner P, Green JH, Galasko CSB (in press). Back pain in children. Spine

Wilkinson RH (1980) Hip arthrography in children. In: Dalinka MK (ed), Arthrography. Springer-Verlag, New York Heidelberg Berlin, pp 119–126

Wilson DJ, Green DJ, MacLarnon JC (1984) Arthrosonography of the painful hip. Clin Radiol 35:17–19

Wilson DJ, McLardy-Smith PD, Woodham CH, MacLarnon JC (1987) Diagnostic ultrasound in haemophilia. J Bone Joint Surg [Br] 69:103–107

28 Osteonecrosis

P.J. Gregg

Introduction 363
Pathology of Osteonecrosis 363
Standard Radiography 364
    Group A: Juxta-articular Lesions 364
    Group B: Head, Neck and Shaft Lesions 366
    Differential Diagnosis 367
Skeletal Scintigraphy 368
Other Investigations 369
References 369

Introduction

The orthopaedic surgeon will be required to initiate investigations of patients suspected of suffering from osteonecrosis in two situations. The first is that of a patient presenting with symptoms – for example pain in a major joint such as the hip, knee or shoulder. The second is that of a patient without symptoms but known to be at risk of developing osteonecrosis. Those at risk include compressed-air workers or deep-sea divers, patients receiving steroid therapy, and patients who have sustained a dislocation of the hip or intracapsular fracture of the neck of the femur.

Pathology of Osteonecrosis

It is necessary to review briefly the pathology of osteonecrosis for a proper understanding of the indications and limitations of the available imaging techniques which are currently used for the diagnosis and management of this condition. The primary event in osteonecrosis is the death of cells within bone as an organ, for example the femoral head. These cells are the osteocytes and haematopoietic and fat cells of the marrow. Following death these cells undergo lysis. At this stage of the process there will be no change in density on plain radiographs because the total mineral content of the bone remains unchanged unless the patient is immobilized for a period of time (for example on traction after sustaining an injury of the hip). In these circumstances the rest of the skeleton will undergo disuse osteoporosis but the osteonecrotic area will not be affected because of the absence of a blood supply. This results in a relative increase in density of the affected part.

Following the primary event of cellular death there may be a series of secondary events which constitute a repair phase. Cells in the surrounding normal bone may proliferate and invade the osteonecrotic area. Some of these cells differentiate into osteoblasts which lay down seams of new bone on the surface of pre-existing dead trabeculae. The result is an absolute increase in the amount of mineral present within the affected area and it is this which may lead to an absolute increase in density observed on a standard radiograph. In parts the cells differentiate into osteoclasts which resorb pre-existing dead trabeculae prior to the laying down of new bone. It is this which may lead to areas of decreased density observed on a plain radiograph.

At any one time in the development of this condition all of these processes may be present in different parts of the affected area. Thus, for example, within the femoral head as a whole there may be areas of bone and marrow necrosis which are unchanged following the primary event; areas which have been revascularized and invaded by live cells but in which there is as yet no new bone formation; areas of dead bone covered with seams of new living bone; and areas of bone resorption. These different processes cannot be identified on plain radiographs. It is important to emphasize this point because it is not accurate to use terms such as "alive", "dead", "revascularized" or "repaired" on the basis of the appearances observed on plain radiographs.

At some stage during the repair process a fracture may occur within the affected bone. This fracture may be situated in the sub-chondral region or deeper within the articulating end of a long bone, in which case there usually is an extension into the sub-chondral region. It is this fracture which ultimately leads to the onset of symptoms, joint surface incongruity and secondary degenerative osteoarthritis.

Plain radiographs cannot distinguish normal living bone from dead bone before any repair process has begun or from revascularized dead bone before new bone formation has taken place. Therefore, dense does not always equal dead!

Table 28.1. Radiographic classification of osteonecrosis

A.	**Juxta-articular lesions**
1.	Dense areas with an intact articular cortex
2.	Spherical segmental opacities
3.	Linear opacity
4.	Structural failure
	(a) Transradiant subcortical band
	(b) Collapse of the articular cortex
	(c) Sequestration of part of the cortex
5.	Secondary osteoarthritis
B.	**Head, neck and shaft lesions**
1.	Dense areas
2.	Irregular calcified areas
3.	Transradiant areas and "cysts"

Standard Radiography

Radiography is still the standard method for confirming the diagnosis of osteonecrosis of bone causing symptoms and for the detection of symptomless areas of osteonecrosis. The basic radiographic abnormality is one of altered bone density; this is usually in the nature of an increase in density but less often it may be a decrease. The radiographic changes which can be seen as a result of osteonecrosis are basically the same whatever the initial cause of the necrosis. These changes were well described by Phemister in 1930. An area of dead bone itself cannot be recognized radiographically. If, however, the affected bone is placed at rest, as in the treatment of a fracture, then the surrounding living bone will undergo disuse osteoporosis which will not be shared by the dead bone. Thus the dead bone eventually appears denser than the surrounding living bone. If and when revascularization of the dead bone occurs, the dead bone may be partially or wholly resorbed and replaced with less dense new bone, resulting in an area of decreased density on the radiograph. In rare instances decreased density results from resorption of dead bone not associated with a simultaneous deposition of new living bone. It is, however, more usual during revascularization for new living bone to be laid down on the surface of dead bone without prior resorption of the latter. This leads to an overall increase in the amount of bone present and so to

an absolute increase in radiographic density. Other factors which may contribute to changes in radiographic density are:

1. Calcification and ossification of the fibrous walls which seem to develop around areas of osteonecrosis, especially those which are present in the bone and marrow of the medullary cavity of long bones.

2. Structural failure of bone in the affected area, in the form of trabecular fracture, which may lead to radiolucent lines.

3. Increased density occurring as a consequence of trabecular collapse and impaction. As a result of these changes several distinct patterns may be seen on the radiographs of patients with osteonecrosis. In the author's opinion the most useful classification of these changes is that proposed by the Medical Research Council Decompression Sickness Panel (McCallum and Walder 1966). Although this classification was originally devised in connection with men suffering from caisson disease of bone it is readily applicable to other causes of osteonecrosis. In this classification there are two groups, A and B, each of which has several sub-groups (Table 28.1).

Group A: Juxta-articular Lesions

Lesions in group A are juxta-articular in position and may occur just beneath the articular surface of the ends of long bones. The usual sites are the humeral head, femoral head, femoral condyles and talus.

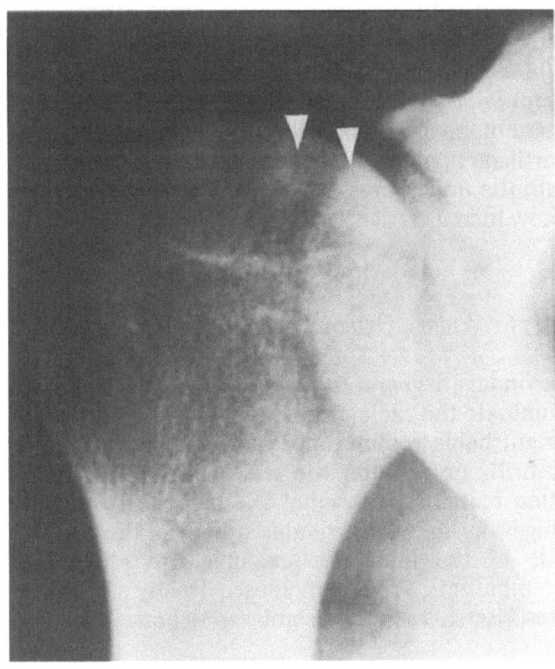

Fig. 28.1. A1 lesions of the humeral head (*arrows*).

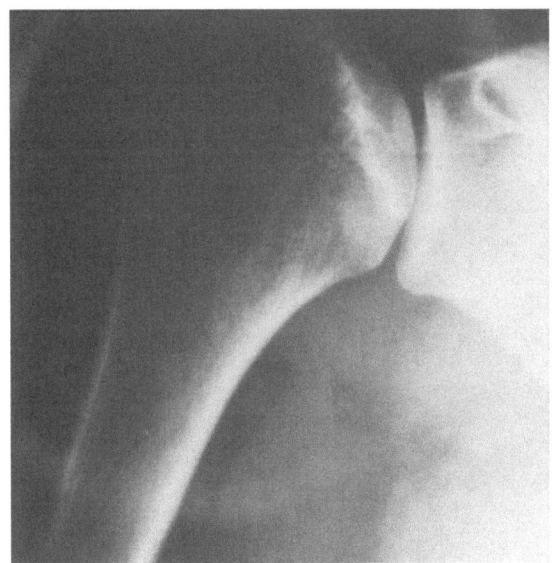

Fig. 28.2. A3 lesion of the humeral head.

A1 : Dense Areas with an Intact Articular Cortex

These dense areas measure from a few millimetres up to 2 cm in diameter and are often multiple. They are found more commonly in the humeral than in the femoral head. Their margins, unlike those of bone islands, are irregular and the trabeculae passing through them appear thickened and fused (Fig. 28.1).

A2 : Spherical Segmental Opacities

These opacities are shaped like a segment of a sphere and abut directly the articular surface. Again they are more commonly found in the humeral head than in the femoral head. They have been likened to a "snow cap" by Poppel and Robinson (1956).

A3 : Linear Opacity

This appearance is common in the humeral head and rare in the femoral head. The linear density, which is usually a few millimetres in width, is seen crossing the sub-chondral bone in a horizontal or

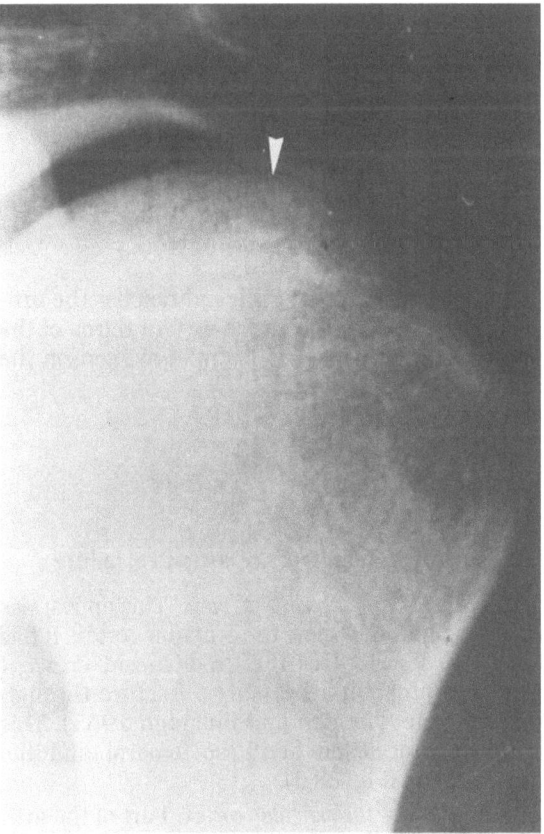

Fig. 28.3. A4(a) lesion of the humeral head (*arrow*).

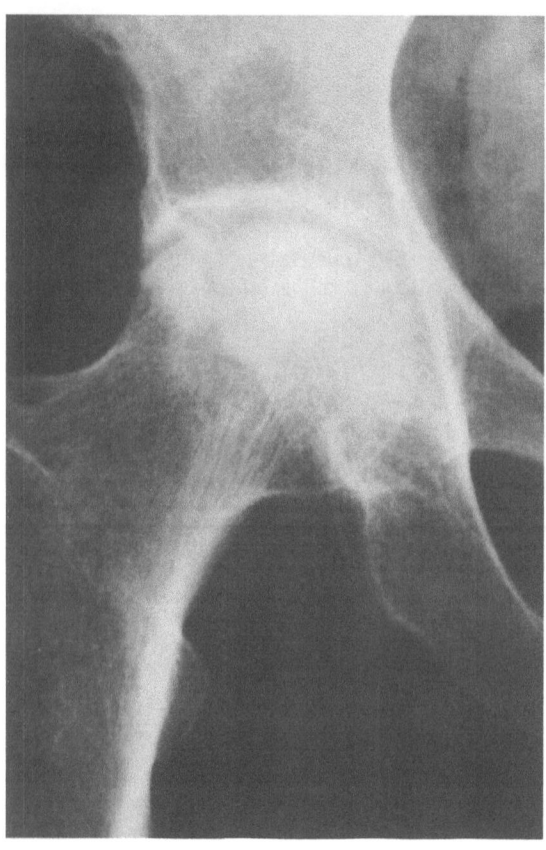

Fig. 28.4. A4(b) lesion of the femoral head.

slightly curved manner. Each end reaches the articular surface so that as much as two thirds of the joint surface may be included by it as seen on the radiograph (Fig. 28.2).

A4: Structural Failure

There are three main types of structural failure:

(a) *Transradiant sub-cortical band.* This appears as a transradiant line below the articular cortex. It has also been described as the "radiolucent crescent sign" and probably represents a fracture through necrotic bone (Norman and Bullough 1963). This lesion may occur in both the femoral and the humeral head (Fig. 28.3).

(b) *Collapse of the articular cortex.* Part of the articular cortex collapses into the underlying bone, with or without the formation of a "step" at the

junction with normal articular cortex. There usually is increased density of the neighbouring bone (Fig. 28.4).

(c) *Sequestration of part of the cortex.* A large segment of the articular cortex and overlying articular cartilage apparently separates but is not depressed into the underlying bone; neighbouring bone may show increased density.

A5: Secondary Osteoarthritis

Secondary degenerative changes have occurred and dominate the radiographic picture. They are indistinguishable from the appearances in primary osteoarthritis except that the width of the joint space often remains reasonably unchanged in the early stages, as does the articular surface of the opposite side of the joint (for example the glenoid or acetabulum). Areas of increased density are usually seen elsewhere in the neighbouring bone.

Group B: Head, Neck and Shaft Lesions

Group B lesions are situated in the articulating end of a long bone (away from the joint surface), neck or shaft of the bone. They are frequently bilateral.

B1: Dense Areas

These lesions are usually multiple. They are commonly found in the neck and upper shaft of the femur and humerus, and less commonly in the distal shaft of the femur or proximal shaft of the tibia. The areas are usually small and ill defined.

B2: Irregular Calcified Areas

Common sites for these lesions are the distal shaft of the femur, proximal shaft of the tibia and proximal shaft of the humerus. They are only found in the medullary cavity and not in the cortex of the shaft. They are often multiple. They consist of irregular areas of increased density which are of various sizes and shapes. In some cases they take the form of a circular cluster and in others a continuous broad strip several centimetres in length with a wavy edge which may be more or less clearly defined (Fig. 28.5).

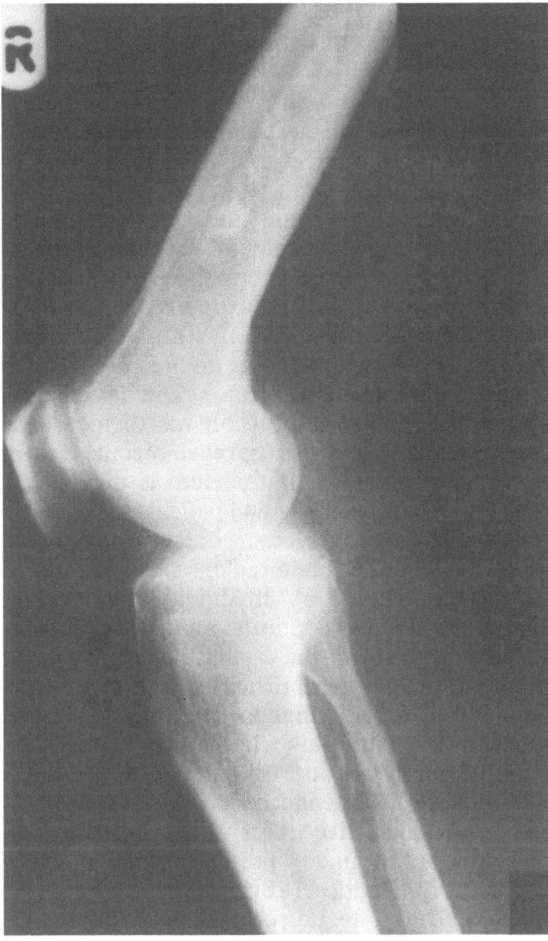

Fig. 28.5. B2 lesion of the distal femoral and upper tibial shafts.

B3: Transradiant Areas and "Cysts"

Transradiant areas, which may be surrounded by a sclerotic margin, may be found in the head of the humerus and the head of the femur. These must not be confused with the "cysts" sometimes seen along the line of attachment of the capsule of the humeral neck or femoral neck. These are thought to be synovial herniations and not the result of osteonecrosis (Golding 1966).

Differential Diagnosis

It has already been mentioned that the radiographic changes of bone necrosis are similar whatever the initial cause. There are some lesions which may resemble osteonecrosis on the radiograph and should be considered:

1. Primary osteoarthritis
2. Enchondroma
3. Normal variants of trabecular pattern, e.g. bone islands
4. Fibrous dysplasia
5. Solitary osteoblastic metastases

When presented with a patient who may be suffering from osteonecrosis, whether this be symptomatic or asymptomatic, standard radiographic views of the bones should be obtained in the first instance. In the case of patients who may be suffering from caisson disease of bone (compressed-air workers and commercial divers) or steroid-associated osteonecrosis, there may be more than one bone or part of a bone affected and a radiographic survey will be indicated. Each radiographic survey should consist of antero-posterior radiographs of both shoulder, hip and knee joints, and lateral radiographs of the distal femoral and proximal tibial shafts. The actual radiographic techniques were well described by Davidson (1976). Often these initial plain radiographs will show the characteristic radiographic changes of osteonecrosis and, in patients with symptoms, evidence of fracture of the sub-chondral bone resulting in joint surface incongruity with or without secondary degenerative osteoarthritis. In these circumstances no further investigations are required, unless the treating surgeon wishes to obtain biopsy material for histological confirmation.

In some cases the plain radiographs may be completely normal despite the fact that the patient is suffering from osteonecrosis. This is because there often is a long delay between the causal incident and the appearance of an abnormality which can be seen on a radiograph. In men at risk of developing caisson disease of bone, the earliest that bone changes indicative of osteonecrosis have been seen on a radiograph is 3–4 months after the individual's first exposure to a hyperbaric environment. But in many cases this time interval is much longer by many months or even years (Medical Research Council Decompression Sickness Central Registry, 1976, personal communication). It is also well known that there may be a delay of up to 3–4 years in the appearance of the radiographic abnormalities of osteonecrosis of the femoral head following intracapsular fracture of the proximal femur. The reason for this long delay is probably that a considerable alteration in bone mineral content, particularly in cancellous bone, must develop before a radiographic change may be detected (Borak 1942; Bachman and Sproul 1955; Edelstyn et al. 1967).

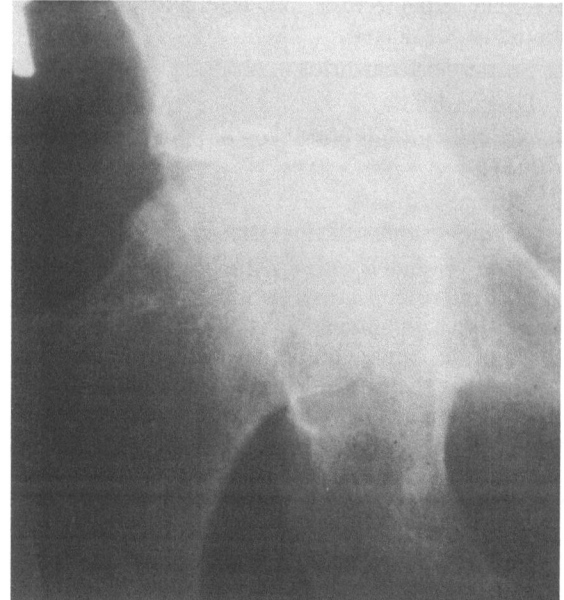

a

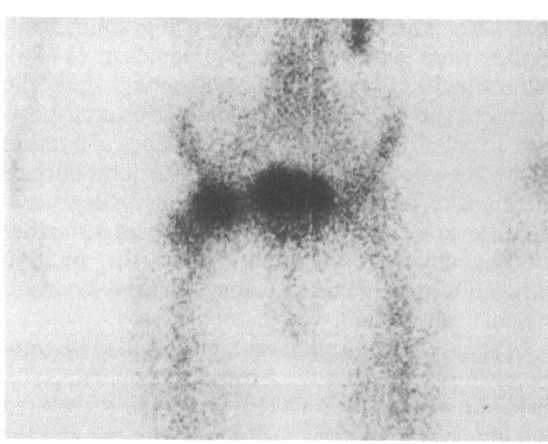

b

Fig. 28.6. a Normal radiograph of the hip of a patient with alcohol-associated osteonecrosis of the femoral head. b Scintigram of both hips. Note the increased uptake of ⁹⁹ᵐTc-labelled methylene diphosphonate in the right femoral head.

Skeletal Scintigraphy

Gregg has shown, in an experimental animal model, that it is possible to detect areas of bone and marrow necrosis by skeletal scintigraphy using ^{99m}Tc-labelled phosphate compounds and a gamma camera. It also was possible to detect abnormalities on the scintigram at a much earlier stage than was possible using standard radiographs (Gregg 1977; Gregg and Walder 1980). The abnormality observed on a scintigram was an area of increased uptake of the radioactive tracer. The pathological basis for this "hot spot" probably was the new bone formation associated with the repair of some of these lesions (Gregg 1977). It therefore is of value to obtain a skeletal scintigram of patients suspected of suffering from osteonecrosis, whatever the underlying cause, when the plain radiographs are found to be normal (Fig. 28.6). It should, however, be emphasized that the abnormal scintigram probably is also dependent on the establishment of a repair process in the nature of revascularization and subsequent new bone formation, and that if this does not occur the scintigram will remain normal. Thus a normal scintigram does not rule out the possibility of the presence of osteonecrosis.

Because radioactive tracer uptake in bone probably only occurs in the presence of an adequate blood supply (Hughes 1980) it is possible that, in the presence of osteonecrosis where revascularization has not occurred, a "cold spot" may be detected on the scintigram due to lack of uptake of the tracer. It may be useful, therefore, to obtain a scintigram in the early stages following an insult which may be associated with the development of osteonecrosis (for example traumatic dislocation of the hip or a fracture of the neck of the talus). However, in the author's experience these cold spots are often ill defined when compared with the more obvious "hot spot" associated with an area of repairing osteonecrosis (Fig. 28.7) and false positive and false negative scintigrams are, therefore, not uncommon. This aspect of the use of scintigraphy in the evaluation of osteonecrosis requires further study. Scintigraphy may also be useful in demonstrating "cold spots" in the capital femoral epiphysis of patients presenting with an irritable hip. The presence of cold spots may be detected before the development of characteristic radiographic abnormalities in those patients subsequently developing Perthes' disease (Calver et al. 1981; Chap. 13). In cases where plain radiographs are normal but abnormalities are found on the scintigram, a biopsy will usually be required to confirm the diagnosis.

If revascularization occurs it may not be associated with any new bone formation, or the new bone may be insufficient to increase the local mineral content to an extent that it can be recognized as an abnormality on the radiograph. It is well known, for example, that even after an area of osteonecrosis has been "repaired" fully, including extensive new bone formation, no abnormality may be detected on the radiograph (McCallum and Walder 1966). For these reasons additional investigations are required in the presence of a normal initial plain radiograph.

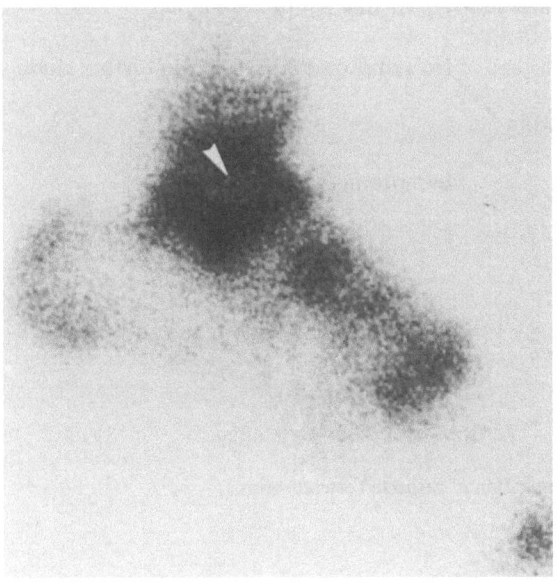

Fig. 28.7. Lateral scintigram of the ankle of a patient with a fracture of the neck of the talus. Note the generalized increased uptake of ^{99m}Tc-labelled methylene diphosphonate (normal response to fracture) and a possible "cold spot" in the centre of the body of the talus (*arrow*).

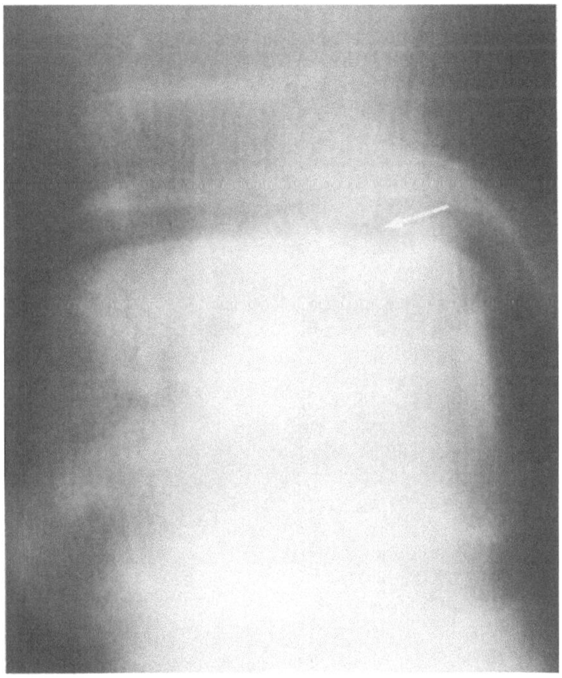

Other Investigations

In the author's experience, patients with osteonecrosis are never symptomatic unless structural failure has occurred in the sub-chondral bone leading to joint surface incongruity. The sub-chondral fracture and resulting joint surface incongruity are not always well defined on standard radiographs and may lead the treating clinician into believing that the joint surface is intact. In these circumstances high-quality tomograms and, on occasions, arthrograms will usually reveal the sub-chondral fracture (Fig. 28.8).

The possible role of computed tomography and magnetic resonance imaging in the routine investigation of osteonecrosis has not yet been clearly defined, but there is evidence that both techniques can provide reliable information.

The investigation of patients with suspected osteonecrosis of bone by imaging techniques is summarized in Fig. 28.9 (p. 370).

Fig. 28.8. Arthrogram of the ankle of a commercial diver presenting with pain in the ankle. Standard radiographs were normal. Note the "wedge-shaped" area of increased density and sub-chondral fracture with defect of the articular surface (*arrow*) seen on the tomogram.

References

Bachman Al, Sproul EE (1955) Correlation of radiographic and autopsy findings in suspected metastases in the spine. Bull NY Acad Med 31:146–148

Borak J (1942) Relationship between clinical and roentgenological findings in bone metastases. Surg Gynecol Obstet 75:599–604

Calver R, Venugopal V, Dorgan J, Bentley G, Gimlette T (1981) Radionuclide scanning in the early diagnosis of Perthes' disease. J Bone Joint Surg [Br] 63:379–382

Davidson JK (1976) Dysbaric osteonecrosis. In: Davidson JK (ed) Aseptic necrosis of bone. Excerpta Medica, Amsterdam, pp 147–209

Edelstyn GA, Gillespie PJ, Grebbell FS (1967) The radiological demonstration of osseous metastases: experimental observations. Clin Radiol 18:158–162

Gregg PJ (1977) Caisson disease of bone. Studies relating to the aetiology, early diagnosis and natural history of caisson disease of bone. MD Thesis, University of Newcastle-upon-Tyne

Gregg PJ, Walder DN (1980) Scintigraphy versus radiography in the early diagnosis of experimental bone necrosis; with special reference to caisson disease of bone. J Bone Joint Surg [Br] 62:214–221

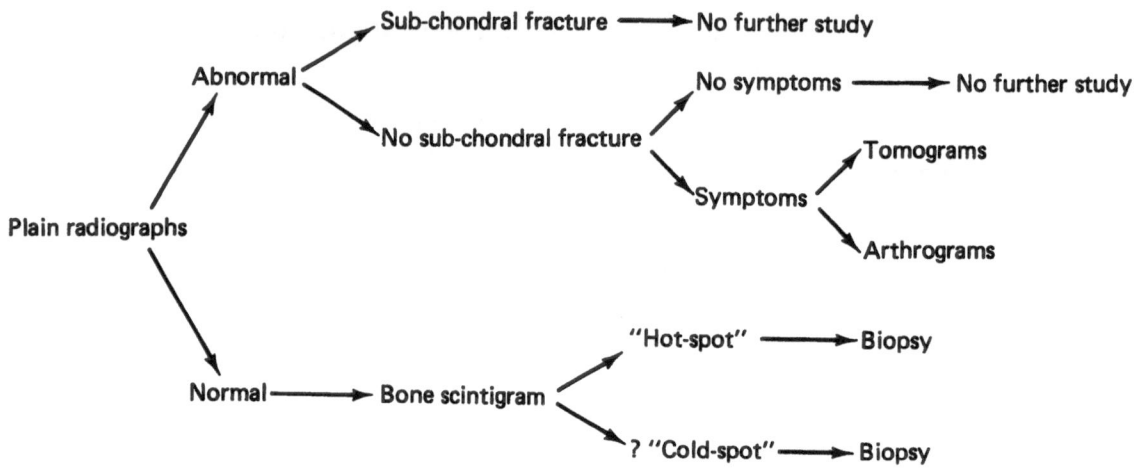

Fig. 28.9. Imaging techniques in the investigation of suspected osteonecrosis.

Hughes SPF (1980) Radionuclides in orthopaedic surgery. J Bone Joint Surg [Br] 62:141–150

McCallum RI, Walder DN (1966) Bone lesions in compressed air workers. J Bone Joint Surg [Br] 48:207–235

Norman A, Bullough P (1963) The radiolucent crescent line – an early diagnostic sign of avascular necrosis of the femoral head. Bull Hosp Jt Dis Orthop Inst 24:99–104

Phemister DB (1930) Repair of bone in the presence of aseptic necrosis resulting from fractures, transplantations and vascular obstruction. J Bone Joint Surg 12:769–787

Poppel MH, Robinson WT (1956) The roentgen manifestations of caisson disease. AJR 76:74–80

Subject Index

Abel views 55–6
Abscess 139
Acetabulum 11
  radiography 67
Achilles tendon 238
Achondroplasia 318, 320, 321
Acquired canal stenosis 129
Acquired lesions 24
Acromio-clavicular joint 9
Acromion 9
Adrenocortical tumour 322
Americium-241 254
Angiography
  appendicular skeleton 19–34
  axial skeleton 95–105
  conventional techniques 19–20
  spine 152
  techniques 148
  tumours 24, 151–2
  see also Arteriography; Venography
Angiosarcoma 285
Ankle joint
  arthrography 45–6
  radiography 13–14
  standard projections 13
Ankylosing spondylitis 215–17
  skeletal scintigraphy 195–6
Annular fissuring 111–12
Anterior spinal artery of
      Adamkiewicz 98
Antero-posterior projection 52–3, 53,
      57
Arterial occlusion 149
Arteriography 19–28, 95–102
  appearances on 21–2
  diagnostic applications
    acquired lesions 24
    congenital lesions 22
  indications for 95
  spinal cord 98
  therapeutic applications 25–8
Arteriovenous fistula 149
Arteriovenous malformations 22,
      95–7, 99
  magnetic resonance imaging
      (MRI) 173
Arteriovenous shunts 32
Arthritides, skeletal
      scintigraphy 192–6

Arthritis, septic 200
Arthrography 35–49, 209–10
  ankle 45–6
  elbow 44
  evaluation of total joint
      replacement 46–7
  facet 47, 117–22
    clinical studies 120–2
    technique 119–20
  foot 46–7
  hand 45
  hip
    in adults 44
    in children 43
  knee 36–40
  shoulder 40–3
  traction 47
  wrist 44–5
Arthroscopy 40
Ascending phlebography 28–32
Avascular necrosis 204, 304

Back pain 225, 325–34
  acute 327
  as clinical problem 331
  diagnostic groups 326–34
  identification of single segment
      failure 330–1
  in childhood 359–61
  low 124, 217
  management of 326
  multi-operated case 331–2
Battered baby syndrome 322
Bicipital groove 8
Bicipital tendon lesions 42
Billing projection 12
Bladder displacement 138
Bone
  metabolic disease of 201–4
  radiographic morphometry 243–5
  radiography 67–74
  tumours 190–2
  ultrasound 238
Bone density disorders 322
Bone graft 204
Bone ischaemia 170
Bone loss, age-related 247
Bone marrow disease, magnetic

  resonance imaging (MRI) 176
Bone measurement,
      radiography 243–9
Bone mineral analysis 141–2
Bone tumours 339–41
  benign 284–5
  computed tomography (CT) 340
  in childhood 356–8
  malignant 285–9
  skeltal scintigraphy 340
Brachial plexus 87, 88
Brewerton's projection 5
Brodie's abscess 199–200
Bulging annulus 126–30
Bursography 48

Caffey's disease 322
Calcaneus 14
Capsulitis 42
Carpal tunnel 6
Carpus
  radiography 5
  standard projections 5
Cast radiography 156
Cellulitis 198, 238–9
Centerolateral disc herniation 84–5
Cerebellar tonsils 80–1
Cervical disc herniations 86
Cervical discography 112–13
Cervical displacement 138
Cervical fusion 114
Cervical meningioma 82
Cervical spine 59, 320–2
  abnormal appearances in
      developmental disorders 321–2
  injuries 273–5
  myelography 80, 320–2
  normal appearances in the
      child 320–1
Cervical spondylosis 86, 88
Cervico-thoracic junction 57–8
Cesium-137 254
Child abuse 352
Childhood disorders 345–62
Chondral fracture 38
Chondroma 137
Chondromalacia patellae 38
Chondrosarcoma 234, 284

Chromosomal abnormalities 313
Chymopapaine
    chemonucleolysis 328–9
Clavicle, radiography 9
Compression of vessels 22
Computed tomography (CT) 114,
    123–43
  advantages of 123–4
  bone tumours 285–9, 340
  clinical applications 124–42
  disadvantages of 124
  fractures 281
  future developments 142
  hip joint 140, 279–80
  indications for 142
  metastatic tumours 298
  methods 124
  musculoskeletal infection 139–40
  musculoskeletal tumours 135–9
  pelvic ring 279–80
  pelvis 140
  sacro-iliac joint 140
  soft tissue tumours 289–90
  spinal anatomy 338
  spinal cord lesions 341
  spinal injuries 272–7
  spine 124–35
  spondylolisthesis 327–8
  spondylolysis 327–8
  technical aspects 123–4
  see also Quantitative computed
    tomography (QCT)
Computed tomography/myelography
    (CTM) 125
Congenital anomalies 173
Congenital deformities 338–9
Congenital dislocation of the
    hip 345–8
Congenital lesions 22
Congenital spinal canal stenosis 129
Connective tissue diseases 217
Contrast medium 21, 22, 77–8, 110,
    124, 148
Coracoid process 9
Cortical integrity, radiography 70
Cortical/total area ratio (CA/TA) 244
Cranio-cervical junction 80
Cruciate ligament tears 38

Deep vein thrombosis 32
Deformity in childhood 360
Degenerative disc disease, magnetic
    resonance imaging (MRI) 171
Degenerative joint disease 218
Desmoid tumour 288
Diastrophic dwarfism 320, 321
Diastrophic dysplasia 316
Digital imaging techniques 145
Digital radiography,
    instrumentation 152–6
Digital subtraction angiography
    (DSA) 20–1, 145
  contrast sensitivity 147–8
  for direct and indirect
    venography 32
  instrumentation 146–7
  intra-arterial 150, 155

performance parameters 147–8
  post processing 148–9
  quantitative 149
  spatial resolution 147
  utilization in clinical orthopaedic
    radiography 149–52
Digital tomosynthesis 157–8
Digital vascular imaging (DVI) 20
Disc degeneration 111–12
Disc prolapse 173
  intra-osseous 112
  trans-annular 112
Disc-space infection, magnetic resonance
    imaging (MRI) 171–2
Discitis 135, 200, 332
Discography 107–15
  advantages of 114
  cervical 112–13
  choice of 113–14
  contra-indications to 113–14
  current status of 114
  disadvantages of 114
  history 107–9
  indications for 113
  mid-line approach 109–10
  oblique extra-thecal approaches 110
  radiological appearances 110–12
  techniques 109–10
Discoid meniscus 38
Displacement of veins 32
Displacement of vessels 22
Distal anterior tibio-fibular
    ligament 45
Dorsal disc herniations 85
Dorsal kyphosis 82
Dorsal spine, myelography (see also
    Thoracic Spine) 79
Dorsolumbar spine 319–20
Down's syndrome 320, 321
Dual energy radiography 156
Dual photon absorbtiometry 210,
    254–7, 260
Dural-based arteriovenous
    malformation 102
Dysplasias, in childhood 360

Elbow
  arthrography 44
  injuries 355
  radiography 6
  standard projections 6–7
Embolization 26–8
  indications for 27–8
  materials used 26
Encasement 22
Enlargement of vessels 22
Epidemiology, ultrasound 225–8
Epidural venous plexus 97
Epidurography 89–93
  accuracy of 89
  combined diagnostic and therapeutic
    procedure 89
  comparison with radiculography 93
  contraindications 89
  in orthopaedic surgery 89
  indications 89
  results 89–93

Ewing's sarcoma 286
Extension 56, 61
Extradural compression 83

Facet
  arthrography 47, 117–22
    clinical studies 120–2
    techniques 119–20
  radiography 64–6
Femur
  anteversion 238
  grading trabecular architecture 246
  neck fractures 247, 248
  radiography 12
  standard projections 12
Film processing 4
Flexion 56, 61
Floppy baby 237
Fluoroscopic screening 62
Foot
  arthrography 46–7
  radiography 14–15
  standard projections 14
Forearm
  radiography 6
  standard projections 6–7
Foreign body 132
Fractures 215
  age-specific incidence of 247
  dislocation 131, 132
  in childhood 352–6
  osteoporotic 260
  radiography 70–3
  skeletal scintigraphy 204
"Frog" lateral 11

Gadolinium-153 210, 254
Gadolinium-DTPA 171–3
Gallium 209
Gamma-ray sources 210–11
Ganglia 44, 47
Ganglionography 47
Giant cell tumours 334
Gleno-humeral dislocations 42–3
Gout, scintigraphy 196

Haemangioblastomas 102–4
Haemangioma 28, 168
Haemangiopericytoma 233
Haematoma 234, 236, 237
Haemophilic arthropathy,
    scintigraphy 196
Hallux 14
Hand
  arthrography 45
  Brewerton's view 5
  radiography 4–5
  standard projections 4
  tenography 48
Hip dislocation, congenital 345–8
Hip disorders
  in childhood 238, 345–52
  irritable hip 350–2
Hip joint
  arthrography 43–4

in adults 44
in children 43
computed tomography (CT) 140
radiography 11–12
skeletal dysplasias 315–16
standard projections 11
trauma 277–80
Histiocytoma 234, 289
Humerus
lateral condyle fracture 355
medial epicondyle fracture 355
radiography 7
standard projections 7
Hybrid subtraction technique 149
Hyperlordosis 73, 74
Hyperparathyroidism 202

Idiopathic juvenile osteoporosis 322
Ilium 10
Implants, infection 200–1, 309–10
Indium-113m 208
Infection 307–11
implants 200–1, 309–10
in childhood 361
skeletal scintigraphy 196–201
Inflammatory spondylitis 64
Infraspinatus 8
Infusion of chemotherapeutic
agents 25–6
Inherited disorders 313
Integrated remask 148
Intra-arterial DSA (ia DSA) 20–1
Intradural extramedullary
compression 83
Intradural intramedullary
compression 83–4
Intradural tumours 334
Intramedullary parenchymal
arteriovenous
malformation 102
Intraosseous phlebography 32
Intra-spinal tumours 134
Intravenous digital subtraction
angiography (iv DSA) 20
Iodine-131 210
Irradiation, metastatic tumours,
response to treatment 304
Irritable hip 350–2
Isotopes 207–20, 254
tumour localizing (see also
Radionuclides) 302
Isthmic spondylolisthesis 224

Joint disorder
magnetic resonance imaging
(MRI) 169–70
radiography 67–74
Joints of Luschka 53, 55

Knee 13
arthrography 36–40
malalignment 317
normal blood-pool of 212
Kniest syndrome 320, 321
Kyphosis 343
plus scoliosis 343

Large abnormal draining veins 32
Lateral condyle fracture 355
Lateral disc protrusion 105
Lateral ligament tears 45
Lateral pelvimetry 10
Lateral projection 53, 55, 58
Leg
radiography 12–13
standard projections 13
Leprosy, scintigraphy 196
Leukaemia 322
Ligament
lateral tears 45
medial (deltoid) tear 45
Limb length measurement in
childhood 360
Lipoma 136, 236
Liposarcoma 166
Loose bodies 39, 45–6, 141
Low Back Pain Syndrome 124
Lower limb
length measurement 15–16, 360
malalignment 317–18
Lumbago 327
Lumbar disc disease 125–6
Lumbar disc herniations 84–6
Lumbar disc prolapse 89
Lumbar discogram 110–11
Lumbar spine 61
injuries 275–7
myelography 78–9
Lumbar spondylosis 85–6
Lumbo-sacral junction 61
Lunate 5

McGregor's line 53
Magnetic resonance imaging
(MRI) 114, 159–79, 275, 285
arteriovenous malformations 173
bone marrow disease 176
bone tumours 285–9
degenerative disc disease 171
disc-space infection 171–2
future aspects 176
image acquisition 160–2
instrumentation 159–60
joint disease 169–70
muscle disease 171
musculoskeletal infection 166–7
musculoskeletal pathology 165–71
normal anatomy 163–4
radiofrequency magnetic field
effects 162–3
safety issues 162–3
scoliosis 342
soft tissue tumours 289–90
spine 164, 171–6, 341
spondylolisthesis 327–8
spondylolysis 327–8
static main magnetic field
effects 162
syringomyelia 175
technical aspects 159–63
time varying (gradient) magnetic field
effects 162
trauma 167–9, 173

tumours 165–6, 173
vascular lesions 167
Magnetic resonance spectroscopy
(MRS) 176
Malalignment 72–3
Malformation syndromes 313
Malignant fibrous histiocytoma 153
Mammary carcinoma 185, 189, 300, 301
Marquet method 16
Massive central disc herniations 84
Medial (deltoid) ligament tears 45
Medial epicondyle fracture 355
Meniscal cysts 38
Meniscal ossicles 38
Metabolic disease of bone 201–4
Metacarpals, radiographic
morphometry 244–5
Metaphyseal chondrodysplasia 318
Metastatic tumours 138, 293–306
assessment of extent of
dissemination 300–2
clinical features 293–5
computed tomography (CT) 298
diagnosis of symptomatic
lesion 293–300
radiography 295–7
renal cell carcinoma 154
response to treatment 303
scintigraphy 190, 297–8
staging of 302–5
Metatropic dwarfism 316, 319, 320, 321
Methane hydroxydiphosphonate
(HMDP) 209
Methylene diphosphonate (MDP) 209, 212, 214
Mini-scanogram 16
Monteggia fracture dislocation 355
Morquio's syndrome 316, 318–21
Multiple epiphyseal dysplasia 315–17
Multiple myeloma 333
Muscle disease, magnetic resonance
imaging (MRI) 171
Musculoskeletal infection, computed
tomography (CT) 139–40
Musculoskeletal pathology, magnetic
resonance imaging
(MRI) 165–71
Musculoskeletal system, magnetic
resonance imaging
(MRI) 163–4
Musculoskeletal trauma 271–82
Musculoskeletal tumours 283
computed tomography (CT) 135–9
Myelography 77–93
arteriovenous malformation 101
cervical spine 80
computed tomography (CTM) 125
dorsal spine 79
history 77
lumbar spine 78–9
pathological appearances 81–7
post-myelographic care 81
scoliosis 342
spinal compression 81–4
spinal cord lesions 341
techniques 77–8

Needle biopsy 333
Neovascularity 22
Neural foraminal stenosis 130
Neurofibroma 128, 134
Neurofibromatosis 22
Neurogenic claudication 224
Neuromuscular deformaties 338
Neuromuscular disease 235–8
  in childhood 358–9
Neuropathetic arthropathy 196
Neutron sources 211
Norgaard's ("ball-catching")
    projection 4–5

Oblique projection 57
Occiput
  C1 and C2 52–3
  C3 to C7 53–7
Occlusion 22
Odontoid hypoplasia 321
Odontoid process 320
Off lateral projection 56
Orthopaedic radiography 156–8
Orthopaedic surgery, epidurography
    in 89
Osteoarthritis, skeletal
    scintigraphy 195
Osteoblastoma 138, 333–4
Osteochondral fractures 38
Osteochondritis dissecans 38, 46
Osteoclastoma 29
Osteogenesis imperfecta 322
Osteoid osteoma 194, 288
Osteomalacia 202
Osteomyelitis 167, 332
  acute 196–8
  chronic 198–9, 309
  in childhood 361
  radiography 307
  scintigraphy 307–8
  subacute 308
Osteonecrosis 363–70
  pathology of 363–4
  radiography 364–8
  skeletal scintigraphy 368
Osteoporosis 187, 203, 215, 260
Osteosarcoma 137, 138, 165, 191,
    195, 287

PACS system 155
Paget's disease 183, 184, 189, 201–2,
    334
Painful heel syndrome 196
Pantopaque 77
Paraspinal pleural 60
Paravertebral masses 60
Paravertebral muscle spasm 74
Pars interarticularis 65
Patella 13
Pelvic ring trauma 277–80
Pelvis
  acetabulum 67
  computed tomography (CT) 140
  ilium 10
  lateral pelvimetry 10
  radiography 9, 11–12, 62, 67

standard projections 9–11
  symphysis pubis 10
Peroneal tenography 47–8
Pertechnetate 208
Perthes' disease 348–9
Pharmacoangiography 21
Photon absorptiometry 251–7
  comparison with quantitative
    computed tomography 264–5
Pigmented villonodular synovitis 40,
    44, 196
Pixel shift 149
Planar electron tube (PET scope) 158
Plantar fasciitis, scintigraphy 196
Polyarthritis, skeletal
    scintigraphy 194–5
Polyarthropathy 182
Polymyositis 239
Popliteal cyst 40
Post-meniscectomy arthrogram 38
Post-operative fibrosis 132–3
Post-operative laminectomy 133
Post-operative spine 132–4
Post-traumatic disability 44
Post-traumatic syrinx 132
Primary vascular abnormalities 22
Primary orthopaedic abnormalities 22
Prolapsed intervertebral disc 127,
    327–9
Prostatic carcinoma 296
Pseudoachondroplasia 316, 318, 320,
    321
Pseudoaneurysm 149
Pseudomeningocoele 134
Psoas abscess 139
Pyogenic spondylitis 200

Quantitative computed tomography
    (QCT) 259–68
  accuracy 264–5
  clinical applications 265–6
  comparison with photon
    absorptiometry 264–5
  dual energy scanning 264
  future developments 266
  precision 264–5
  radiation dose 264–5
  scanning technique 263–5
  single energy scanning 263–4
  technical aspects 261–3
Quantitative digital radiography
    (QDR) 261
Quantum mottle 148

Radial neck fractures 355
Radiculography, comparison with
    epidurography 93
Radiography
  acetabulum 67
  additional 62–7
  ankle joint 13–14
  appendicular skeleton 3–34
  axial skeleton 51–75
  bone disorder 67–74
  bone measurement 243–9
  cancer staging 302
  carpus 5

clavicle 9
cortical integrity 70
elbow 6
errors due to inadequate or
    incomplete 74
errors due to inherent deficiencies
    of 75
facet 64–6
femur 12
film processing 4
foot 14–15
forearm 6
fracture 70–3
hand 4–5
hip joint 11–12
humerus 7
joint disorder 67–74
leg 12–13
metastatic tumours 295–7
    response to treatment 303–4
osteomyelitis 307
osteonecrosis 364–8
pelvis 9, 62
scapula 8
scoliosis 67, 342
shoulder 7
shoulder girdle 7
spinal cord lesions 341
spondylolysis 63–4
sternum 9
wrist 5
Radionuclides 184, 194, 207–20, 254
  americium-241 254
  cesium-137 254
  gadolinium-153 210, 254
  gallium 209
  indium-113m 208
  iodine-131 210
  pertechnetate 208, 215
  technetium 208, 212
  tumour localising 302
  xenon-133 210
Rectal carcinoma 193
Rectus femoris tendon 168
Rectus sheath haematomas 235
Reflex sympathetic dystrophy syndrome
    (RSDS) 205, 217–18
Reiter's disease, scintigraphy 196
Remask technique 148
Renal cell carcinoma 154
Renal osteodystrophy 202–3
Repair 72
Retropharyngeal haematoma 56
Rheumatoid arthritis 39, 43, 44,
    211–15
  extra-articular manifestations 215
Romanus lesion 66
Rotation 72

Sacral meningocoele 175
Sacro-iliac joint 10–11, 61–2, 72
  computed tomography (CT) 140
Sacrum 61
Salter–Harris classification 352
Scanography 16
Scaphoid 5
Scapula, radiography 8

Schmorl's nodes 112
Sciatica 124
Scintigraphy (*see* Skeletal scintigraphy)
Scoliosis 74, 134, 341–2
 in childhood 360
 magnetic resonance imaging
  (MRI) 342
 myelography 342
 plus kyphosis 343
 radiography 67, 156, 342
 skeletal scintigraphy 342
Screening 62
Septic arthritis 200, 309
Sheaths of hand and wrist,
  tenography 48
Shoulder
 arthrography 40–3
 radiography 7
 standard projections 7
Shoulder girdle
 radiography 7
 standard projections 7
Single photon absorptiometry 210,
  252–4, 260
Sitting horizontal beam lateral
  projection 11–12
Skeletal dysplasias 313–23
 classification 313–14
 clinical appearances and age at
  diagnosis 315
 diagnosis 314–15
 hip joints 315–16
Skeletal metastases (*see* Metastatic
  tumours)
Skeletal scintigraphy 181–206
 abnormal scintigram 189–90
 ankylosing spondylitis 195–6
 artefacts 188–9
 arthritides 192–6
 bladder uptake 187
 bone tumours 340
 cancer staging 302–3
 future of 205
 in adult 187
 in child and adolescent 187
 indications for 190–205
 infection 196–201, 327–8
 mechanism of uptake of
  radionuclides 184
 metabolic disease of bone 201
 metastatic tumours 190, 297–8
  response to treatment 304
 miscellaneous conditions 196,
  204–5
 normal scintigram 184–9
 osteoarthritis 195
 osteonecrosis 368
 polyarthritis 194–5
 renal uptake of 187
 scoliosis 342
 synovial uptake of radionuclides 194
 tumours 190–2
Skeletal tumours 137–9
Slipped upper femoral epiphysis 350
Smith–Petersen projection 11
Sodium pertechnetate 215
Soft tissue injuries 281
Soft tissue sarcoma 136, 232

Soft tissue trauma 233–5
Soft tissue tumours 135–7, 289–90
 in childhood 357–8
Spasm 74
Spasm curve 342
Special axial projection (Stripp axial) 8
Spinal canal 78, 225–8
Spinal canal stenosis 130
Spinal cord 79, 83, 84
 arteriography 98
 vascular supply 97
Spinal cord compression 343
 myelography 81–4
Spinal cord lesions 340–1
 computed tomography (CT) 341
 myelography 341
Spinal deformity 335–43
 bone detail 336
 congenital 338–9
 curve evaluation 337
 erect views 335–6
 evaluation for treatment 337
 fusion evaluation 337
 large curves 337
 neuromuscular 338
 pain evaluation 337
 routine evaluation of 335
Spinal disorders, magnetic resonance
  imaging (MRI) 171–6
Spinal dysraphism 83, 134, 175, 339
Spinal fusion 109, 114, 133, 337
Spinal infection
 acute 332
 chronic 332–3
Spinal injuries 272–7
Spinal lesions 95
 magnetic resonance imaging
  (MRI) 341
Spinal muscle measurement,
  ultrasound 225
Spinal myeloma 139
Spinal neoplasm 333–4
Spinal stenosis 89, 329–30
 central 329–30
 lateral 329
Spinal trauma 84, 130–2
Spine
 anatomy 325–6
 angiography 152
 computed tomography (CT) 124–35
 magnetic resonance imaging
  (MRI) 164
Spondyloepiphyseal dysplasia
  congenita 316, 319–21
Spondyloepiphyseal dysplasia
  tarda 316
Spondylolisthesis 128, 130, 184,
  326–7
Spondylolysis 130, 204, 326–7
 radiography 63–4
Spondylosis 84–6
Standing axial projection (Harris)
  projection 15
Stereoradiography 16–17
Sterno-clavicular joints 9
Sternum, radiography 9
STIR (Short Tau Inversion
  Recovery) 173

Stryker's projection 7–8
Subchondral cortical integrity 72
Subtalar joint 15, 140
Supine horizontal beam lateral 11
Supracondylar fractures 355
Suprascapular fossa 9
Supraspinatus 8
Symphysis pubis 10
Synovial lesions 39–40
Synovial rupture, scintigraphy 196
Syringomyelia 83
 magnetic resonance imaging
  (MRI) 175

Tears of glenoid labrum 43
Tears of menisci 36
Tears of rotator cuff 41–2
Technetium 208
Technetium-99m 212
Temporal/energy subtraction 149
Tendonitis 238
Tendons, ultrasound 238
Tenography 47–8
 sheaths of hand and wrist 48
Teres minor 8
Therapeutic embolization 99
Thoracic aortic injury 152
Thoracic spine (*see also* Dorsal spine)
  58–60
Thoracic spine injuries 275–7
Thoraco-lumbar injuries 275–7
Thoraco-lumbar junction 60, 66
Thrombosis 32
Tibial torsion 238
Tomography 62–3, 72, 80
 spinal anatomy 339
Tracers 207–11
 bone-seeking 209
Traction, arthrography 47
Transient osteoporosis 204
Transient synovitis 350–2
Trapezium 5
Trauma
 acute diagnosis 24
 delayed effects 24
 extremity angiography 149–51
 iatrogenic 24
 magnetic resonance imaging
  (MRI) 167–9, 173
Traumatic nerve root avulsion 87
Tuberculosis 200, 310
 in childhood 361
Tuberculous disease of the dorsal
  spine 82
Tumour blush 22
Tumours
 angiography 24, 151–2
 bone 190–2
 in childhood 356–8
 invasion of veins 32
 magnetic resonance imaging
  (MRI) 165–6, 173
 skeletal scintigraphy 190–2
 ultrasound 232–3
Turner's syndrome 322
Two-dimensional Fourier transform
  (2DFT) 161

Ultrasound
    accuracy   221
    anatomical relevance   221–3
    appendicular skeleton   231–9
    axial skeleton   221–9
    clinical relevance   223–5
    epidemiology   225–8
    hip disorders in children   238
    intra-operative   224–5
    normal condition   232
    patient management   223–4
    precision   221
    reproducibility   221
    spinal muscle measurement   225
    technique   231–2
    tumours   232–3

Valsalva manoeuvre   32
Vascular lesions, magnetic resonance
        imaging (MRI)   167
Vascular spinal tumour   101–2
Vastus lateralis   236
Vastus medialis   237
Veins, abnormal draining   32
Vena cava filters   32
Venography   28–34
    appearances on   32
    direct   32
    epidural   102–5
    indications for   32–4
    indirect   32
    lower extremity   28–32
    technique   28–32

    upper limb   32
    use of DSA for   32
Vertebral body wedging and
        collapse   245–6

Wrist
    arthrography   44–5
    radiography   5
    standard projections   5
    tenography   48

Xenon-133   210
X-ray fluorescence analysis   210–11
X-ray (or photon) densitometry   251–2